AF822527

The Art and Science of Contemporary Surgical Endodontics

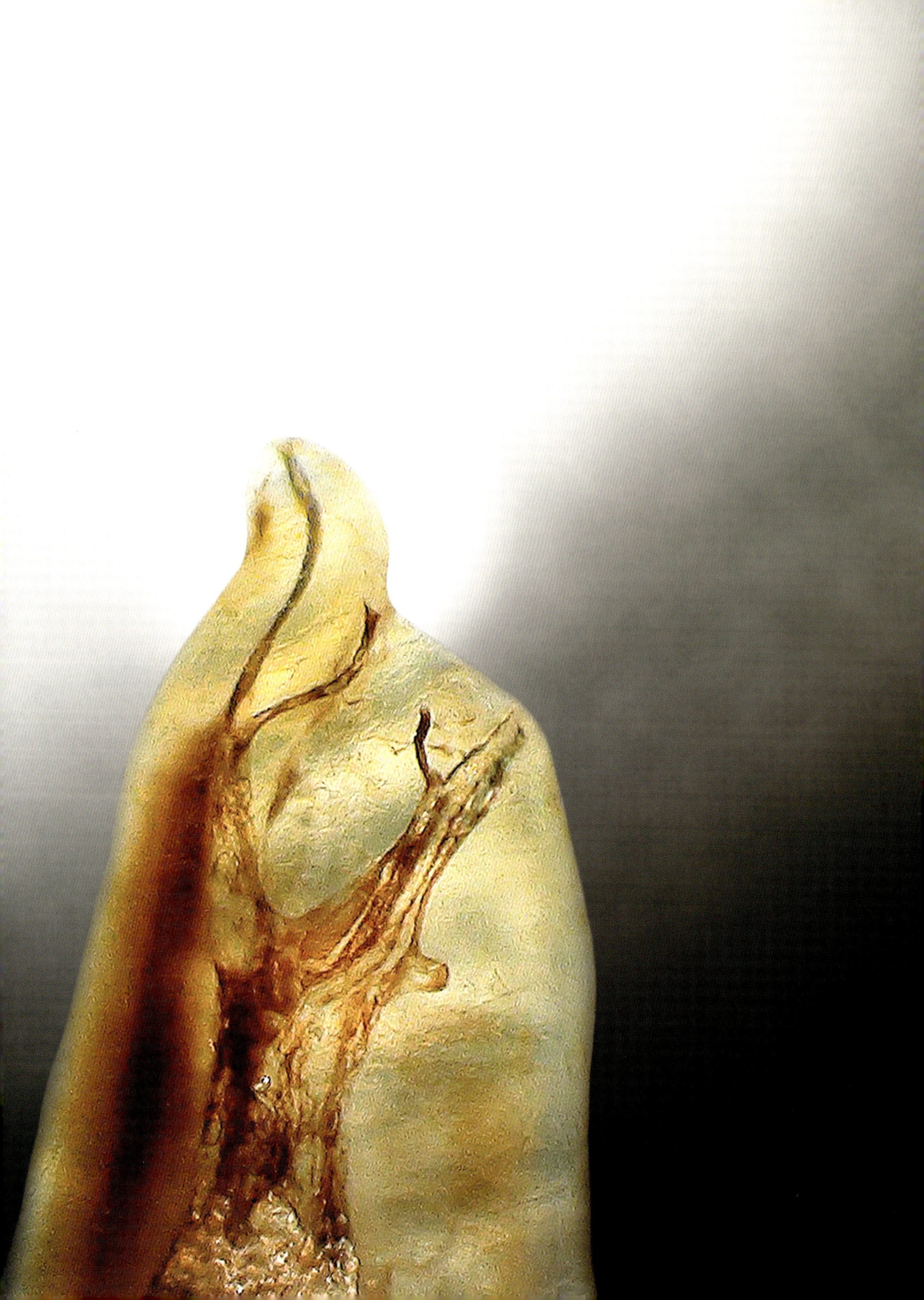

The Art and Science of
CONTEMPORARY SURGICAL ENDODONTICS

Mahmoud Torabinejad, DMD, MSD, PhD

Ronald E. Buell Professor of Endodontics
Director of Advanced Program in Endodontics
School of Dentistry
Loma Linda University
Loma Linda, California

Richard Rubinstein, DDS, MS

Adjunct Clinical Associate Professor
Department of Cariology, Restorative Sciences and Endodontics
University of Michigan School of Dentistry
Ann Arbor, Michigan

Private Practice Limited to Endodontics
Farmington Hills, Michigan

QUINTESSENCE PUBLISHING

Berlin, Barcelona, Chicago, Istanbul, London, Milan, Moscow, New Delhi, Paris,
Prague, São Paulo, Seoul, Singapore, Tokyo, Warsaw

Library of Congress Cataloging-in-Publication Data

Names: Torabinejad, Mahmoud, editor. | Rubinstein, Richard, 1946- editor.
Title: The art and science of contemporary surgical endodontics / edited
by Mahmoud Torabinejad, Richard Rubinstein.
Description: Hanover Park, IL : Quintessence Publishing Co Inc, [2017] |
Includes bibliographical references and index.
Identifiers: LCCN 2017003236 (print) | LCCN 2017005621 (ebook) | ISBN
9780867157314 (hardcover) | ISBN 9780867157550 (ebook)
Subjects: | MESH: Dental Pulp Diseases--surgery | Dental Pulp--diagnostic
imaging | Pulpectomy--methods
Classification: LCC RK351 (print) | LCC RK351 (ebook) | NLM WU 230 | DDC
617.6/342059--dc23
LC record available at https://lccn.loc.gov/2017003236

QUINTESSENCE PUBLISHING
USA

© 2017 Quintessence Publishing Co, Inc

Quintessence Publishing Co, Inc
4350 Chandler Drive
Hanover Park, IL 60133
www.quintpub.com

5 4 3 2 1

All rights reserved. This book or any part thereof may not be reproduced, stored in a retrieval system, or transmitted in any form or by any means, electronic, mechanical, photocopying, or otherwise, without prior written permission of the publisher.

Editor: Leah Huffman
Design: Erica Neumann
Production: Sue Robinson

Printed in China

Contents

Foreword

In February of 1969, I published a paper in the *Journal of the New Jersey Dental Association* titled "Surgical Endodontics, A Conservative Approach." According to the *Random House Dictionary*, *conservative* is defined as "disposed to preserving existing conditions." At that time, popular dental semantics referred to the two courses of endodontic action as *conservative* and *surgical*. This implies that the surgical approach is radical and the nonsurgical approach is conservative. However, both of these methods try to "preserve existing conditions" by retaining teeth, and therefore both must be considered conservative. In fact, modern endodontic surgery may be more conservative than disassembly, retreatment, and re-restoration. Despite advances in surgical endodontics, this conversation still takes place today.

In 1969, Donald E. Arens was teaching surgical endodontics to graduate students at Indiana University and requested reprints of my paper for the residents. This began a lifelong professional association and a personal friendship. When he decided to codify his teaching materials into a textbook, he joined with William Adams and Roland DeCastro to write *Endodontic Surgery* (Harper & Row, 1981). I was honored to contribute a chapter to this first English-language textbook devoted to surgical endodontics. The basic premise of the text was that "surgical endodontics is an extension of root canal basic therapy to preserve natural dentition."

Ten years later, *Surgical Endodontics* (Blackwell, 1991) by James Gutmann and John Harrison was followed by *Practical Lessons in Endodontic Surgery* (Quintessence, 1991) by the late Donald E. Arens, Mahmoud Torabinejad, Richard Rubinstein, and myself. This trio of textbooks has served our profession well in establishing a scientific basis and offering practical methods for understanding and performing surgical endodontics. In 2001, *Color Atlas of Microsurgery in Endodontics* (Saunders) by Syngcuk Kim, Gabriele Pecora, and Richard Rubinstein introduced the profession to the modern understanding of true endodontic microsurgery.

Since then, there have been few books that have addressed the surgical needs of modern-day dentists who want to adopt contemporary and evidence-based surgical endodontics methods into their practices. *The Art and Science of Contemporary Surgical Endodontics* consists of 17 chapters and 31 videos that span its entire scope. It has been assembled and coauthored by Mahmoud Torabinejad and Richard Rubinstein, two leaders in the field of surgical endodontics. Their professional careers, research, and didactic skills complement each other and have produced the new standard for teaching and studying evidence-based surgical endodontics.

Noah Chivian, DDS
Professor of Endodontics, Rutgers School of Dental Medicine
Adjunct Professor of Endodontics, University of Pennsylvania, School of Dental Medicine
Director Emeritus, Chivian Department of Dentistry, Newark Beth Israel Medical Center

Preface

One of the primary objectives of dentists has always been to prevent tooth loss and save natural dentition. Despite these efforts, many teeth still develop decay or suffer traumatic injury and often require endodontic care. Endodontics is a discipline of dentistry that deals with the morphology, physiology, and pathology of the human dental pulp and periapical tissues, as well as the prevention and treatment of diseases and injuries related to these tissues. The scope of endodontics is wide and includes initial nonsurgical root canal treatment, nonsurgical retreatment of unsuccessful treatment, and/or surgical endodontics. Many advances have been made in endodontic surgery in the past 10 to 20 years. These include enhanced magnification and illumination, ultrasonic tips, microinstruments, newer root-end filling materials, and the use of cone beam computed tomography (CBCT). These advances have significantly improved surgical endodontics and have increased the feasibility and predictability of this procedure to save natural dentition.

Like other dental procedures, the practice of surgical endodontics requires two inseparable components: art and science. The *art* of surgical endodontics consists of executing technical skills during surgical procedures. The *science* of surgical endodontics includes the basic and clinical sciences related to biologic and pathologic conditions that guide the art of procedures involved in surgical endodontics through the principles and practice of evidence-based treatment. In this textbook, the authors have incorporated evidence-based information when available and when appropriate. The textbook is written specifically for advanced students in the field of endodontics, endodontists, and others who would like to incorporate surgical endodontics in their practices.

The Art and Science of Contemporary Surgical Endodontics has been systematically organized to simulate the order of procedures performed in a clinical setting after presenting the necessary information related to the anatomy, histology, and physiology of tissues involved in surgical endodontics, as well as pathologic entities simulating lesions of pulpal origin. The first four chapters are dedicated to the basic sciences of tissues involved in surgical endodontics, followed by an extensive chapter on diagnosis and treatment planning. Several chapters focus on the most recent advances in the art of surgical endodontics related to CBCT, illumination and magnification, local anesthesia and hemostasis, management of soft tissues, removal of osseous tissue, root-end resection, root-end preparation, and root-end filling materials, as well as suturing and postoperative instructions. Following chapters are dedicated to the maxillary sinus and its relation to surgical endodontics; soft and hard tissue healing based on classic literature; and adjunctive surgical procedures such as management of procedural accidents, resorption, root amputation, hemisection, replantation, transplantation, crown lengthening, and grafting materials. A chapter on the pharmacology of surgical endodontics describes the medications that can be used preoperatively and postoperatively to aid healing and provide patient comfort, and the last chapter assesses the outcomes of surgical endodontics based on current evidence. Unique to this book is a DVD set of video clips showing many of the surgical procedures described in the textbook (see page xi).

Therefore, *The Art and Science of Contemporary Surgical Endodontics* not only teaches the reader how to perform surgical endodontics but also provides him or her with a summary of the science and technology behind technical aspects of surgical endodontics that is concise, current, and easy to follow.

Acknowledgments

We would like to thank the contributing authors for sharing their materials and experiences with us. Their contributions have significantly increased the feasibility and predictability of surgical endodontics and have resulted in saving natural dentition. We would also like to express our appreciation to the editorial staff at Quintessence Publishing, whose collaboration and dedication have made this textbook possible. In addition, we would like to acknowledge the contribution of our colleagues who provided cases that have improved the quality of this textbook. Finally, we would like to thank Mr Daryl Osborne from Educational Support Services at the Loma Linda University School of Dentistry for editing the video clips for our textbook.

Mahmoud Torabinejad
Richard Rubinstein

Contributors

Hamid Abedi, BDS

Lecturer
Department of Endodontics
School of Dentistry
Loma Linda University
Loma Linda, California

Bruno C. Azevedo, DDS, MS

Assistant Professor
Department of Oral and Maxillofacial Radiology
School of Dentistry
University of Louisville
Louisville, Kentucky

Mohamed I. Fayad, DDS, MS, PhD

Clinical Associate Professor
Department of Endodontics
Director of Research
College of Dentistry
University of Illinois at Chicago
Chicago, Illinois

Sarandeep S. Huja, BDS, DDS, MDS, MS, PhD

Associate Dean and Professor, Orthodontics Graduate Program Director
Department of Orthodontics
College of Dentistry
University of Kentucky
Lexington, Kentucky

Bradford R. Johnson, DDS, MHPE

Professor of Endodontics
Department Head and Director of Postgraduate Endodontics
College of Dentistry
University of Illinois at Chicago
Chicago, Illinois

Kathryn A. Jurosky, DDS, MS

Private Practice
Palo Alto, California

Karl Keiser, DDS, MS

Adjunct Associate Professor
Department of Endodontics
School of Dentistry
University of Texas Health Science Center at San Antonio
San Antonio, Texas

Tord Lundgren, DDS

Professor and Chair
Department of Periodontics
School of Dentistry
Loma Linda University
Loma Linda, California

Zhongrong Luo, MD, PhD

Assistant Professor
Department of Pathology and Human Anatomy
School of Medicine
Loma Linda University
Loma Linda, California

Masoud Parirokh, DMD, MSc

Distinguished Professor and Chair of Endodontics
School of Dentistry
Kerman University
Kerman, Iran

Ove A. Peters, DMD, MS, PhD

Professor and Co-chair
Department of Endodontics
Arthur A. Dugoni School of Dentistry
University of the Pacific
San Francisco, California

Bonnie Retamozo, DDS, MSD

Assistant Professor
Department of Endodontics
School of Dentistry
Loma Linda University
Loma Linda, California

Dwight D. Rice, DDS

Associate Professor
Department of Radiologic and Imaging Sciences
Department of Dental Research
School of Dentistry
Loma Linda University
Loma Linda, California

W. Eugene Roberts, DDS, PhD

Professor Emeritus of Orthodontics
Indiana University School of Dentistry

Adjunct Professor of Mechanical Engineering
Purdue University
Indianapolis, Indiana

Richard Rubinstein, DDS, MS

Adjunct Clinical Associate Professor
Department of Cariology, Restorative Sciences and Endodontics
University of Michigan School of Dentistry
Ann Arbor, Michigan

Private Practice Limited to Endodontics
Farmington Hills, Michigan

Erik Sahl, DDS, MSD

Assistant Professor, Director of Advanced Program in Periodontics
Department of Periodontics
School of Dentistry
Loma Linda University
Loma Linda, California

Nasser Said-Al-Naief, DDS, MS

Professor and Chair, Director of Oral and Maxillofacial Pathology Laboratory
Department of Pathology and Radiology
School of Dentistry
Oregon Health & Science University
Portland, Oregon

Shahrokh Shabahang, DDS, MS, PhD

Associate Professor of Endodontics
School of Dentistry
Loma Linda University
Loma Linda, California

Dimitris N. Tatakis, DDS, PhD

Professor and Director of Postdoctoral Program
Division of Periodontology
Assistant Dean for Global Initiatives
College of Dentistry
The Ohio State University
Columbus, Ohio

Roderick W. Tataryn

Private Practice Limited to Endodontics
Spokane, Washington

Mahmoud Torabinejad, DMD, MSD, PhD

Ronald E. Buell Professor of Endodontics
Director of Advanced Program in Endodontics
School of Dentistry
Loma Linda University
Loma Linda, California

Peter Velvart, Dr med dent

Private Practice Limited to Endodontics
Zurich, Switzerland

Thomas von Arx, Prof Dr med dent

Associate Professor and Vice Chairman
Department of Oral Surgery and Stomatology
School of Dental Medicine
University of Bern
Bern, Switzerland

Shane N. White, BDentSc, MA, MS, PhD

Professor of Endodontics
School of Dentistry
University of California, Los Angeles
Los Angeles, California

Kenneth R. Wright, PhD

Associate Professor, Graduate Program Director
Division of Human Anatomy
School of Medicine
Loma Linda University
Loma Linda, California

List of Videos

Description	Duration (min)
Chapter 5	
5-1 Gow-Gates block injection	1:57
5-2 Vazirani-Akinosi block injection	1:05
5-3 Second division block injection	0:49
5-4 Infraorbital block	1:55
5-5 Intraosseous injection	2:49
5-6 Periodontal ligament injection	1:41
5-7 Incision and drainage	4:54
5-8 Irretrievable filling materials 1	4:09
5-9 Irretrievable filling materials 2	7:41
5-10 Irretrievable filling materials 3	7:21
5-11 Symptomatic cases during root canal therapy	10:40
5-12 Symptomatic cases after root canal therapy	7:36
5-13 Exploratory surgery	8:05
Chapter 9	
9-1 Full-thickness flap	2:52
9-2 Palatal root surgery	10:33
9-3 Ochsenbein Luebke flap	1:48
9-4 Papilla base flap	5:37
Chapter 13	
13-1 Simple interrupted suture	1:18
13-2 Figure-eight suture	1:05
13-3 Interrupted simple sling suture	1:36
13-4 Continuous independent sling suture	2:13
13-5 Horizontal mattress suture	1:05
13-6 Simple interrupted suture removal	0:29
13-7 Continuous sling suture removal	0:37
Chapter 15	
15-1 Repair of external resorption by tooth replantation	7:03
15-2 Tooth replantation	5:20
15-3 Transplantation	7:56
15-4 Root amputation	5:26
15-5 Hemisection	1:45
15-6 Crown lengthening	7:04
15-7 Guided tissue regeneration	8:54

The authors have attempted to present a complete collection of surgical videos representative of all regions of the mouth, but they recognize that there are emerging technologies, methods, and approaches that are too expansive to be included at this time. Future editions of this textbook will include videos reflecting new advances and developments in surgical endodontics.

Chapter One

Anatomical Zones in Endodontic Surgery

Kenneth R. Wright, Dwight D. Rice, Zhongrong Luo

The oral environment is a complex region formed of a mixture of hard and soft tissues. Its functions include chewing, swallowing, and speech, as well as acting as an accessory airway. Maintenance of a healthy dentition is imperative to the overall well-being of the individual and proper functioning of the alimentary system. An in-depth understanding of the structure and function of the oral apparatus is required to provide proper care to oral structures and tissues.

In addition to posing the risk of damaging parts of the tooth, endodontic procedures also risk damaging tissues and anatomical structures surrounding the tooth root.[1] It is therefore essential to have a thorough understanding of the anatomy of the jaws and in particular the parts of these bones housing neurovascular structures or pneumatic spaces. In this chapter, we examine the anatomy of the maxillary sinus, the mandibular canal with its branches (the mental canal/foramen and the incisive canal), and the incisive canal and palatine foramina of the maxilla, as well as their relationships to the roots of teeth. But first we examine the anatomy of the oral region in general.

The Bony Framework

Maxilla

The maxilla forms much of the midportion of the face, the borders of the nasal aperture, part of the margin of the orbits, and most of the hard palate and the support for the upper lip and teeth (Fig 1-1). Branches from the maxillary artery supply most of the maxillary region, and sensory innervation is provided by the maxillary division of the trigeminal nerve, designated as cranial nerve V2.

Associated with the nasal cavity are four sets of paranasal sinuses, found in the frontal, maxillary, sphenoid, and ethmoid bones. The largest of the paranasal sinuses, the maxillary sinus, is housed in the body of the maxilla (Fig 1-2). This pneumatic space is roughly pyramid shaped, with the base of the pyramid formed by the medial wall of the sinus, which is also the lateral wall of the nasal cavity. The medial wall of the sinus is actually formed by parts of five bones—the maxilla, the lacrimal bone, the

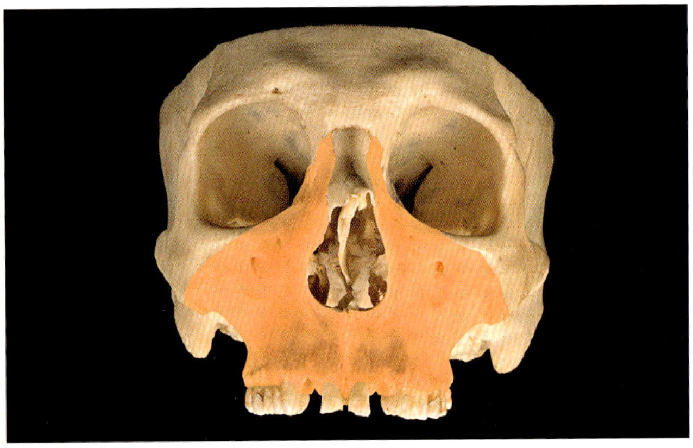

Fig 1-1 The maxilla shown from an anterior angulation. Borders of the maxilla include the floor of the orbit, the zygomatic bone, and the lateral borders of the nasal cavity. The alveolar process forms the inferior boundary.

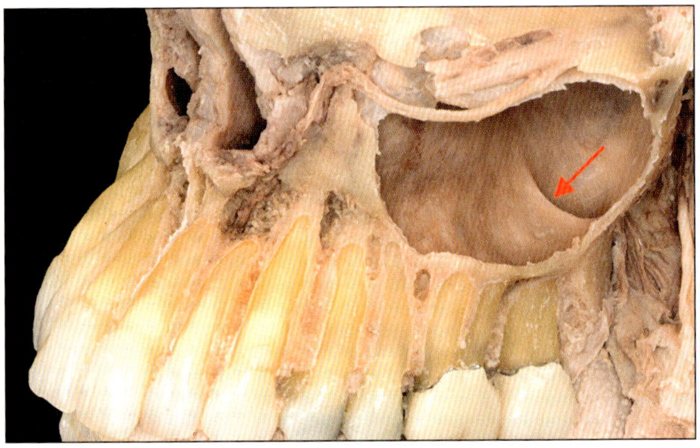

Fig 1-2 The maxillary sinus is housed in the body of the maxilla. This pneumatic space is roughly pyramid shaped, with the base of the pyramid formed by the medial wall of the sinus, which is also the lateral wall of the nasal cavity. Note the presence of a sinus septum *(arrow)*.

inferior nasal concha, the perpendicular plate of the palatine bone, and the uncinate process of the ethmoid bone. The ostium of the sinus drains to the middle meatus, the space inferior to the middle nasal concha, on the lateral nasal wall (Fig 1-3). The posterior wall of the sinus faces the maxillary tuberosity, the roof forms the floor of the orbit, and the floor of the sinus extends inferiorly into the alveolar ridge of the maxilla, most commonly in the area of the second premolar and first and second molars. Innervation of the mucosa lining the maxillary sinus is provided by the posterior, middle, and anterior superior alveolar nerves and the infraorbital nerve, all branches of V2. The blood supply is primarily from branches of the maxillary artery accompanying these nerve branches, as well as the descending palatine artery, which accompanies the greater and lesser palatine nerves, and sometimes the posterior superior alveolar artery. During endodontic surgery, it is important to be aware of the position of the posterior superior alveolar nerve to avoid damaging it.

The maxillary sinus, like all the paranasal sinuses, is lined by respiratory mucosa, comprising pseudostratified ciliated columnar epithelium with goblet cells overlying a rather thin lamina propria that adheres to the periosteum covering underlying bone (mucoperiosteum). The mucosa covering the floor of the sinus—the sinus membrane—is often somewhat thickened and is sometimes referred to as the *Schneiderian membrane* clinically (Figs 1-4 and 1-5).

The alveolar process or ridge is the portion of the maxilla that houses the roots of the teeth. The cortical plate forming the outer walls of this ridge is relatively thin, allowing the infiltration of anesthetics. Below the midpoint of the inferior orbital rim, an infraorbital foramen provides passage for the infraorbital nerve, a continuation of the maxillary nerve (V2), along with infraorbital vessels. A canine eminence shows the location of the root of the canine tooth. Medial to this eminence is an incisive fossa, and lateral to the eminence is a canine fossa (Fig 1-6).

The hard palate is formed primarily by the two lateral palatine processes of the maxilla, which fuse in the midline to form the intermaxillary, or median palatine, suture. Two transverse palatine sutures separate the posterior borders of the palatine processes of the maxilla from the horizontal plates of the palatine bones, which form the posterior third of the hard palate. These sutures are sometimes incomplete laterally, forming greater palatine foramina that transmit the greater palatine nerves and vessels. Posterior to the greater palatine foramina are smaller lesser palatine foramina, located within the pyramidal processes of the palatine bones and transmitting the lesser palatine nerves and vessels. Just posterior to the maxillary central incisors lies the incisive fossa, into which open incisive canals by way of incisive foramina, transmitting the nasopalatine nerves and sphenopalatine vessels from the nasal cavity (Fig 1-7).

The oral portion of the maxilla is covered by mucosa. The buccal or vestibular surface of the maxilla is covered by alveolar mucosa, which transitions to attached gingiva at the mucogingival junction. On the palatal side, the mucosa covering the hard palate transitions to the gingiva covering the tooth-bearing alveolar process. Much of the hard palate is covered by a mucoperiosteum, characterized by the attachment of collagen fibers in the lamina propria that blend with the underlying periosteum, without an intervening submucosa. A median palatine mucosal raphe indicates the location of the median palatine suture. Anteriorly, immediately posterior to the

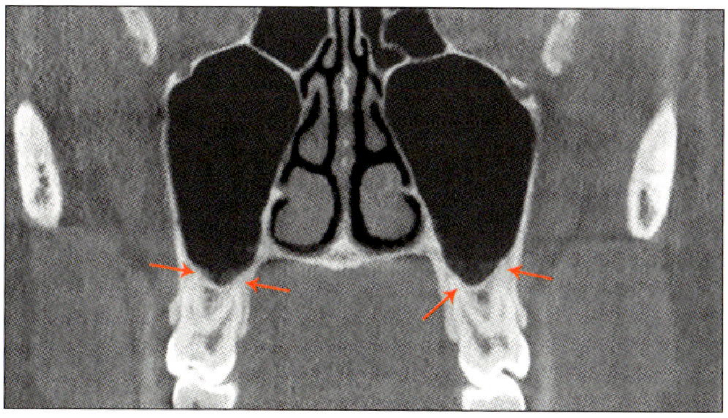

Fig 1-3 A coronal section of the maxillary sinus using cone beam computed tomography (CBCT) imaging. Note the close proximity of the root tips to the floor of the sinus *(red arrows)*.

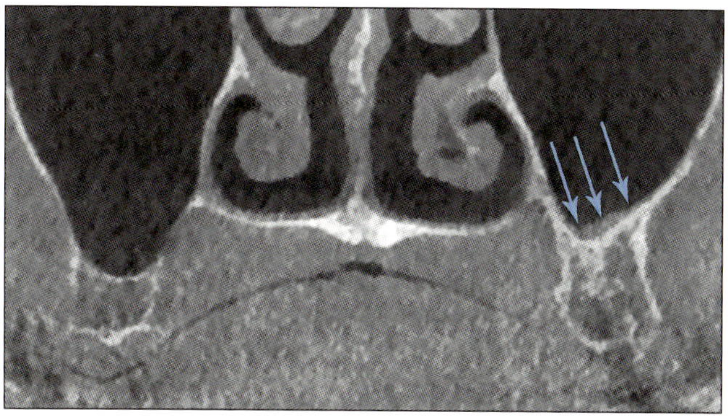

Fig 1-4 Coronal CBCT image of a slightly thickened sinus membrane *(arrows)*.

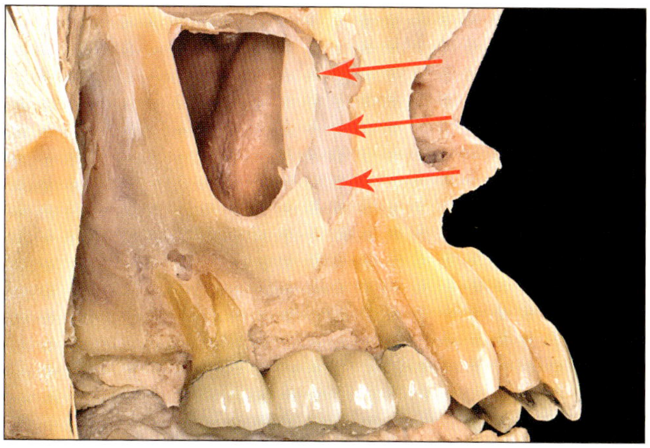

Fig 1-5 The mucosa covering the floor and walls of the sinus is sometimes referred to as the *Schneiderian membrane* clinically. The *arrows* point to a section left during the dissection. Notice its thin, delicate nature.

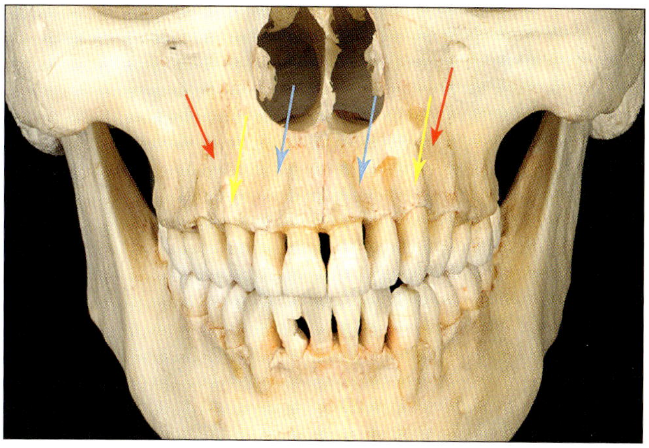

Fig 1-6 The canine eminence *(yellow arrows)* shows the location of the root of the canine tooth. Medial to this eminence is an incisive fossa *(blue arrows)*, and lateral to the eminence is a canine fossa *(red arrows)*.

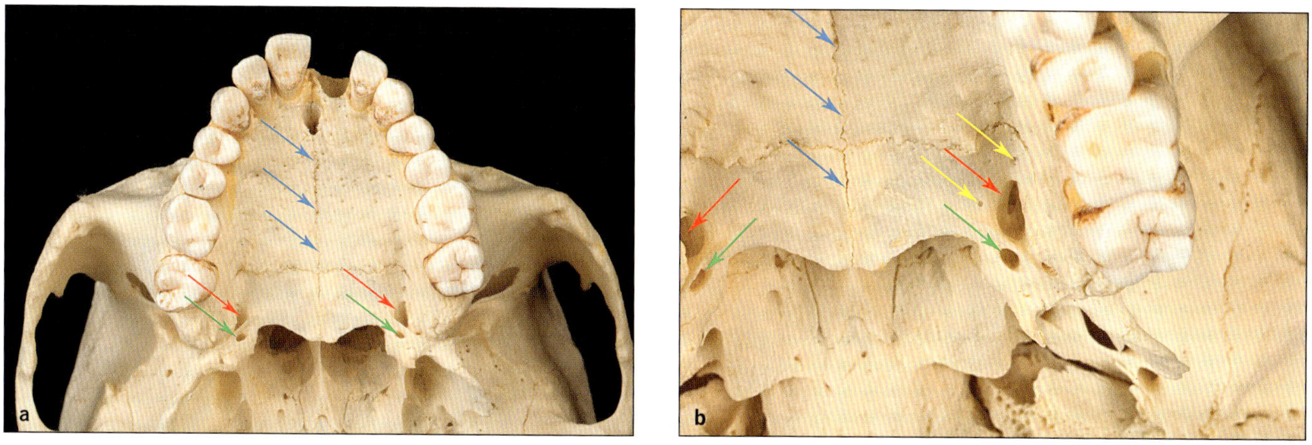

Fig 1-7 *(a and b)* Remarkable features of the hard palate include the intermaxillary suture *(blue arrows)*, greater palatine foramina *(red arrows)*, and lesser palatine foramina *(green arrows)*. Note the supplemental foramina *(yellow arrows)* in the posterior region *(b)*.

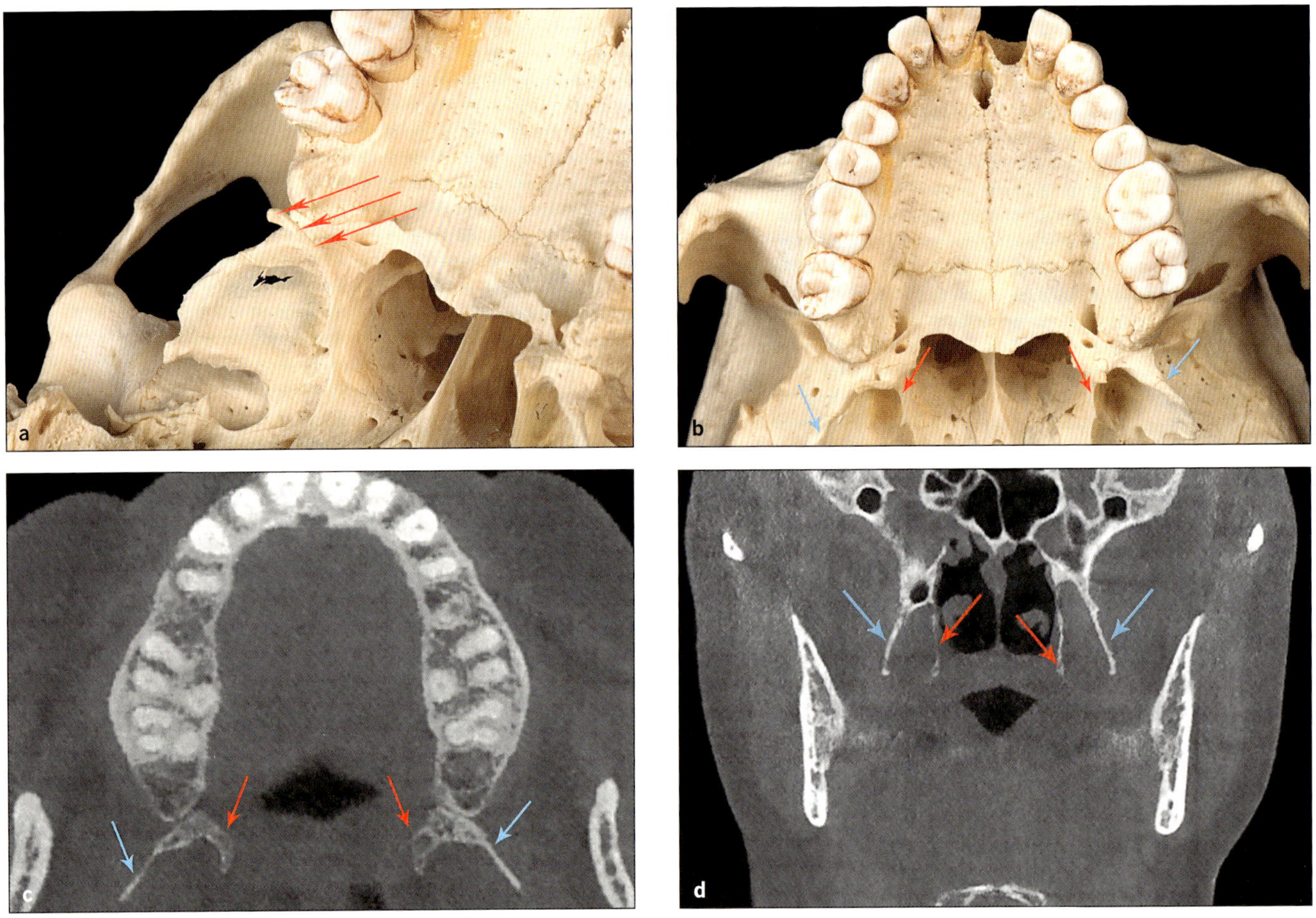

Fig 1-8 *(a)* At the inferior tip of the medial pterygoid plate, just posterior to the lateral aspect of the hard palate, is a hooklike process called the *hamulus (red arrows)*. *(b and c)* The medial *(red arrows)* and lateral *(blue arrows)* pterygoid plates of the sphenoid bone seen in axial view in dry skull and CBCT images. *(d)* Coronal CBCT image showing the medial *(red arrows)* and lateral *(blue arrows)* pterygoid plates.

central incisors, a small midline incisive papilla indicates the location of the incisive fossa, and projecting laterally from the midline is a series of mucosal ridges called *palatine rugae*. Posterior to this lies a fatty region underlying the mucosa as well as a glandular region that contains numerous mucoserous minor salivary glands, or *palatine glands*. The mucosa of the hard palate transitions to the mucosa covering the soft palate, a muscular and glandular structure that blends laterally into the palatoglossal and palatopharyngeal folds, or anterior and posterior pillars of the *fauces*, the opening of the oral cavity into the oropharynx. The soft palate, also called the *palatine velum*, terminates posteriorly in the midline by a small muscular projection, the *uvula*, which serves to close off the oropharynx from the nasopharynx during swallowing.

The posterolateral border of the hard palate, just posterior to the greater and lesser palatine foramina, articulates or fuses with the pterygoid process of the sphenoid bone. This process is made up of medial and lateral pterygoid plates, which run vertically just posterior to the hard palate. Between the two pterygoid plates lies the pterygoid fossa, and above that is a small scaphoid fossa. The lateral and medial pterygoid muscles have attachments to the lateral pterygoid plate, and the tensor veli palatini muscle attaches to the scaphoid fossa of the medial pterygoid plate. At the inferior tip of the medial pterygoid plate, just posterior to the lateral aspect of the hard palate, is a hooklike process called the *hamulus* (Fig 1-8). The tendon of tensor veli palatini hooks over the hamulus before inserting into the soft palate. The hamulus also serves as a point of attachment for the pterygomandibular raphe and for the superior pharyngeal constrictor. Overactive pterygoid muscles can generate myofascial pain, which can mimic endodontic symptoms.

Neurovascular supply to the maxilla

Blood supply. The maxilla with its associated soft tissues and teeth are supplied primarily by the maxillary artery, a terminal artery that branches from the external carotid artery deep to the ramus of the mandible and travels through the infratemporal fossa, where it gives off branches to the muscles of mastication and surrounding structures. The inferior alveolar artery originates from this portion of the maxillary artery. The maxillary artery then passes through the pterygomaxillary fissure to provide blood supply to the palate via the descending palatine artery; the walls of the nasal cavity and anterior palate via branches of the sphenopalatine artery; the mucosa of the maxillary sinus and the maxillary teeth via the posterior, middle, and anterior superior alveolar arteries; and the floor of the orbit and part of the face via the infraorbital artery. The blood supply to this region is supplemented by the facial/angular artery and its superior labial and lateral nasal branches, as well as the ascending palatine and tonsillar branches.

Nerve supply. The maxillary region of the face and oral cavity are both supplied primarily by branches of the maxillary division of the trigeminal nerve (V2). This nerve branches from the trigeminal ganglion in the middle cranial fossa and passes through the foramen rotundum to enter the upper part of the pterygopalatine fossa. In this fossa, the maxillary nerve is connected to the pterygopalatine ganglion, a parasympathetic ganglion, by two small pterygopalatine (sphenopalatine) nerves. These little nerves conduct sensory fibers to the ganglion, from which they are distributed to the nasal and oral regions. Preganglionic parasympathetic fibers from the superior salivatory nucleus in the pontine tegmentum of the brain stem travel with the facial nerve to the geniculate ganglion, where they leave the facial nerve as the greater petrosal nerve. This nerve travels in a small groove on the floor of the middle cranial fossa, joining with the deep petrosal nerve, which is composed of postganglionic sympathetic fibers from the superior cervical ganglion. Together, the greater and deep petrosal nerves combine to form the nerve of the pterygoid canal (Vidian nerve), which passes through the pterygoid canal to enter the pterygopalatine fossa. The preganglionic parasympathetic fibers synapse in the pterygopalatine ganglion, from which postganglionic fibers are distributed with sensory fibers from V2 to the nasal and oral regions. Postganglionic sympathetic fibers from the deep petrosal nerve accompany the postganglionic parasympathetic and sensory fibers. Major branches from the pterygopalatine ganglion include lateral nasal branches, the nasopalatine nerve, greater and lesser palatine nerves, posterior superior alveolar nerves, and the infraorbital nerve, which gives rise to the middle and anterior superior alveolar nerves. A small zygomatic branch divides into zygomaticotemporal and zygomaticofacial nerves, which supply skin and soft tissues in the zygomatic region of the face. From the zygomatic nerve, a small communicating branch carries postganglionic fibers to the lacrimal nerve, a branch of the ophthalmic division of the trigeminal nerve, to provide stimulation for lacrimal gland secretion. The posterior, middle, and anterior superior alveolar nerves supply the pulps and periodontium of maxillary teeth and the mucosa of the maxillary sinus.

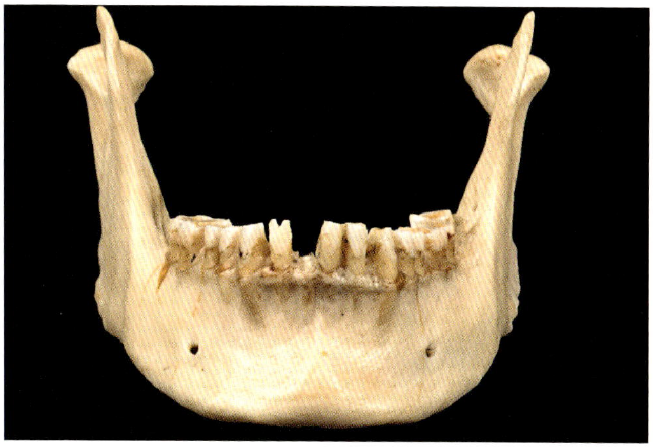

Fig 1-9 Anterior view of the mandible.

Mandible

The mandible, a horseshoe-shaped bone forming the chin and lower jaw, is the only movable bone in the head (other than the ossicles in the middle ear) (Fig 1-9). The body of the mandible is the horizontal portion of the bone supporting the teeth, and the ramus is the more vertical posterior portion articulating with the temporal bone. Anteriorly in the midline is the symphysis menti, a site of fusion of two mandibular primordia during the embryologic development of the mandible that forms much of the chin. Extending outward and downward from the midline is a triangular-shaped mental protuberance; its two inferior angles are known as *mental tubercles*. Two incisive fossae are found just superior to the tubercles. A mental foramen is located laterally about midway between the lower margin of the body of the mandible and the alveolar crest, at approximately the level of the first premolar or slightly more posteriorly, although the position is variable. An oblique line begins partway back along the body, starting near the inferior border and terminating as the anterior border of the ramus and leading up to the triangle-shaped coronoid process. The posterior border of the ramus meets the inferior border of the body of the mandible at the (gonial) angle of the mandible.

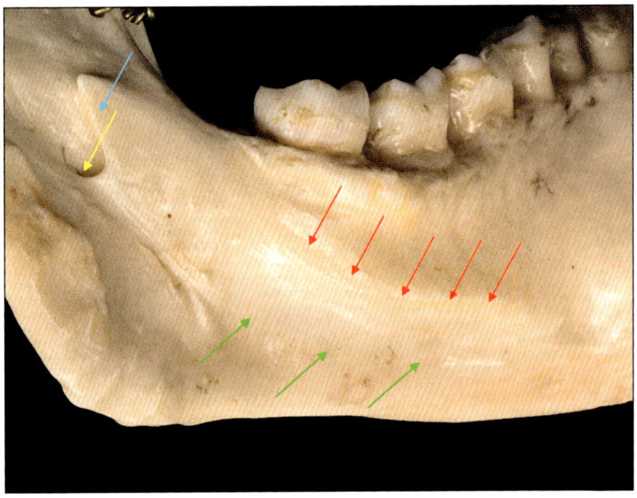

Fig 1-10 The internal or deep surface of the mandible. Note the submandibular fossa *(green arrows)*, the mylohyoid line *(red arrows)*, the lingula *(blue arrow)*, and the mandibular foramen *(yellow arrow)*.

The area just anterior and superior to the angle is roughened, indicating the area of attachment for the masseter muscle. Superior to the posterior border of the ramus is the condylar process, formed of the rounded condyle that articulates with the mandibular or glenoid fossa of the temporal bone, with a narrow neck of the mandible just proximal to the condyle. Just inferior to the medial aspect of the condyle is the pterygoid fovea, a point of attachment for the lateral pterygoid muscle. The depression along the superior border of the ramus, between the condyle and coronoid process, is the mandibular notch, which allows passage of the masseteric nerve and vessels going to supply the masseter muscle.

On the medial or deep surface of the ramus of the mandible, roughly midway between the inferior border of the mandible and the mandibular notch and approximately midway between the anterior and posterior borders of the ramus, is the mandibular foramen through which the inferior alveolar nerve and vessels enter the mandible to be distributed to the mandibular teeth and soft tissues. Just anterosuperior to the mandibular foramen, a triangular bony protuberance, the lingula, serves as an attachment for the sphenomandibular ligament as well as a landmark for administration of inferior alveolar nerve blocks. In the midline of the anterior aspect of the mandible, on its deep surface, the genial tubercles or spines serve as attachments for the genioglossus and geniohyoid muscles. Extending posteriorly along the body of the mandible is the oblique mylohyoid line, which serves as the attachment for the mylohyoid muscle. Superoanterior to the mylohyoid line is the sublingual fossa, and inferoposterior to the mylohyoid line is the submandibular fossa. These two fossae house the major salivary glands with the same names. Extending anteroinferiorly from the mandibular foramen is the mylohyoid groove, which accommodates the nerve going to the mylohyoid and anterior digastric muscles. A roughened area on the inner surface of the angle of the mandible is the attachment of the medial pterygoid muscle (Fig 1-10).

The muscular tongue fills most of the oral cavity proper (the space interior to the dental arches) and is separated from the mandibular dental arch by the sublingual sulcus (floor of the mouth). The mucosa of the sulcus overlies several important structures: the submandibular duct, the lingual nerve, and more inferiorly the hypoglossal nerve, in addition to the vena comitans of the hypoglossal nerve. In the anterior region of the floor of the mouth are the sublingual glands, one on either side of the tongue, forming sublingual folds (plicae). The tongue is attached to the floor of the mouth and dental arch by the midline lingual frenulum. The mucosa of the floor of the mouth, as with the maxilla, transitions to gingiva on the medial aspect of the alveolar process of the mandible. Each lip also has a midline frenulum that attaches the lip to the alveolar bone of its associated dental arch. An overactive frenulum can cause mucogingival defects, which can have implications for esthetics and for endodontic implant placement.

Neurovascular supply to the mandible and associated structures

Blood supply. The mandibular region is supplied primarily by branches from the facial, lingual, and maxillary arteries. The facial artery is a branch of the external carotid artery, entering the facial region by curving around the inferior border of the mandible about midway between the mental tubercle and the angle of the mandible, and then running diagonally toward the corner of the mouth and then just lateral to the nose, where it becomes the angular artery. The facial artery gives off submental, inferior, and superior labial branches and a lateral nasal branch. The lingual artery supplies the tongue by way of deep lingual and dorsal lingual branches. The sublingual artery supplies the floor of the mouth, the sublingual salivary gland, and surrounding muscles.

The inferior alveolar artery originates from the maxillary artery in the infratemporal fossa and travels with the inferior alveolar nerve through the mandibular foramen into the mandibular canal, where it gives off branches to the pulp and periodontium of mandibular teeth. A mental artery branches off, passes through the mental foramen with the mental nerve, and supplies the lower lip and chin area. A buccal artery, also from the maxillary artery, supplies much of the buccal region, anastomosing with the facial artery.

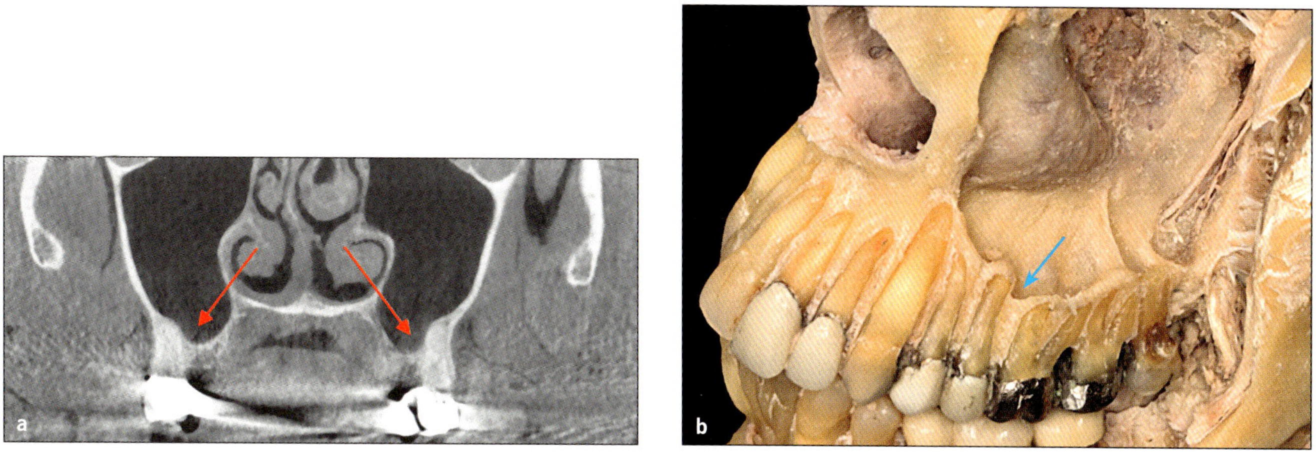

Fig 1-11 *(a)* Coronal CBCT image showing roots extending well superior to the floor of the sinus *(red arrows)*. *(b)* The dissection also shows the floor of the sinus dropping down between the root apices *(blue arrow)*.

Nerve supply. The primary nerve supply to the mandibular region is via the mandibular division of the trigeminal nerve (V3). Branches from this nerve supply both sensory and motor innervation. The mandibular nerve (V3) emerges from the trigeminal ganglion by passing through the foramen ovale into the infratemporal fossa, where it gives off motor branches to the muscles of mastication along with tensor tympani and tensor veli palatini, and supplies the mylohyoid muscle and the anterior belly of the digastric muscle. The lingual nerve supplies general sensation to the anterior two-thirds of the tongue, the mucosa covering the floor of the mouth, and lingual gingiva associated with mandibular teeth. The buccal nerve supplies the skin of the buccal region and the buccal mucosa and buccal gingiva for both mandibular and maxillary teeth. The inferior alveolar branch travels through the mandibular foramen, giving off branches to tooth pulp and periodontium, and terminates by giving off mental and incisive branches, which supply the chin, lower lip, and gingiva in the region of the mandibular incisors.

Anatomical Danger Zones in Endodontic Surgery

In performing endodontic surgery, a number of anatomical, histologic, and neurovascular structures are vulnerable to damage. In order to avoid damaging these structures, a thorough understanding of the anatomy and histology associated with the areas adjacent to the roots of the teeth is imperative. The remainder of this chapter focuses on these "danger areas," while chapter 2 focuses on the histology of the oral cavity.

Maxillary sinus (antrum of Highmore)

The maxillary sinus is one of the first of the paranasal sinuses to form during fetal development.[2] As a person ages, the maxillary sinus expands laterally and inferiorly, until its floor finally lies about 4 to 5 mm inferior to the level of the floor of the nasal cavity.[3–5] In edentulous areas, the sinus floor can drop to become nearly level with the height of the alveolar ridge; this pneumatization of the sinus has implications for oral surgical procedures such as implant and apical endodontic surgery. As the floor of the sinus continues to descend, it comes to lie in proximity to the apices of maxillary teeth (Fig 1-11), primarily the second premolar and the first and second molars.[3] In rare cases, the floor of the sinus can extend as far anteriorly as the canine root.[3] With time, the bone forming the floor of the sinus can thin considerably, allowing the roots to protrude into the sinus[3] (Fig 1-12). Eberhardt et al[6] showed in a CT study that the apex of the mesiobuccal root of the maxillary second molar was closest to the sinus floor. This relationship can often be adequately seen with panoramic radiography, but CT provides better resolution[7] (Fig 1-13). Nimigean et al[4] reported that alveolar recesses (depressions between root apices) were present in 52% of cases, increasing the risk of penetration into the antrum during surgical procedures. They described three different relationships between tooth roots and the floor of the sinus: *(1)* one in which there is a thick layer of bone between the root and the floor, *(2)* one in which there is only a very thin layer of bone between root and antrum, and *(3)* one in which the root apices penetrate into the floor of the sinus, with the roots being covered only by the sinus membrane.[8–11] In the study by Nimigean et al,[4] the buccal roots of the first and second molars were most likely to penetrate the sinus floor.

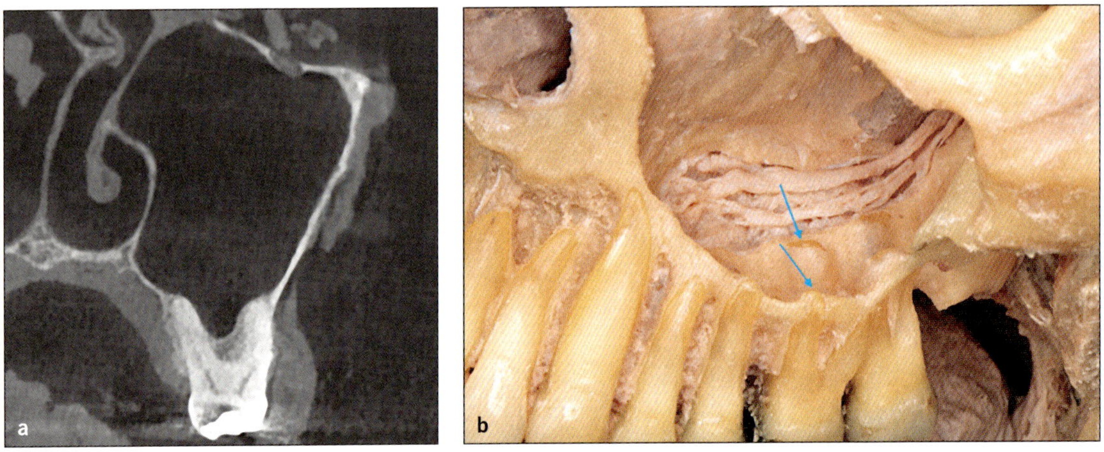

Fig 1-12 *(a and b)* Notice the small fenestrations into the floor of the sinus; in addition, one can appreciate the close proximity of the greater palatine nerve to the palatal roots of the maxillary second and third molars *(blue arrows)*. The CBCT image is aligned in the coronal plane of the first molar, showing the mesial buccal and palatal root.

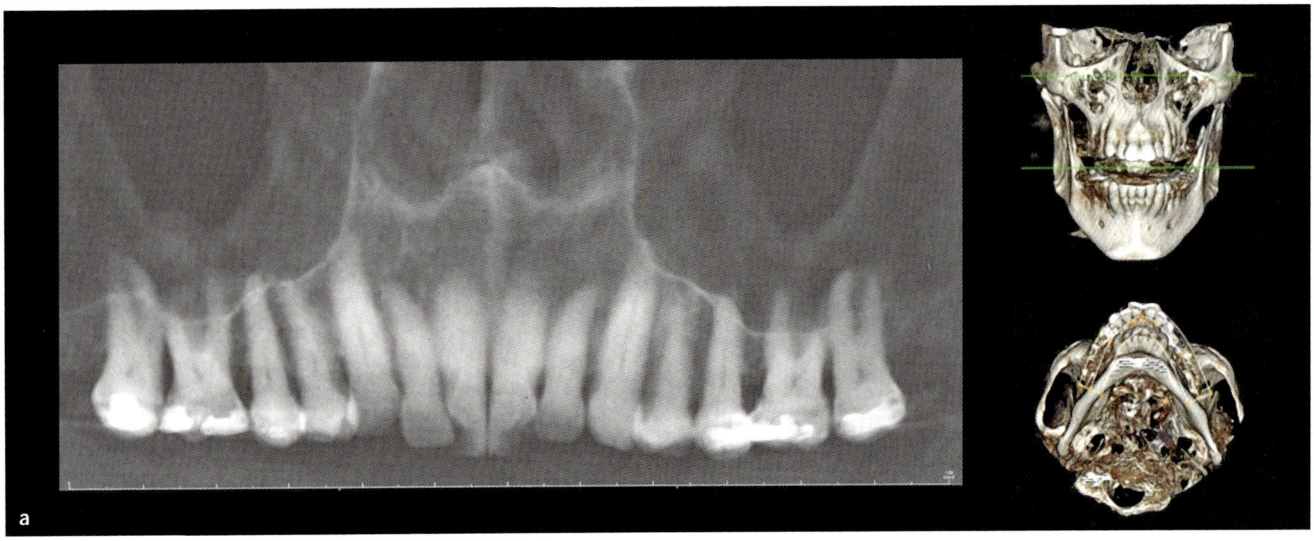

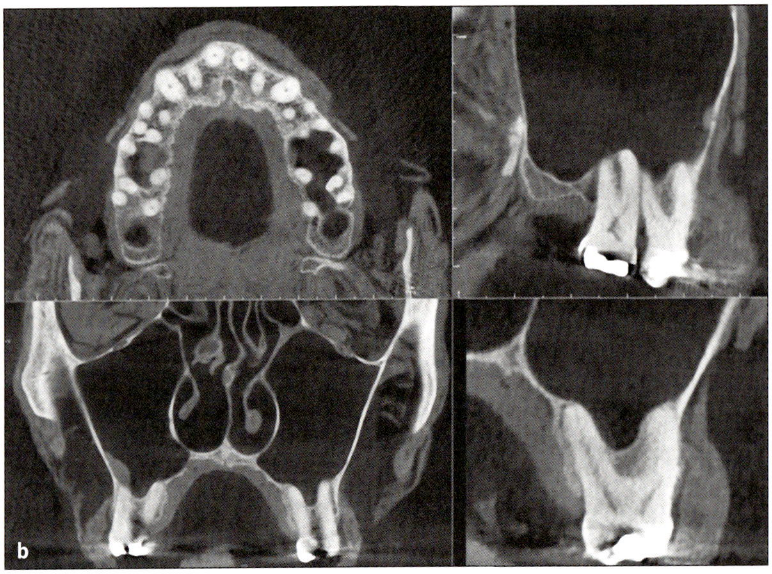

Fig 1-13 *(a)* Panoramic reconstruction from a CBCT scan showing the relationship between the sinus floor and root apices. *(b)* CBCT image showing a multiplanar reconstruction (MPR).

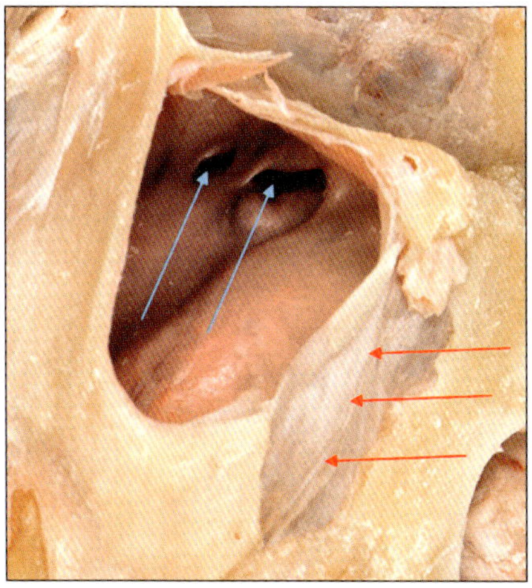

Fig 1-14 A portion of the sinus membrane *(red arrows)* was left on the anterior floor of the maxillary sinus. Note the double ostium *(blue arrows)* in the posterior superior portion of the sinus.

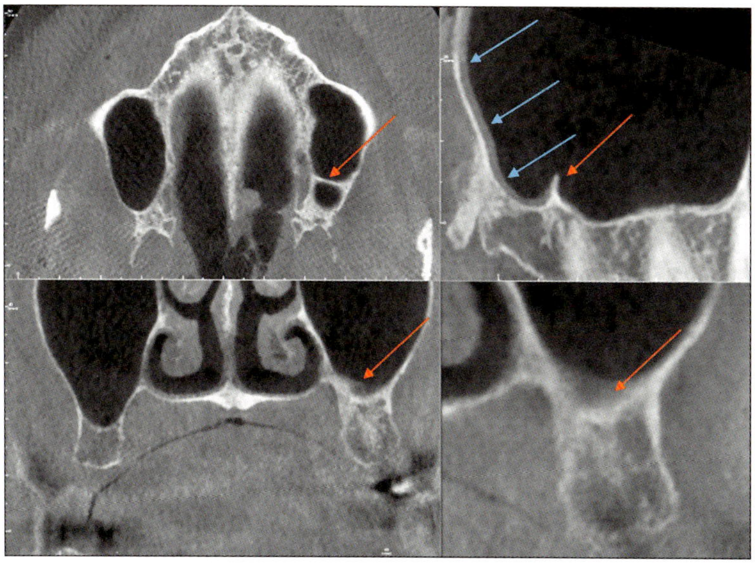

Fig 1-15 A small sinus septum is present on this CBCT image *(red arrows)*. The sinus membrane is also visible on this reconstruction *(blue arrows)*.

The sinus membrane, the mucosa lining the maxillary sinus (Fig 1-14), is formed of an epithelial layer of pseudostratified ciliated columnar tissue (respiratory epithelium) sitting on a lamina propria; it is attached to the periosteum lining the bone, which forms the walls of the sinus. While Testori[12] states that the normal thickness of this membrane is 0.13 to 0.5 mm, Janner et al[13] reported that the thickness varies from 0.16 to 34.61 mm, with the mucosa being thicker in men than in women, and suggested that any thickening greater than 2 mm is pathologic. Srouji et al[14] showed that the deeper layer of the membrane contains osteoprogenitor cells that could potentially be stimulated to differentiate into osteoblasts, which could then build up the sinus floor. When procedures affecting the floor of the maxillary sinus are performed (eg, for placing implants), the sinus membrane is often elevated from the floor of the sinus, so that it remains intact during the procedure. It has been shown that damage to the membrane can make the sinus more susceptible to infection and other complications.[15] Yildirim et al[16] showed that in cases where the floor of the sinus is indented by maxillary teeth, the mucosa tends to be thicker than the floors of sinuses without indentations.

Many maxillary sinuses are partially or completely divided into smaller compartments by bony septa, often called *Underwood's septa*[12,17–21] (see Fig 1-2). Maestre-Ferrin et al[17] report that between 13% and 35.3% of sinuses have some sort of septum. Krennmair et al[20] suggest that these septa often result from bone resorption of the floor of the sinus after tooth loss or from increased pneumatization over time. According to Krennmair et al,[20] these septa tend to form most frequently in the anterior part of the sinus, but other studies reported prevalence in other locations.[22–25] Most of the septa are oriented vertically, but Gülşen et al[19] report on two cases showing horizontal septation of the sinus and suggest that this will affect the ability to elevate the sinus membrane to place implants. It is important to examine the sinus radiographically for septa before performing procedures that could disturb the floor or membrane of the maxillary sinus. Partial blockage of the ostium, anthroliths in the sinus, and other benign to aggressive pathologies might be present on CBCTs and should be evaluated whenever the sinus is present in the scan (Fig 1-15).

The function of the paranasal sinuses remains largely unknown. Theories include roles such as humidification and warming of inspired air, assisting in regulating intranasal pressure, increasing the surface area of the olfactory membrane, lightening the skull to maintain proper head balance, imparting resonance to the voice, absorption of shocks to the head, contributing to facial growth, and perhaps as evolutionary remains of useless air spaces.[3] When radiographic imaging includes these areas, any abnormalities should be noted.

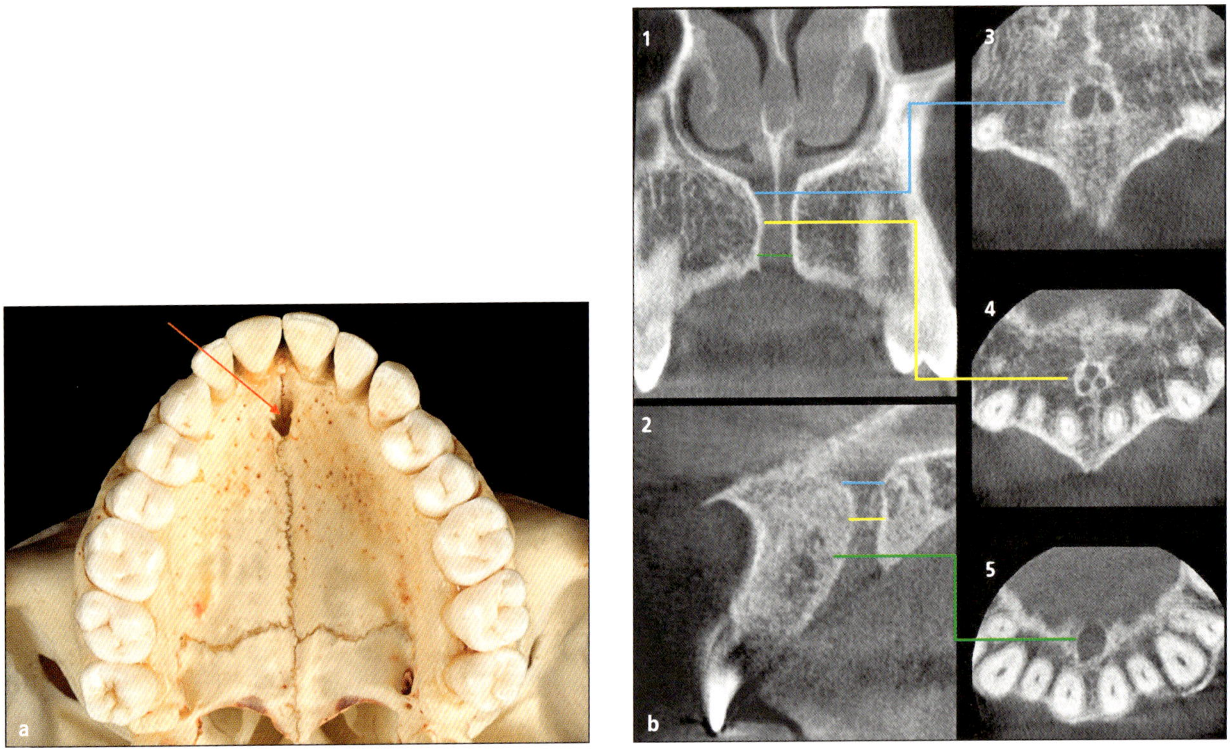

Fig 1-16 *(a)* The incisive canal opens in the hard palate just posterior to the central incisors by way of the incisive fossa *(red arrow)*. *(b)* CBCT image of the incisive canal and foramen. 1, coronal; 2, sagittal; 3, superior axial; 4, middle axial; 5, inferior axial.

Maxillary incisive fossa and canals

The maxillary incisive canal (Fig 1-16), so named because of its proximity to the maxillary incisors, is a cylindric or funnel-shaped tube connecting the nasal cavity with the oral cavity and transmitting the nasopalatine nerve. The sphenopalatine artery, a terminal branch of the maxillary artery, anastomoses with the greater palatine artery in the canal. The incisive canal opens in the hard palate just posterior to the central incisors by way of the incisive fossa. The incisive canals are larger, and the bone anterior to the canal is thicker in men than in women.[26–28] The bone anterior to the canal thins with age, even in dentulous patients. The canal is shorter in edentulous patients than in dentulous patients.[27] Careful attention should be paid when performing apical surgery, root canal therapy, or implant surgery in close proximity to this area.

Greater palatine foramen

While traditional textbooks[29] describe the greater palatine foramen as being at the lateral extremity of the transverse palatine suture or opposite the maxillary second molar, it is actually more posteriorly located—either opposite or posterior to the third molar, about 1.5 cm from the median suture, and about 0.2 cm from the posterior border of the hard palate[30–32]; it can be as far as 0.47 cm from the posterior margin of the hard palate in some ethnic groups.[31] The opening is most often in an inferior or vertical position and less commonly in an anterior or horizontal position,[30] although this varies with ethnicity.[32] A bony projection similar to the lingula is occasionally present along the posterior boundary of the foramen, separating it from the lesser palatine foramen.[30]

The lesser palatine foramen is located posterior to the greater palatine foramen. Although there is typically only one on each side, there can be two or more foramina per side. The most common position of the lesser palatine foramen is at the junction of the palatine bone and the inner lamella of the pterygoid plate.[31]

The greater palatine foramen is the opening for the greater palatine canal (Fig 1-17), which transmits the greater and lesser palatine nerves and the descending palatine artery, which then branches into greater and lesser palatine arteries before exiting their respective foramina. The walls of the greater palatine canal are formed anteriorly by the infratemporal surface of the maxilla, posteriorly by the pterygoid process of the sphenoid bone, and medially by the perpendicular plate of the palatine

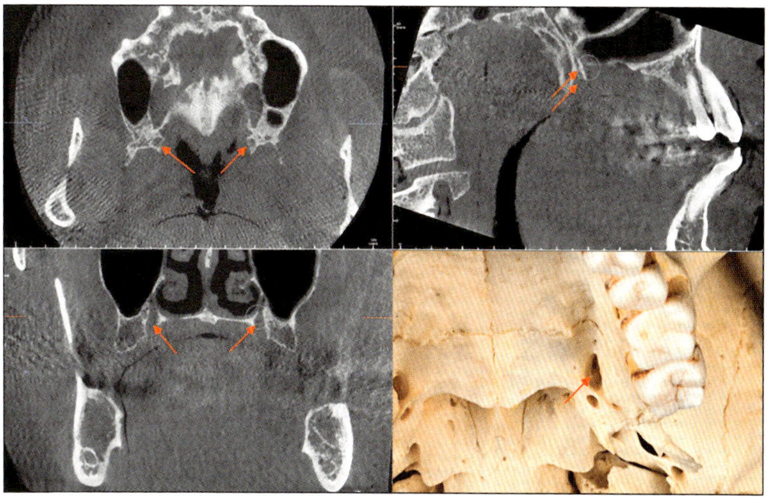

Fig 1-17 The greater palatine canal is in close proximity to the maxillary palatal root of the second molar and should be given great care in surgical planning and treatment. The *red arrows* indicate the position of the canal and foramen in multiplanar CBCT imaging as well as dry skull anatomy.

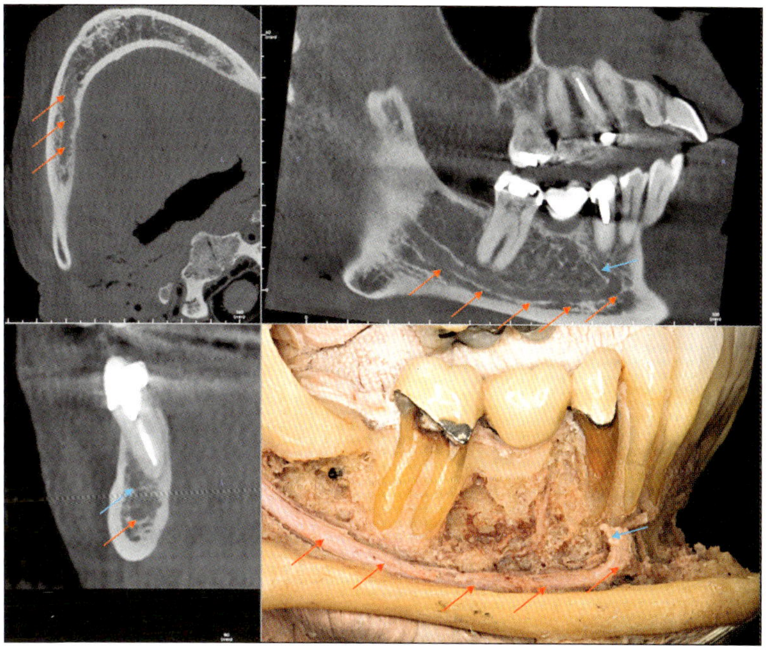

Fig 1-18 The mandibular canal shown in MPR CBCT reconstruction as well as dissection. The *red arrows* show the course of the canal and nerve. In this case, the canal loops in the anterior region *(blue arrow)*. This looping must be considered for surgical treatments in this area.

process.[33] The close proximity of these structures, especially when dealing with palatal surgical approaches to the maxillary second and third molars (see Fig 1-12), requires vigilant attention to minimize possible postsurgical complications.

Greater palatine nerve

Before or after exiting the greater palatine foramen, the greater palatine nerve splits into several branches that supply sensory and secretory fibers to the mucous membranes of the hard palate and palatal gingiva.[34] Because of this branching pattern, one should avoid incisions without first dissecting out these vital structures.

Mandibular canal

The mandibular canal begins at the mandibular foramen on the inner surface of the ramus of the mandible and continues downward and forward in the body of the mandible, approximately midway between the superior and inferior borders of the mandible (Fig 1-18). However, there is variation in the vertical position of the canal.[35] In one study,[36] it was reported that the average distance between the inferior border of the mandible and the mandibular canal was 10.52 mm. The mean maximum diameters of the mandibular canal, inferior alveolar nerve, inferior alveolar artery, and inferior alveolar vein were 2.52, 1.84, 0.42, and 0.58 mm, respectively.[36] Gowgiel[37] reported that the canal was located near the lingual cortical plate and

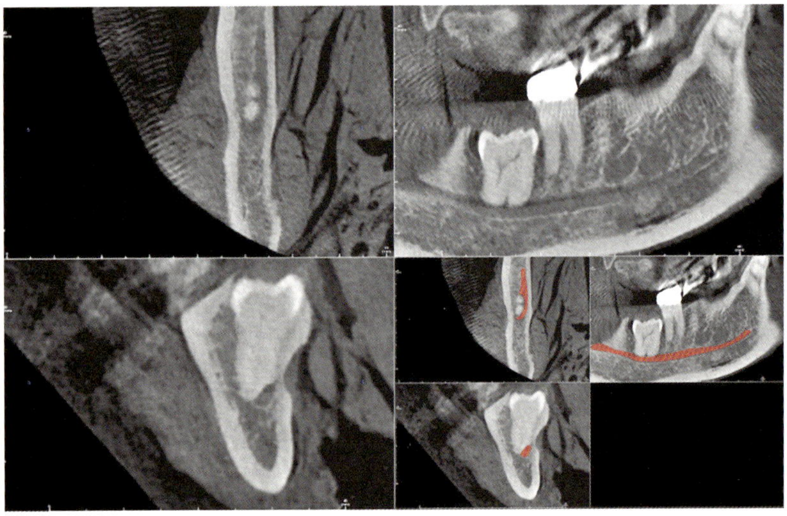

Fig 1-19 Impacted third molar. The roots can cause deviation or narrowing of the canal. *Red highlighting* emphasizes the proximity of the roots to the canal. This MPR CBCT reconstruction shows that care must be taken when planning treatment.

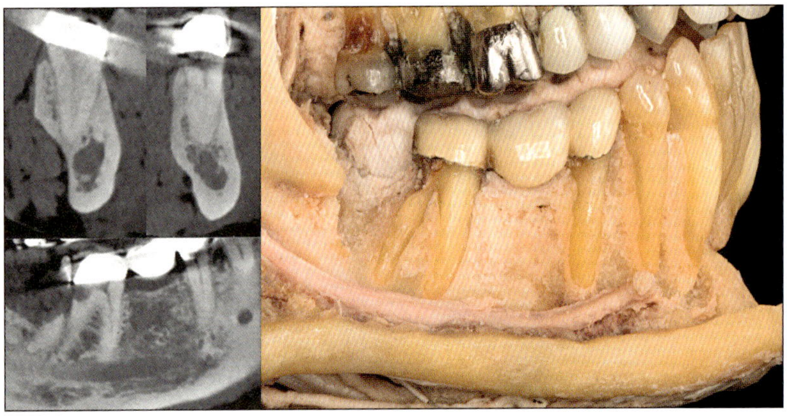

Fig 1-20 CBCT imaging and dissection showing root apex location in relationship to the mandibular nerve and canal.

that there was thicker cortical and trabecular bone on the buccal side of the canal than on the lingual side. Monaco et al[38] showed that the roots of third molar teeth can be located either buccal or lingual to the mandibular canal or that the canal can pass between the roots. They also showed that with an impacted third molar (Fig 1-19), the roots can cause a deviation or a narrowing of the canal.[39] On radiographs, the mandibular canal often appears as a pair of parallel white lines with a dark region between them. On CBCT scans, the canal often appears as round or oval in cross section but sometimes is not readily visible. Wadu et al[40] reported that there is a lot of variation in the radiographic appearance of the canal, as well as the actual composition of the canal wall—what appears to be radiopaque cortical bone on radiographs often turns out to be porous and trabecular in dissections.

The roots of molars can be located lingual or buccal to the canal, or the canal can be located apical to the roots. In some cases the canal passes between the roots, and in rare cases the roots go around the canal and then rejoin.[41] In some cases the canal runs in the lower half of the body of the mandible, and in some cases the upper half.[42] The canal is often found on the lingual side of the mandible posteriorly and then moves toward the vestibular side of the mandible in the anterior portion. Factors like age, race, and sex can affect the course of the canal and the structures within it.[43] The canal often bifurcates or even trifurcates. The inferior alveolar nerve (IAN) typically gives off mental and incisive branches. There can be duplicate canals.[43] Wadhwani et al[44] suggested that if there is difficulty achieving anesthesia of the lower lip and chin area, it could be due to anatomical variation such as additional mandibular canals and IAN branches. He proposes that during embryologic development, the IAN is actually made up of three separate nerves supplying the posterior, middle, and anterior teeth and that these three nerves fuse to form the IAN. Failure of these nerves to fuse could be the cause of the multiple canals. In addition, there is variation in the location of neurovascular structures within the canal. It is difficult to detect bifid canals on panoramic radiographs, whereas with CBCTs they are much more easily detectable. In two-dimensional (2D) images, the mylohyoid groove can imitate an extra canal.[45] Atieh[39] used three radiographic features to indicate the relationship between molar roots and the canal: darkening of the root, interruption of the radiopaque borders, and diversion of the mandibular canal. If these features are identifiable, then panoramic radiography is adequate.

Juodzbalys et al[43] report that the inferior alveolar artery is most frequently on the lingual side and slightly superior to the nerve. Hsu et al[46] measured distances from the lingual and buccal cortical plates to the canal and from the top of the canal to the superior surface of the alveolar ridge. They also measured the average thickness of the cortical bone at the upper surface. They found that the cortical bone was thicker near the second premolar than the first molar.

Relationship of roots to canal

The roots of molar and premolar teeth are often in close proximity to the mandibular canal. Bürklein et al[47] showed that in multirooted teeth, the distal roots of molars were closer to the mandibular canal compared with the mesial roots (Fig 1-20). A direct relationship between the root tips and the mandibular canal was found in 3.2% of second premolars, 2.9% of first molars, 15.2% of second molars, and 31.3% of third molars.[47] In women, roots tended to be closer to the canal than in men. The right and left sides tended to be symmetric. The distance between root tips and the canal is increased in young adulthood. Burklein et al[47] provided evidence that extrusion of filling materials from root tips during endodontic procedures can cause nerve damage. Abdulla[48] showed that the mesial roots of first and second molars are nearer to the canal than the distal roots and that the second molar roots are closer to the canal than first molar roots. One group[49] identified nine radiographic features that showed the relationship between tooth roots and the mandibular canal:

1. *Radiolucent band:* Increased radiolucency of the root(s) of the mandibular third molar where the mandibular canal crosses it
2. *Loss of mandibular border:* Interruption of the radiopaque lines that represent the superior and inferior borders of the mandibular canal where it crosses the root(s) of the third molar
3. *Change in mandibular canal direction:* Significant change in the direction of the mandibular canal where it is superimposed on or is in contact with the root(s) of the mandibular third molar
4. *Mandibular canal narrowing:* Narrowing of the mandibular canal where it is superimposed on or is in contact with the root(s) of the mandibular third molar
5. *Root narrowing:* Narrowing of the root(s) of the mandibular third molar where the mandibular canal crosses it
6. *Root deviation:* Abrupt deviation in form (dilaceration) of the root(s) of the mandibular third molar where it is superimposed on or is in contact with the mandibular canal
7. *Bifid apex:* Bifid and dark apex of the root(s) of the mandibular third molar where the mandibular canal crosses it
8. *Superimposed:* Superimposition of the root(s) of the mandibular third molar and the mandibular canal
9. *Contact mandibular canal:* Root(s) of the mandibular third molar in contact with the superior border of the mandibular canal

Many studies suggested that 3D imaging (CBCT) is much more effective in showing the relationship between roots and the canal and avoiding damage than 2D imaging (panoramic radiography).[42,45,47,49–51] If there is any question regarding the relationship of the canal in an area where surgical intervention will take place, CBCT imaging is highly recommend if not required.

Branching and other aspects of the nerve

Ikeda et al[52] reported that there are typically three main nerve branches from the IAN: the ramus retromolaris, the rami molares, and the ramus incisivus (Fig 1-21). Starkie and Stewart[53] showed that there are often nerve plexuses branching from the IAN. They have identified a postero-internal alveolar plexus and an anteroexternal incisor plexus. Within the mandible, the IAN has dental and interdental branches. The dental branches form the dental plexus and innervate the teeth; the interdental branches innervate the alveolar bone, the periodontium, and the gingiva.[54] Wadu et al[40] demonstrated that the main nerve divides into its incisive and mental branches in the molar area well before reaching the mental foramen and that the incisive branch supplies the canine and incisors. They also demonstrated that a molar branch leaves the main IAN soon after entering the mandibular canal and gives off oblique branches to the root tips. Fibers from this branch sometimes reach as far mesially as the second premolar. Wadu et al[40] report cross innervation of the incisive branches, with a dominance of the right side supporting the left.

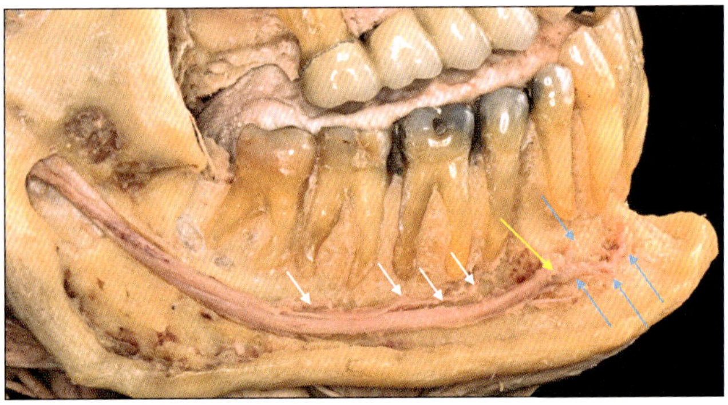

Fig 1-21 Branching of the IAN. Branches indicated by *white arrows* supply teeth and surrounding tissues. The *yellow arrow* indicates the origin of the mental nerve, and the *blue arrows* show an incisor plexus.

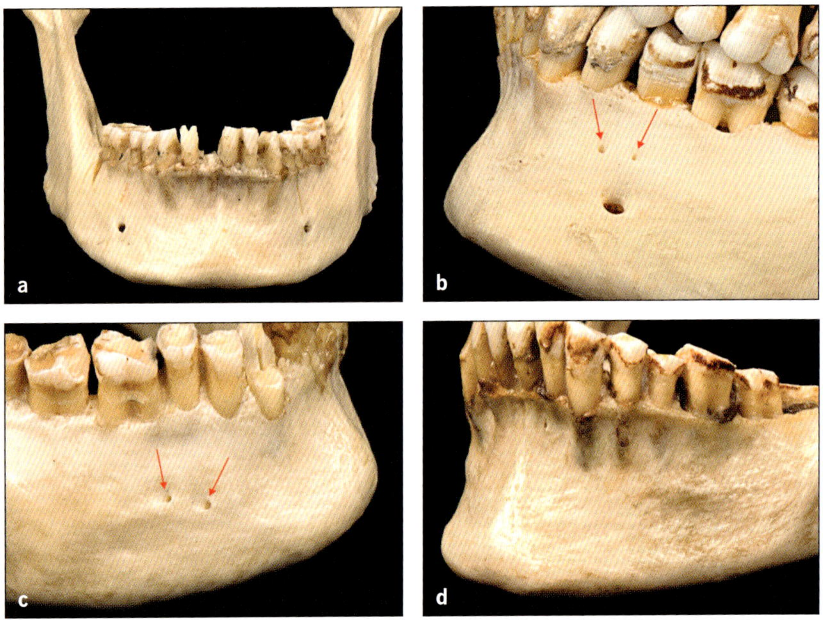

Fig 1-22 Variations in the mental foramina. *(a)* Normal presentation. *(b)* Main foramen with two supplemental foramina *(arrows)*. *(c)* Two smaller foramina *(arrows)*. *(d)* No visible foramen present.

Mental foramen

The mental foramina are two openings in the body of the mandible through which pass the mental nerves and accompanying vessels (Fig 1-22). Hiatt and Gartner[55] locate them at the level of the mandibular second premolar, inferior to the interproximal region between the first and second premolars. During mandibular growth, the position and orientation of the mental foramina change from facing forward to facing upward and backward.[29] However, there is variation in position from subcanine to submolar[51,56] as well as in number—normally there is one on either side, but there are sometimes multiple foramina, or in rare cases the foramen is absent. So there is interindividual variation in size, shape, number, location, symmetry, and orientation of the mental foramen as well as variations between ethnic groups.[51,57–65] Based on recent studies,[56] the incidence of multiple foramina seems highest in Japanese populations and lowest in white persons. Iwanaga et al[59] investigated the size and location of accessory mental foramina and showed that most of these house a branch of the mental nerve, with only a few cases showing arteries exiting from the accessory foramina. Sisman et al[66] refers to these accessory foramina as accessory buccal foramina.

The mental nerve is often described as having three branches, two of which form an incisor plexus labial to the teeth, supplying the gingiva and possibly the periosteum. The third branch supplies the skin of the chin and lower lip.[67] Iwanaga et al[59] identified four branches: a mental branch, a medial inferior labial branch, a lateral inferior labial branch, and an angular branch. There is often an anterior loop of the mental nerve present within the bone mesial to the mental foramen.[51,56,68] However, reports of the incidence and length of the loop and its visibility on radiographs varies widely.[51] The nerve can be damaged in this area if the clinician is unaware of its presence. While the mental foramen is often detectable on

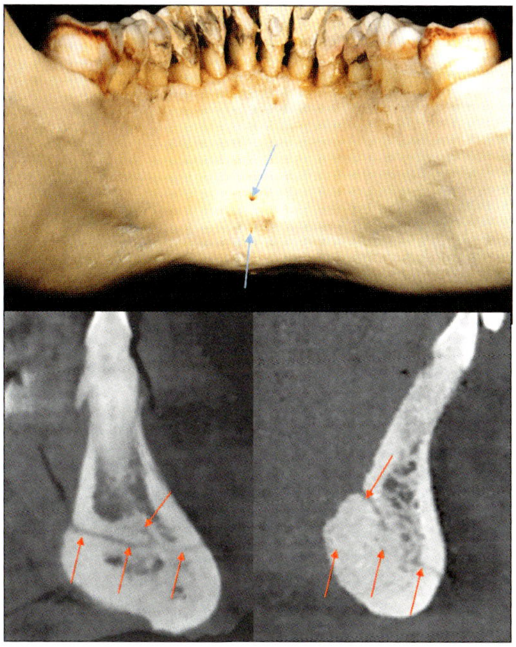

Fig 1-23 Lingual foramina *(blue arrows)* on the inner aspect of the mandible in the midline. These are typically situated above or between the mental spines (genial tubercles). The lingual canal *(red arrows)* can have single or multiple branches.

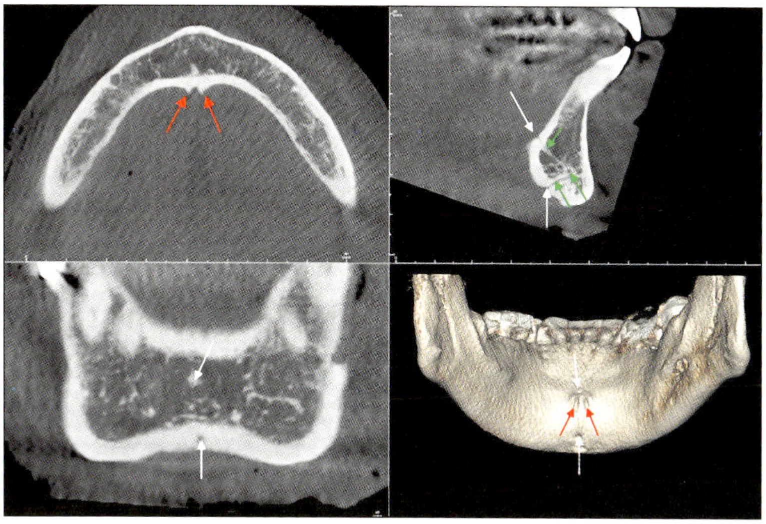

Fig 1-24 Genial tubercles *(red arrows)* with multiple lingual foramina *(white arrows)* and a V-shaped lingual canal *(green arrows)*.

panoramic radiographs, it is often not clearly visible.[69,70] Again, CBCT scans provide better information than conventional 2D images.

According to Mohammadi,[54] periapical infections, overfilling, and apical surgery are endodontic causes for paresthesia of the mental and incisive nerves. Irrigation with sodium hypochlorite can irritate the nerve periapically. The location of the mental foramen should be determined before apical surgery. Its location can change treatment planning.

Mandibular incisive canals

The mandibular canal housing the IAN and vessels is described as terminating by bifurcating into *(1)* a mental canal leading to the mental foramen and *(2)* an incisive canal transmitting nerves and vessels to the mandibular canines and incisors[71,72] and occasionally first premolars.[73] These incisive branches have been described as forming a delicate plexus that is undetectable in radiographs.[74] Mraiwa et al[75] demonstrated mandibular incisive canals both by imaging and by dissection in the bone of the chin area. Most of these canals showed a well-corticalized border located in the central region of the bone near the symphysis menti. The canals showed a slight downward course from their origin to their termination. The authors concluded that the mandibular incisive nerve typically extends closer to the midline than previously reported.[71] Yovchev et al[73] demonstrated that the canals traveled medial to the mental foramina and between the lingual and vestibular cortical plates of the anterior mandible. Raitz et al[76] showed that exclusively using panoramic radiography causes serious underestimation of the presence of an incisive canal, whereas CBCT is much more effective in identifying the canal. With CBCT, Yovchev et al[73] estimated the prevalence of mandibular incisive canals at more than 92%. Their data also suggest that the mandibular incisive canal is wider in men than in women and also wider on the right side of the body. As with other anatomical structures, there is variation in size, shape, and location.[77]

Lingual foramen and canal

An examination of the inner aspect of the mandible in the midline reveals one or more small foramina, typically situated above or between the mental spines (genial tubercles) (Fig 1-23). Tepper et al[78] showed that while 100% of examined mandibles had midline foramina, a large percentage also had foramina located lateral to the midline. They also demonstrated that many mandibles had multiple lingual foramina (Fig 1-24). They cite a number of studies where hemorrhages occurred following implant placement because clinicians were unaware of the presence of these tiny canals that conduct blood vessels within the mandible and between the mandible and the lingual mucosa. McDonnell et al[79] demonstrated by dissection that an anastomosis between sublingual arteries formed a vessel that entered the lingual foramen. They further showed that this vessel traveled through the canal associated with the lingual foramen. Mraiwa et al[75] explained that spiral CT is more effective than either standard intraoral radiographs or panoramic radiographs in demonstrating the presence of these foramina/canals.

Acknowledgment

The author would like to thank Pedro Nava, PhD, for his feedback on the chapter.

References

1. Gluskin AH. Mishaps and serious complications in endodontic obturation. Endod Top 2005;12:52–70.
2. Shah RK, Dhingra JK, Carter BL, Rebeiz EE. Paranasal sinus development: A radiographic study. Laryngoscope 2003;113:205–209.
3. Hauman CH, Chandler NP, Tong DC. Endodontic implications of the maxillary sinus: A review. Int Endod J 2002;35:127–141.
4. Nimigean V, Nimigean VR, Măru N, Sălăvăstru DI, Bădiță D, Tuculină MJ. The maxillary sinus floor in the oral implantology. Rom J Morphol Embryol 2008;49:485–489.
5. Scuderi AJ, Harnsberger HR, Boyer RS. Pneumatization of the paranasal sinuses: Normal features of importance to the accurate interpretation of CT scans and MR images. AJR Am J Roentgenol 1993;160:1101–1104.
6. Eberhardt JA, Torabinejad M, Christiansen EL. A computed tomographic study of the distances between the maxillary sinus floor and the apices of the maxillary posterior teeth. Oral Surg Oral Med Oral Pathol 1992;73:345–346.
7. Shakhawan MA, Hawramy FA, Mahmood KA. The relation of maxillary posterior teeth roots to the maxillary sinus floor using panoramic and computed tomography imaging in a sample of Kurdish people. Tikrit J Dent Sci 2012;1:81–88.
8. Ok E, Güngör E, Colak M, Altunsoy M, Nur BG, Ağlarci OS. Evaluation of the relationship between the maxillary posterior teeth and the sinus floor using cone-beam computed tomography. Surg Radiol Anat 2014;36:907–914.
9. Jung YH, Cho BH. Assessment of the relationship between the maxillary molars and adjacent structures using cone beam computed tomography. Imaging Sci Dent 2012;42:219–224.
10. Hussein ZA, Al-Nakib LH. Assessment of the relationship between maxillary sinus floor and maxillary posterior teeth root apices using spiral CT scan. J Baghdad Coll Dent 2013;25(3):80–86.
11. Kilic C, Kamburoglu K, Yuksel SP, Ozen T. An assessment of the relationship between the maxillary sinus floor and the maxillary posterior teeth root tips using dental cone-beam computerized tomography. Eur J Dent 2010;4:462–467.
12. Testori T. Maxillary sinus surgery: Anatomy and advanced diagnostic imaging. J Implant Reconstr Dent 2011;3:18–25.
13. Janner SF, Caversaccio MD, Dubach P, Sendi P, Buser D, Bornstein MM. Characteristics and dimensions of the Schneiderian membrane: A radiographic analysis using cone beam computed tomography in patients referred for dental implant surgery in the posterior maxilla. Clin Oral Implants Res 2011;22:1446–1453.
14. Srouji S, Kizhner T, Ben David D, Riminucci M, Bianco P, Livne E. The Schneiderian membrane contains osteoprogenitor cells: In vivo and in vitro study. Calcif Tissue Int 2009;84:138–145.
15. Sakkas A, Konstantinidis I, Winter K, Schramm A, Wilde F. Effect of Schneiderian membrane perforation on sinus lift graft outcome using two different donor sites: A retrospective study of 105 maxillary sinus elevation procedures. GMS Interdiscip Plast Reconstr Surg DGPW 2016;5:Doc11.
16. Yildirim D, Eroglu M, Salihoglu M, Yildirim A, Karagoz H, Erkan M. The relationship between dental indentation and maxillary sinusitis. Open J Medical Imaging 2013;3(2):65–68.
17. Maestre-Ferrín L, Galán-Gil S, Rubio-Serrano M, Peñarrocha-Diago M, Peñarrocha-Oltra D. Maxillary sinus septa: A systematic review. Med Oral Patol Oral Cir Bucal 2010;15(2):e383–e386.
18. Rancitelli D, Borgonovo AE, Cicciù M, et al. Maxillary sinus septa and anatomic correlation with the Schneiderian membrane. J Craniofac Surg 2015;26:1394–1398.
19. Gülşen U, Mehdiyev i, Üngör C, Şentürk MF, Ulaşan AD. Horizontal maxillary sinus septa: An uncommon entity. Int J Surg Case Rep 2015;12:67–70.
20. Krennmair G, Ulm CW, Lugmayr H, Solar P. The incidence, location, and height of maxillary sinus septa in the edentulous and dentate maxilla. J Oral Maxillofac Surg 1999;57:667–671.
21. Malec M, Smektala T, Tutak M, Trybek G, Sporniak-Tutak K. Maxillary sinus septa prevalence and morphology—Computed tomography based analysis. Int J Morphol 2015;33:144–148.
22. Underwood AS. An inquiry into the anatomy and pathology of the maxillary sinus. J Anat Physiol 1910 Jul;44(pt 4):354–369.
23. Velásquez-Plata D, Hovey LR, Peach CC, Alder ME. Maxillary sinus septa: A 3-dimensional computerized tomographic scan analysis. Int J Oral Maxillofac Implants 2002;17:854–860.
24. Kim MJ, Jung UW, Kim CS, et al. Maxillary sinus septa: Prevalence, height, location, and morphology. A reformatted computed tomography scan analysis. J Periodontol 2006;77:903–908.
25. González-Santana H, Peñarrocha-Diago M, Guarinos-Carbó J, Sorní-Bröker M. A study of the septa in the maxillary sinuses and the subantral alveolar processes in 30 patients. J Oral Implantol 2007;33:340–343.
26. Al-Amery SM, Nambiar P, Jamaludin M, John J, Ngeow WC. Cone beam computed tomography assessment of the maxillary incisive canal and foramen: Considerations of anatomical variations when placing immediate implants. PLoS One 2015;10(2):e0117251.
27. Tözüm TF, Güncü GN, Yıldırım YD, et al. Evaluation of maxillary incisive canal characteristics related to dental implant treatment with computerized tomography: A clinical multicenter study. J Periodontol 2012;83:337–443.
28. Güncü GN, Yıldırım YD, Yılmaz HG, et al. Is there a gender difference in anatomic features of incisive canal and maxillary environmental bone? Clin Oral Implants Res 2013;24:1023–1026.
29. Berkovitz BKB, Moxham BJ. A Textbook of Head and Neck Anatomy. Chicago: Year Book Medical Publishers, 1988.
30. Westmoreland EE, Blanton PL. An analysis of the variations in position of the greater palatine foramen in the adult human skull. Anat Rec 1982;204:383–388.
31. Piagkou M, Xanthos T, Anagnostopoulou S, et al. Anatomical variation and morphology in the position of the palatine foramina in adult human skulls from Greece. J Craniomaxillofac Surg 2012;40(7):e206–e210.
32. Chrcanovic BR, Custódio AL. Anatomical variation in the position of the greater palatine foramen. J Oral Sci 2010;52:109–113.
33. Howard-Swirzinski K, Edwards PC, Saini TS, Norton NS. Length and geometric patterns of the greater palatine canal observed in cone beam computed tomography. Int J Dent 2010;2010.pii:292753.
34. Hafeez NS, Ganapathy S, Sondekoppam R, Johnson M, Merrifield P, Galil KA. Anatomical variations of the greater palatine nerve in the greater palatine canal. J Can Dent Assoc 2015;81:f14.
35. Nortjé CJ, Farman AG, Grotepass FW. Variations in the normal anatomy of the inferior dental (mandibular) canal: A retrospective study of panoramic radiographs from 3612 routine dental patients. Br J Oral Surg 1977;15:55–63.
36. Kilic C, Kamburoğlu K, Ozen T, et al. The position of the mandibular canal and histologic feature of the inferior alveolar nerve. Clin Anat 2010;23:34–42.
37. Gowgiel JM. The position and course of the mandibular canal. J Oral Implantol 1992;18:383–385.
38. Monaco G, Montevecchi M, Bonetti GA, Gatto MR, Checchi L. Reliability of panoramic radiography in evaluating the topographic relationship between the mandibular canal and impacted third molars. J Am Dent Assoc 2004;135:312–318.
39. Atieh MA. Diagnostic accuracy of panoramic radiography in determining relationship between inferior alveolar nerve and mandibular third molar. J Oral Maxillofac Surg 2010;68:74–82.

40. Wadu SG, Penhall B, Townsend GC. Morphological variability of the human inferior alveolar nerve. Clin Anat 1997;10(2):82–87.
41. Schneider T, Filo K, Kruse AL, Locher M, Grätz KW, Lübbers HT. Variations in the anatomical positioning of impacted mandibular wisdom teeth and their practical implications. Swiss Dent J 2014;124:520–538.
42. Xu GZ, Yang C, Fan XD, et al. Anatomic relationship between impacted third mandibular molar and the mandibular canal as the risk factor of inferior alveolar nerve injury. Br J Oral Maxillofac Surg 2013;51(8):e215–e219.
43. Juodzbalys G, Wang HL, Sabalys G. Anatomy of mandibular vital structures. Part I: Mandibular canal and inferior alveolar neurovascular bundle in relation with dental implantology. J Oral Maxillofac Res 2010;1(1):e2.
44. Wadhwani P, Mathur RM, Kohli M, Sahu R. Mandibular canal variant: A case report. J Oral Pathol Med 2008;37:122–124.
45. Correr GM, Iwanko D, Leonardi DP, Ulbrich LM, Araújo MR, Deliberador TM. Classification of bifid mandibular canals using cone beam computed tomography. Braz Oral Res 2013;27:510–516.
46. Hsu JT, Huang HL, Fuh LJ, et al. Location of the mandibular canal and thickness of the occlusal cortical bone at dental implant sites in the lower second premolar and first molar. Comput Math Methods Med 2013;2013:608570.
47. Bürklein S, Grund C, Schäfer E. Relationship between root apices and the mandibular canal: A cone-beam computed tomographic analysis in a German population. J Endod 2015;41:1696–1700.
48. Abdulla AG. Relationship of inferior alveolar canal to the apices of lower molar teeth radiographically. Tikrit Med J 2008;14:124–126.
49. Koong B, Pharoah MJ, Bulsara M, Tennant M. Methods of determining the relationship of the mandibular canal and third molars: A survey of Australian oral and maxillofacial surgeons. Aust Dent J 2006;51:64–68.
50. Bagherpour A, Rezaei MM, Nasseri S. Spatial relationship between mandibular third molars and inferior alveolar nerve using a volume rendering software. J Dent Materials Techniques 2013;2:1–5.
51. Greenstein G, Tarnow D. The mental foramen and nerve: Clinical and anatomical factors related to dental implant placement: A literature review. J Periodontol 2006;77:1933–1943.
52. Ikeda K, Ho KC, Nowicki BH, Haughton VM. Multiplanar MR and anatomic study of the mandibular canal. AJNR Am J Neuroradiol 1996;17:579–584.
53. Starkie C, Stewart D. The intra-mandibular course of the inferior dental nerve. J Anat 1931;65(pt 3):319–323.
54. Mohammadi Z. Endodontics-related paresthesia of the mental and inferior alveolar nerves: An updated review. J Can Dent Assoc 2010;76:a117.
55. Hiatt JL, Gartner LP. Textbook of Head and Neck Anatomy, ed 3. Philadelphia: Lippincott Williams & Wilkins, 2002:70,81.
56. Hasan T. Characteristics of the mental foramen in different populations. Internet J Biol Anthropol 2010;4(2):1–7.
57. Kieser J, Kuzmanovic D, Payne A, Dennison J, Herbison P. Patterns of emergence of the human mental nerve. Arch Oral Biol 2002;47:743–747.
58. Mbajiorgu EF, Mawera G, Asala SA, Zivanovic S. Position of the mental foramen in adult black Zimbabwean mandibles: A clinical anatomical study. Cent Afr J Med 1998;44(2):24–30.
59. Iwanaga J, Watanabe K, Saga T, et al. Accessory mental foramina and nerves: Application to periodontal, periapical, and implant surgery. Clin Anat 2016;29:493–501.
60. Sawyer DR, Kiely ML, Pyle MA. The frequency of accessory mental foramina in four ethnic groups. Arch Oral Biol 1998;43:417–420.
61. Ilayperuma I, Nanayakkara G, Palahepitiya N. Morphometric analysis of the mental foramen in adult Sri Lankan mandibles. Int J Morphol 2009;27:1019–1024.
62. Igbigbi PS, Lebona S. The position and dimensions of the mental foramen in adult Malawian mandibles. West Afr J Med 2005;24:184–189.
63. Singh R, Srivastav AK. Study of position, shape, size and incidence of mental foramen and accessory mental foramen in Indian adult human skulls. Int J Morphol 2010;28:1141–1146.
64. Afkhami F, Haraji A, Boostani HR. Radiographic localization of the mental foramen and mandibular canal. J Dent (Tehran) 2013;10:436–442.
65. Ikiz I, Erem T. Relation of the mental foramen to teeth on the mandibles belonging to the Byzantium period. Int J Anthropol 1997;12:1–4.
66. Sisman Y, Sahman H, Sekerci A, Tokmak TT, Aksu Y, Mavili E. Detection and characterization of the mandibular accessory buccal foramen using CT. Dentomaxillofac Radiol 2012;41:558–563.
67. Standring S (ed). Gray's Anatomy: The Anatomical Basis of Clinical Practice, ed 40. Edinburgh: Churchill Livingstone/Elsevier, 2008:519.
68. Solar P, Ulm C, Frey G, Matejka M. A classification of the intraosseous paths of the mental nerve. Int J Oral Maxillofac Implants 1994;9:339–344.
69. Jacobs R, Mraiwa N, Van Steenberghe D, Sanderink G, Quirynen M. Appearance of the mandibular incisive canal on panoramic radiographs. Surg Radiol Anat 2004;26:329–333.
70. Yosue T, Brooks SL. The appearance of mental foramina on panoramic radiographs. I. Evaluation of patients. Oral Surg Oral Med Oral Pathol 1989;68:360–364.
71. De Andrade E, Otomo-Corgel J, Pucher J, Ranganath KA, St George N Jr. The intraosseous course of the mandibular incisive nerve in the mandibular symphysis. Int J Periodontics Restorative Dent 2001;21:591–597.
72. Rosa MB, Sotto-Maior BS, Machado Vde C, Francischone CE. Retrospective study of the anterior loop of the inferior alveolar nerve and the incisive canal using cone beam computed tomography. Int J Oral Maxillofac Implants 2013;28:388–392.
73. Yovchev D, Deliverska E, Indjova J, Zhelyazkova M. Mandibular incisive canal: A cone beam computed tomography study. Biotechnol Biotechnol Equipment 2013;27:3848–3851.
74. Kohavi D, Bar-Ziv J. Atypical incisive nerve: Clinical report. Implant Dent 1996; 5:281–283.
75. Mraiwa N, Jacobs R, Moerman P, Lambrichts I, van Steenberghe D, Quirynen M. Presence and course of the incisive canal in the human mandibular interforaminal region: Two-dimensional imaging versus anatomical observations. Surg Radiol Anat 2003;25:416–423.
76. Raitz R, Shimura E, Chilvarquer I, Fenyo-Pereira M. Assessment of the mandibular incisive canal by panoramic radiograph and cone-beam computed tomography. Int J Dent 2014;2014:187085.
77. Juodzbalys G, Wang HL, Sabalys G. Anatomy of mandibular vital structures. Part II: Mandibular incisive canal, mental foramen and associated neurovascular bundles in relation with dental implantology. J Oral Maxillofac Res 2010;1(1):e3.
78. Tepper G, Hofschneider UB, Gahleitner A, Ulm C. Computed tomographic diagnosis and localization of bone canals in the mandibular interforaminal region for prevention of bleeding complications during implant surgery. Int J Oral Maxillofac Implants 2001;16:68–72.
79. McDonnell D, Reza Nouri M, Todd ME. The mandibular lingual foramen: A consistent arterial foramen in the middle of the mandible. J Anat 1994;184(pt 2): 363–369.

Chapter Two

Histology of Tissues Involved in Surgical Endodontics

Kenneth R. Wright

In the practice of endodontic surgery, it is important to have an understanding of not only the gross anatomy of the structures involved during different stages of surgery (see chapter 1) but also the histology of these tissues. An awareness of the properties of these tissues and their capacity for healing and repair assists the dental practitioner in performing procedures with minimal damage and optimal healing. A number of studies have correlated histologic findings to outcomes of endodontic surgical procedures.[1–12] Endodontic surgical procedures require an understanding of periodontal and periradicular tissues. This chapter is not an exhaustive examination of periodontal and periradicular tissues but provides basic and essential information regarding tissues involved during endodontic surgery.

Oral Mucosa

The oral mucosa is the tissue lining the oral cavity. A mucosa, or mucous membrane, is a wet tissue that contains glands that secrete a somewhat viscous liquid called *mucus*, along with a watery serous fluid. Some erroneously call the oral mucosa a type of skin, but this is incorrect. Skin has its own set of properties that differ significantly from those of a mucosa. The term *mucosa* has come to refer to any wet tissue lining a body passageway, such as the digestive, respiratory, and urogenital tracts. While the oral mucosa is continuous with skin at the lips, it is a different entity. This membrane forms a barrier against infection but also serves in secretion, sensation, temperature regulation,[13] and immunologic protection.[14] The saliva, a portion of which is secreted by minor salivary glands embedded in the mucosa, mixes with food to help break it down and digest it and also aids in speaking.

A mucosa is composed of two distinct layers: an epithelium and an underlying and supporting layer of connective tissue termed the *lamina propria*. Most mucosae lie upon yet another layer of connective tissue called the *submucosa*, but this layer is sometimes reduced or absent where the mucosa covers bone.[13]

The epithelium lining essentially the entire oral cavity is a stratified squamous epithelium, similar to that forming the epidermal layer of the skin. In the skin, the epidermis is made of morphologically and functionally distinct

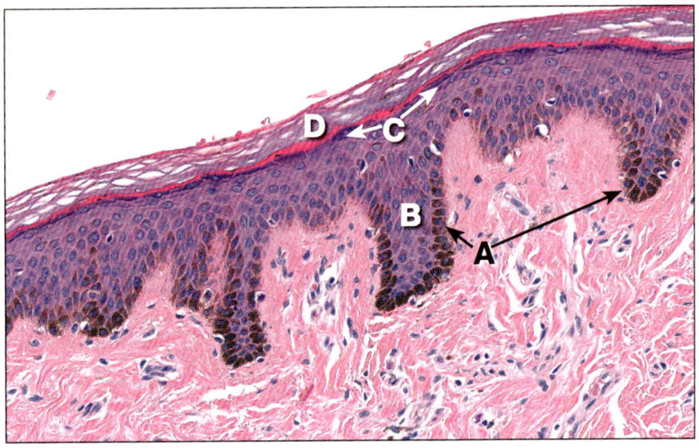

Fig 2-1 Heavily pigmented epidermis (thin skin). A, stratum basale (note the abundance of melanin produced by melanocytes); B, stratum spinosum; C, stratum granulosum (*arrows* point to cells containing dark purple keratohyalin granules); D, stratum corneum.

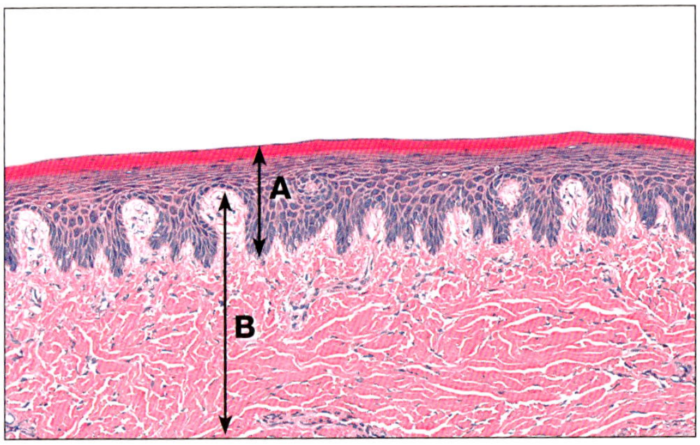

Fig 2-2 Oral epithelium. A, nonkeratinized stratified squamous epithelium; B, lamina propria.

layers of cells. The stratum basale, or basal layer, typically only a single cell thick, is the deepest layer of cells and is formed of a population of cells that act as stem cells, undergoing frequent mitoses to produce the cells of the more superficial layers. Also found in this basal layer, in pigmented epithelia, are melanocytes, which produce the pigment melanin, a dark substance that protects the DNA of the epithelial cells from ultraviolet radiation. These cells account for about 5% of the cells of the epidermis.[14] The stratum spinosum, or "prickle cell" layer, is made up of cells that, because of their attachment to adjacent cells by desmosomes, appear to have spiny projections on their surfaces. As the cells in the stratum spinosum move toward the surface of the epithelium, their shape changes from rounded to slightly flattened, and their cytoplasm fills with keratohyalin granules. These granule-filled cells form the stratum granulosum. The superficial layer of the epidermis, the stratum corneum, consists of dead cells filled with filamentous keratin, which eventually detach and are shed at the surface (Fig 2-1).

Most of the stratified squamous epithelium lining the oral cavity is nonkeratinized (Fig 2-2), which means that the layers of cells are modified from those forming the epidermis. The stratum basale and stratum spinosum are similar to those of the epidermis, but as the cells from the stratum spinosum migrate toward the surface, they do not become filled with keratohyalin granules (which are involved in the keratinization process), so the next layer is called the *stratum intermedium*. The surface layer is made up of cells that are not keratinized and contain viable organelles. This surface layer is called the *stratum superficiale*.

There are regional variations in the oral mucosa. Lining mucosa is the most widespread type, covering the inner surface of the lip, the buccal region, the soft palate, the undersurface of the tongue, the alveolar region, and the floor of the mouth. The epithelium is nonkeratinized and generally thicker than in other regions of the oral cavity. The lamina propria is also somewhat thicker than in other parts of the mouth and is composed of lax, irregularly distributed collagen fibers intermingled with elastic fibers, allowing for stretching of the tissue (Fig 2-3).

Masticatory mucosa typically covers bone in places like the hard palate and the attached gingiva, where the mucosa is exposed to shearing forces such as when masticating food. The epithelium of this mucosa tends to be orthokeratinized, or at least parakeratinized. In the first case, there is a stratum granulosum and a stratum corneum similar to what we see in the skin. In the second case, the surface cells, while containing some keratin, still have pyknotic nuclei, and a stratum granulosum is not well developed.[13] Masticatory mucosa is able to withstand abrasive forces and is much less distensible than lining mucosa. The collagen fibers in the lamina propria are grouped into tight bundles, providing much less give than the lamina propria of lining mucosa. In the case of masticatory mucosa, there is generally little, if any, submucosa. Collagen fibers from the lamina propria attach to the periosteum covering the underlying bony structures, which are invested by the masticatory mucosa, thus anchoring the mucosa and reducing its flexibility (Fig 2-4).

The mucosa covering the dorsum of the tongue is sometimes referred to as a *specialized mucosa*,[13] because although much of the epithelium is keratinized, the mucosa remains flexible and is associated not only with mechanical function but also with general sensation and with the sense of taste by way of numerous taste buds associated with various papillae. Filiform papillae, the most abundant type of papillae, are keratinized and cone-shaped and serve a mechanical function, holding food particles and crushing them against the hard palate (Fig 2-5a). These papillae are not furnished with taste buds. The fun-

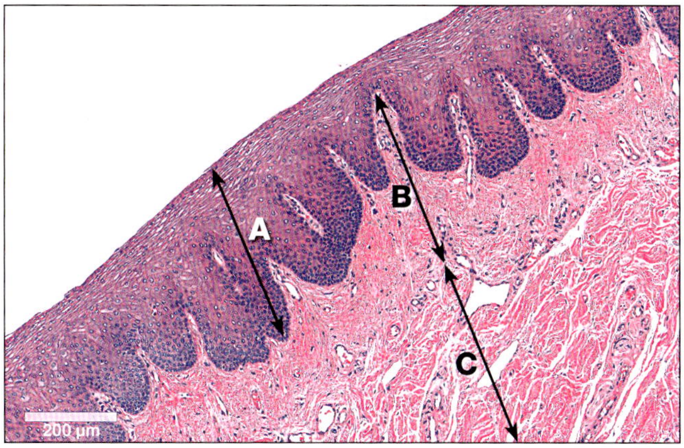

Fig 2-3 Lining mucosa (lip). A, nonkeratinized stratified squamous epithelium; B, papillary layer of lamina propria; C, reticular layer of lamina propria.

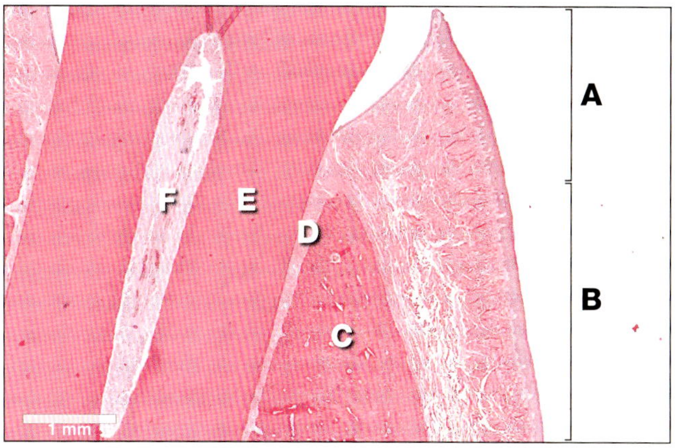

Fig 2-4 Masticatory mucosa (gingiva). A, free (marginal) gingiva (nonkeratinized); B, attached gingiva (parakeratinized); C, alveolar bone (alveolar crest); D, periodontal ligament; E, root dentin; F, pulp chamber.

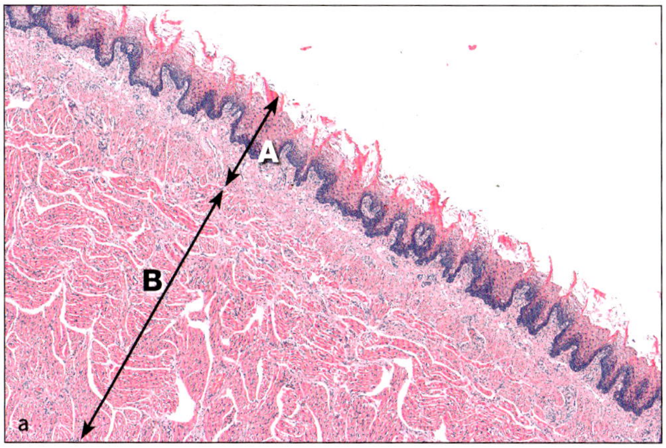

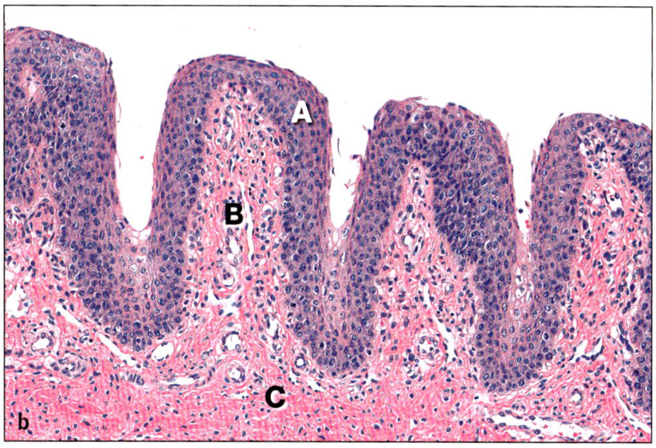

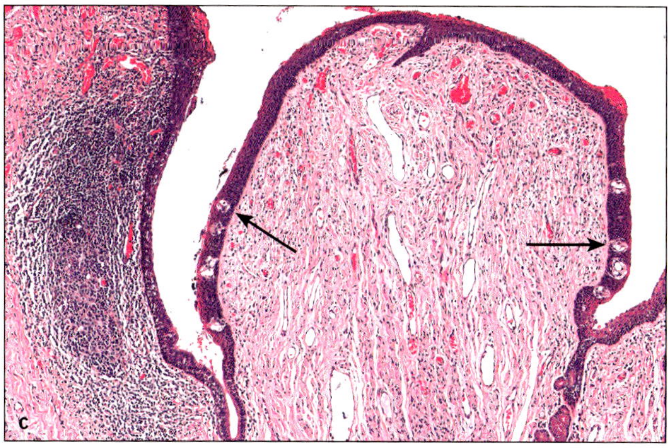

Fig 2-5 Papillae of the tongue. *(a)* Filiform papillae. A, mucosa; B, submucosa formed primarily of skeletal muscle. *(b)* Foliate papillae. A, stratified squamous nonkeratinized epithelium; B, each papilla has a lamina propria core; C, papillary layer of lamina propria. *(c)* Circumvallate papilla. *Arrows* indicate taste buds.

giform papillae, on the other hand, are rounded and nonkeratinized and supplied with taste buds. Foliate papillae, more abundant in other mammals than in humans, can be found along the lateral margins of the tongue in rows, have a leaflike shape, and have taste buds along their sides (Fig 2-5b). Circumvallate papillae are located in the posterior part of the tongue, are surrounded by a deep sulcus, are keratinized on their upper surface, and contain taste buds along their sides (Fig 2-5c). Special minor salivary glands (of von Ebner) drain into the sulci surrounding the papillae.

Mucosal Junctions

A mucocutaneous junction is a transition zone between the skin and a mucosa. In the oral region, this occurs at the lips, where the skin of the outer lip region transitions to the mucosa of the inner lip at the red (vermilion) zone, what most people consider as "the lip" proper. While the red zone is keratinized, it lacks the hair follicles and sweat glands present in the skin of the outer lip, but it usually retains a few sebaceous glands, especially at the corners of the mouth. This vermilion zone is red because the dermal papillae extend close to the surface and contain capillary loops, giving this zone its coloration. As the skin and vermilion zone transition to oral mucosa, the epithelium goes from keratinized to parakeratinized to nonkeratinized.[13] The glands transition from sweat and sebaceous in the skin to sebaceous in the vermilion zone to mucous and serous in the oral mucosa.

The mucogingival junction is a fairly abrupt transition from alveolar mucosa to the attached gingiva. This is evidenced by a change in color from a deep reddish-pink of the alveolar mucosa to a pale pink with stippling of the attached gingiva. There is a faint mucogingival groove indicating where the transition occurs. At this junction, the epithelium transitions from the gingival keratinized or parakeratinized epithelium to the mucosal nonkeratinized epithelium. The lamina propria of the gingiva contains large bundles of collagen fibers that attach to the underlying periosteum. This produces the stippled appearance of the attached gingiva. The lamina propria of the alveolar mucosa, by contrast, contains a looser arrangement of collagen fibers and abundant elastic fibers, allowing the mucosa to return to its original form after stretching. A free gingival groove separates the attached gingiva from the free gingiva coronally and indicates the point of attachment of the free gingiva.

The term *alveolar mucosa* refers specifically to the soft tissue covering the alveolar processes of the maxilla and mandible. This tissue is of the lining mucosa type and is continuous with buccal and labial mucosa as well as the mucosa forming the floor of the mouth. It transitions to attached gingiva at the mucogingival junction.

The dentogingival junction, the interface between gingiva and the crown of the tooth, is discussed below.

Attached Gingiva

The attached gingiva, anchored to the alveolar bone, transitions to free gingiva (marginal gingiva), which extends above the alveolar crest. The buccal/labial side of the free gingiva is keratinized, but the epithelium on the coronal side of the free gingiva, facing into the gingival sulcus (the space between the free gingiva and the crown of the tooth), in nonkeratinized. A healthy gingival sulcus is between 0.5 and 3 mm deep. A deeper sulcus results from gingival recession and is called a *periodontal pocket*. The sulcus ends where the gingival epithelium lining the sulcus, called *sulcular epithelium*, transitions to an epithelium that is attached to the crown of the tooth, called *junctional epithelium*. This area of attachment is called a *dentogingival junction*. This junctional epithelium is unusual in that an epithelium normally attaches to an underlying collagen-based connective tissue by way of an intervening basal lamina. Here, an epithelial tissue attaches to a calcified tissue—enamel—by way of hemidesmosomes. Between the surface epithelial cells and the enamel (or cementum in the case of gingival recession) is what is called an "inner" basal lamina. (The "outer" basal lamina lies between the deep layer of epithelium and its underlying lamina propria.) This epithelium is a unique modification of stratified squamous nonkeratinizing epithelium.

Junctional epithelium tends to have a chronic low level of inflammation, releasing fluid containing inflammatory cells and cytokines into the gingival sulcus.

Palatal Mucosa

Because the masticatory mucosa is subject to abrasion and shearing forces during chewing and other activities, there must be a mechanism that tightly binds the epithelium to the underlying lamina propria and then the lamina propria to the underlying periosteum. As with the dermis of the skin, papillae of lamina propria project upward into the epithelial layer, providing a great overlap between epithelium and connective tissue. At the same time, rete pegs, downward projections of the epithelium, lie between the papillae of the lamina propria. The combination of papillae and pegs serves to increase the surface interface between epithelium and lamina propria, thus anchoring the epithelium so that it will not separate from the lamina propria when forces are applied to it. The lamina propria is in its turn bound to the underlying periosteum by collagen bundles so that the entire mucosa is able to withstand shearing forces. In the lateral regions of the hard palate, a submucosa containing fat and glands is interposed between the mucosa and the periosteum, providing cushioning against the mechanical forces due to chewing and action of the tongue.

Lamina Propria

The lamina propria is a layer of connective tissue that underlies and supports the epithelial layer of a mucosa. The term refers to the mucosa's "own layer," implying that

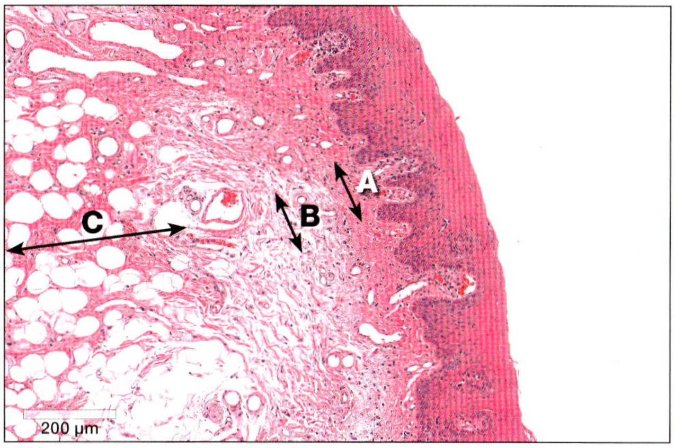

Fig 2-6 Lamina propria. A, papillary layer; B, reticular layer; C, submucosa.

the lamina propria is inseparable from its overlying epithelium. The lamina propria is separated from, yet firmly attached to, the overlying epithelium by a basal lamina. The lamina propria is subdivided into two somewhat indistinct yet separate layers: *(1)* a superficial *papillary layer*, so called because papillae extend upward into the region of the epithelium from this layer, and *(2)* a thicker and denser *reticular layer*, named for the fact that the larger and more densely packed collagen fibers appear to form a reticulum (Fig 2-6). The papillary layer is characterized by thin, loosely arranged collagen fibers and capillary loops that extend up into the papillae, and the reticular layer lies deep to it. The lamina propria, unlike the epithelium, is richly supplied with vessels and nerves. An amorphous ground substance fills the spaces between cells, fibers, and neurovascular elements.

The typical cells found in the lamina propria include the fibroblast, the most abundant cell type that is responsible for the secretion and turnover of ground substance and fibers; the macrophage, a member of the mononuclear phagocytic system that is responsible for phagocytosis of debris and foreign cells and that acts as an antigen-presenting cell; the mast cell, a basophilic cell containing histamine, heparin, and other substances involved in inflammation; and lymphocytes, plasma cells, and neutrophils, all involved with immune function in the case of infection.

Blood Supply

Large blood vessels that supply the oral mucosa are found in the submucosa running parallel to the surface epithelium. In the case of a mucoperiosteum, the vessels are found in the reticular layer of the lamina propria. The vessels derive primarily from the maxillary or facial arteries. Branches from these mucosal arteries extend upward through the lamina propria, forming capillary networks in the papillary layer.

Nerve Supply

The nerve supply to the oral mucosa comes primarily from the maxillary and mandibular divisions of the trigeminal nerve, but with contributions from the facial, glossopharyngeal, and vagus nerves. Most of the innervation is sensory, both general and special (taste). Efferent fibers provide sympathetic innervation to vessels and glands.

Interdental Gingiva

The gingiva located between adjacent teeth takes the form of a *col*, a depression with buccal and lingual peaks. The epithelium is essentially junctional epithelium. Inflammation tends to be chronic in this area because of the difficulty of eliminating debris and bacteria.

Periodontal Ligament

The periodontal ligament (PDL) is a strong connective tissue that anchors each tooth to its socket, or *alveolus*. The PDL develops from ectomesenchymal tissue concurrently with the development of the root of the tooth. As the root grows and as the tooth erupts, the collagen fibers within the PDL are remodeled to compensate for the changing forces on the tooth. Once the tooth reaches full occlusion, the pattern of periodontal fibers remains stable unless other forces cause a change in fiber orientation (eg, due to tooth movement, occlusal wear, etc). The role of the collagen fibers in the PDL is to provide maximal resistance to occlusal and interproximal forces being applied to the tooth as well as to anchor and stabilize the tooth. The fibers therefore assume a specific orientation and attachment to surrounding tissues. In examining his-

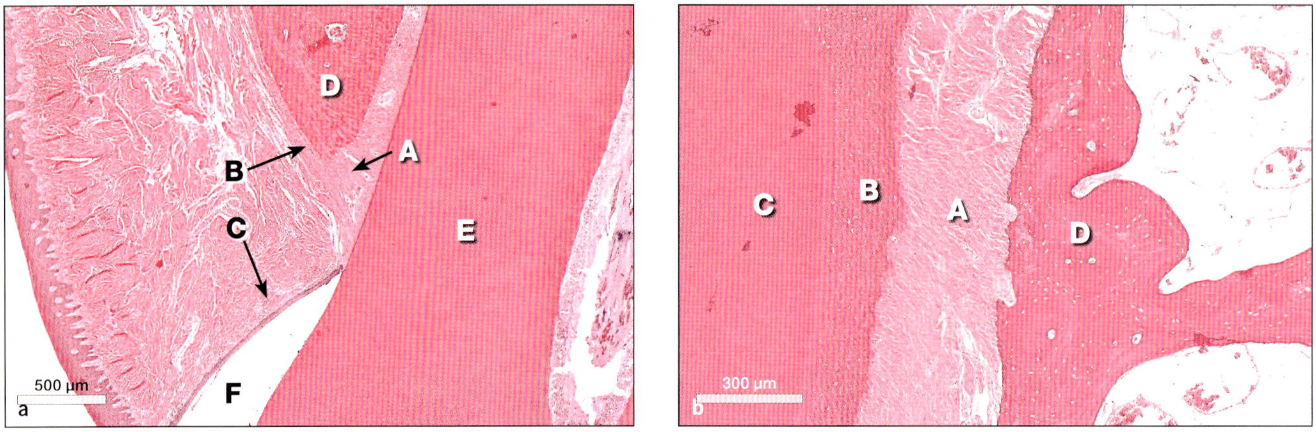

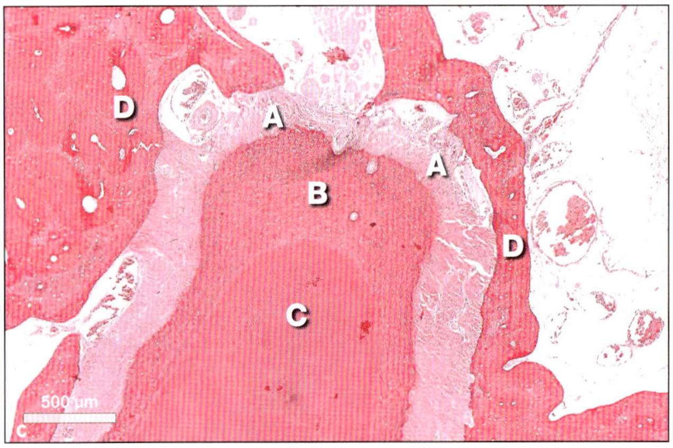

Fig 2-7 PDL fiber groups. *(a)* A, alveolar crest fibers; B, dentoperiosteal fibers; C, dentogingival fibers; D, alveolar crest; E, dentin; F, gingival sulcus. *(b)* A, oblique fiber group; B, cellular cementum; C, dentin; D, alveolar bone. *(c)* A, apical fibers; B, apical cellular cementum; C, root dentin; D, alveolar bone.

tologic sections of the PDL, it is possible to identify these specific groups of periodontal fibers. The fibers can be divided into two broad categories: *(1)* the *dentoalveolar group*, consisting of fibers attaching the tooth to the bone of the tooth socket, and *(2)* the *gingival fiber group*, made up of fibers connecting the tooth to the gingiva.[13] Within each group, five subgroups have been described. In the dentoalveolar group, alveolar crest fibers link the bone forming the crest of the tooth socket to the upper region of the tooth root; horizontal fibers run in a horizontal orientation along the sides of the root, from the root to the wall of the alveolus; oblique fibers, like horizontal fibers, attach the root to the wall of the alveolus but run in an oblique orientation; apical fibers attach the apex of the root to the adjacent alveolar bone; and interradicular fibers, found only in multirooted teeth, attach the furcation zone of the tooth to the alveolus. Within the gingival group, dentogingival fibers anchor the free gingiva to the upper part of the root; alveologingival fibers bind the free gingiva to the alveolar crest area without attaching directly to the tooth; dentoperiosteal fibers originate in the cementum of the upper root, run above the alveolar crest, and insert into the mucoperiosteum of the attached gingiva; transseptal fibers run from the root of one tooth over the alveolar crest to the root of an adjacent tooth, without attaching to bone; and circular fibers run entirely in the free gingiva, encircling the tooth without attaching to it (Fig 2-7).

The primary cell type in the PDL is the fibroblast. This cell retains the ability to both secrete and resorb collagen fibers and ground substance, so that the PDL undergoes frequent remodeling. There are ectomesenchymal cells in the PDL that can give rise to new fibroblasts, and thus the PDL has great reparative/regenerative capacity.

Alveolar Bone

Both the maxilla and the mandible have alveolar processes—ridges of bone that house the roots of the teeth in sockets called *alveoli*. A lingual-buccal or lingual-labial cut through each of these processes reveals that each alveolar process consists of an external cortical plate, formed of lamellar compact bone, and an internal layer of cancellous or spongy bone, formed of small bony trabeculae that, like the compact bone, have a lamellar construction. The spaces between trabeculae are filled with marrow and blood vessels. Extending inward from the crest of each alveolar process are the alveoli. The walls of the

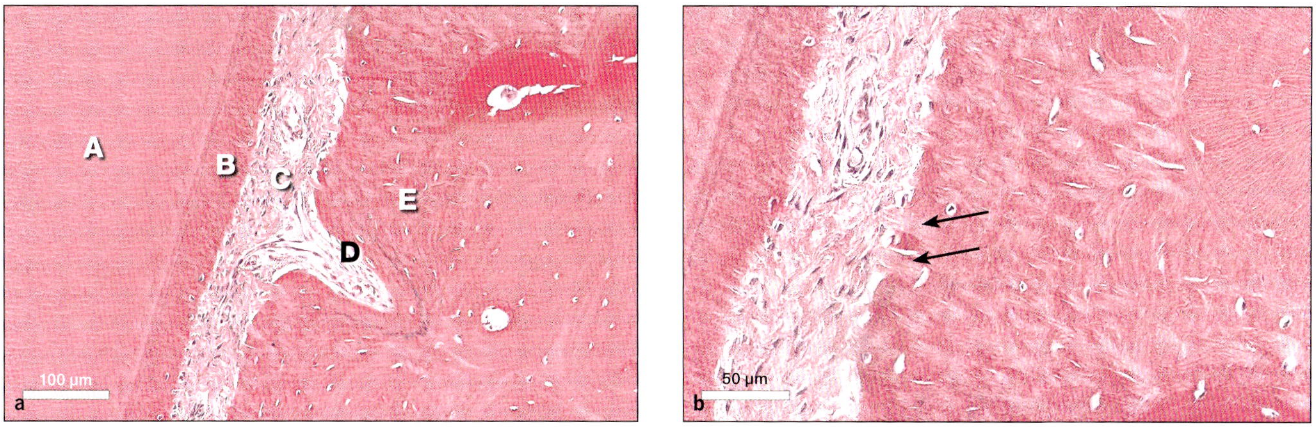

Fig 2-8 Alveolar bone proper. *(a)* Cribriform plate. A, dentin; B, cementum; C, PDL; D, bony canal transmitting small blood vessels between bone and PDL (these openings give this layer of bone its name); E, alveolar bone (note the immature "woven" appearance). *(b)* Bundle bone. Alveolar bone proper is frequently referred to as *bundle bone* because of the presence of bundles of collagen (Sharpey fibers) from the PDL inserting into the bone matrix *(arrows)*.

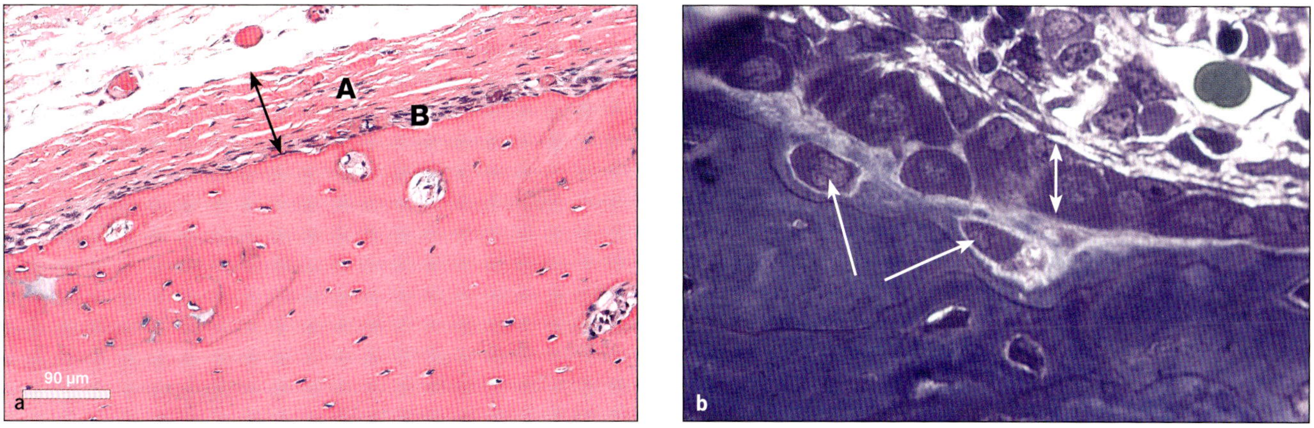

Fig 2-9 *(a)* Periosteum. *Double-headed arrow* indicates the full thickness of the periosteum. A, fibrous layer; B, osteogenic layer. *(b)* Endosteum (rat). Osteoblasts *(double-headed arrow)* form this portion of the endosteum of a long bone; *single-headed arrows* indicate two osteoblasts, which upon embedding themselves in bone matrix will become osteocytes.

alveoli are formed of a dense layer of bone known as *alveolar bone proper*. Radiographically, this bone tends to be a little more radiopaque than the surrounding bone, so it has been given the name *lamina dura*, literally "hard plate." This layer of bone is important in serving as an attachment for the PDL by means of Sharpey fibers—collagen fibers from the PDL that become partially embedded in the bone matrix as it mineralizes. The cementum lining the external surface of the tooth root also contains Sharpey fibers, so that the tooth is anchored to the alveolar bone proper. Because of the bundles of collagen seen embedded in the alveolar bone lining the tooth socket, this bone is sometimes called *bundle bone*. This bone is also perforated with tiny canals or foramina that allow the passage of blood vessels and nerves between the bone and the PDL. These perforations have earned this layer of bone the name *cribriform plate*, cribriform meaning sieve-like or porous. Alveolar bone proper is a dynamic tissue undergoing frequent remodeling because of changing forces applied to the bone during mastication and clenching. Therefore, the bone often has a somewhat immature appearance compared with other bone in the region, with frequent reversal lines giving evidence of remodeling (Fig 2-8).

The external surfaces of the cortical plates of the alveolar processes are covered by a dense layer of connective tissue called the *periosteum*. The periosteum is made up of two distinct layers of material: *(1)* an outer fibrous layer, composed of collagen fibers and ground substance secreted by fibroblasts, and *(2)* an inner layer adjacent to the bone surface formed of osteoprogenitor cells, which under the right conditions will differentiate into osteoblasts. So we say that the periosteum is formed of a fibrous layer and an osteogenic layer. The inner surfaces of bone, adjacent to the bone marrow, are lined by a cellular layer called the *endosteum*. This layer is composed primarily of osteoblasts, along with flattened bone-lining cells that are thought to be cells of the osteoblast lineage[15] (Fig 2-9). Osteoblasts are large bone matrix–producing cells, while lining cells are flattened and more metabol-

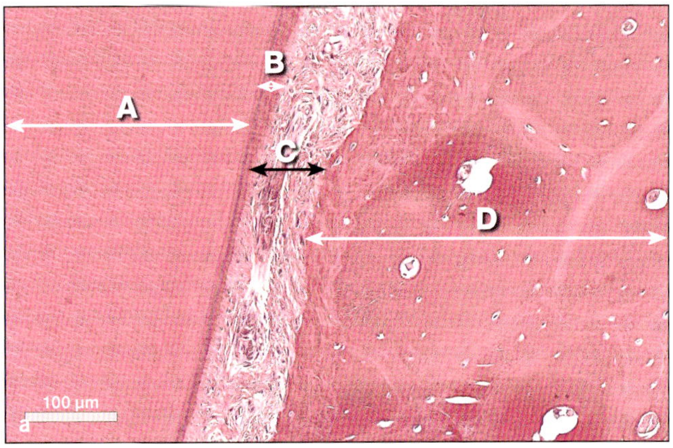

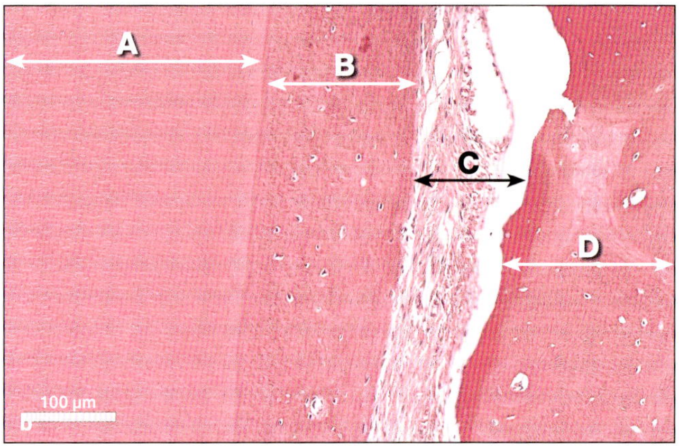

Fig 2-10 *(a)* Acellular cementum. A, dentin; B, acellular cementum covering root dentin; C, PDL; D, alveolar bone. *(b)* Cellular cementum. A, dentin; B, cellular cementum covering root dentin; C, PDL; D, alveolar bone.

ically quiescent. Osteoclasts—bone-resorbing cells—are occasionally seen in the endosteal layer in areas where bone remodeling is occurring.

Cementum

Of the four normal calcified tissues—enamel, dentin, bone, and cementum—cementum is the least mineralized, with about 45% to 50% mineral content. Dentin is sensitive to painful stimuli, so it is important to keep it covered—by enamel in the crown and by cementum in the root. As the root is being formed, cementoblasts differentiate and begin to secrete matrix on the outer surface of the root. In the cervical region, the layer of cementum is thin and acellular. The layer of cementum thickens progressively as the root grows apically and becomes cellular in the apical part of the root. Two main types of cementum have been identified. The first is called *acellular extrinsic fiber cementum*, or primary cementum. This is the cementum that is first produced as the root is just beginning to form and is anywhere from 0 to 50 micrometers in thickness, depending on how apical the measurement is, which tooth it is, and how old the tooth is. About halfway down the root, the cementum transitions to *cellular intrinsic fiber cementum* (secondary cementum). Embedded within the matrix of this cementum are cementocytes in lacunae, which connect to one another by processes lodged in canaliculi. Collagen fibers from the PDL become embedded in the cementum just like they do in bone, thus anchoring the tooth root to the alveolar bone (Fig 2-10).

Apical Foramen

As the root of a tooth takes shape during tooth development, a foramen forms at the root tip that allows passage of neurovascular structures between the pulp of the tooth and the PDL (Fig 2-11). These nerves and vessels are branches of the superior alveolar nerve and artery (maxilla) or the inferior alveolar nerve and artery (mandible). The foramina range in size from 0.3 to 0.6 mm, with the palatal roots of maxillary molars and the distal roots of mandibular molars having the largest diameters.[13] However, there is considerable variation in the location, size, and shape of apical foramina (Fig 2-12).

There is typically an apical constriction, defined as "the apical part of the root canal with the narrowest diameter."[16] It is important to be aware that both the shape and the location of the apical constriction are quite variable.[16] The apical foramen typically does not extend to the very apex of the root. Martos et al[17] found that the mean distance between the major apical foramen and the root apex was 0.69 mm, with a greater distance in posterior teeth than anterior teeth. They also showed that the foramen often deviates buccally or distally. There is also variability in the shape and size of the apical foramen.[18] In addition to the major foramen, many teeth have minor or accessory canals and foramina (Fig 2-13). These have been shown to be quite variable in number, location, and size.[19] In roots with multiple canals, the canals are often connected to each other through one (Fig 2-14) or multiple isthmi, which can complicate surgical endodontic procedures[20] (Fig 2-15).

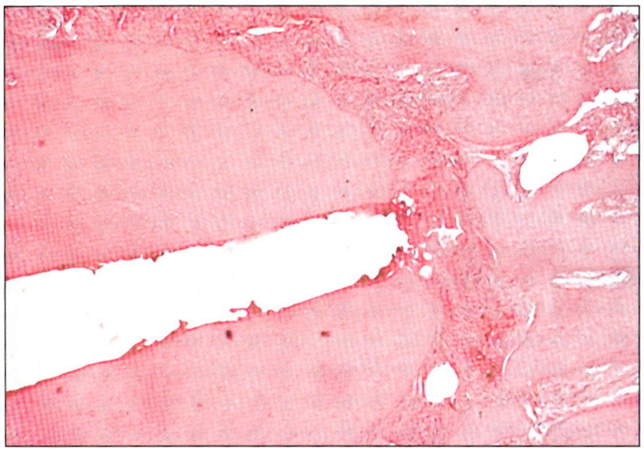

Fig 2-11 The apical foramen is the pathway of communication between the root canal of the tooth and the PDL. (Courtesy of Dr Mahmoud Torabinejad, Loma Linda, California.)

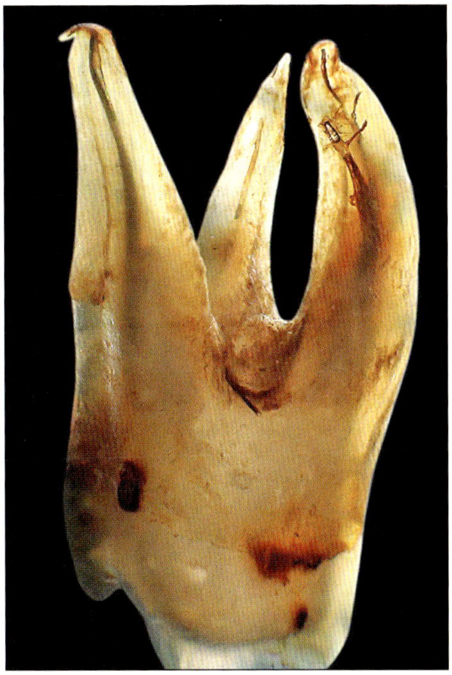

Fig 2-12 A cleared maxillary first molar showing the complex canal anatomy of the mesiobuccal and palatal roots. (Courtesy of Dr Craig Barrington, Waxahachie, Texas.)

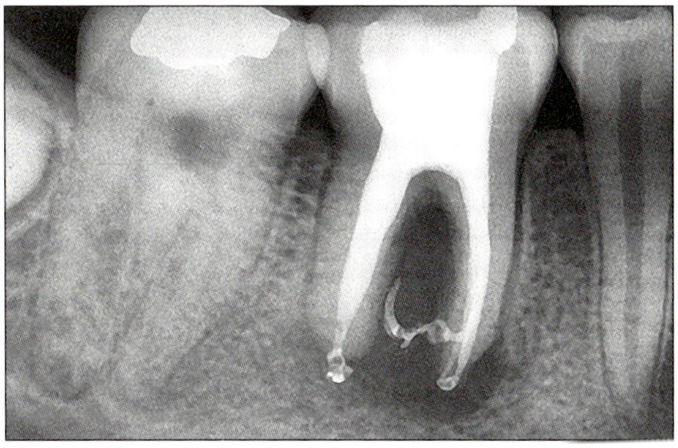

Fig 2-13 A radiograph showing multiple accessory canals and foramina in the mesiobuccal root of a mandibular first molar after root canal treatment. (Courtesy of Dr Mahmoud Torabinejad, Loma Linda, California.)

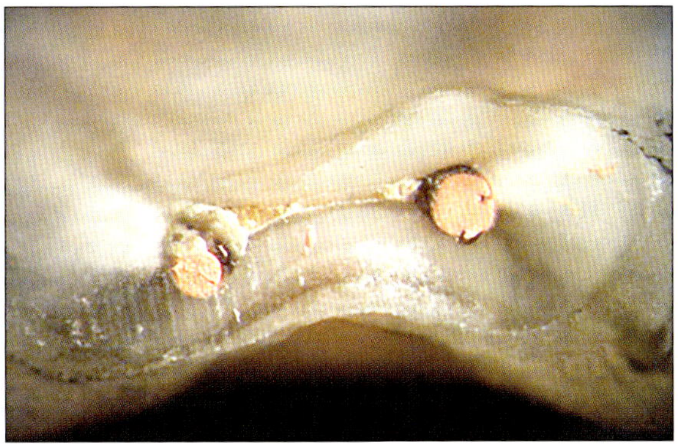

Fig 2-14 A large isthmus exists between the mesiobuccal and mesiolingual of a mandibular first molar after resection of the mesial root. (Courtesy of Dr Steve E. Senia, San Antonio, Texas.)

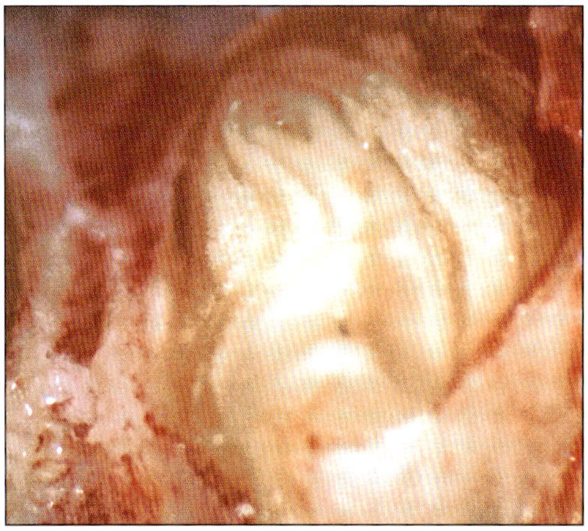

Fig 2-15 Multiple isthmi observed between the apical foramina of the mesiobuccal root of a maxillary first molar after resection of this root during an apical surgery. (Courtesy of Dr Richard Rubinstein, Farmington Hills, Michigan.)

Acknowledgments

The author would like to thank John Hough for providing the images and Resa Chase, MD, for proofreading the chapter.

References

1. Andreasen JO, Rud J. A histobacteriologic study of dental and periapical structures after endodontic surgery. Int J Oral Surg 1972;1:272–281.
2. Block RM, Bushell A, Rodrigues H, Langeland K. A histopathologic, histobacteriologic, and radiographic study of periapical endodontic surgical specimens. Oral Surg Oral Med Oral Pathol 1976;42:656–678.
3. Çalışkan MK, Kaval ME, Tekin U, Ünal T. Radiographic and histological evaluation of persistent periapical lesions associated with endodontic failures after apical microsurgery. Int Endod J 2016;49:1011–1019.
4. Chueh LH, Chiang CP. Histology of irreversible pulpitis premolars treated with mineral trioxide aggregate pulpotomy. Oper Dent 2010;35:370–374.
5. Enriquez FJJ, Vieyra JP, Ocampo FP. Relationship between clinical and histopathologic findings of 40 periapical lesions. Endod Pract US 2015;8(4):36–40.
6. Khayat A. Histological observations of periradicular healing following root canal treatment. Aust Endod J 2005;31:101–105.
7. Lia RC, Garcia JM, Sousa-Neto MD, Saquy PC, Marins RH, Zucollotto WG. Clinical, radiographic and histological evaluation of chronic periapical inflammatory lesions. J Appl Oral Sci 2004;12:117–120.
8. Nosrat A, Ryul Kim J, Verma P, S Chand P. Tissue engineering considerations in dental pulp regeneration. Iran Endod J 2014;9:30–39.
9. Parvathy V, Kumar R, James EP, George S. Ultrasound imaging versus conventional histopathology in diagnosis of periapical lesions of endodontic origin: A comparative evaluation. Indian J Dent Res 2014;25:54–57.
10. Ramachandran Nair PN, Pajarola G, Schroeder HE. Types and incidence of human periapical lesions obtained with extracted teeth. Oral Surg Oral Med Oral Pathol Oral Radiol Endod 1996;81:93–102.
11. Torabinejad M, Faras H. A clinical and histological report of a tooth with an open apex treated with regenerative endodontics using platelet-rich plasma. J Endod 2012;38:864–868.
12. Wais FT. Significance of findings following biopsy and histologic study of 100-periapical lesions. Oral Surg Oral Med Oral Pathol 1958;11:650–653.
13. Nanci A. Ten Cate's Oral Histology, ed 8. St. Louis: Mosby, 2013.
14. Pawlina W. Histology: A Text and Atlas with Correlated Cell and Molecular Biology, ed 7. Philadelphia: Wolters Kluwer, 2016.
15. Matic I, Matthews BG, Wang X, et al. Quiescent bone lining cells are a major source of osteoblasts during adulthood. Stem Cells 2016;34:2930–2942.
16. Alothmani OS, Chandler NP, Friedlander LT. The anatomy of the root apex: A review and clinical considerations in endodontics. Saudi Endod J 2013;3:1–9.
17. Martos J, Ferrer-Luque CM, González-Rodríguez MP, Castro LA. Topographical evaluation of the major apical foramen in permanent human teeth. Int Endod J 2009;42:329–334
18. Abarca J, Zaror C, Monardes H, Hermosilla V, Muñoz C, Cantin M. Morphology of the physiological apical foramen in maxillary and mandibular first molars. Int J Morphol 2014;32:671–677.
19. Arora S, Tewari S. The morphology of the apical foramen in posterior teeth in a North Indian population. Int Endod J 2009;42:930–939.
20. Weller RN, Niemczyk SP, Kim S. Incidence and position of the canal isthmus. Part 1: Mesiobuccal root of the maxillary first molar. J Endod 1995;21:380–383.

Chapter Three

Bone Physiology and Metabolism in Endodontic Surgery

Sarandeep S. Huja, W. Eugene Roberts

Bones have fascinated human beings since the dawn of time. Much of what is known about the evolution of vertebrates is based on the ordered recovery of bones and teeth from the soil. Over the millennia, these structures tended to be well preserved. Compared with living bone, teeth are relatively inert structures. Accretion capability at the dentin-pulp interface (secondary dentin) is limited, and some turnover of the cementum occurs because of root resorption and cementum repair processes. The enamel is a hard and inert structure, but bone is a dynamic structure that constantly adapts to its environment. As a reservoir of calcium, bone remodeling (physiologic turnover) performs a critical life support role in mineral metabolism (Fig 3-1). In addition, the skeleton is the structural scaffold of the body. Collectively bones are essential elements for locomotion, antigravity support, and life-sustaining functions such as mastication. Adaptation of bone is the physiologic basis of clinical practice. A detailed knowledge of the dynamic nature of bone physiology is essential for modern clinical practice.

Osteology

Differential osteology of the maxilla and mandible

Although equal and opposite functional loads are delivered to the maxilla and mandible, the maxilla transfers stress to the entire cranium, whereas the mandible must absorb the entire load. Consequently, the mandible is much stronger and stiffer than the maxilla. A midsagittal section through the incisors (Fig 3-2) and a frontal section through the molar region (Fig 3-3) show the distinct differences in the osseous morphology of the maxilla and mandible. The maxilla has relatively thin cortices that are interconnected by a network of trabeculae. Because it is loaded primarily in compression, the maxilla is structurally similar to the body of a vertebra. The mandible, however, has thick cortices and more radially oriented trabeculae. The structural array is similar to the

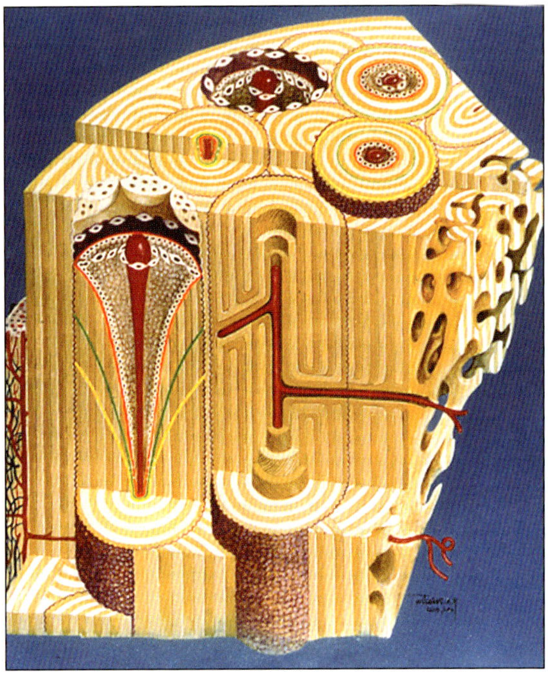

Fig 3-1 Artist's rendering of the dynamic principles of cortical bone remodeling by renowned dental illustrator Rolando De Castro. Remodeling is a vascularly mediated process of bone turnover that maintains the integrity of structural support and is a source of metabolic calcium. Osteoblasts are derived from preosteoblasts circulating in the blood, and perivascular mesenchymal cells give rise to osteoblasts. Note the three colored chevrons *(yellow, green, and orange)* progressively marking the mineralization front of the evolving second osteon that is moving superiorly on the left. (Reprinted from Roberts et al[1] with permission.)

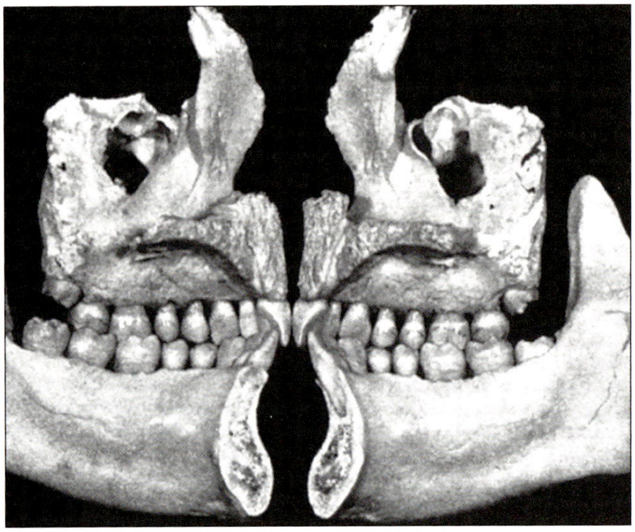

Fig 3-2 Midsagittal section of a human skull shows that the maxilla is composed primarily of trabecular (spongy) bone. The opposing mandible has thick cortices connected by relatively coarse trabeculae. (Reprinted from Atkinson[2] with permission.)

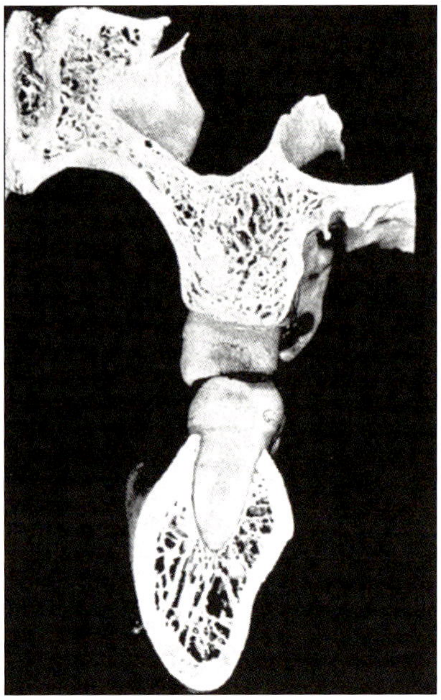

Fig 3-3 Frontal section of the maxilla and mandible in the plane of the first molars. Because it transmits masticatory loads to the entire cranium, the maxilla has thin cortices connected by relatively fine trabeculae. The mandible, however, is loaded in bending and torsion; it is therefore composed of thick cortical bone connected by coarse, oriented trabeculae. (Reprinted from Atkinson[2] with permission.)

shaft of a long bone and indicates that the mandible is loaded predominantly in bending and torsion. This biomechanical impression based on osteology is confirmed by in vivo strain-gauge studies in monkeys. Hylander[3,4] demonstrated substantial bending and torsion in the body of the mandible associated with normal masticatory function (Fig 3-4). A clinical correlation consistent with this pattern of surface strain is the tendency of some human beings to form tori in the areas of maximal bending and torsion (Fig 3-5). The largest tori are on the side on which the individual habitually chews (preferential working side).

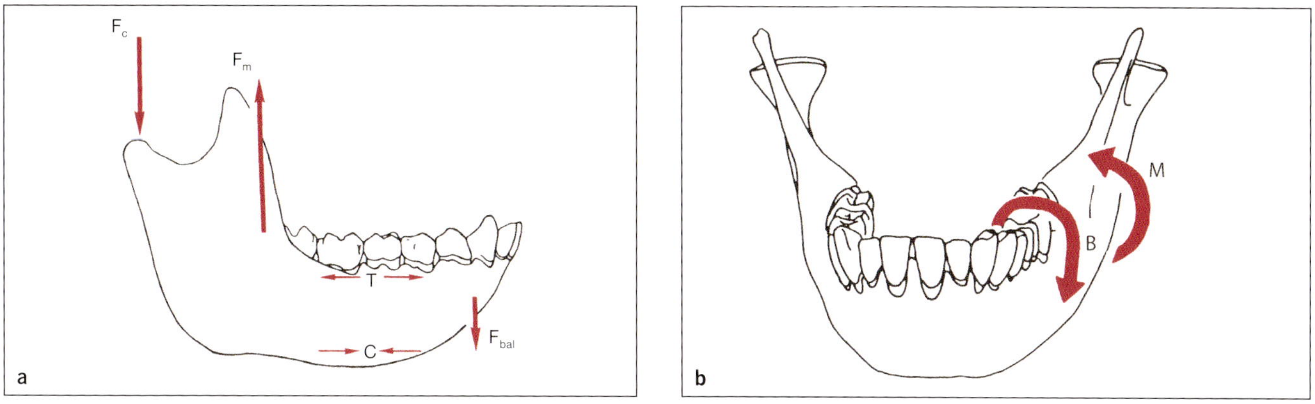

Fig 3-4 Stress patterns in the primate mandible during unilateral mastication. F_c and F_m are the condylar reaction and the resultant muscle forces on the balancing side, respectively. F_{bal} is the force transmitted through the symphysis from the balancing to the working side. T and C indicate the location of tensile stress and compressive stress, respectively. *(a)* During the power stroke, the mandibular corpus on the balancing side is bent primarily in the sagittal plane, resulting in tensile stress along the alveolar process and compressive stress along the inferior border of the mandible. *(b)* On the working side, the corpus is twisted primarily about its long axis (it also experiences direct shear and is slightly bent). The muscle force on this side tends to evert the inferior border of the mandible and invert the alveolar process *(curved arrow* M*)*. The twisting movement associated with the bite force has the opposite effect *(curved arrow* B*)*. The portion of the corpus between these two twisting movements experiences maximal twisting stress. (Reprinted from Hylander[4] with permission.)

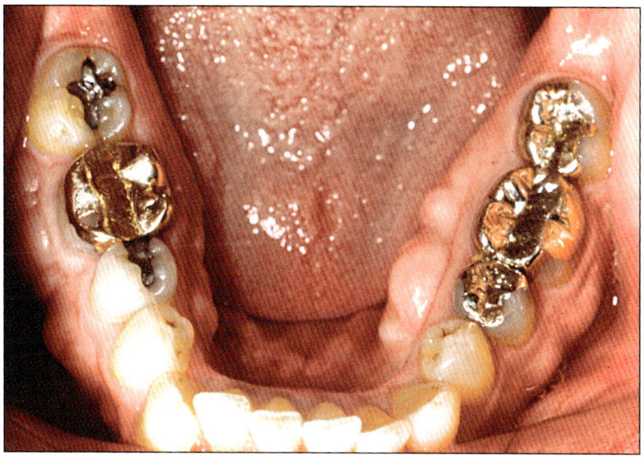

Fig 3-5 Occlusal view of the mandibular dentition of a male patient with extensive buccal and lingual tori. Note that the exostoses are most extensive in the area of the second premolar and first molar, the area of maximal torsion in the posterior segment of the mandible.

Bone Physiology

Classification of bone tissue

During bone adaptation and growth, different bone types can be observed histologically, and the practitioner should have knowledge of these bone types.

Woven bone

Woven bone varies considerably in structure; however it is relatively weak, disorganized, and poorly mineralized. Woven bone serves a crucial role in wound healing by *(1)* rapidly filling osseous defects, *(2)* providing initial continuity for fractures and osteotomy segments, and *(3)* strengthening a bone weakened by surgery or trauma. The first bone formed in response to healing is usually woven bone (Fig 3-6). Woven bone is not found in the adult skeleton under normal, steady-state conditions; rather, it is compacted to form composite bone, remodeled to lamellar bone, or rapidly resorbed if prematurely loaded.[6,7]

Lamellar bone

In contrast to woven bone, lamellar bone, a strong, highly organized, well-mineralized tissue, makes up more than 99% of the adult human skeleton (Figs 3-7a to 3-7c). When new lamellar bone is formed, a portion of the mineral component (hydroxyapatite) is deposited by osteoblasts during primary mineralization (Fig 3-7d). Secondary mineralization, which completes the mineral component, is a physical process (crystal growth) that requires many months. Within physiologic limits, the

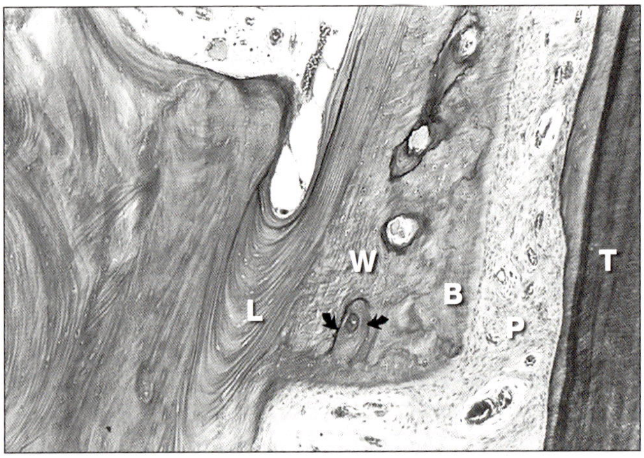

Fig 3-6 A section of human periodontium from the mandibular first molar region shows a typical histologic response to orthodontic tooth movement. With respect to the mature lamellar bone (L) on the left, the tooth (T) is being moved to the right. The first bone formed adjacent to the periodontal ligament (P) is woven bone (W). Subsequent lamellar compaction forms primary osteons of composite bone *(arrows)*. Bundle bone (B) is formed where ligaments such as the periodontal ligament are attached. (Reprinted from Roberts et al[5] with permission.)

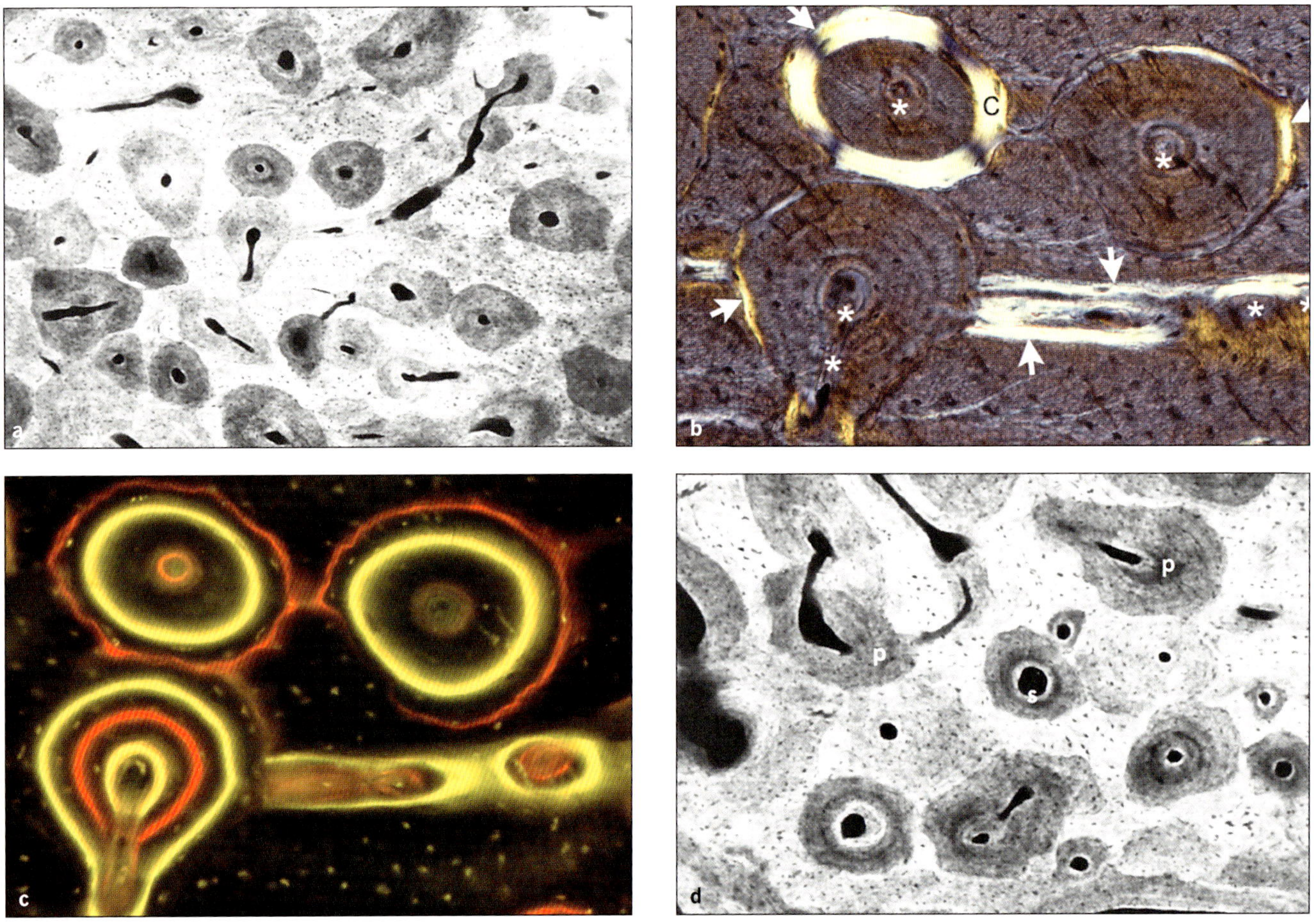

Fig 3-7 *(a)* Microradiograph provides a physiologic index of bone turnover and relative stiffness. The more radiolucent (dark) osteons are the youngest, the least mineralized, and the most compliant. Radiodense (white) areas are the oldest, most mineralized, and most rigid portions of the bone. *(b)* Polarized light microscopy shows the collagen fiber orientation in bone matrix. Lamellae with a longitudinally oriented matrix (C) are particularly strong in tension, whereas a horizontally oriented matrix (dark) has preferential strength in compression—*arrows* mark resorption arrest lines, and *asterisks* mark vascular channels. *(c)* Multiple fluorochrome labels administered at 2-week intervals demonstrate the incidence and rates of bone formation. *(d)* This microradiograph shows an array of concentric secondary osteons (haversian systems) characteristic of rapidly remodeling cortical bone. Primary (p) and beginning secondary (s) mineralization are more radiolucent and radiodense, respectively. (Reprinted from Roberts et al[8] with permission.)

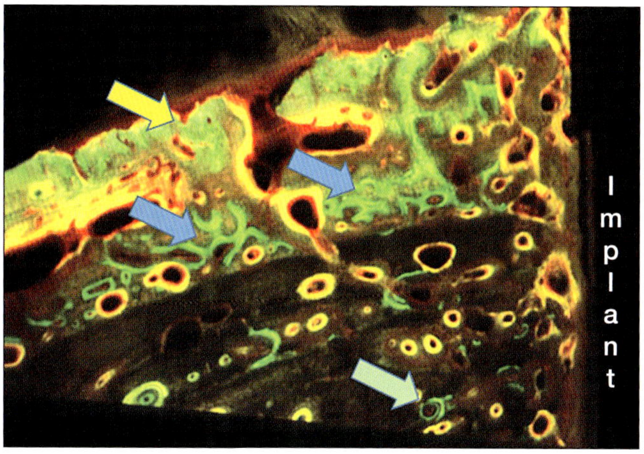

Fig 3-8 Epifluorescent photomicrograph demonstrating healing at an implant interface 12 weeks after implantation in a canine model. The original cortical bone is undergoing secondary osteonal remodeling *(green arrow)* with formation of secondary osteons. A periosteal callus is evident and demonstrates woven bone *(yellow arrow)*. Underneath the woven bone in the older parts of the callus *(blue arrows)*, lamellar compaction is clearly seen with a mix of discrete and diffuse labels, where the woven bone is being replaced with a more lamellar bone.

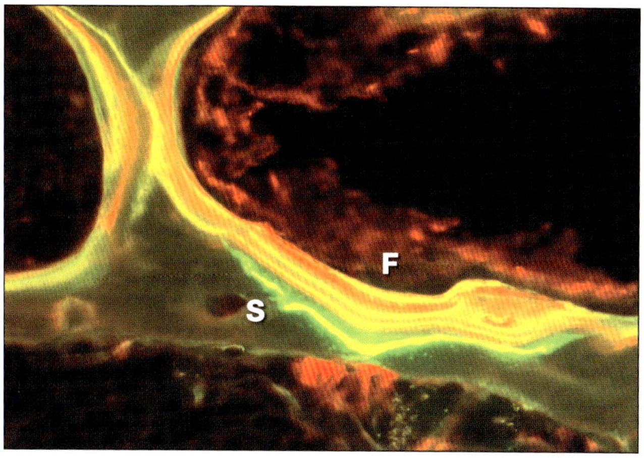

Fig 3-9 Trabecular bone remodeling in the vertebrae in a rat: Multiple fluorochrome labels demonstrate bone formation (F) over a scalloped resorption arrest line (S). (Reprinted from Roberts et al[17] with permission.)

strength of bone is related directly to its mineral content.[9,10] The relative strengths of different histologic types of osseous tissue can be stated thus: Woven bone is weaker than new lamellar bone, which is weaker than mature lamellar bone.[11] Adult human bone is comprised almost entirely of the remodeled variety: secondary osteons and spongiosa.[5,10,12]

Composite bone

Composite bone is an osseous tissue formed by the deposition of lamellar bone within a woven bone lattice (Fig 3-8), a process called *cancellous compaction*.[13,14] This process is the quickest means of producing relatively strong bone.[15] Composite bone is an important intermediary type of bone in the physiologic response to mechanical loading, and it usually is the predominant osseous tissue for stabilization during the early process of postoperative healing. When the bone is formed in the fine compaction configuration, the resulting composite of woven and lamellar bone forms structures known as *primary osteons*. Although composite bone may be high-quality load-bearing osseous tissue, it eventually is remodeled into secondary osteons.[5,11]

Bundle bone

Bundle bone is a functional adaptation of lamellar structure to allow attachment of tendons and ligaments. Perpendicular striations called *Sharpey fibers* are the major distinguishing characteristics of bundle bone. Distinct layers of bundle bone usually are seen adjacent to the periodontal ligament (see Fig 3-6) along physiologic bone-forming surfaces.[16] Bundle bone is the mechanism of ligament and tendon attachment throughout the body.

Skeletal Adaptation: Remodeling and Modeling

Bone remodeling

Bone remodeling is a coupled sequential process of bone resorption followed by bone formation (see Fig 3-7). Bone remodeling occurs in both cortical bone (see Fig 3-7) and trabecular bone (Fig 3-9) compartments of the skeletal system. However, histologic sections reveal important differences between bone remodeling in the cortical versus trabecular bone at a tissue level. Histologically, when viewed in transverse sections of long bones, the end result of bone remodeling in cortical bone is the production of a new, circular-shaped osteon typically 200 to 300 microns in diameter (see Fig 3-7c). This type of cortical bone remodeling can also be described as intracortical secondary osteonal bone remodeling. Thus, the remodeling occurs within the substance of the cortical bone (in the intracortical compartment) and away from the periosteal and endosteal surfaces. In addition, the osteons that result from the bone remodeling process are secondary osteons.[18] These osteons have a reversal line,

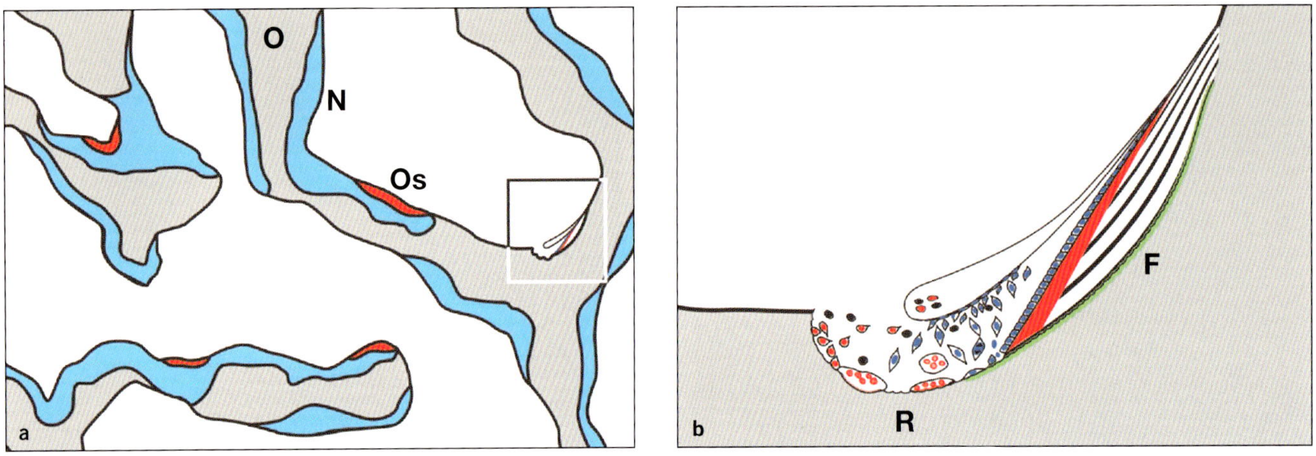

Fig 3-10 *(a)* A schematic drawing of trabecular bone remodeling over a 1-year interval shows the pattern of new bone formation (N) relative to old bone (O) and osteoid seams (Os). The box marks an area of active trabecular resorption, which is magnified in part *b*. *(b)* A detailed drawing of an active remodeling site shows a hemicutting/filling cone with a similar perivascular array of resorptive (R) and formative (F) cells as shown for cortical bone remodeling. The osteoclastic and osteoblastic cell lines are red and blue, respectively. An unmineralized osteoid seam *(solid red line)* marks the bone-forming surface. (Reprinted from Roberts et al[17] with permission.)

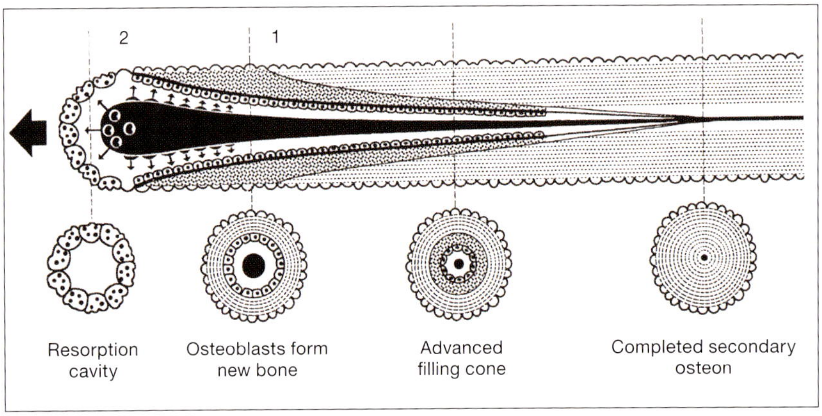

Fig 3-11 The cutting/filling cone has a head of osteoclasts that cut through the bone and a tail of osteoblasts that form a new secondary osteon. The velocity through bone is determined by measuring between two tetracycline labels (1 and 2) administered 1 week apart. (Adapted from Roberts et al[14] with permission.)

unlike primary osteons[19] that lack one because no bone resorption occurs in their development. In essence, primary osteons are produced by bone formation and thus not by a coupled process of bone resorption and bone formation. In trabecular bone, the bone tissue structure is frequently not wide enough to accommodate osteons 200 to 300 microns in size. Thus, only "hemi-osteonal" surface bone remodeling (Fig 3-10) occurs in trabecular bone.[20] However, the bone remodeling is identical to that of cortical bone as it follows the same coupled resorption and formation process. A schematic drawing (see Fig 3-10a) of adult trabecular bone illustrates the pattern of turnover associated with continuous remodeling to support calcium homeostasis. An individual remodeling site is shown in Fig 3-10b. The A→R→F process is similar to the cutting/filling cones of cortical bone remodeling (Fig 3-11). The trabecular bone remodeling mechanism is essentially a hemicutting/filling cone.[18] At a cellular level, though very complex interactions exist, the resorption is carried out by osteoclasts, and the formation is effected by the osteoblasts.[21] To restate, bone remodeling in both cortical and trabecular bone involves the coordinated, coupled activity of osteoclasts and osteoblasts.

Bone remodeling is a homeostatic process. It results in the rejuvenation and replacement of old bone that has served its purpose. It is unique to bone and does not occur within the substance of other mineralized tissues such as enamel, dentin, and cementum. This provides a distinct advantage to bone and makes it a tissue that is capable of regeneration. The bone remodeling also underlies the immense adaptive potential of this mineralized and hard tissue, both terms otherwise implying limited adaptability.[22] From a functional standpoint, bone remodeling provides for calcium and thus helps in precisely regulating calcium levels in the body.[18] From an evolutionary perspective, bone acts as a calcium reservoir, allowing for life forms to move away from the sea water. Without such a reservoir and a method for mobilization of calcium stores, calcium in the immediate environment (eg, sea water) was essential for various cellular functions.

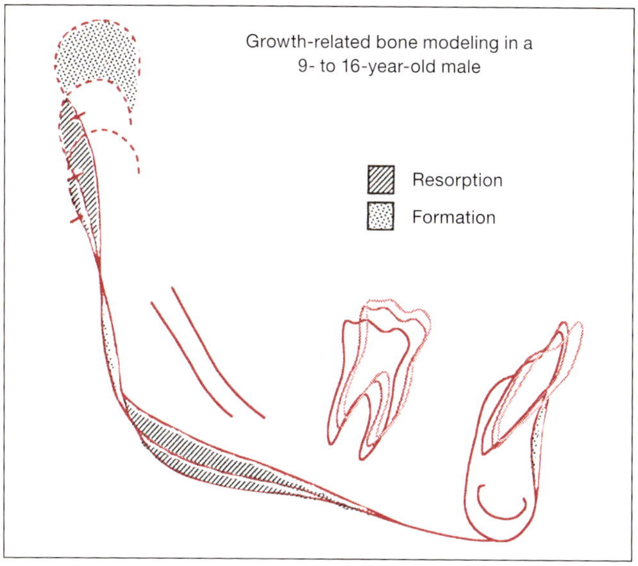

Fig 3-12 Orthopedic bone modeling related to growth in an adolescent male involves several site-specific areas of bone formation and resorption. Although extensive bone remodeling (ie, internal turnover) is also underway, it is not evident in cephalometric radiographs superimposed on stable mandibular structures.

There are two terms used to further describe the type of bone remodeling: *stochastic* and *targeted*.[23] Stochastic remodeling occurs somewhat uniformly throughout the body (ie, the continuous repair and regeneration process). There are multiple sites (about 1 million by some estimates) in both trabecular and cortical bone at which stochastic bone remodeling is occurring at any one time. These remodeling sites also provide for metabolic calcium. During calcium deprivation,[24] bone remodeling is enhanced, and the bone remodeling rate is increased with more "cutting/filling cones" or osteons being produced (see Fig 3-11). Targeted remodeling occurs at a specific site of injury and not throughout the entire body. A relevant and easily understandable example is the bone-implant interface. In placing an implant, microdamage (small linear cracks) are created within the bone due to the insertion of the screw.[25] The microdamage, a manifestation of tissue injury in a mineralized tissue, is repaired by bone remodeling.[26] Thus, microdamage production stimulates bone remodeling at the site of damage (ie, close to the interface) and repairs the damaged bone. Another form of bone injury is manifestation of diffuse damage.[27] This damage is not as clearly visible in histologic sections as microdamage. Injury of both hard and soft tissue produces a localized insult, and repair is targeted to that specific area.

Bone modeling

Bone modeling is a distinct and different process from *bone remodeling*. These two processes are frequently confused even though they can be readily distinguished at a histologic level. Histologic sections labeled with intravital dyes can clearly distinguish bone remodeling and modeling.[28,29] This contrast is not trivial, and the underlying process and controls of bone remodeling and modeling are different. It is not uncommon to find bone modeling being measured in studies and being mistaken for bone remodeling. This then leads to confusion in the literature and more unfortunately to incorrect interpretations.

Bone modeling is a surface-specific activity and results in a change in shape and size.[18] It is an uncoupled process, and the bone resorption and formation are not linked or coupled in a sequential manner (Fig 3-12). The bone formation and resorption mediated by the osteoblasts and osteoclasts respectively do not occur on the same bone surface and occur independently of each other. One example of the end result of bone modeling that can occur over a duration of years is the difference in the diameter of the dominant arm of a tennis player from the contralateral nondominant arm.[30] The bone of the dominant arm has a diameter about 1.6-fold greater than the nondominant arm. The change in size occurs over a period of years and due to modeling events on the periosteal surface (and endosteal surface) of the arm. This does not mean that bone remodeling cannot occur within the cortical bone (intracortical compartment) independently or simultaneously; however, they are two different processes with different control mechanisms.[31] There are numerous other examples of bone modeling, including the formation of a callus after fracture of a bone (or insertion of an endosseous implant) and changes seen on the surfaces of bone (changes in shape and size) during growth (see Fig 3-12). The surface changes are modeling, but there is no doubt that remodeling is concurrently occurring within the bone. In fact, modeling occurs primarily during growth (on periosteal and endosteal bone surfaces) and

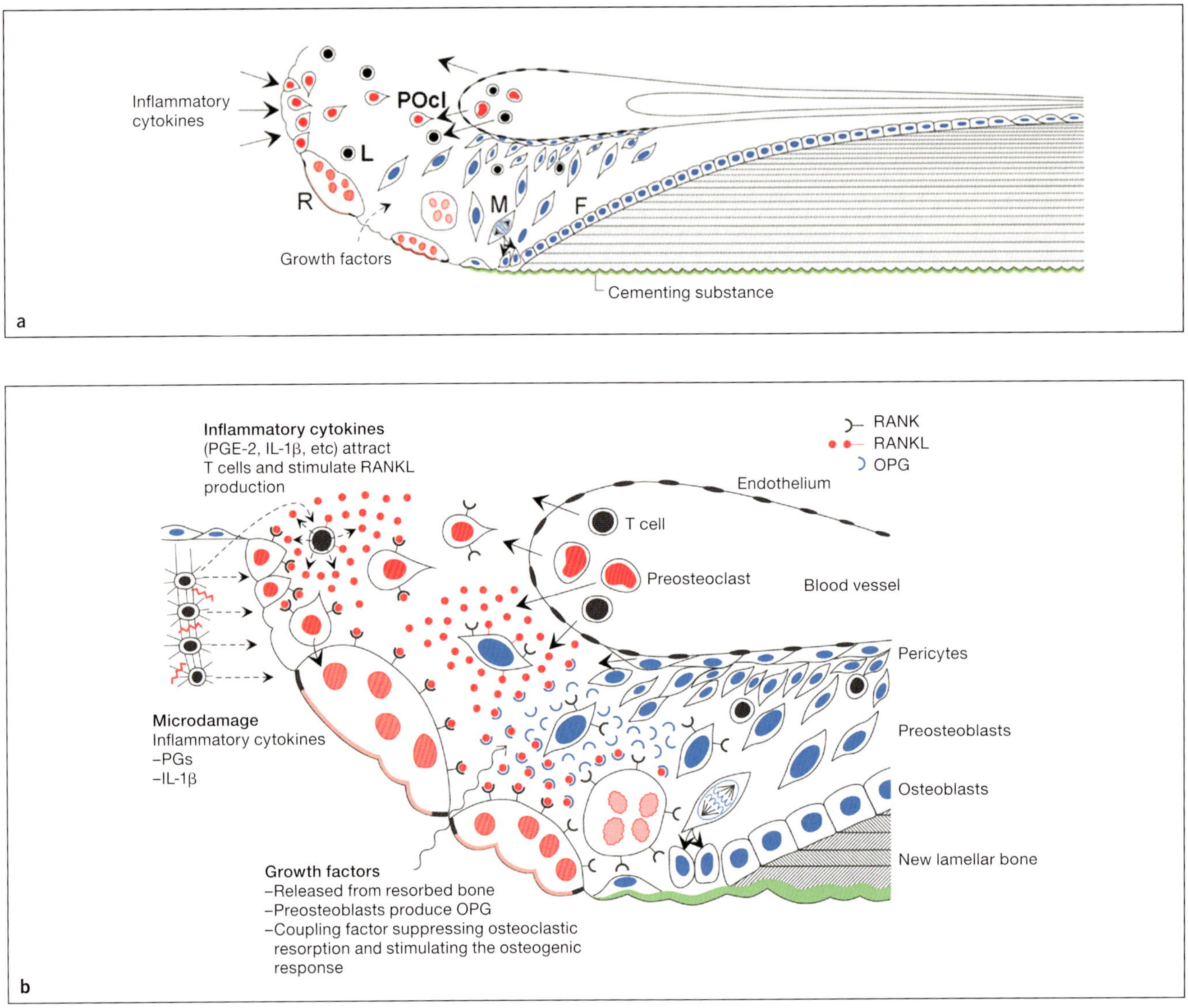

Fig 3-13 *(a)* A hemisection of a cutting/filling cone moving to the left demonstrates the intravascular and perivascular mechanisms for coupling bone resorption (R) to formation (F) during the remodeling process. Lymphocytes (L) are attracted from the circulation by inflammatory cytokines. They help recruit preosteoclasts (POcl) from the circulation. See text for details. *(b)* A magnified view of the head of a hemicutting/filling cone illustrates the proposed mechanism for coupling bone resorption to formation via the genetic RANK/RANKL/OPG mechanism. The cutting head is stimulated by inflammatory cytokines produced by osteocytes in damaged bone *(left)*. Preosteoclasts have RANK receptors that are bound and activated by RANKL, probably produced or mediated by T cells (lymphocytes) near the resorption front. Growth factors from resorbed bone *(bottom)* stimulate production of preosteoblasts, which then produce OPG to block the RANK receptors on osteoclasts; the latter then withdraw from the scalloped surface and degenerate. Relatively flat mononuclear cells *(bottom center)* form cementing substance to form a resorption arrest line. Osteoblasts *(bottom right)* produce new lamellar bone to fill the resorption cavity. PG, prostaglandin; IL, interleukin. (Reprinted from Roberts et al[17] with permission.)

then decreases after maturity. It is activated again during healing and other pathologic biologic processes (eg, bony cyst producing expansion).

Modeling changes can be seen on radiographs (eg, bony expansion or protuberance with tori), but remodeling events, which usually occur at the same time, are apparent only at the tissue level of examination. True remodeling is not imaged on clinical radiographs.[32] Constant remodeling (internal turnover) mobilizes and redeposits calcium by means of coupled resorption and formation: Bone is resorbed and redeposited at the same site. Osteoblasts, osteoclasts, and possibly their precursors are thought to communicate by chemical messages known as *coupling factors*. Transforming growth factor β is released from bone during the resorption process; this cytokine helps stimulate subsequent bone formation to fill resorption cavities.[33] It is currently thought that growth factors released from bone mediate the coupling process via a genetic mechanism for activating and suppressing osteoclasts. Thus, receptor activator of nuclear factor kappa-B (RANK), RANK ligand (RANKL), and osteoprotegerin (OPG) are gene products that control the remodeling sequence of bone resorption followed by formation. This ubiquitous genetic mechanism appears to be involved in the inflammatory induction of bone resorption and the coupling of bone formation at the same site[34,35] (Fig 3-13).

Cortical Bone Growth and Maturation

Cutting and filling cones

The rate at which cutting and filling cones progress through compact bone is an important determinant of turnover. The progression is calculated by measuring the distance between initiation of labeled bone formation sites along the resorption arrest line in longitudinal sections.[14] In a study using two fluorescent labels administered 2 weeks apart in adult dogs, the velocity was 27.7 ± 1.9 mm/day (mean ± SEM [standard error of the mean], n = 4 dogs, 10 cutting and filling cones sampled from each). At this speed, evolving secondary osteons travel about 1 mm in 36 days. Newly remodeled secondary osteons (formed within the experimental period of the dog study) contained an average of 4.5 labels (administered 2 weeks apart); the incidence of resorption cavities is about one-third the incidence of labeled osteons.[36] These data are consistent with a remodeling cycle of about 12 weeks in dogs[36] compared with 6 weeks in rabbits[14] and 17 weeks in human beings.[12,14] This relationship is useful for extrapolating animal data to human applications. More recent experimental studies have shown that new secondary osteons may continue to fix bone labels for up to 6 months, indicating that terminal filling of the lumen is slow.[37]

Traumatic or surgical wounding usually results in intense but localized modeling and remodeling responses. After an osteotomy or placement of an endosseous implant, callus formation and resorption of necrotic osseous margins are modeling processes; however, internal replacement of the devitalized cortical bone surrounding these sites is a remodeling activity. In addition, a gradient of localized remodeling disseminates through the bone adjacent to any invasive bone procedure. This process, called the *regional acceleratory phenomenon* (RAP), is an important aspect of postoperative healing.[12,38]

Modeling and remodeling are controlled by an interaction of metabolic and mechanical signals. Bone modeling is largely under the integrated biomechanical control of functional applied loads. However, hormones and other metabolic agents have a strong secondary influence, particularly during periods of growth and advanced aging. Paracrine and autocrine mechanisms, such as local growth factors and prostaglandins, can override the mechanical control mechanism temporarily during wound healing.[39] Remodeling responds to metabolic mediators such as parathyroid hormone (PTH) and estrogen primarily by varying the rate of bone turnover. Bone scans with 130Te-bisphosphate, a marker of bone activity, indicate that the alveolar processes, but not the basilar mandible, have a high remodeling rate.[40,41] Uptake of the marker in alveolar bone is similar to uptake in trabecular bone of the vertebral column. The latter is known to remodel at a rate of about 20% to 30% per year, compared with most cortical bone that turns over at a rate of 2% to 10% per year.[29] Metabolic mediation of continual bone turnover provides a controllable flow of calcium to and from the skeleton.

Bone remodeling rate

It is well known that cortical bone remodels at 2% to 10% per year while turnover in the trabecular bone is 30% to 35% per year.[20,23] Trabecular bone is metabolically active and is the source of serum calcium. Interestingly, in the alveolar bone that supports the tooth, the physiologic rate of cortical bone turnover can be as high as 35% per year, which is 3- to 10-fold higher than cortical bone elsewhere (eg, in the long bones) in the body.[42,43] In implant adjacent bone, the rate of bone turnover can be as high as 100% to 500% per year, suggesting intense cortical bone remodeling in implant adjacent bone.[44] It is likely that this elevated turnover is required to maintain a compliant zone of bone and to buffer for the modulus mismatch between the implant and bone.

Regional acceleratory phenomenon

RAP was first described by Dr Harold Frost[38] as a complex reaction to diverse noxious stimuli. He indicated that it is an "SOS" mechanism and acceleration of normal vital tissue processes. In humans, it lasts 4 months in bone and somewhat less in soft tissues. Importantly, RAP is a process of intermediary organization of tissues and organs and is not revealed in isolated cells. This statement is very important because it means that a conclusion that RAP is occurring in an experimental system based on isolated cells is incorrect as originally defined. Initially RAP was described in cortical tissues and later in trabecular bone. RAP is not typically accompanied by osteopenia in the cortical[45] and trabecular[46] bone.

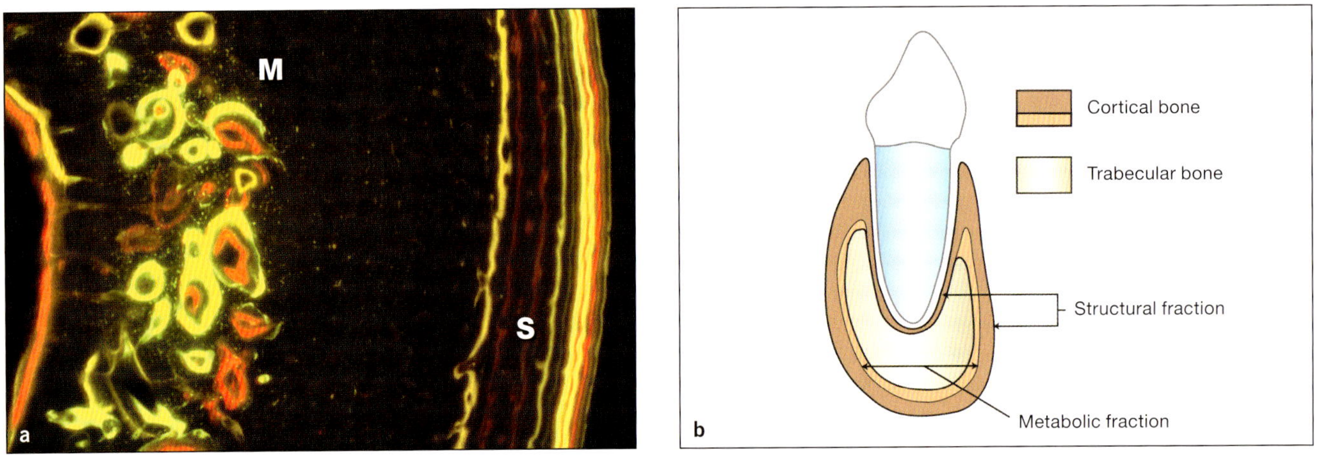

Fig 3-14 *(a)* The structural (S) and metabolic (M) fractions of cortical bone are revealed by multiple fluorochrome labeling of a rabbit femur during the late growth and early adult periods. Continuing periosteal bone formation *(right)* contributes to structural strength, and high remodeling of the endosteal half of the compacta provides a continual supply of metabolic calcium. *(b)* Structural and metabolic fractions of bone in the mandible. (Adapted from Roberts et al[8] with permission.)

Structural and metabolic fractions

The structural fraction of cortical bone is the relatively stable outer portion of the cortex; the metabolic fraction is the highly reactive inner aspect (Fig 3-14a). The primary metabolic calcium reserves of the body are found in trabecular bone and the endosteal half of the cortices, and thus these regions constitute the metabolic fraction. Diaphyseal rigidity is quickly enhanced by adding a circumferential lamella at the periosteal surface. Even a thin layer of new osseous tissue at the periosteal surface greatly enhances bone stiffness because it increases the diameter of the bone. In engineering terms, cross-sectional rigidity is related to the second moment of the area. Thus, when a relatively rigid material (bone shaft) is doubled in diameter, the stiffness increases 16 times.

The addition of new osseous tissue at the endosteal (inner) surface has little effect on overall bone strength. Structurally, the long bones and mandible are modified tubes—an optimal design for achieving maximal strength with minimal mass.[9] Within limits, loss of bone at the endosteal surface or within the inner third of the compacta has little effect on bone rigidity. The inner cortex can be mobilized to meet metabolic needs without severely compromising bone strength (Fig 3-14b); this is the reason why patients with osteoporosis have bones with a normal diameter but thin cortices. Even under severe metabolic stress, the body follows a cardinal principle of bone physiology: maximal strength with minimal mass.[47]

Methods to Quantify Bone Adaptation and Healing

The morphology of bone has been well described, but its physiology is elusive because of the technical limitations inherent in the study of mineralized tissues. Accurate assessment of the mechanical response to applied loads requires time markers (bone labels) and physiologic indices (DNA labels, histochemistry, and in situ hybridization) of bone cell function. Systematic investigation with these advanced methods has defined new concepts of clinically relevant bone physiology. Specific assessment methods include the following:

- Polarized light birefringence detects the preferential orientation of collagen fibers in the bone matrix.[5]
- Fluorescent labels (eg, tetracycline) permanently mark all sites of bone mineralization at a specific point in time (anabolic markers).[5,43]
- Microradiography assesses mineral density patterns in the same sections.[6]
- Autoradiography detects radioactively tagged precursors (eg, nucleotides and amino acids) used to mark physiologic activity.[48–50]
- Nuclear volume morphometry differentially assesses osteoblast precursors in a variety of osteogenic tissues.[51]
- Cell kinetics is a quantitative analysis of cell physiology based on morphologically distinguishable events in the

Fig 3-15 Calcium metabolism is a complex physiologic process. Maintaining zero calcium balance requires optimal function of the gut, parathyroid glands, bone, liver, and kidneys. PTH and the active metabolite of vitamin D, 1,25-dihydroxycholecalciferol, are the major hormones involved. ECF, extracellular fluid. (Adapted from Roberts et al[8] with permission.)

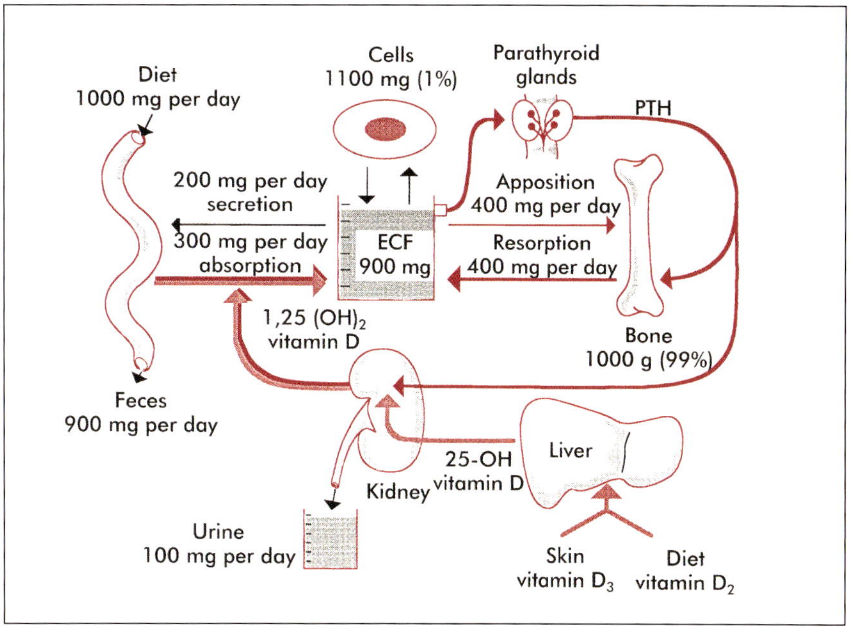

cell cycle (ie, DNA synthesis [S] phase, mitosis, and differentiation-specific change in nuclear volume).[51,52]

- Finite element modeling is an engineering method of calculating stresses and strains in all materials, including living tissue.[8,53–55]
- Backscatter emission is a variation of electron microscopy that assesses relative mineral density at the microscopic level in a block specimen.[56]
- Microcomputed tomography is an in vitro imaging method for determining the relative mineral density of osseous tissue down to a resolution of about 5 μm (about the size of an osteoblast nucleus).[57]
- Microindentation testing is a method for determining the mechanical properties of bone at the microscopic level.[58–61]

Bone Metabolism

Bone metabolism is an important aspect of clinical dentistry, and this section discusses the fundamentals of bone metabolism with respect to clinical practice.

The skeletal system is composed of highly specialized mineralized tissues that have structural and metabolic functions. Structurally, lamellar, woven, composite, and bundle bone are unique types of osseous tissue adapted to specific functions. Bone modeling and remodeling are distinct physiologic responses to integrated mechanical and metabolic demands. Because of the interaction of structure and metabolism, a thorough understanding of osseous structure and function is fundamental to patient selection, risk assessment, and treatment planning.[47,62]

Bone is the primary calcium reservoir in the body (see Fig 3-14). About 99% of the calcium in the body is stored in the skeleton. The continual flux of bone mineral responds to a complex interaction of endocrine, biomechanical, and cell-level control factors that maintain the serum calcium level at about 10 mg/dL.

Calcium homeostasis is the process by which mineral equilibrium is maintained. Maintenance of serum calcium levels at about 10 mg/dL is an essential life-support function. Life is thought to have evolved in the sea; calcium homeostasis is the mechanism of the body for maintaining the primordial mineral environment in which cellular processes evolved.[63] Calcium metabolism is one of the fundamental physiologic processes of life support. When substantial calcium is needed to maintain the critical serum calcium level, bone structure is sacrificed (Fig 3-15). The alveolar processes and basilar bone of the jaws are also subject to metabolic bone loss.[64] Even in cases of severe skeletal atrophy, the outer cortex of the alveolar process and the lamina dura around the teeth are preserved. This preservation is analogous to the thin cortices characteristic of osteoporosis.

Calcium homeostasis is supported by three temporally related mechanisms: *(1)* rapid (instantaneous) flux of calcium from bone fluid (which occurs in seconds); *(2)* short-term response by osteoclasts and osteoblasts (which extends from minutes to days); and *(3)* long-term control of bone turnover (over weeks to months). Precise regulation of serum calcium levels at about 10 mg/dL is essential for nerve conductivity and muscle function. A low serum calcium level can result in tetany and death. A sustained high serum calcium level is often a manifestation of hyperthyroidism and some malignancies. Hypercalcemia may lead to kidney stones and dystrophic calcification of soft tissue. Normal physiology demands precise control of the serum calcium level.[62–64]

Calcium Conservation

Calcium conservation is the aspect of bone metabolism that involves preservation of skeletal mass. A failure in calcium conservation stemming from a single problem or a combination of metabolic and biomechanical problems may leave a patient with inadequate bone mass for reconstructive dentistry. The kidney is the primary calcium conservation organ in the body. Positive calcium balance normally occurs during the growing period and for about 10 years thereafter. Peak skeletal mass is attained between 25 and 30 years. Zero calcium balance (see Fig 3-15) is the ideal metabolic state for maintaining skeletal mass. Preservation of bone requires a favorable diet, endocrine balance, and adequate exercise.[47,62]

Endocrinology

Peptide hormones (eg, PTH, growth hormone, insulin, and calcitonin) bind receptors at the cell surface and may be internalized with the receptor complex. Steroid hormones (eg, vitamin D, androgens, and estrogens) are lipid soluble and pass through the plasma membrane to bind receptors in the nucleus.[47,62] PTH increases serum calcium by direct and indirect vitamin D–mediated effects. Clinically, a major effect of 1,25-dihydroxycholecalciferol is induction of active absorption of calcium from the gut. Sex hormones have profound effects on bone. Androgens (testosterone and other anabolic steroids) build and maintain musculoskeletal mass. The primary hypertrophic effect of androgens is an increase in muscle mass. The anabolic effect on bone is a secondary biomechanical response to increase loads generated by the enhanced muscle mass. Estrogen, however, has a direct effect on bone; it conserves skeletal calcium by suppressing the activation frequency of bone remodeling.[65] At menopause, enhanced remodeling activation increases turnover.[66] Because a slight negative calcium balance is associated with each remodeling event, a substantial increase in the turnover rate can result in rapid bone loss, leading to symptomatic osteoporosis. Even young women are susceptible to significant bone loss if the menstrual cycle (menses) stops.[15] Bone loss is a common problem in women who have low body fat and who exercise intensely (eg, running or gymnastics) and in women who are anorexic.[67]

Estrogen replacement therapy (ERT) was widely recommended for calcium conservation and the prevention of osteoporosis in postmenopausal women.[68,69] However, the increased incidence and progression of breast cancer have greatly decreased the use of ERT.[70] The antiestrogen tamoxifen is used to treat some forms of breast cancer. Fortunately, in postmenopausal women tamoxifen has a beneficial effect on bone similar to that of estrogen.[71] Raloxifene (Evista, Eli Lilly) has been shown to reduce the risk of osteoporosis and heart disease without increasing the risk of breast cancer. Some studies have even shown a substantial anticancer protective effect.

Metabolic Bone Disease

Osteoporosis is a generic term for very low bone mass (osteopenia). The most important risk factor for the development of osteoporosis is age: After the third decade, osteopenia is related directly to longevity. Other high-risk factors are *(1)* a history of long-term glucocorticoid treatment, *(2)* slight stature, *(3)* smoking, *(4)* menopause or dysmenorrhea, *(5)* lack of or little physical activity, *(6)* low-calcium diet, *(7)* excessive consumption of alcohol, *(8)* vitamin D deficiency, *(9)* kidney failure, *(10)* liver disease (cirrhosis), and *(11)* a history of fractures. These risk factors are effective in identifying 78% of those with the potential for osteopenia.[72,73] This is a good screening method for skeletally deficient dental patients. However, one must realize that more than 20% of individuals who eventually develop osteoporosis have a negative history for known risk factors. Any clinical signs or symptoms of low bone mass (eg, low radiographic density of the jaws, thin cortices, or excessive bone resorption) are grounds for referral. A thorough medical workup, including a bone mineral density measurement, usually is necessary to establish the diagnosis of osteopenia. The term *osteoporosis* usually is reserved for patients with evidence of fracture or other osteoporotic symptoms. The treatment of metabolic bone diseases such as osteoporosis depends on the causative factors. Medical management of these often complex disorders is best handled by physicians specifically trained in bone metabolism.[47,62]

An increasing number of adults are seeking dental treatment. All health care practitioners can play an important role in screening patients with high-risk lifestyles. Arresting the progression of metabolic bone disease is preferable to treating the condition after debilitating symptoms appear. A carefully collected history is the best screening method for determining which patients should be referred for a thorough metabolic workup. Clinicians must assess carefully the probability of metabolic bone disease.[47,62]

In addition to osteoporosis, clinicians should be particularly vigilant for osteomalacia, a disease of poor bone mineralization associated with vitamin D deficiency,[29] and for renal osteodystrophy, a related condition in patients with compromised kidney function.[74]

Dental treatment is usually contraindicated in patients with active metabolic bone disease because of excessive resorption and poor rates of bone formation. However, if the metabolic problems (particularly negative calcium balance) are resolved with medical treatment, these patients can be treated, assuming that sufficient skeletal structure remains. In fact, some individuals with osteoporosis retain near-normal jaw and alveolar bone, probably because they have healthy oral structures that are loaded normally. Apparently, under these circumstances, the disease preferentially attacks bone and other parts of the body with a less optimal mechanical environment.[47,62,75] A study of all adult female dental patients at Indiana University School of Dentistry showed that about 65% were at high risk for developing osteoporosis (these women were estrogen deficient or had at least two other risk factors).[76]

Osteoporosis is the most common metabolic bone disease, but patients can be affected by many other osseous pathologies, such as renal osteodystrophy, hyperparathyroidism, hypoparathyroidism, hyperthyroidism, and osteomalacia osteogenesis imperfecta. In addition, bone can be compromised by a number of other systemic diseases.

With the use of more potent bisphosphonates to treat osteoporotic patients including Reclast (Novartis), the question has arisen whether tooth movement is retarded or, even more important, whether osteonecrosis of the jaw (ONJ)[77] will develop after tooth extractions. Animal studies suggest that while potent bisphosphonates such as zoledronic acid greatly suppress bone remodeling,[78,79] they do not abolish the formation of new osteons at a site of injury. In other words, bone remodeling at a tissue level does occur in response to injury in an animal model that has received potent and high-dose bisphosphonates. However, the risks of drug-induced ONJ should be taken into consideration prior to any dental treatment in patients receiving intravenous bisphosphonates.

Mechanical Loading

Mechanical loading is essential to skeletal health. An important element of bone biomechanics is the inflammatory control of bone development, the adaptation to applied loads, and the response to pathologic challenges. The physiologic mechanism for controlling bone morphology involves inherent (genetic) and environmental (epigenetic) factors. There are three genetic mechanisms: *(1)* growth and ischemic factors, *(2)* vascular induction and invasion, and *(3)* mechanically induced inflammation. The latter two are influenced by two major physical influences: *(1)* diffusion limitation for maintaining viable osteocytes and *(2)* mechanical loading history[80] (Fig 3-16).

Control of most bone modeling and some remodeling processes is related to strain history, which is usually defined in microstrain (με) (deformation per unit length × 10^{-6}).[81] Repetitive loading generates a specific response, which is determined by the peak strain.[82–86] In an attempt to simplify the often conflicting data, Frost[87] proposed the mechanostat theory. Reviewing the theoretic basis of this theory, Martin and Burr[10] proposed that *(1)* subthreshold loading of less than 200 με results in disuse atrophy, manifested as a decrease in modeling and an increase in remodeling; *(2)* physiologic loading of about 200 to 2,500 με is associated with normal, steady-state activities; *(3)* loads exceeding the minimal effective strain (about 2,500 με) result in a hypertrophic increase in modeling and a concomitant decrease in remodeling; *(4)* after peak strains exceed about 4,000 με, the structural integrity of bone is threatened, resulting in pathologic overload. Figure 3-17 is a representation of the mechanostat. Many of the concepts and microstrain levels are based on experimental data.[10,88] The strain range for each given response probably varies between species and may be site specific in the same individual.[8,10,83–86] However, the mechanostat provides a useful clinical reference for the hierarchy of biomechanical responses to applied loads.

Normal function helps build and maintain bone mass. Suboptimally loaded bones atrophy as a result of increased remodeling frequency and inhibition of osteoblast formation.[89] Under these conditions, trabecular connections are lost and cortices are thinned from the endosteal surface. Eventually the skeleton is weakened until it cannot sustain normal function. An increasing number of adults with a history of osteopenia caused by metabolic bone disease are seeking dental treatment as the population ages.

When flexure (strain) exceeds the normal physiologic range, bones compensate by adding new mineralized tissue at the periosteal surface. Adding bone is an essential compensating mechanism because of the inverse relationship between load (strain magnitude) and the fatigue resistance of bone.[90] When loads are less than 2,000 με, lamellar bone can withstand millions of loading cycles, more than a lifetime of normal function. However, increasing the cyclic load to 5,000 με, about 20% of the ultimate strength of cortical bone, can produce fatigue failure in 1,000 cycles, which is achieved easily in only a few weeks of normal activity. Repetitive overload at less than one-fifth of the ultimate strength of lamellar bone (25,000 με, or 2.5% deformation) can lead to skeletal failure, stress fractures, and shin splints.

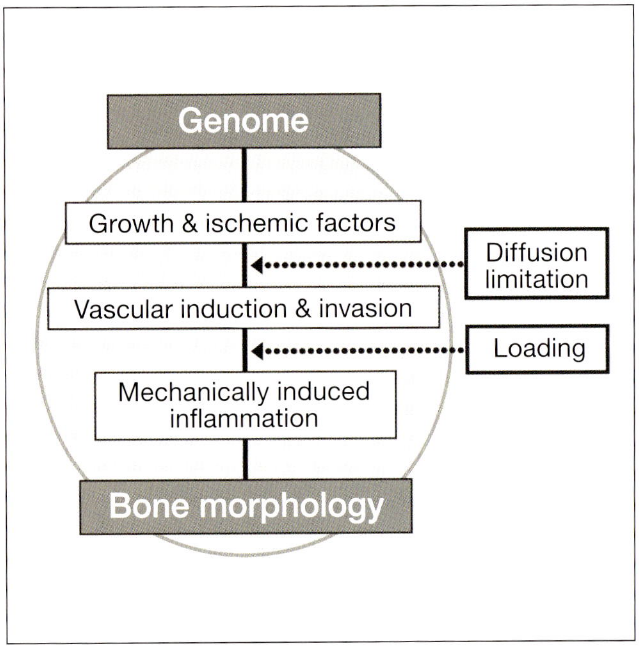

Fig 3-16 The genome dictates bone morphology by a sequence of three genetic mechanisms: *(1)* growth and ischemic factors, *(2)* vascular induction and invasion, and *(3)* mechanically induced inflammation. The latter two are influenced by two major physical influences: *(1)* diffusion limitation for maintaining viable osteocytes and *(2)* mechanical loading history. (Reprinted from Roberts and Hartsfield[80] with permission.)

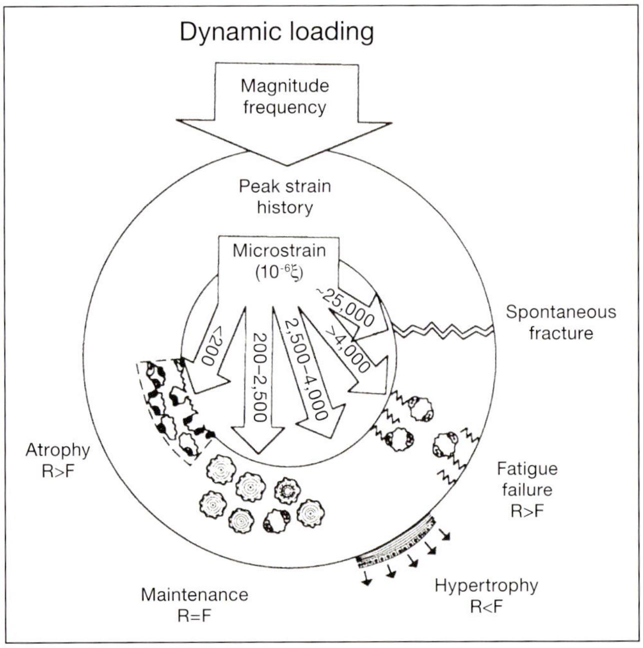

Fig 3-17 The mechanostat concept of Frost as defined by Martin and Burr. Bone formation (F) and resorption (R) are the modeling phenomena that change the shape and/or form of a bone. The peak strain history determines whether atrophy, maintenance, hypertrophy, or fatigue failure occurs. Note that the normal physiologic range of loading (Maintenance R=F) is only at less than 10% of maximal bone strength (spontaneous fracture). Fatigue damage can accumulate rapidly at greater than 4,000 $\mu\varepsilon$.

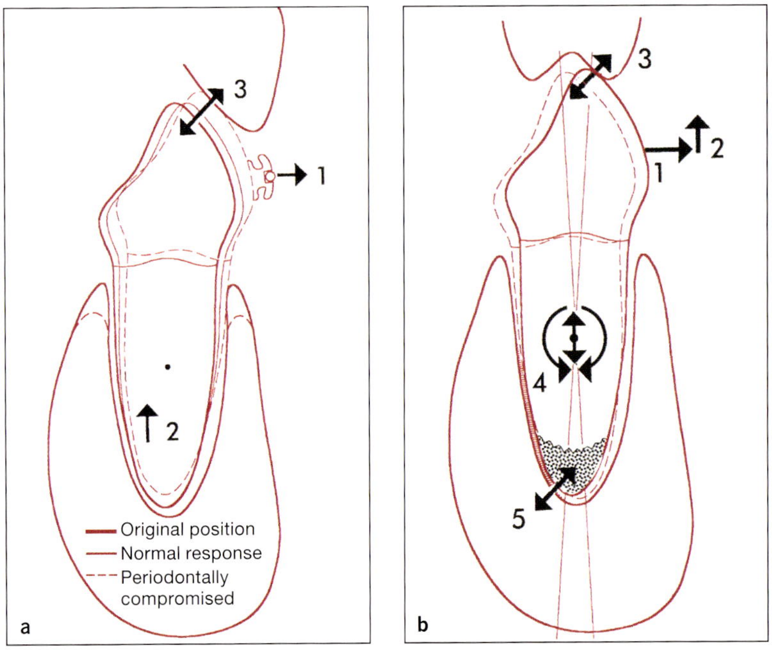

Fig 3-18 *(a)* A moderate load in the buccal direction results in tipping displacement of the crown (1). In the absence of vertical constraint, a normal healthy tooth would be expected to extrude slightly because of the inclined plane effect of the root engaging the tapered alveolus (2). As a result of diminished bone support and destruction of restraining collagen fibers at the alveolar crest, a periodontally compromised tooth may tip and extrude considerably more. Depending on the occlusion, this displacement may cause an occlusal prematurity (3). *(b)* Orthodontic tipping (1) with an extrusive component (2) may produce an occlusal prematurity (3) and mobility (4). An individual tooth in chronic occlusal trauma is expected to fatigue the root apex continuously. This combination of physical failure in a catabolic environment may lead to progressive root resorption (5).

From a dental perspective, occlusal prematurities or parafunction may lead to compromise of periodontal bone support. Localized fatigue failure may be a factor in periodontal clefting, alveolar recession, tooth ablation (cervical ditching), or temporomandibular joint arthrosis. Guarding against occlusal prematurities and excessive tooth mobility, while achieving an optimal distribution of occlusal loads, is an important objective for dental treatment. The human masticatory apparatus can achieve a biting strength of more than 2,200 N, or more than 500 lbs of force.[91,92] Because of the high magnitude and frequency of oral loads, functional prematurities used during dental or orthodontic treatment could contribute to isolated incidences of alveolar clefting (Fig 3-18a) and root resorption (Fig 3-18b). Excessive tooth mobility should be monitored carefully during dental treatment. Prevention of occlusal prematurities is a particular concern in treating periodontally compromised teeth.

Remodeling/Repair of Root

Remodeling is the physiologic term for internal turnover of a mineralized tissue without a change in its overall form. Pioneer histologic studies by Dr Kaare Reitan have demonstrated that root resorption cavities are usually repaired (filled) with secondary cementum. In effect, this is "repair" of the root of a tooth. This cementum repair is very similar but not identical to remodeling of trabecular bone. The similarities between bone remodeling and root resorption are striking: Kimura and coworkers[93] concluded that the "odontoclasts" of root resorption have an intravascular origin similar to the osteoclasts of bone remodeling. Considering all available evidence, it appears that root resorption is a portion of the turnover process to replace damaged root structure. Continuous forces, particularly if they are associated with traumatic occlusion, may result in permanent loss of root structure[18] if multiple sites of root resorption communicate before the initiation of their respective cementum repair phases.

Osteoblast Histogenesis and Bone Formation

Osteoblasts are derived from paravascular connective tissue cells (Fig 3-19). The less differentiated precursor and committed osteoprogenitor cells are associated closely with blood vessels. Their progeny (preosteoblasts) migrate away from the blood vessels. The major rate-limiting step in the histogenesis sequence occurs as the cells move through an area of low cell density about 30 mm from the nearest blood vessel.[95] The osteoblast histogenesis sequence (Fig 3-20) was determined by in situ morphologic assessment of three distinct events in cell physiology: *(1)* DNA S phase, *(2)* mitosis, and *(3)* the increase in nuclear volume (A′ → C shift) that accomplishes differentiation to a preosteoblast.[97]

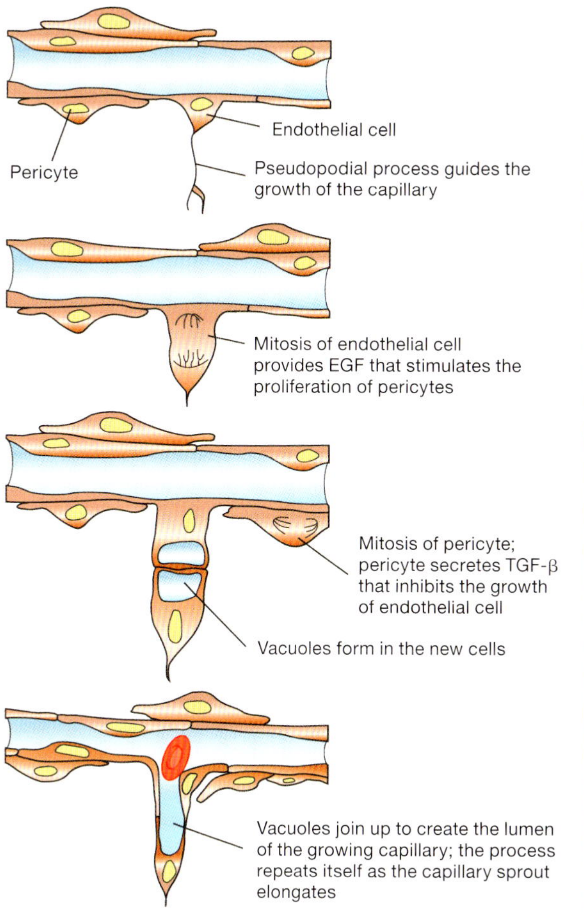

Fig 3-19 Angiogenesis involves a well-defined sequence of capillary budding followed by an extension of the perivascular network of pericytes, which are the source of osteoprogenitor cells. EGF, epidermal growth factor; TGF-β, transforming growth factor β. (Redrawn after Chang et al.[94])

Careful cell kinetic analysis of mechanically induced osteogenesis[51] demonstrated that the initial mechanically mediated step in osteoblast histogenesis is the differentiation of preosteoblasts from less differentiated precursor cells (Fig 3-21). Subsequent studies further classified the less differentiated precursor cells into committed osteoprogenitor (A′) cells and self-perpetuating precursor (A) cells.[96] The morphologic marker for this key step in osteoblast differentiation (change in genomic expression) is an increase in nuclear volume—preosteoblasts have larger nuclei than their precursors.

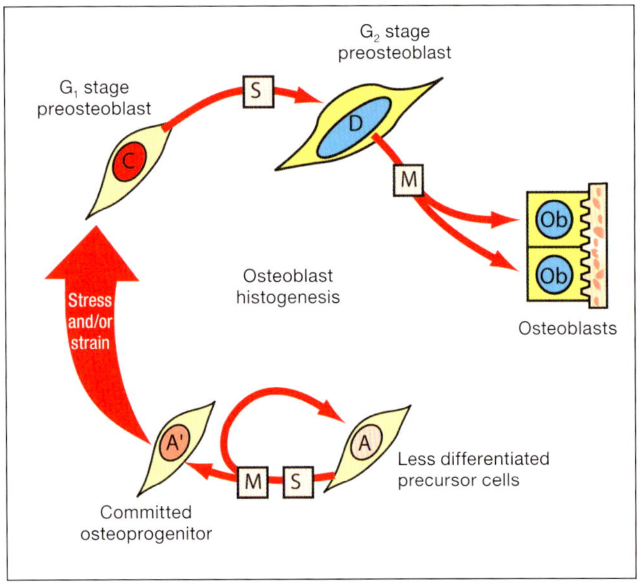

Fig 3-20 Frequency distribution of nuclear volume for fibroblast-like cells in unstimulated rat periodontal ligament. A, A', C, and D cells are a morphologic classification based on peaks in the distribution curve. The osteoblast histogenesis sequence is a progression of five morphologically and kinetically distinguishable cells. The process involves two DNA S phases and two mitotic (M) events. (Redrawn after Roberts and Morey[96] with permission.)

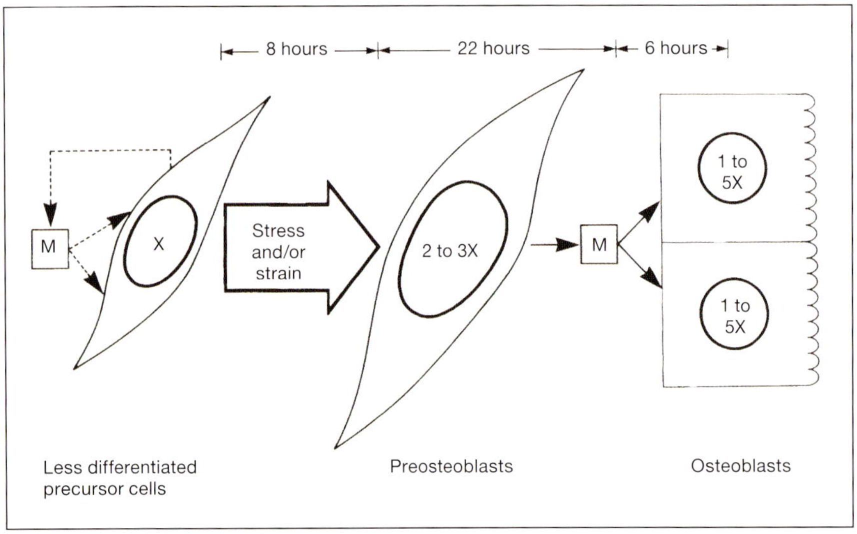

Fig 3-21 Differentiation of less differentiated precursor cells to preosteoblasts involves an increase in nuclear volume mediated by stress, strain, or both. The increase in nuclear size is a morphologic manifestation of change in genomic expression (differentiation). (Reprinted from Roberts et al[51] with permission.)

Osteoclast Recruitment and Bone Resorption

The osteoclast resorption rate is largely controlled by metabolic factors, particularly PTH.[98,99] No direct evidence exists to suggest that osteoclasts are produced in the periodontal ligament (PDL) or at any other bone surface. Preosteoclasts derived from the marrow enter the PDL and adjacent bone through the blood circulation.[52,100,101]

Roberts and Ferguson[52] compared the cell kinetics of metabolic and mechanical induction of PDL resorption. As shown in Fig 3-22, the number of osteoclasts per millimeter of bone surface is maximal about 9 hours after a single injection of parathyroid extract. Mechanical stimulation produces a slow but more sustained response that requires almost 50 hours to reach the same osteoclast density.

Because osteoclasts originate in the marrow, production of osteoclast precursor cells is under systemic (metabolic) and local (hematopoietic) control. The reservoir of circulating osteoclast precursors is controlled systemically. However, the localization of resorptive sites in the PDL is regulated mechanically. Metabolic stimuli such as PTH produce a relatively nonspecific resorption response along previously resorbing surfaces.[102] Mechanical induction is a specific response that occurs only in the direction of tooth movement. The current challenge is to understand the mechanical and biologic components of the resorptive mechanism.

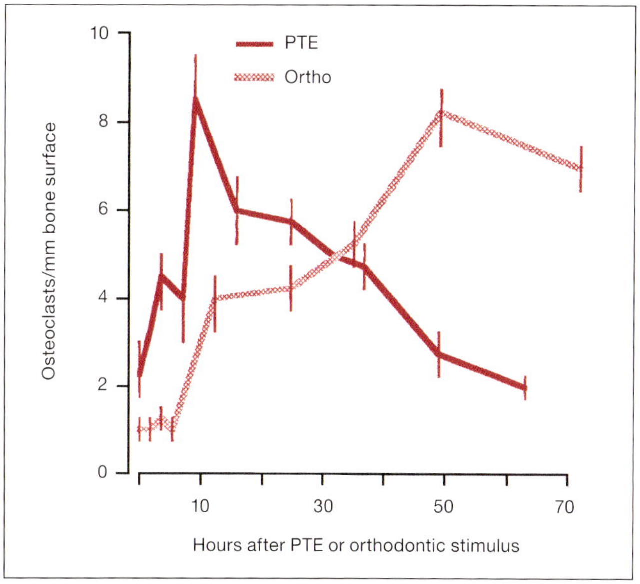

Fig 3-22 Metabolic (parathyroid extract [PTE]) versus mechanical stimulation of PDL osteoclastic activity. (Reprinted from Roberts and Ferguson[52] with permission.)

Because osteoblasts and their precursors have a more complete complement of bone-related receptors (ie, PTH, growth hormone, and estrogen), they may play a role in controlling osteoclasts.[52,103,104] The intricate bone modeling and remodeling responses require close coordination of osteoblastic and osteoclastic function.[105]

Bone and Wound Healing in Endodontics—Application of Principles of Bone Physiology

The principles of bone biology outlined earlier in the chapter can be directly applied to understanding osseous healing after periradicular surgery. There are vast similarities between the healing after endodontic surgeries and the healing after other corticotomies and osteotomies that are performed for other purposes such as orthognathic surgery, implant placement, or distraction osteogenesis, because the fundamental process of bone healing is very similar. In addition, the healing in the periradicular region is also similar to that produced by a critical size defect,[106] which is a frequent model to study enhanced materials, drugs, and strategies to promote healing in large bony defects.

Wound healing after periradicular surgery has primarily been studied in canine or monkey models because the bone physiology and healing of these animals is very similar to that which occurs in humans. Both models possess secondary osteonal bone remodeling, which was described earlier in this chapter. In addition, the bone modeling response to repair is well demonstrated in these animal models. There are advantages and limitations of each animal model; however, the three Rs (replacement, reduction, refinement) are critical for any ethical animal research.[107]

The healing response for an osseous excisional wound has been described in a primate and canine model with[108] and without[109] root resection (Fig 3-23a). The defects are initially filled with a coagulum consisting of disorganized fibrin, which is then replaced by granulation tissue. The granulation tissue consists of an extracellular matrix generated by fibroblasts, immune cells such as neutrophils, and macrophages. Abundant vascularization is key in active bone-formation areas (Fig 3-23b). At the remaining cortical and trabecular bone edges, osteocytes forming a thin layer are devoid of nuclei, suggesting that the bone beneath the surface has been damaged; this is typically seen as a deeply stained "basophilic" area. This deeply stained area is likely the exposed mineralized matrix that is absorbing the histologic stain and has accumulated some diffuse damage at the ultrastructural level.[27,110]

At a tissue level, in both cortical and trabecular bone, microdamage,[26] best seen as linear cracks within the bone, is a known stimulus for bone remodeling to occur through a process described earlier in the chapter. At the bone fronts on the endosteal surfaces, growth of trabecular bone takes place from the periphery to the center of the excisional wound. Here pericytes from the endothelium of the blood vessels, undifferentiated mesenchymal cells, and fibroblast-like cells differentiate into osteoblasts and form small islands of bone. These islands then enlarge and include metabolically active osteocytes (see Fig 3-23b) in new islands of woven bone. These woven bone surfaces can be lined by active osteoblasts that are laying osteoid—the unmineralized matrix deposited by

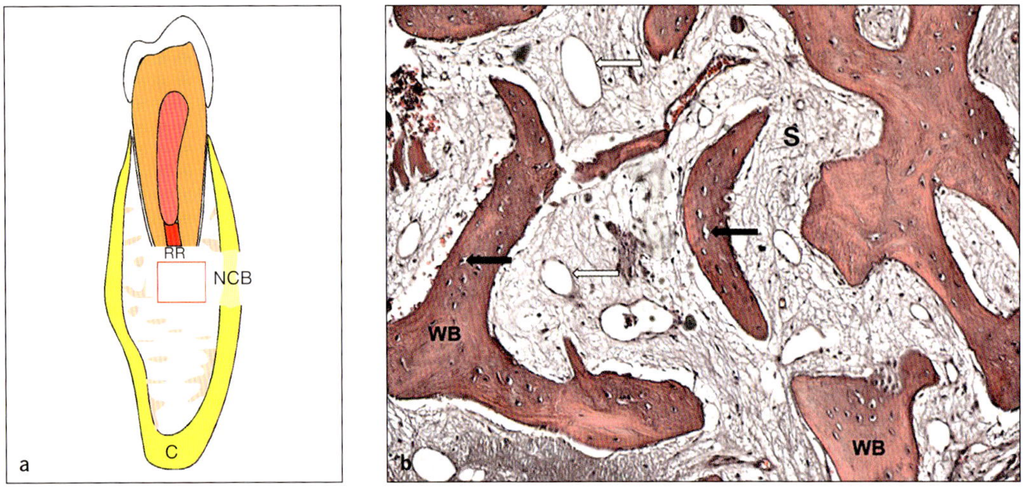

Fig 3-23 *(a)* Schematic of bone healing after periradicular surgery on a mandibular premolar. RR, resected root; C, cortical bone; NCB, new cortical bone forming at the site of access from the buccal plate. *(b)* Inset of part a *(red box)*. Histologic events of bone healing in bone within the marrow cavity of the mandible. This cavity is highly vascularized *(white arrows)* and contains a dense connective tissue stroma (S) composed of fibroblasts, mesenchymal cells, and blood vessels, which give rise to pericytes that differentiate into osteoblasts. The new woven bone (WB) islands have densely stained and large osteocytes *(black arrows)*.

the osteoblasts that will later be mineralized. Eventually, the woven bone will undergo lamellar compaction and be remodeled into lamellar trabecular bone.

On the cortical bone fronts, bone formation will take place by apposition on the surfaces and by secondary osteonal remodeling within the substance of the bone, by processes described earlier in this chapter. The woven bone will grow toward the connective tissue underlying the mucoperiosteum at the site of surgical access. The entire bone healing process takes approximately 3 to 4 months at a tissue level. Beyond that, trabecular bone remodels at a rate of 20% to 30% per year. Thus, it is anticipated that the newly formed bone will be remodeled and revitalized every 2 to 3 years.

In an excisional wound, the buccal bone is removed by disease or by intent. There is extensive orthopedic literature of bone healing[45,46] such as that which occurs at the monocortical buccal plate. The repair across a corticotomy or osteotomy site has been described to be akin to a fracture healing process. However, because significant micromotion does not exist, the typical callus to stabilize the discontinuous segment does not form, nor does a cartilaginous intermediate template as in long bones. Bone formation de novo occurs at the site of injury. The bone between the ends of the cut cortical bone plate is filled in below the periosteum, and the facial/buccal surface is restored. It will also eventually be remodeled by intracortical osteonal remodeling. At the resected end of the root, cementum will be laid down by apposition, and the PDL will reestablish at the apical end of the root.

During the surgical procedure, the diseased tissues are removed by rotary instruments. Depending on the type of instrument used, its sharpness, and the use of coolant, bone damage can be minimized. It is desirable to limit the amount of necrosis and damage to the bone and its osteocytes. Should a large area of necrosis exist, osteoclasts will have to resorb bone prior to formation of new bone. It has been shown that direct bone apposition can occur over a thin layer of altered "basophilic" bone during the reparative process.

In summary, by understanding bone remodeling, modeling, and the process of bone healing and adaptation, periapical osseous healing can be appreciated as a specialized regeneration of localized tissues.

Summary

Bone physiologic, metabolic, and cell kinetic concepts have important clinical applications. The application of fundamental concepts is limited only by the knowledge and imagination of the clinician. Modern clinical practice is characterized by a continual evolution of methods based on fundamental and applied research.

Acknowledgments

WER was supported by the National Institute of Dental Research (National Institutes of Health [NIH]) grants DE09237 and DE09822), NASA-Ames grants NCC 2-594 and NAG 2-756, and private donors through Indiana University Foundation. The author gratefully acknowledges the assistance of faculty and staff members at the University of the Pacific School of Dentistry and Indiana University School of Dentistry. SSH was supported by the American Association of Orthodontists Foundation, NIH R03, Delta Dental, and funds from the Ohio State University and University of Kentucky.

References

1. Roberts WE, Arbuckle GR, Simmons KE. What are the risk factors of osteoporosis? Assessing bone health. J Am Dent Assoc 1991;122:59–61.
2. Atkinson SR. Balance: The magic word. Am J Orthod 1964;50:189.
3. Hylander WL. Mandibular function in *Galago crassicaudatus* and *Macaca fascicularis:* An in vivo approach to stress analysis of the mandible. J Morphol 1979; 159:253–296.
4. Hylander WL. Patterns of stress and strain in the macaque mandible. In: Carlson DS (ed). Craniofacial Biology. Ann Arbor, MI: University of Michigan, 1981:1–37.
5. Roberts WE, Turley PK, Brezniak N, Fielder PJ. Implants: Bone physiology and metabolism. J Calif Dent Assoc 1987;15:54–61.
6. Roberts WE, Chase DC. Kinetics of cell proliferation and migration associated with orthodontically-induced osteogenesis. J Dent Res 1981;60:174–181.
7. Keeting PE, Scott RE, Colvard DS, Han IK, Spelsberg TC, Riggs BL. Lack of a direct effect of estrogen on proliferation and differentiation of normal human osteoblast-like cells. J Bone Miner Res 1991;6:297–304.
8. Roberts WE, Garetto LP, Katona TR. Principles of orthodontic biomechanics: Metabolic and mechanical control mechanisms. In: Carlson DS, Goldstein SA (eds). Bone Biodynamics in Orthodontic and Orthopaedic Treatment. Ann Arbor: University of Michigan, 1992:189–256.
9. Currey J. The Mechanical Adaptations of Bone. Princeton, NJ: Princeton University, 1984:80–87.
10. Martin RB, Burr DB. Structure, Function and Adaptation of Compact Bone. New York: Raven, 1989.
11. Roberts WE, Garetto LP, Simmons KE. Endosseous implants for rigid orthodontic anchorage. In: Bell WH (ed). Surgical Correction of Dentofacial Deformaties. Philadelphia: Saunders, 1992.
12. Roberts WE. Bone tissue interface. J Dent Educ 1988;52:804–809.
13. Enlow DH. Facial Growth. Philadelphia: Saunders, 1990.
14. Roberts WE, Smith RK, Zilberman Y, Mozsary PG, Smith RS. Osseous adaptation to continuous loading of rigid endosseous implants. Am J Orthod 1984;86:95–111.
15. Drinkwater BL, Nilson K, Chesnut CH 3rd, Bremner WJ, Shainholtz S, Southworth MB. Bone mineral content of amenorrheic and eumenorrheic athletes. N Engl J Med 1984;311:277–281.
16. Colditz GA, Stampfer MJ, Willett WC, Hennekens CH, Rosner B, Speizer FE. Prospective study of estrogen replacement therapy and risk of breast cancer in postmenopausal women. JAMA 1990;264:2648–2653.
17. Roberts WE, Roberts JA, Epker BN, Burr DB, Harsfield JK. Remodeling of mineralized tissues, part I: The Frost legacy. Semin Orthod 2006;12:216–237.
18. Roberts WE. Bone physiology, metabolism, and biomechanics in orthodontic practice. In: Graber TM, Vanarsdall RL Jr, Vig KWL (eds). Orthodontics: Current Principles and Techniques, ed 5. St Louis: Mosby, 2012:287–343.
19. Martin RB, Burr DB, Sharkey NA. Skeletal Tissue Mechanics. New York: Springer, 1998.
20. Parfitt AM. Osteonal and hemi-osteonal remodeling: the spatial and temporal framework for signal traffic in adult human bone. J Cell Biochem 1994;55:273–286.
21. Robling AG, Castillo AB, Turner CH. Biomechanical and molecular regulation of bone remodeling. Annu Rev Biomed Eng 2006;8:455–498.
22. Huja SS. Are we any closer to understanding the mechanisms of expedited tooth movement? In: Kapila SD, Nervina J, Hatch N (eds). Expedited Orthodontics: Improving the Efficiency of Orthodontic Treatment Through Novel Technologies, vol 51, Craniofacial Growth Series. Ann Arbor: University of Michigan, 2015:47–64.
23. Parfitt AM. Targeted and nontargeted bone remodeling: Relationship to basic multicellular unit origination and progression. Bone 2002;30:5–7.
24. Midgett RJ, Shaye R, Fruge JF Jr. The effect of altered bone metabolism on orthodontic tooth movement. Am J Orthod 1981;80:256–262.
25. Shank SB, Beck FM, D'Atri AM, Huja SS. Bone damage associated with orthodontic placement of miniscrew implants in an animal model. Am J Orthod Dentofacial Orthop 2012;141:412–418.
26. Burr DB, Martin RB, Schaffler MB, Radin EL. Bone remodeling in response to in vivo fatigue microdamage. J Biomech 1985;18:189–200.
27. Huja SS, Hasan MS, Pidaparti R, Turner CH, Garetto LP, Burr DB. Development of a fluorescent light technique for evaluating microdamage in bone subjected to fatigue loading. J Biomech 1999;32:1243–1249.
28. Parfitt AM, Drezner MK, Glorieux FH, et al. Bone histomoprhometry: Standardization of nomenclature, symbols, and units. Report of the ASBMR Histomorphometry Nomenclature Committee. J Bone Min Res 1987;2:595–610.
29. Parfitt AM. The physiologic and clinical significance of bone histomorphometric data. In: Recker RR (ed). Bone Histomorphometry: Techniques and Interpretation. Boca Raton, FL: CRC, 1983:143–223.
30. Jones HH, Priest JD, Hayes WC, Tichenor CC, Nagel DA. Humeral hypertrophy in response to exercise. J Bone Joint Surg Am 1977;59:204–208.
31. Frost HM. Wolff's law and bone's structural adapatation to mechanical usage: An overview for clinicians. Angle Orthod 1994;64:175–188.
32. Roberts WE, Marshall KJ, Mozsary PG. Rigid endosseous implant utilized as anchorage to protract molars and close an atrophic extraction site. Angle Orthod 1990;60:135–152.
33. Mundy GR, Bonewald LF. Transforming grwoth factor beta. In: Gowen M (ed). Cytokines and Bone Metabolism. Boca Raton, FL: CRC, 1992:93–107.
34. Boyle WJ, Simonet WS, Lacey DL. Osteoclast differentiation and activation. Nature 2003;423:337–342.
35. Amizuka N, Shimomura J, Li M, et al. Defective bone remodelling in osteoprotegerin-deficient mice. J Electron Microsc (Tokyo) 2003;52:503-513.
36. Roberts WE, Helm FR, Marshall KJ, Gongloff RK. Rigid endosseous implants for orthodontic and orthopedic anchorage. Angle Orthod 1989;59:247–256.
37. Brockstedt H, Bollerslev J, Melsen F, Mosekilde L. Cortical bone remodeling in autosomal dominant osteopetrosis: A study of two different phenotypes. Bone 1996;18:67–72.
38. Frost HM. The regional acceleratory phenomenon: A review. Henry Ford Hosp Med J 1983;31:3–9.
39. Roberts WE, Garetto LP. Physiology of osseous and fibrous integration. Alpha Omegan 1992;85(4):57–60.
40. Jeffcoat MK, Williams RC, Kaplan ML, Goldhaber P. Nuclear medicine techniques for the detection of active alveolar bone loss. Adv Dent Res 1987;1:80–84.
41. Reddy MS, English R, Jeffcoat MK, Tumeh SS, Williams RC. Detection of periodontal disease activity with a scintillation camera. J Dent Res 1991;70:50–54.
42. Tricker ND, Dixon RB, Garetto LP. Cortical bone turnover and mineral apposition in dentate bone mandible. In: Garetto LP, Turner CH, Duncan RL, Burr DB (eds). Bridging the Gap Between Dental and Orthopaedic Implants. Indianapolis: Indiana University School of Dentistry, 2002:226–227.
43. Huja SS, Fernandez SA, Hill KJ, Li Y. Remodeling dynamics in the alveolar process in skeletally mature dogs. Anat Rec A Discov Mol Cell Evol Biol 2006;288:1243–1249.
44. Garetto LP, Tricker ND. Remodeling of bone surrounding at the implant interface. In: Garetto LP, Turner CH, Duncan RL, Burr DB (eds). Bridging the Gap Between Dental and Orthopaedic Implants. Indianapolis, IN: School of Dentistry, Indiana University, 2002:89–100.
45. Mueller M, Schilling T, Minne HW, Ziegler R. A systemic acceleratory phenomenon (SAP) accompanies the regional acceleratory phenomenon (RAP) during healing of a bone defect in the rat. J Bone Miner Res 1991;6:401–410.
46. Bogoch E, Gschwend N, Rahn B, Moran E, Perren S. Healing of cancellous bone osteotomy in rabbits—Part I: Regulation of bone volume and the regional acceleratory phenomenon in normal bone. J Orthop Res 1993;11:285–291.
47. Roberts WE, Garetto LP, Arbuckle GR, Simmons KE, DeCastro RA. What are the risk factors of osteoporosis? Assessing bone health. J Am Dent Assoc 1991; 122:59–61.
48. Roberts WE. Advanced techniques for quantitative bone cell kinetics and cell population dynamics. In: Jaworski ZFG (ed). Proceedings of the First Workshop on Bone Morphometry [28–31 March 1973, Ottawa, ON, Canada]. Ottawa: University of Ottawa, 1976:310–314.
49. Roberts WE, Chase DC, Jee SS. Counts of labelled mitoses in the orthodontically-stimulated periodontal ligament in the rat. Arch Oral Biol 1974;19:665–670.
50. Roberts WE, Jee WS. Cell kinetics of orthodontically-stimulated and non-stimulated periodontal ligament in the rat. Arch Oral Biol 1974;19:17–21.
51. Roberts WE, Mozsary PG, Klingler E. Nuclear size as a cell-kinetic marker for osteoblast differentiation. Am J Anat 1982;165:373–384.
52. Roberts WE, Ferguson DJ. Cell kinetics of the periodontal ligament. In: Norton LA, Burstone CJ (eds). The Biology of Tooth Movement. Boca Raton, FL: CRC, 1989: 56–67.
53. Katona TR, Paydar NH, Akay HU, Roberts WE. Stress analysis of bone modeling response to rat molar orthodontics. J Biomech 1995;28:27–38.
54. Rapperport DJ, Carter DR, Schurman DJ. Contact finite element stress analysis of porous ingrowth acetabular cup implantation, ingrowth, and loosening. J Orthop Res 1987;5:548–561.

55. Siegele D, Soltesz U. Numerical investigations of the influence of implant shape on stress distribution in the jaw bone. Int J Oral Maxillofac Implants 1989;4:333–340.
56. Huja SS, Roberts WE. Mechanism of osseointegration: Characterization of supporting bone with indentation testing and backscattered imaging. Semin Orthod 2004;10:162–173.
57. Yip G, Schneider P, Roberts WE. Micro-computed tomography: High resolution imaging of bone and implants in three dimensions. Semin Orthod 2004;10:174–187.
58. Huja SS, Katona TR, Moore BK, Roberts WE. Microhardness and anisotropy of the vital osseous interface and endosseous implant supporting bone. J Orthop Res 1998;16:54–60.
59. Huja SS, Hay JL, Rummel AM, Beck FM. Quasi-static and harmonic indentation of osteonal bone. J Dent Biomech 2010:736830.
60. Huja SS, Katona TR, Roberts WE. Microhardness testing of bone. In: An YH, Draughn RA (eds). Mechanical Testing of Bone and the Bone-Implant Interface. Boca Raton, FL: CRC, 2000:247–256.
61. Huja SS, Phillips CA, Fernandez SA, Li Y. Tissue level mechanical properties of cortical bone in skeletally immature and mature dogs. Vet Comp Orthop Traumatol 2009;22:210–215.
62. Roberts WE, Simmons KE, Garetto LP, DeCastro RA. Bone physiology and metabolism in dental implantology: Risk factors for osteoporosis and other metabolic bone diseases. Implant Dent 1992;1:11–21.
63. Midgett RJ, Shaye R, Fruge JF Jr. The effect of altered bone metabolism on orthodontic tooth movement. Am J Orthod 1981;80:256–262.
64. Rhodes WE, Pflanzer R. Human Physiology. Philadelphia: WB Saunders, 1989.
65. Frost HM. Bone Remodeling and Its Relationship to Metabolic Bone Diseases. Springfield, IL: Charles C Thomas, 1973.
66. Heaney RP. Estrogen-calcium interactions in the postmenopause: A quantitative description. Bone Miner 1990;11:67–84.
67. Rigotti NA, Neer RM, Skates SJ, Herzog DB, Nussbaum SR. The clinical course of osteoporosis in anorexia nervosa. A longitudinal study of cortical bone mass. JAMA 1991;265:1133–1138.
68. Consensus conference report on osteoporosis. J Am Dent Assoc 1984:254–799.
69. Eriksen EF, Mosekilde L. Estrogens and bone. In: Heersche JNM, Kanis JA (eds). Bone and Mineral Research, ed 7. New York: Elsevier, 1990:273–311.
70. Henrich JB. The postmenopausal estrogen/breast cancer controversy. JAMA 1992;268:1900–1902.
71. Love RR, Mazess RB, Barden HS, et al. Effects of tamoxifen on bone mineral density in postmenopausal women with breast cancer. N Engl J Med 1992; 326:852–856.
72. Heaney RP. Calcium, dairy products and osteoporosis. J Am Coll Nutr 2000;19(2 suppl):83S–99S.
73. Johnston CC Jr. Osteoporosis—Extent and cause of the disease. Proc Soc Exp Biol Med 1989;191:258–260.
74. Malluche H, Faugere MC. Renal bone disease 1990: An unmet challenge for the nephrologist. Kidney Int 1990;38:193–211.
75. Calciolari E, Donos N, Park JC, Petrie A, Mardas N. A systematic review on the correlation between skeletal and jawbone mineral density in osteoporotic subjects. Clin Oral Implants Res 2016;27:433–442.
76. Becker AR, Handick KE, Roberts WE, Garetto LP. Osteoporosis risk factors in female dental patients. A preliminary report. Ind Dent Assoc J 1997;76:15–19.
77. Khan AA, Morrison A, Hanley DA, et al; International Task Force on Osteonecrosis of the Jaw. Diagnosis and management of osteonecrosis of the jaw: A systematic review and international consensus. J Bone Miner Res 2015;30:3-23.
78. Helm NB, Padala S, Beck FM, D'Atri AM, Huja SS. Short-term zoledronic acid reduces trabecular bone remodeling in dogs. Eur J Oral Sci 2010;118:460–465.
79. Huja SS, Kaya B, Mo X, D'Atri AM, Fernandez SA. Effect of zoledronic acid on bone healing subsequent to mini-implant insertion. Angle Orthod 2011;81:363–369.
80. Roberts WE, Hartsfield JK Jr. Bone development and function: Genetic and environmental mechanisms. Semin Orthod 2004;10:100–122.
81. Cowin SC. Bone Mechanics. Boca Raton, Florida: CRC Press, 1989.
82. Riggs BL. Overview of osteoporosis. West J Med 1991;154:63–77.
83. Lanyon LE. Control of bone architecture by functional load bearing. J Bone Miner Res 1992;7(2, suppl):S369–S375.
84. Rubin CT, Lanyon LE. Regulation of bone mass by mechanical strain magnitude. Calcif Tissue Int 1985;37:411–417.
85. Rubin CT, Lanyon LE. Osteoregulatory nature of mechanical stimuli: Function as a determinant for adaptive remodeling in bone. J Orthop Res 1987;5:300–310.
86. Rubin CT, McLeod KJ, Bain SD. Functional strains and cortical bone adaptation: Epigenetic assurance of skeletal integrity. J Biomech 1990;23(suppl 1):43–54.
87. Frost HM. Skeletal structural adaptations to mechanical usage (SATMU): 2. Redefining Wolff's law: The remodeling problem. Anat Rec 1990;226:414–422.
88. Robling AG, Burr DB, Turner CH. Skeletal loading in animals. J Musculoskelet Neuronal Interact 2001;1:249–262.
89. Carter DR. Mechanical loading history and skeletal biology. J Biomech 1987;20: 1095–1109.
90. Frost HM. Intermediary Organization of the Skeleton. Boca Raton, FL: CRC, 1986.
91. Brunski JB. Forces on dental implants and interfacial stress transfer. In: Laney WR, Tolman DE (eds). Tissue Integration in Oral, Orthopedic, and Maxillofacial Reconstruction [Proceedings of the Second International Congress on Tissue Integration in Oral, Orthopedic, and Maxillofacial Reconstruction, 23–27 September 1990, Rochester, MN]. Chicago: Quintessence, 1992:108–124.
92. Brunski JB, Skalak R. Biomechanical considerations. In: Worthington P, Brånemark PI (eds). Advanced Osseointegration Surgery. Chicago: Quintessence, 1992.
93. Kimura R, Anan H, Matsumoto A, Noda D, Maeda K. Dental root resorption and repair: Histology and histometry during physiological drift of rat molars. J Periodontal Res 2003;38:525–532.
94. Chang HN, Garetto LP, Katona TR, Potter RH, Roberts WE. Angiogenic induction and cell migration in an orthopaedically expanded maxillary suture in the rat. Arch Oral Biol 1996;41:985–994.
95. Roberts WE, Wood HB, Chambers DW, Burk DT. Vascularly oriented differentiation gradient of osteoblast precursor cells in rat periodontal ligament: Implications for osteoblast histogenesis and periodontal bone loss. J Periodontal Res 1987; 22:461–467.
96. Roberts WE, Morey ER. Proliferation and differentiation sequence of osteoblast histogenesis under physiological conditions in rat periodontal ligament. Am J Anat 1985;174:105–118.
97. Deguchi T, Takano-Yamamoto T, Yabuuchi T, Ando R, Roberts WE, Garetto LP. Histomorphometric evaluation of alveolar bone turnover between the maxilla and the mandible during experimental tooth movement in dogs. Am J Orthod Dentofacial Orthop 2008;133:889–897.
98. Chambers TJ, McSheehy PM, Thomson BM, Fuller K. The effect of calcium-regulating hormones and prostaglandins on bone resorption by osteoclasts disaggregated from neonatal rabbit bones. Endocrinology 1985;116:234–239.
99. Holtrop ME, Raisz LG, Simmons HA. The effects of parathyroid hormone, colchicine, and calcitonin on the ultrastructure and the activity of osteoclasts in organ culture. J Cell Biol 1974;60:346–355.
100. Roberts WE. Cell population dynamics of periodontal ligament stimulated with parathyroid extract. Am J Anat 1975;143:363–370.
101. Roberts WE, Goodwin WC Jr, Heiner SR. Cellular response to orthodontic force. Dent Clin North Am 1981;25:3–17.
102. Roberts WE. Cell kinetic nature and diurnal periodicity of the rat periodontal ligament. Arch Oral Biol 1975;20:465–471.
103. Rodan GA, Martin TJ. Role of osteoblasts in hormonal control of bone resorption—A hypothesis. Calcif Tissue Int 1981;33:349–351.
104. Sims NA, Walsh NC. Intercellular cross-talk among bone cells: New factors and pathways. Curr Osteoporos Rep 2012;10:109–117.
105. Zhao N, Lin J, Kanzaki H, et al. Local osteoprotegerin gene transfer inhibits relapse of orthodontic tooth movement. Am J Orthod Dentofacial Orthop 2012; 141:30–40.
106. Cooper GM, Mooney MP, Gosain AK, Campbell PG, Losee JE, Huard J. Testing the critical size in calvarial bone defects: Revisiting the concept of a critical-size defect. Plast Reconstr Surg 2010;125:1685–1692.
107. Russell WMS, Burch RL. The Principles of Humane Experimental Technique. London: Methuen, 1959.
108. Corcoran JF, Sieraski SM, Ellison RL. Osseous healing kinetics after apicoectomy in monkeys: II. A quantitative histological appraisal. J Endod 1985;11:269–274.
109. Harrison JW, Jurosky KA. Wound healing in the tissues of the periodontium following periradicular surgery. III. The osseous excisional wound. J Endod 1992; 18:76–81.
110. Huja SS, Katona TR, Burr DB, Garetto LP, Roberts WE. Microdamage adjacent to endosseous implants subjected to bending fatigue loads. Bone 1999;25: 217–222.

Chapter Four

Radiolucent Periapical Pathosis

Nasser Said-Al-Naief

Although 300 bacterial colonies or more can be harbored in the oral cavity, only selective species are responsible for causing dental decay (dental caries) and periodontal disease, including *Streptococcus mutans*, *Atopobium*, *Propionibacterium*, *Lactobacillus*, and *Actinomyces*, among others.[1,2] If caries lesions are neglected and not appropriately managed, bacteria will enter and invade the dentinal tubules of the tooth, where metabolic byproducts and cell walls can trigger and propagate pulpal inflammation, ultimately causing pulpal necrosis.[3,4] The outcome of pulpal inflammation mostly depends on the invading microorganisms and host immune response.[5–8] The presence of impaired cellular immunity, coupled with byproducts generated from immune responses and immune complexes, would further propagate pulpal inflammation. *S mutans*, *Streptococcus sobrinus*, and *Lactobacillus* species, among others, play a significant role in the initiation and progression of caries.[9] These organisms are acidogenic and aciduric, capable of producing an acidic environment with enamel and dentin demineralization while maintaining a survival advantage.[10–14] Additionally, these organisms are capable of binding to type I collagen in dentin after intratubular invasion.[9,15–17] Compared with mild pulp trauma caused by abrasion, slow caries, or superficial filling procedures, where the pulp cells maintain healthy status, viability, and the capability of producing a layer of protective dentin, odontoblastic layer destruction is seen secondary to advanced caries, bacterial toxins, irritating restorative materials, necrotic cells, or enzymes generated secondary to extracellular matrix degradation.[17–19] Matrix metalloproteinases, generated after the demineralization of dentin, are also of significance in the advancement of dental caries.[17]

The presence of pain represents an initial sign of inflammation in the dental pulp, which can eventually lead to total pulp destruction and development of periapical pathology.[11,20–25] Pulpal pain is produced in response to bacterial infiltration and advancement through carious dentin, where the predominance of anaerobic bacteria and their significance in initiation of the inflammatory cascade are well documented.[26,27] Much attention has also been directed to the significance of the bacterial ecology, their interaction, and the synergistic or negative relationship with developing periapical disease of varying severity.[26] Endodontic infections can be separated into extraradicular or intraradicular, according to their anatomical location; intraradicular infections may be further divided into primary, secondary, or persistent infections, depending on the time participating microorganisms established themselves within the root canal.[26]

The composition of the microbiota may also vary depending on the different types of infection and different forms of apical periodontitis. Further, culture-independent molecular biology techniques have shed light on the recognition of several new pathogens and are considered to be a great asset to what has already been confirmed with culture-dependent studies, where several candidate endodontic pathogens were recognized.[28] Advanced culture and molecular biology techniques have highlighted the polymicrobial nature of endodontic infections, which would generally fall into nine phyla, namely Firmicutes, Bacteroidetes, Spirochaetes, Fusobacteria, Actinobacteria, Proteobacteria, Synergistetes, TM7, and SR1, as well as several other bacterial types that are yet to be categorized.[29] Gram-negative bacteria are beyond doubt considered to be the most common microorganisms implicated in primary endodontic infections, including *Dialister* (eg, *Dialister invisus* and *Dialister pneumosintes*), *Fusobacterium* (eg, *Fusobacterium nucleatum*), *Porphyromonas* (eg, *Porphyromonas endodontalis* and *Porphyromonas gingivalis*), *Prevotella* (eg, *Prevotella intermedia*, *Prevotella nigrescens*, *Prevotella baroniae*, and *Prevotella tannerae*), *Tannerella* (eg, *Tannerella forsythia*), and *Treponema* (eg, *Treponema denticola* and *Treponema socranskii*), but Gram-positive bacteria such as *Actinomyces* (eg, *Actinomyces israelii*), *Filifactor* (eg, *Filifactor alocis*), *Olsenella* (eg, *Olsenella uli*), *Parvimonas* (eg, *Parvinomas micra*), *Peptostreptococcus* (eg, *Peptostreptococcus anaerobius* and *Peptostreptococcus stomatis*), *Pseudoramibacter* (eg, *Pseudoramibacter alactolyticus*), *Streptococcus* (eg, *Streptococcus anginosus* group), and *Propionibacterium* (eg, *Propionibacterium propionicum* and *Propionibacterium acnes*) as well as several uncultivated species have been implicated.[26,28–30]

The periapical region represents the interface between the dentition and the body's defense system. An orchestrated and collective cascade of events that encompass invading microorganisms, host tissue response, and the biologic events that accompany both[31–34] contribute to propagation of pulpal inflammation and subsequent spread to the periradicular region.[19,27,35–38] Bacteria, predominantly anaerobic[27,38] and less commonly spirochetes, fungi, and viruses, the latter species predominantly encountered in immunocompromised patients, contributes to the development of periapical pathology in association with necrotic and diseased root canals.[39–42] Acid and bacterial byproducts are major factors in the initiation, propagation, and progression of pulpal inflammation and accompanying symptoms. Bacterial fermentations of carbohydrate and liberated organic acids, including lactic acid and propionic acid, may fail to excite alpha nerves and simultaneously reversibly suppress important impulses elicited by other stimuli, which may partially explain the lack of thermal sensitivity in teeth with deep caries and high *Lactobacilli* count.[43–45] Ammonia is probably the most important among the algegenic (pain producing) molecules, followed by urea and indole, which are liberated secondary to ammonia acid fermentation.[44] Lipoteichoic acid (LTA) is produced in large quantities by cariogenic bacteria in the presence of sucrose and accentuates pulpal inflammatory responses when released extracellularly by Gram-positive bacteria.[46,47] The allogeneic metabolites from anaerobic Gram-negative bacteria in deep caries could partially explain why *Bacteroides* spp, *P intermedia*, and the amount of lipopolysaccharide (LPS) in caries positively correlates to the presence of heat sensitivity or pain.[48,49] LPS activates the Hageman factor, leading to bradykinin production, a potent pain inducer.[49–51] LPS and lipoteichoic acid activate in a similar fashion on the immune system via binding to CD14, activating signaling by Toll-like receptors[52,53] and inducing proinflammatory cytokines such as tumor necrosis factor-α (TNF-α), interleukin-1 (IL-1), interleukin-8 (IL-8), interleukin-12 (IL-12), and anti-inflammatory cytokine interleukin-10 (IL-10).[9,54,55]

Classification of Periapical Lesions

Periapical pathosis has undergone many different classifications, some of which concentrated on the clinical features while others focused on the overall clinicopathologic and histomorphologic features. Nevertheless, none was comprehensive enough to include and account for structural aspects of periapical lesions.[35,36,56] An optimal classification of periapical pathosis would encompass the correlation between clinical and histomorphologic features. Nair,[56] for example, classified these lesions into acute apical periodontitis (primary or secondary), chronic apical periodontitis, apical abscess (acute and chronic subtypes), and periapical cyst, dividing the latter into true or pocket cysts based on the distribution and type of inflammatory cells present within the lesions, the identification or lack of epithelial cell lining, and whether the lesion had transformed into a cyst. He also took into consideration the relationship of the cystic cavity to the apical foramen of the root canal. The classification followed by the original World Health Organization[57] separated the lesions into acute or chronic periapical periodontitis, periapical abscess with sinus tract, periapical abscess without sinus tract, and radicular cysts.

Acknowledging the lack of correlation between histomorphologic features, clinical signs and symptoms, and duration of the lesion, Torabinejad and Shabahang[58] in 2014 simplified the classification of periapical lesions into six main groups: normal periapical tissues, symptomatic (acute) apical periodontitis, asymptomatic (chronic) apical periodontitis, acute and chronic apical abscess-

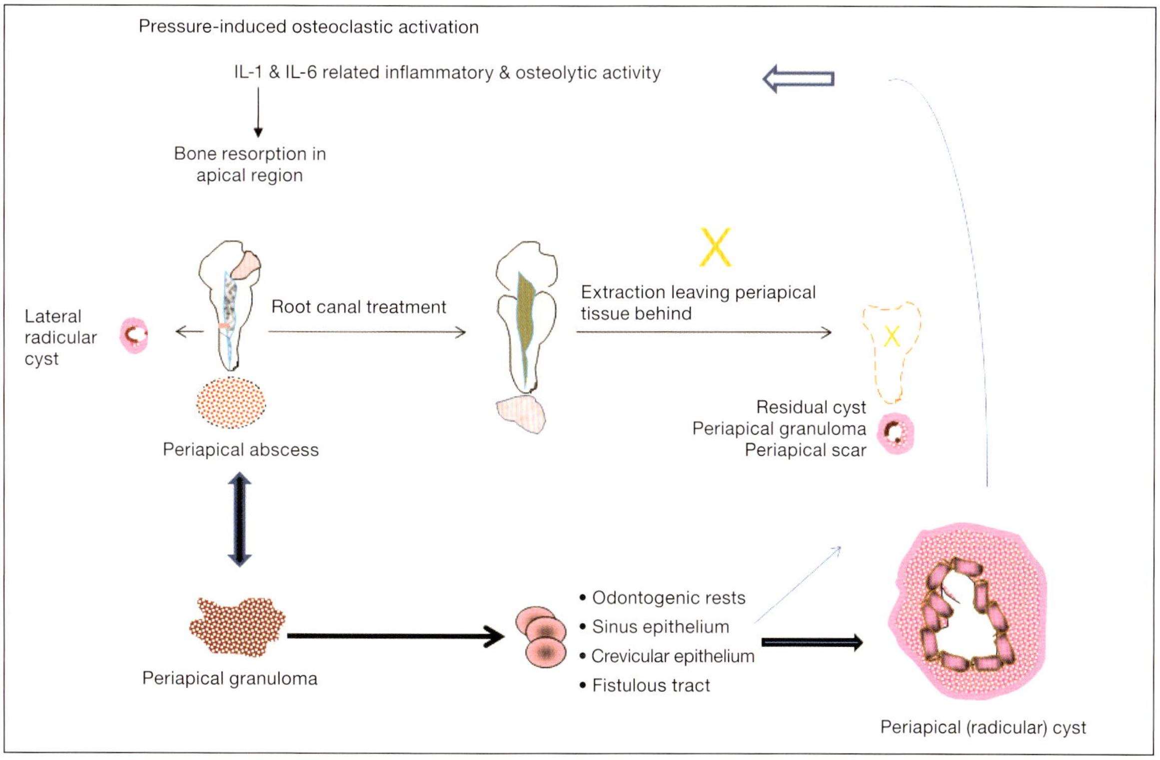

Fig 4-1 A summary of events leading to periapical pathology. The presence of deep caries that involves the pulp results in the formation of a periapical abscess, which will eventually be replaced by granulation tissue (periapical granuloma). The periapical granuloma may potentially revert back to abscess formation. Alternatively, the inflammation present in the periapical granuloma will stimulate the growth and proliferation of the epithelium from different sources to form the radicular cyst. The presence of a lateral pulpal canal facilitates dissemination of bacteria to the periodontal ligament (PDL) and stimulation of the proliferation of the epithelial rests with the PDL to form the lateral radicular cyst. The cyst increases in size due to several factors and is associated with pressure-induced osteoclastic activation as well as inflammatory mediator–related osteolytic activity, which will collectively result in resorption of the apical bone. The majority of the periapical radiolucencies that persist following root canal therapy represent periapical scars. Further, tissues that are left behind after extraction of the teeth may present residual cysts, periapical granuloma, and/or scars.

es, and condensing osteitis. Acute (symptomatic) lesions are associated with pain and swelling, whereas chronic (asymptomatic) lesions are associated with few or mild symptoms. In symptomatic apical periodontitis, the patient suffers from spontaneous pain and discomfort with sensitivity to pressure or percussion. The tooth is responsive to cold, heat, and electric testing. If and when the pulp is necrotic, it will respond positively (with pain) to percussion but negatively (no pain) to vitality testing. Histologic examination reveals a sea of neutrophils and macrophages supported by a liquefactive necrotic background (abscess). The identification of radiographic evidence of resorption would be minimal, if any, at this stage.[35,58,59]

In asymptomatic apical periodontitis, the pulp undergoes total necrosis and thus is nonresponsive to electric or thermal stimuli. Further, the tooth also shows little or no response to percussion. Histologically, examination of the periapical lesion shows periapical granulomas or cysts.[35,58,59]

There is considerable inconsistency regarding the incidence of various classes of endodontic-related lesions.[60] Variations may be due to the sampling methods and/or histologic criteria adopted in establishing the diagnosis. The majority of studies have shown that close to 60% of the practical pathologies represent granulomas, 22% represent cysts, and a lesser percentage (12%) reveal periapical scars.[58]

The classification adopted in this chapter is simplified into the following categories: acute and chronic periapical abscess (with potential fistulous tract formation), periapical granuloma, periapical cyst, and periapical scar (Fig 4-1). It also describes the distinction between those entities of pulpal origin and etiopathogenesis and those that are classified as periapical pathology mimickers, which lack any relationship to pulpal etiology and origin. In a recent review, Sullivan et al[61] reviewed a large series of periapical lesions and reported the overall incidence of periapical pathology of endodontic origin to be 97.2%, with the majority (60%) representing periapical granulomas, followed by radicular cysts (36.7%), periapical scars (0.27%), and periapical abscesses (0.23%). In another review of a large series,[62] the incidence of periapical granulomas and cysts was reported to be around 73%.

Periapical Pathosis of Pulpal Origin

Periapical abscess

The periapical abscess represents the initial accumulation of inflammation and bacteria in the apical region, secondary to advanced pulpal disease. Patients often present with tooth pain, purulent discharge, and potential accompanying fever and cervical lymphadenopathy. In the early abscess, radiographic examination may not be helpful prior to the first 10 days' occurrence.[63,64] Clinically, patients suffering from acute and chronic abscesses will experience pain with pressure, sensitivity to percussion, and extrusion of teeth from sockets without swelling of the surrounding tissue. Patients may also experience shivers, malaise, and difficulty chewing. Radiographically, thickening of the apical PDL with an ill-defined radiolucency may be seen at midstage of the disease; this is associated with significant apical bone resorption.

Acute periapical abscess

An acute periapical abscess is a localized liquefactive lesion that represents the direct extension of inflammatory changes from the pulp to the periradicular tissue, with subsequent destruction of that area. The pathogenesis of periapical abscesses is multifactorial.[65] Following infection of the root canal, bacteria may proceed to involve the periradicular tissue via the apical and/or lateral canals or secondary to root perforation. This will further proceed to acute or chronic periapical inflammation.[65,66] The potential of bacteria spreading to other anatomical sites and producing cellulitis is also a possibility.[67] Clinically, the tooth is characterized by spontaneous, rapid-onset pain with potential accompanying moderate to severe discomfort and pain, malaise, headaches, trismus, lymphadenopathy, and nausea.[65] The patient may also develop Ludwig's angina, which may contribute to life-threatening airway obstruction,[68–70] or cavernous sinus thrombosis, an even more dangerous life-threatening situation in which blood accumulates in the cavernous sinus secondary to pressure related to the spread of infection into the midfacial area and edema.[71,72] In extreme circumstances, a periapical abscess may lead to further and more serious complications, including brain abscess, septicemia, orbital abscess, and necrotizing fasciitis, among others.[65,73–81] Evidence of swelling may not be obvious in the beginning, especially when the infection is confined to the bone. Patients may also experience high temperature and leukocytosis. The tooth is typically negative for electric and thermal pulp tests, but it will be painful upon percussion and palpation. Early radiographic examination may not be impressive and reflects simple widening of the immediate periapical region, but occasionally well-defined radiolucencies in the epochal region are detected.[58]

The extravasation of neutrophils, which occurs as a result of the infiltration of microorganisms from the diseased pulp to the periapical region, is triggered by the process of chemotaxis, which is in turn related to tissue injury, bacterial products (lipopolysaccharides), as well as complement factor C.[31] Neutrophils act with a dual function: They neutralize microorganisms while releasing leukotrienes and prostaglandins as part of a defense mechanism. While the leukotrienes attract more neutrophils and macrophages into the area, the prostaglandins activate osteoclasts, leading to the resorption of bone in that region.[82] The process of resorption could be initially halted by the application of indomethacin[83,84] and inhibiting cyclooxygenase. The death of neutrophils leads to the release of enzymes and destruction of the extracellular matrix, which not only limits the amount of destruction to the localized area but also attracts the influx of additional inflammatory cells to combat this inflammatory cascade. Activated macrophages will also produce a variety of interleukins, including IL-1, IL-6, TNF-α, and IL-8 chemotactic factors. These cytokines intensify local angiogenesis and osteoclasts and therefore facilitate bone resorption and degradation of the extracellular matrices, among other functions,[58,84,85] thus suppressing prostaglandin synthesis.

The development and progression of acute periapical abscesses are multifactorial. Routine culture, polymerase chain reaction (PCR), and gene-sequencing studies[86–90] have collectively demonstrated, with variable sensitivity and specificity, several bacterial species including *Firmicutes* (eg, genera *Streptococcus*, *Dialister*, *Filifactor*, and *Pseudoramibacter*), *Bacteroidetes* (eg, genera *Porphyromonas*, *Prevotella*, and *Tannerella*), *Fusobacteria* (eg, genera *Fusobacterium* and *Leptotrichia*), *Actinobacteria* (eg, genera *Actinomyces* and *Propionibacterium*), *Spirochaetes* (eg, genus *Treponema*), *Synergistetes* (eg, genus *Pyramidobacter* and some as-yet-uncultivated phenotypes), and *Proteobacteria* (eg, genera *Campylobacter* and *Eikenella*). Regardless of the study and method of identification, *Firmicutes* and *Bacteroidetes* together contribute to more than 70% of the species found in periapical abscesses. Representatives of *Spirochaetes* and *Synergistetes* have been revealed only by culture-independent molecular methods. Diverse groups of Gram-negative and Gram-positive bacteria have been identified.[26–30,65]

The significance and relevance of host-related factors on the severity of the periapical pathology have also been studied with interest. Systemic conditions such as diabetes, herpes infection, stress, and autoimmune status, in addition to the genetic background (eg, genetic polymorphism) may also be relevant to the severity of the disease.[65,75,77,91] Ferreira et al[91] investigated the expres-

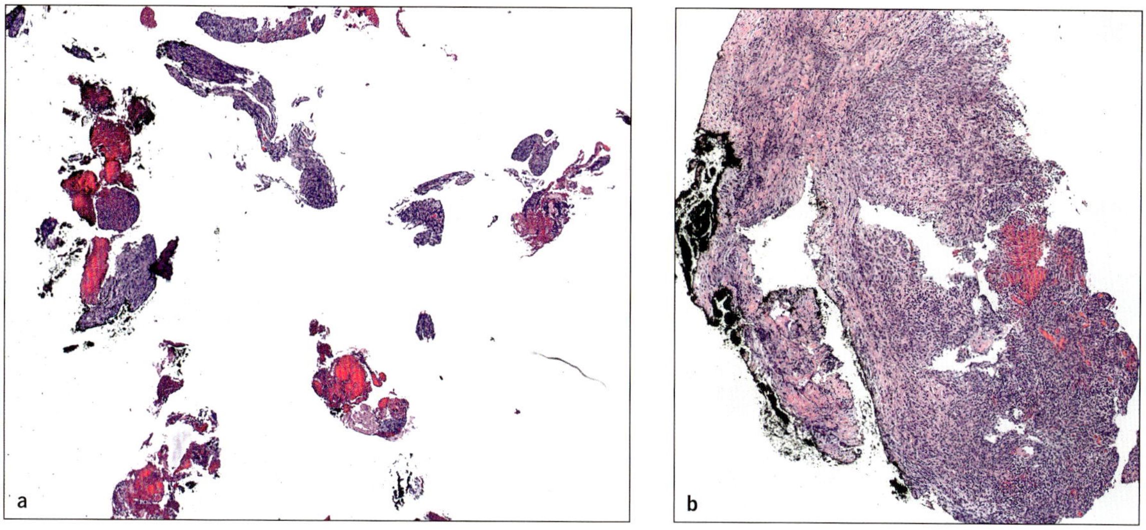

Fig 4-2 *(a)* Histomorphologic examination of an acute periapical abscess in a 15-year-old boy, curetted from the apical region of a symptomatic mandibular right first molar, which was painful to percussion and tested nonvital with thermal and electric pulp testing. *(b)* Higher-power photomicrograph showing dense inflammatory cell infiltrate admixed with hemorrhage (hematoxylin-eosin [h&e] stain; original magnification ×20).

sion of IL-17 in periapical abscesses and granulomas and demonstrated that abscesses, predominantly due to the rich neutrophilic components, showed higher expression of IL-17 than granulomas. They emphasized the role of the cytokine in the pathogenesis of the periapical lesions, especially in the acute stage of the process. IL-17α is a member of the IL-17 cytokine family, which is directly associated with the initiation and propagation of inflammatory stimuli in several diseases, including rheumatoid arthritis, psoriasis, and multiple sclerosis.[91,92] The main source of IL-17α in the abscesses and granulomas seems to be the $CD4^+$ cells. However, the levels of expression are lower in periapical granulomas than in abscesses, which may be explained by the higher percentage of $CD8^+$ cells, T lymphocytes, and neutrophils in abscesses compared with granulomas.[91,93–95]

Histologically, acute periapical abscesses are characterized by the presence of a dense, neutrophilic inflammatory cell infiltrate in a loose and edematous fibrocollagenous connective tissue background. Vascular ectasia is also commonly encountered, and lymphoplasmacytic and eosinophilic inflammatory cell components of variable intensity may also be present (Fig 4-2).

Management. With the goal of eliminating periapical pathosis, the management of acute apical abscesses involves incision for drainage accompanied by root canal treatment or extraction of the involved tooth to remove the source of infection.[96,97] Drainage may be achieved through the root canal or through incision and drainage. The latter is preferred if swelling is detected, because it would provide more rapid improvement in status.[97] Analgesics may help with the symptoms, and antibiotics may be prescribed based on an assessment of the patient's condition and the presence or absence of systemic involvement, including fever, lymphadenopathy, trismus, and/or cellulitis.[65] Penicillin is the first choice for treatment of endodontic infections, because most of the bacterial species involved with endodontic infections, including abscesses, are susceptible to it.[98–101] Amoxicillin is also often prescribed, because it offers a broader spectrum of antimicrobial coverage, may provide more rapid improvement with pain or swelling, and offers longer dosage intervals than penicillin.[102] Clindamycin may also offer equivocal results to penicillin with its strong antimicrobial activity against oral anaerobes.[101,103–105] The combination of early diagnosis and empirical antibiotic therapy with timely surgical intervention is probably a prerequisite to ensuring the successful management of complications of acute dental abscesses.[74]

Chronic periapical abscess and fistulous tract (gum boil)

This occurs as a sequela of healing events that take place in the acute periapical abscess, which is also initiated by direct extension from the inflamed necrotic pulp to the periapical region. The presence of microorganisms in conjunction with the metabolic products and enzymes liberated during the process of extension from pulpal to periapical areas together induce an immunologic response of cellular and humoral immunity, leading to a nonspecific reaction and further contributing to the etiopathogenesis of periapical disease. Lysozymes analyzed in chronic periapical lesions are thought to stimulate the effect of immunoglobulins and may play a specific protective role, affecting the local immunologic reactions in the periapical region.[106,107] Degraded proteins as well as cholesterol may act as antigens to elicit a host response, which can be harmful to periradicular tissues. The interaction of immunocompetent inflammatory cells identified in the periapical tissue with the host may also induce bone resorption. Polymorphonuclear leukocytes (PMNs) and macrophages together migrate to the periapical tissue and target quick phagocytosis of dead neutrophils by macrophages, which further propagate the chronic nature of the lesion. Recently, technical advancements in molecular biology have made it possible to discover the role of inflammatory mediators including antibodies, cytokines, matrix metalloproteinases, growth factors, and arachidonic metabolism to further understand the mechanism of the process. Both T and B lymphocytes play an essential role in the development and propagation of periapical disease, with the T-helper subset producing IL-2 and interferon-γ (IFN-γ) while T-suppressor cells secrete IL-5, IL-6, and IL-10, which regulate this production of antibodies by the plasma cells. B lymphocytes are responsible for antibody production and interact closely with the T-cell population in the process of transformation of B cells to plasma cells. Macrophages have an essential role and produce IL-1, TNF-α, interferon, and growth factors, which further contribute to periapical inflammatory changes.[31,106,108] Additionally, antigen-presenting cells play a crucial role in the polarization of T-helper cells and immune response toward Th1, Th2, Th17, or T-regulatory cells.[109,110]

The Th1 immune response, triggered by IFN-γ and postinflammatory cytokines including IL-1, IL-6, and TNF-α, among others, are involved in the progression of lesions and bone destruction. In comparison, immune-suppressive mechanisms mediated by transforming growth factor-β (TGF-β) and TH2 cytokines (IL-4, IL-5, IL-10) are responsible for the healing process and restriction of inflammatory/immune mechanisms.[111,112] Further, IL-17, which stimulates the production of IL-8, may also play an important role in exacerbating inflammatory changes in periapical lesions.[94] The Th17 immune response seems to play a dominant role in exacerbating inflammation and facilitating osteoclastic bone resorption and destruction of the periapical tissues.[113] Osteoclasts are derived from pro-osteoclasts, which migrate through the blood as monocytes to the periradicular tissues and attach to bone surfaces, where they remain dormant until signaled by osteoblasts to proliferate and cause resorption. The roles of proinflammatory cytokines (including IL-1, IL-6, and IL-8), TNF-α, IFN-γ, colony-stimulating factors, growth factors, and leukotrienes in the pathogenesis and advancement of periapical lesions have been well explained by many investigators.[114–119] Čolić et al[120] have described a positive correlation between the presence of PMNs and the high production of IL-17, which also correlates with the positive expression of IFN-γ. They also described the lack of a correlation with IL-23 production in symptomatic periapical lesions when compared with asymptomatic lesions, which were associated with a predominance of T and B cells, plasma cells, high levels of IFN-γ, high production of IL-12, and a marked presence of macrophages. In 1978, Torabinejad and Bakland[108] highlighted the multifactorial etiology of bone resorption in periapical pathogenesis and also reported that antigen-antibody complex– and immunoglobulin E–mediated reactions could well initiate the preliminary changes seen in the periapical tissues. Additionally, delayed hypersensitivity (ie, cell-mediated immunity) is likely to participate in the process, with significant contribution to the progression of these lesions.[108]

Histology. Inflammatory changes of varying degree, including the presence of neutrophils, lymphoplasmacytic inflammatory cell infiltrate, and a distinct population of histiocytes, are seen in the chronic periapical abscess. The abscess is mostly supported by granulation tissue with generalized acute and chronic inflammation, comprised of lymphoplasmacytic inflammatory cell infiltrate, reactive histiocytosis, a predominance of neutrophils, and plasma cells with a distinct population of Russell bodies (Fig 4-3).

Occasionally, submucosal and/or chronic apical abscess formation may produce symptomatic or asymptomatic gingival swelling that drains peripherally on the gingiva, producing the so-called *gum boil* (parulis, fistulous tract). Radiographic examination demonstrating periapical pathology, along with confirmation of nonvital tooth status, can indicate a parulis of odontogenic origin related to necrotic pulp from a periodontal abscess. Insertion of a gutta-percha point as well as radiographic imaging help to delineate the source of infection. This draining fistula actually represents a good prognostic sign, indicating a competent immune system attempting to eliminate disease status from necrotic pulp.[121,122]

When purulent exudate spreads through the medullary bone to perforate the cortical bone and discharges into the submucosa or subcutaneous soft tissue, localized swelling develops only intraorally. In other situations, acute apical abscesses may not only drain through the buccal or palatal bones into the oral cavity but may also occasionally drain into the maxillary sinus or the nasal cavity. Apical abscesses of mandibular teeth most probably would drain through the buccal or lingual bones into the oral cavity; however, the infectious process may also extend into fascial spaces of the head and neck, resulting in cellulitis and systemic signs and symptoms with more consequent complications.[123]

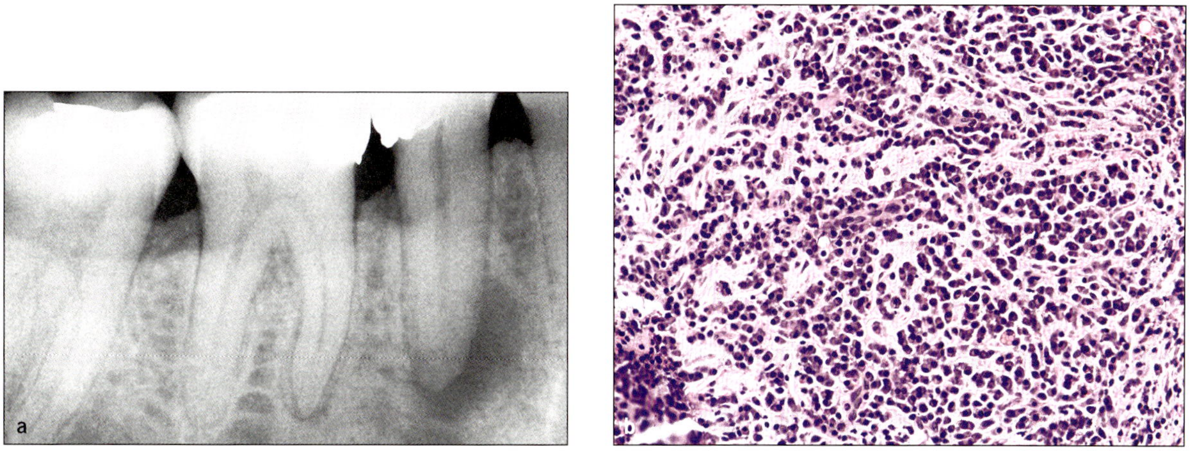

Fig 4-3 *(a)* Periapical radiograph of a chronic periapical abscess showing a well-demarcated radiolucency apical to the mandibular right second premolar, which is symptomatic to percussion and contains a deep amalgam filling. (Courtesy of Dr Lane Thompson, Loma Linda University.) *(b)* Histomorphologic examination reveals a dense mononuclear, predominantly plasmacytic inflammatory cell infiltrate (h&e stain; original magnification ×60).

Periapical granuloma

A periapical granuloma is composed of granulation tissue and arises either as a sequela of a periapical abscess or independently as an initial lesion. Although the term *granuloma* may be considered a misnomer here, since it typically describes a granulomatous type of inflammation (eg, sarcoidosis), using it within the context of periapical pathology is typical of describing the characteristic granulation tissue. Clinically, the initial phase of periapical inflammation is characterized by a dull, constantly throbbing toothache with associated negative or delayed vitality testing. The pain is typically exacerbated by biting or percussion pressure. There is virtually no radiographic evidence seen at this stage, but with progression of the chronic inflammation symptoms may diminish, and radiographic evidence becomes more evident and easily detected. Further, chronic disease may be occasionally detected in the absence of any acute phase of the disease. Radiographic examinations reveal the presence of variably sized, well-defined or ill-defined radiolucencies that may or may not be surrounded by a radiopaque rim. The reliability of radiographic patterns in distinguishing between periapical granuloma and periapical cysts has been questioned, but cone beam computed tomography may provide more accurate and reliable information in distinguishing between the two.[58,121,122]

Histomorphologic examinations of periapical granulomas demonstrate granulation tissue with acute and chronic inflammation, comprised of dense lymphoplasmacytic inflammatory cell infiltrate with a variably dense histiocytic component. Reactive lymphoplasmacytic inflammatory infiltrate with Russell bodies is commonly seen, and aggregates of neutrophils may also be observed. Odontogenic epithelial rests, representing remnants of rests of Malassez, are often observed. Cholesterol clefts with accompanying multinucleated foreign body–type giant reactions are also often present. Hemorrhage and hemosiderin are often encountered (Fig 4-4).

Periapical granulomas arise with a shift from predominantly neutrophilic inflammatory components to a more chronic inflammatory cell infiltrate characterized by a rich, macrophage-lymphoplasmacytic inflammatory cell infiltrate, supported by well-vascularized fibrocollagenous and granulation tissue background. IL-1, IL-6, and TNF-α derived from macrophages are powerful lymphocytic stimulators. Activated T cells also produce a variety of cytokines that downregulate the output of the aforementioned proinflammatory cytokines, which suppress osteoclastic activity and limit the extent of bone resorption. At the same time, T cell–derived cytokines may also instigate connective tissue overgrowth (TGF-β) and subsequent stimulation of the proliferative effect of fibroblasts and microvasculature,[31,82,106,108,124] which halts the process of bone destruction and bone remodeling during the chronic phase of the disease. However, this process may be a recurrent one if and when seepage of the microorganisms recurs from the infected pulp canal to the periapical region.[31] Approximately 45% of all periapical granulomas contain epithelial cells[31] derived from rests of Malassez remnants, with continuous antigen stimulation and coexisting inflammatory and immune responses. These remnants proliferate, leading to the formation of periapical cysts, also called radicular cysts.[125,126]

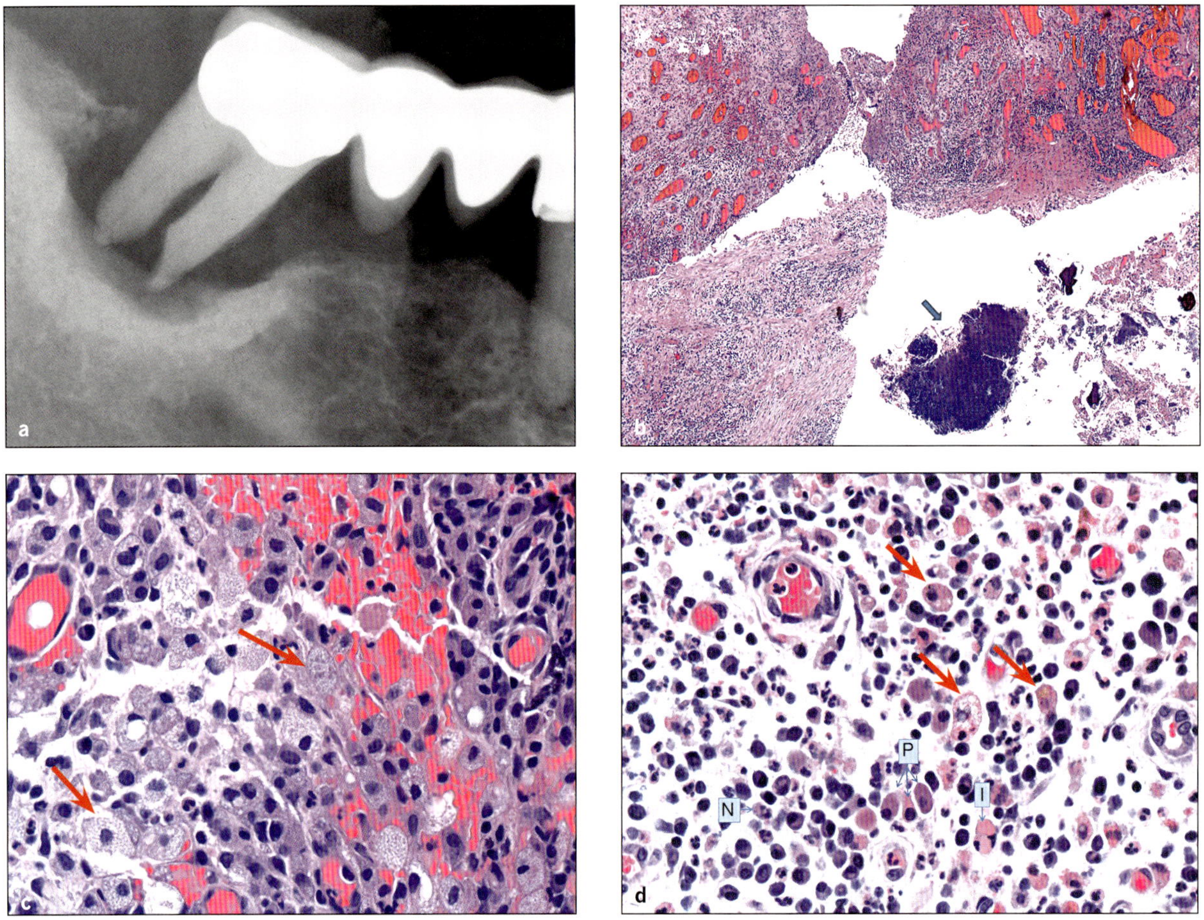

Fig 4-4 *(a)* Periapical radiograph showing a periapical granuloma with prominent apical bone and focal root resorption. (Courtesy of Dr Shawneen Gonzalez, Oregon Health & Science University.) *(b)* Low-power photomicrograph of the periapical granuloma depicting highly vascularized granulation tissue with dense inflammatory cell infiltrate. Actinomycotic bacterial colonies *(arrow)* are also seen. *(c)* A high-power view showing granulation tissue with reactive histiocytosis *(arrows)*. Scattered eosinophils and plasma cells are also present (h&e stain; original magnification ×100). *(d)* A high-power view of the granulation tissue with reactive histiocytes, some of which appear hemosiderin laden *(arrows)*. Lymphocytes, neutrophilic aggregates (N), and plasma cells (P), some of which exhibit immunoglobulin production (I) (Russell bodies), are also present (h&e stain; original magnification ×100).

Neto et al[127] evaluated the differences in expression of tryptase + mast cells in periapical granulomas and cysts and discovered larger numbers of these cells in chronic periapical granulomas than in periapical (radicular) cysts, which may be a reflection of the differences in pathobiology and etiopathogenesis of the two lesions.[128] Studies have demonstrated that tryptase is involved in the activation of fibroblasts and the induction or production of collagen, contributing to wound healing and fibrosis, in addition to the capability of possessing fibrinolytic properties.[129–131] These results also show that the central portion of these lesions bears the highest metabolic activity, while the higher frequency of mast cells in the peripheral portions of radicular cysts and near perilesional bone seems to be indicative of the participation of these cells in lesion expansion and bone resorption.[132,133]

Radicular cyst

Radicular cysts develop in the periapical region following the proliferation of odontogenic epithelial rests—specifically rests of Serres or Malassez—but may also be derived from crystal crevicular epithelium, sinus epithelium, or epithelium lining the sinus tracts.[134]

Clinically, radicular cysts typically present with asymptomatic swelling and mild sensitivity, especially when they attain larger sizes. Tooth mobility may also be noted, and negative response to electric testing, thermal testing, and percussion are typically seen.[58,122] Radiographically, periapical granulomas and radicular cysts may show identical features, namely variably sized radiolucencies, with or without loss of lamina dura, and apical root resorption. Large cysts may be encountered occasionally. The inflam-

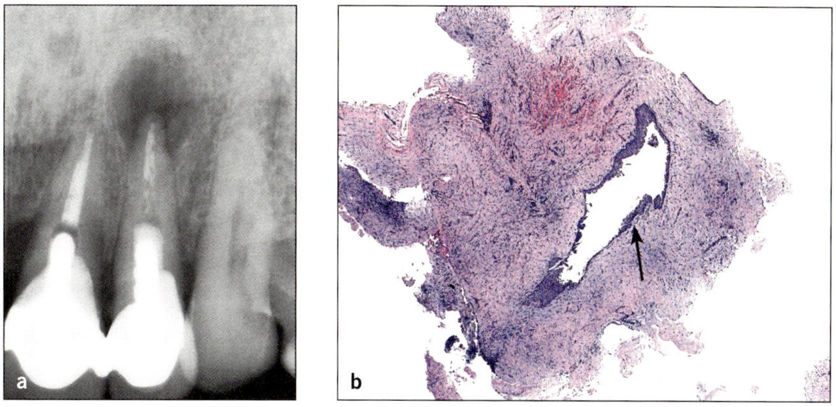

Fig 4-5 *(a)* Periapical radiograph of a maxillary left lateral incisor previously treated with root canal therapy associated with a well-defined periapical radiolucency. (Courtesy of Dr Shawneen Gonzalez, Oregon Health & Science University.) *(b)* A low-power photomicrograph of the excised apical tissue showing a cystic cavity lined by stratified squamous epithelium *(arrow)* covering a dense fibrocollagenous wall that supports a patchy inflammatory cell infiltrate (h&e stain; original magnification ×10).

matory cell infiltrate along with a bacterial load may also seep through the lateral canal, if and when present, resulting in the so-called "lateral radicular cyst" seen in the interradicular position, similar to lateral periodontal cysts. Tooth vitality status along with histomorphologic examination can readily distinguish between lateral radicular and lateral periodontal cysts. Further, many or most examples of the so-called "globular maxillary cyst" are proven to be practically representative of actual radicular cysts.[134] Additionally, if and when the cyst is left behind following extraction of the tooth where the cyst existed, the remaining cyst would be designated as a "residual periapical cyst." Histologic features of all the subtypes—lateral radicular, radicular, and residual cysts—are identical.

Histology

Histologic examination of radicular cysts displays a cystic cavity lined by nonkeratinized inflamed, hyperplastic, and edematous stratified squamous epithelium, covering a dense fibrocollagenous wall. Occasionally, mucous cell prosoplasia, cilia, and/or apocrine-like changes may be identified within the epithelial lining, and cellular debris is often seen within the lumen of the cyst. Rushton body–type calcification may also be observed. These mostly represent aborted keratinization without evidence of calcification.[134–136] Bleeding within the cyst wall may also leave behind cholesterol clefts with accompanying multinucleated foreign body–type giant cell reaction. Granulation tissue with acute and chronic inflammation composed of reactive lymphoplasmacytic and histiocytic inflammatory cell infiltrate with Russell bodies is commonly seen in the background. Pulse granulomas (giant cell hyaline angiopathy) are also often detected within the cystic lining.[58,122,134,137–143] Various reports regarding the true incidence of cysts varied from below 20% to up to 65% of all apical periodontitis cases.[137–146] The majority of cysts occur in the maxilla, specifically in the anterior region[134] (Figs 4-5 to 4-7).

Several investigators have addressed the pathogenesis of radicular cysts.[147–156] Shear et al[150–152] have advocated three stages in their development: *(1)* The dormant epithelial rests of Malassez[157] proliferate in response to growth factors secreted.[31,158] The cysts further develop as a result of stimulation of a focal abscess or secondary to necrotic and degenerative changes occurring as a result of the nutritional deprivation.[31] *(2)* The cystic epithelium becomes well-defined.[159,160] *(3)* The cyst grows secondary to osmotic pressure and/or unexplainable molecular events.[31,161–168]

Bernardi et al[169] have extensively investigated the pathobiology of the cystic epithelial lining and further elucidated the complexity of its development. They highlighted the significance of molecular events, including the role of cell proliferative markers, apoptosis, the contribution and interaction with the extracellular matrix, as well as the significance of inflammatory components and bone metabolic factors in the complexity of the development of these cysts. Analysis of cell proliferative markers Ki-67, AgNOR, and p53 have clearly demonstrated the confinement of the proliferative activity to the basal layer level.[170–173] Analysis of apoptotic regulators indicated a proapoptotic microenvironment in both the epithelium and the supporting stroma, showing lower antiapoptotic markers and higher BAX (proapoptotic) markers, respectively.[173] The mesenchymal epithelial interaction also plays an important role in the development of those cysts.[174–176] The secretion of bone metabolism–related factors may favor an increase in osteolytic activity, facilitating cystic expansion into the adjacent bone tissue.[177–180] Additionally, the contribution of inflammatory cytokines, including IL-1α, IL-1β, and IL-6 in the development of radicular cysts is also emphasized by several studies.[181–183]

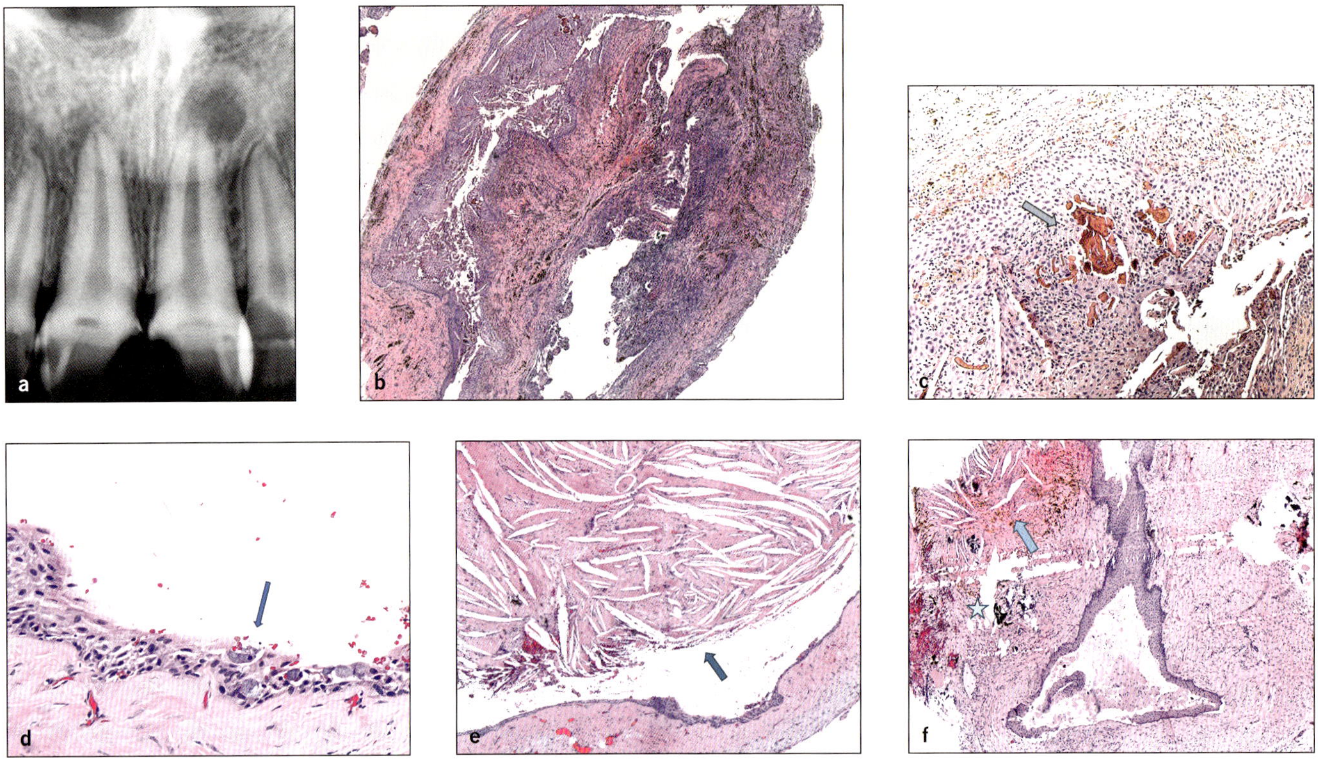

Fig 4-6 *(a)* Periapical radiograph showing carious anterior maxillary teeth. The maxillary left central incisor is associated with a well-defined periapical radiolucency. (Courtesy of the Department of Endodontics, Oregon Health & Science University.) *(b)* A low-power photomicrograph of the excised periapical tissue showing a cystic cavity lined by mostly inflamed hyperplastic stratified squamous epithelium (h&e stain; original magnification ×10). *(c to f)* Variation of histomorphologic findings in radicular cysts, including Rushton bodies *(c, arrow)*, mucous cell prosoplasia *(d, arrow)*, cholesterol clefts with accompanying multinucleated foreign body–type giant cell reaction *(e and f, arrows)*, and the root canal filled with foreign body material *(f, star)*.

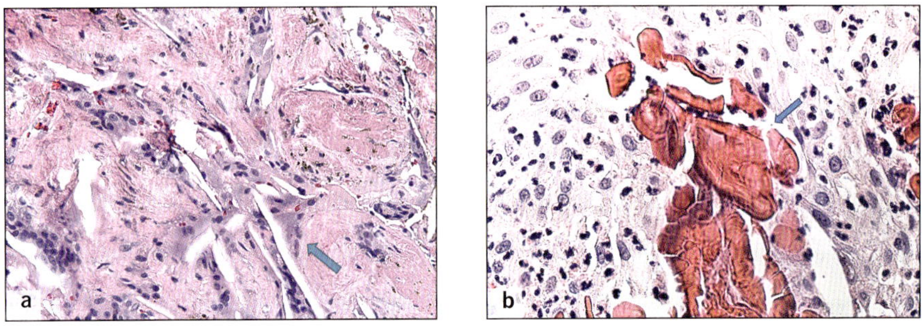

Fig 4-7 A high-power view depicting the presence of cholesterol clefts with accompanying multinucleated foreign body–type giant cell reaction *(a, arrow)* and Rushton bodies within the cystic epithelium *(b, arrow)* (h&e stain; original magnification ×100).

Treatment

Radicular cysts are best managed by root canal therapy and/or extraction of the tooth, with conservative excision of the cyst, eliminating the periapical pathology. Root canal therapy is often followed by surgical endodontics if and when the periapical pathology fails to resolve. Periapical granulomas may, but do not always, develop into radicular cysts.

There are five principal biologic reasons for the persistence of periapical radiolucency following root canal treatment[31]: *(1)* intraradicular infection; *(2)* extraradicular infection, mostly related to Actinomycotic colonies present within these lesions; *(3)* a cystic lesion; *(4)* foreign body reactions and/or material most probably related to endodontic origin and/or bleeding (responsible for cholesterol cleft deposition within the lesions); and *(5)* scar tissue.

Periapical scar

Occasionally, the inflammatory process in the apical region is replaced by a dense, relatively acellular, fibrous

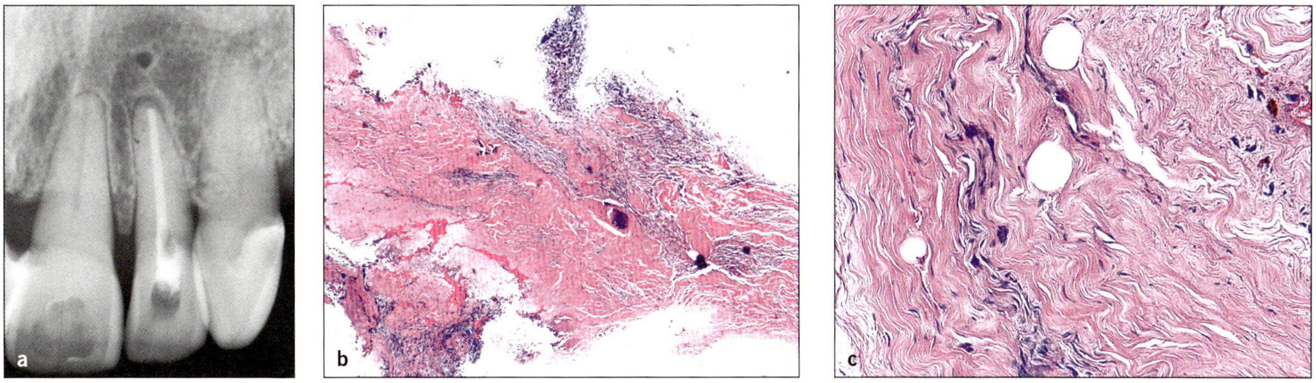

Fig 4-8 *(a)* Periapical radiograph of a maxillary left lateral incisor previously treated with root canal therapy associated with a small periapical radiolucency. (Courtesy of Dr Shawneen Gonzalez, Oregon Health & Science University.) *(b)* A low-power photomicrograph of the excised periapical tissue showing a dense, relatively acellular fibrocollagenous connective tissue scar supporting a patchy mononuclear inflammatory cell infiltrate (h&e stain; original magnification ×10). *(c)* A high-power photomicrograph of the periapical scar demonstrating a dense, relatively acellular fibrocollagenous connective tissue (h&e stain; original magnification ×100).

collagenous connective tissue. This scenario is often seen secondary to root canal therapy in an immunocompetent patient. The development of a periapical scar represents the ultimate healing attempt of the tissue that would be replaced by a dense, fibrotic, collagenous connective tissue background.[184–187] The incidence of periapical scars varies from 6.6% to 12%[188–190] (Fig 4-8).

Periapical Pathosis Mimickers and Radiolucencies Not of Pulpal Origin

Clinicians must always confirm suspected periapical pathology via tissue examination not only to determine the appropriate treatment plan and management of the condition but also to rule out the possibility of periapical pathology mimickers, which are unrelated to pulpal disease.[191–193] The differential diagnosis of periapical radiolucencies should also include lesions of nonodontogenic origin.[194] These include normal anatomical structures such as nutrient canals, unusual arborization of bony trabeculae, and Stafne cysts.[195] Canalis sinosus, which is a poorly recognized anatomical feature representing a neurovascular canal that carries the anterior superior alveolar nerve and vessels, may also be confused with periapical pathology.[196] A wide spectrum of entities have been described under this category of periapical pathology mimickers and are selectively described in this section. A review of the literature reveals a general incidence of periapical pathology mimickers to be within the range of 0.7% to 5%.[193,197]

In general, a misdiagnosis may result from more than one factor, including misperception, misinterpretation, incomplete diagnostic examination,[195] or less than optimal tissue sampling. Therefore, fewer teeth with periapical radiolucencies would be initially treated surgically, with no material available for histomorphologic interpretation.[198] It is agreed upon, with rare exceptions, that all periapical pathology should be examined histologically.[199] Certain circumstances encountered should further motivate the clinician to perform periapical surgery with submission of the tissue for histomorphologic confirmation,[198] especially if the periapical radiolucency is detected in the presence of a vital, caries-free tooth that is also free of deep or larger restorations. Detection of anesthesia of the associated nerve, root resorption, an irregular radiolucent pattern, and failure to respond to endodontic treatment should further warrant investigating the nature of the lesion. It has been reported that approximately 25% of malignant lesions that mimicked periapical pathology and 10.8% of benign lesions that mimicked periapical pathology presented with asymptomatic swelling, while painful swelling was reported in 46.6% of malignant lesions and in only 10.8% of benign lesions that mimicked periapical pathology.[200] Additionally, it is worth mentioning that despite the fact that periapical pathology in a tooth that presents with a negative vitality status should be considered to be of endodontic nature,[201–203] lesions of non-endodontic origin may also devitalize teeth, especially when located in close proximity to the root apices. Therefore, the vitality status should be theoretically viewed and interpreted in the context of general clinical history and radiographic interpretation.[200,204,205]

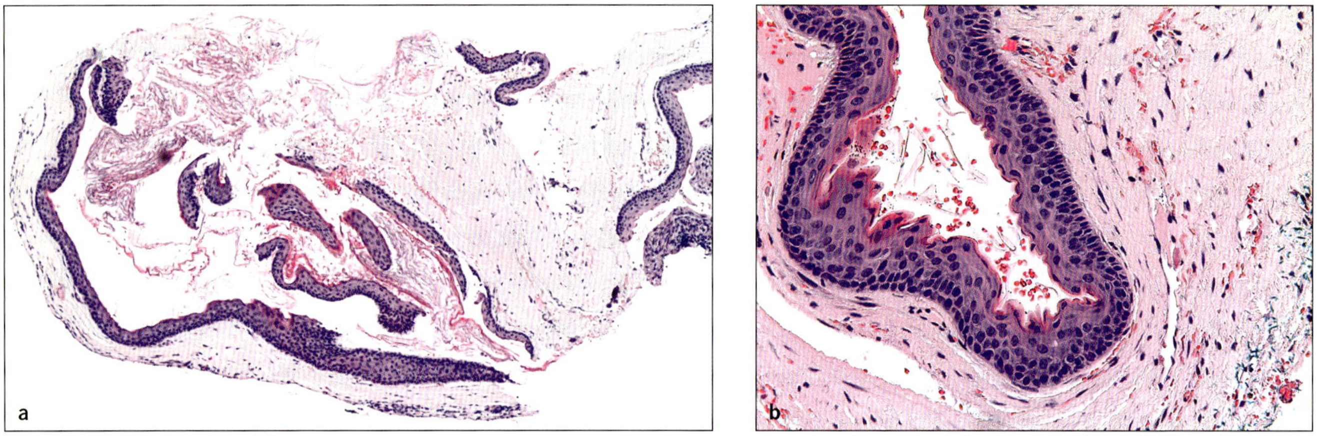

Fig 4-9 *(a)* A low-power photomicrograph of an OKC with a well-defined cystic cavity, lined by an epithelium that demonstrates uniform thickness and surface keratinization (h&e stain; original magnification ×10). *(b)* A high-power photomicrograph of the OKC showing a palisaded basal layer, uniform six- to seven-layer thickness, and a distinct surface parakeratinization (h&e stain; original magnification ×100).

Odontogenic keratocyst and other odontogenic cysts and tumors

The odontogenic keratocyst (OKC), also known as a *keratocystic odontogenic tumor*, is the most common lesion mimicking periapical pathology.[193,197,206–210] Kontogiannis et al[197] reported that OKCs represented close to 35% of all nonperiapical and endodontic-related periapical pathology. The distinction is of great importance, because OKCs exhibit aggressive biologic behavior and are known for their recurrence and massive bone destruction.[211] Radiographically, an OKC may present as a unilocular or, more commonly, a large multilocular radiolucency that may involve a significant portion of the mandibular body or ramus. Cortical expansion and/or perforation is not uncommon, but tumors may, at least initially, spread anteroposteriorly within the medullary space, which may potentially contribute to delays in discovery and diagnosis.[212,213] The radiographic examination, coupled with the characteristic histomorphologic features, can easily differentiate OKCs from periapical pathosis, yet lesions may be deceptively seen in a periapical location as already mentioned. Histologically, an OKC demonstrates characteristic features, namely a cystic cavity lined by uniform thickness; a stratified squamous epithelium with a wavy, parakeratinized surface; a palisaded basal layer; lack of rete ridges; and often prominent separation from the underlying connective tissue (Fig 4-9). The orthokeratinized OKC differs from a traditional OKC in that it has a classic orthokeratinized surface pattern and lacks a basal cell palisaded architecture. It has also been reported in a periapical location mimicking periapical pathosis. This cyst has lower recurrence rates than the traditional OKC and thus also shows less aggressive overall biologic behavior.[212,213]

The calcified odontogenic cyst (COC), or *calcifying cystic odontogenic tumor*, is another odontogenic tumor that may present occasionally in a periapical location and therefore may be mistaken for periapical pathosis.[208,214,215] COC is a rare, benign intraosseous (or less commonly peripheral extraosseous) odontogenic tumor that involves the maxillary and mandibular arches with similar frequency, most commonly seen in the premolar and canine regions.[211,213,215–219] COC is histologically characterized by the presence of ameloblastic-type epithelium with the addition of ghost cells and evidence of calcification,[216] which can also help in the initial radiographic interpretation of the lesion. In 2006, Buchner et al[217] reported that COCs represent approximately 1.6% of all odontogenic tumors.

Ameloblastoma is the second most common odontogenic tumor, has its origin from the odontogenic epithelium, and is most commonly encountered in the posterior mandibular region in patients over 40 years old.[122] It may present as a unilocular or multilocular radiolucency, more often in the posterior mandibular region than other locations, and may also exhibit significant expansion and bone destruction. Typically, ameloblastomas present as a unilocular or, more commonly, a honeycomb or soap-bubble multilocular radiolucency and are commonly associated with significant bone resorption, destruction, and/or cortical perforation.[122,213] The lesion is benign but also notorious for postsurgical recurrence. The presence of periapical ameloblastoma is rare, accounting for approximately 0.7% of all periapical lesions studied by Chapelle et al,[220] and has been reported to occur in the periapical location by many investigators.[192,193,221–230] Despite the presence of histologic variants in ameloblastoma, including granular cell, acanthomatous, and desmoplastic, the histologic pattern is somewhat characteristic, showing islands and nests of odontogenic epithelium rimmed by

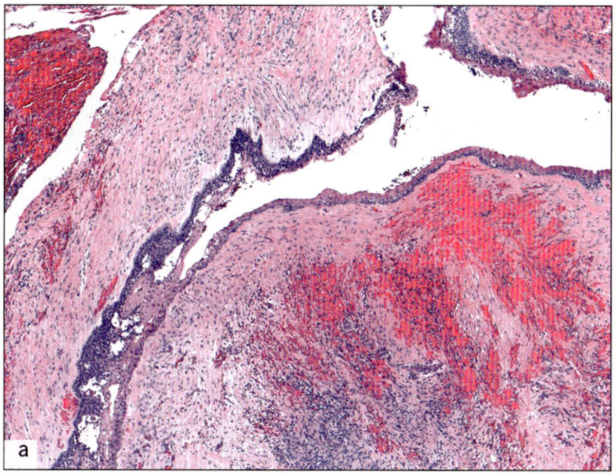

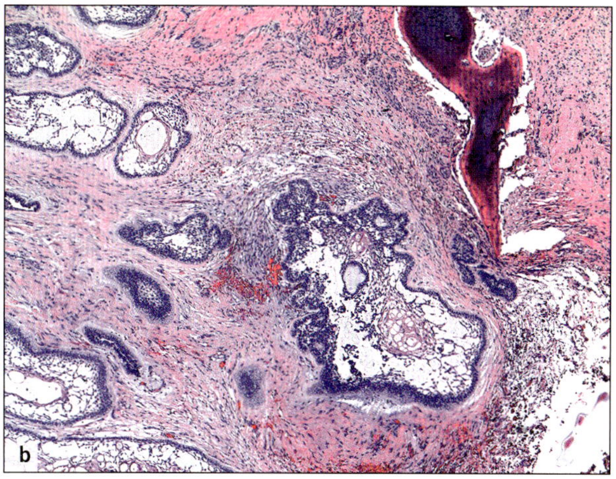

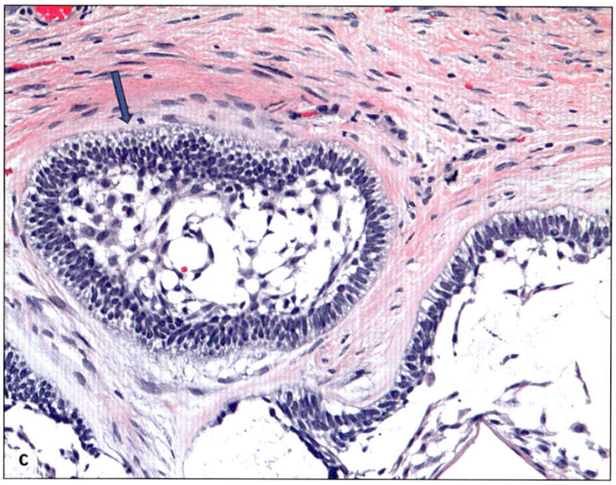

Fig 4-10 *(a)* Low-power view of unicystic ameloblastoma showing the characteristic peripheral, palisaded columnar cells and stellate reticulum pattern but confined within the cystic lining (h&e stain; original magnification ×10). *(b)* Low-power view of the same tumor demonstrating the presence of a solid infiltrative pattern of ameloblastoma within the wall of the unicystic tumor (h&e stain; original magnification ×10). *(c)* A higher-power photomicrograph of a solid ameloblastoma demonstrating the nest, island, and follicles with characteristic peripheral, palisaded columnar epithelial cells showing reverse polarization *(arrow)* and enclosing stellate reticulum–like epithelial tissue (h&e stain; original magnification ×60).

peripheral columnar cells exhibiting reverse polarity and enclosing stellate reticulum-like tissue[213] (Fig 4-10). Unicystic ameloblastoma has been also reported by Gondak et al[224] to mimic periapical pathosis. Treatment of the unicystic type is conservative total surgical enucleation of the cystic area, with lower tendency for postsurgical recurrence when compared with the solid form. Unicystic tumors share the same histomorphologic pattern seen in the solid tumor, albeit confined to a well-defined cystic cavity more commonly in association with a pericoronal impacted tooth location.

The adenomatoid odontogenic tumor (AOT) is most commonly associated with a pericoronal impacted tooth (maxillary and mandibular canines) and is rarely seen in patients over 20 years old. Radiographically, the lesion may mimic a dentigerous cyst or a unicystic ameloblastoma, with the exception of the identification of calcification within the pericoronal radiolucency. AOT has also been rarely reported in an apical location and thus may be mistaken for a periapical pathosis.[227,230] Histologically, AOT also demonstrates diagnostic features, including a pattern of monotonous basophilic odontogenic epithelium arranged in ducts, nests, and spherules with the identification of calcification and amyloid-like material.

Other cysts included in the differential diagnosis of periapical pathosis include traumatic (hemorrhagic) bone cysts and nasopalatine duct cysts (Fig 4-11). A thorough radiographic, clinical, and vitality status examination coupled with histomorphologic analysis should easily delineate these entities from periapical pathosis. Hemorrhagic bone cysts (HBCs) typically display a homogenous unilocular radiolucency that scallops in between the roots of vital mandibular teeth. HBC is typically diagnosed when clinicians attempt to biopsy the lesion, only to discover a virtually empty content. Exploratory biopsy also leads to an expected bony filling and healing within several weeks of the procedure. Nasopalatine duct cysts are typically discovered as a heart-shaped midline nasal

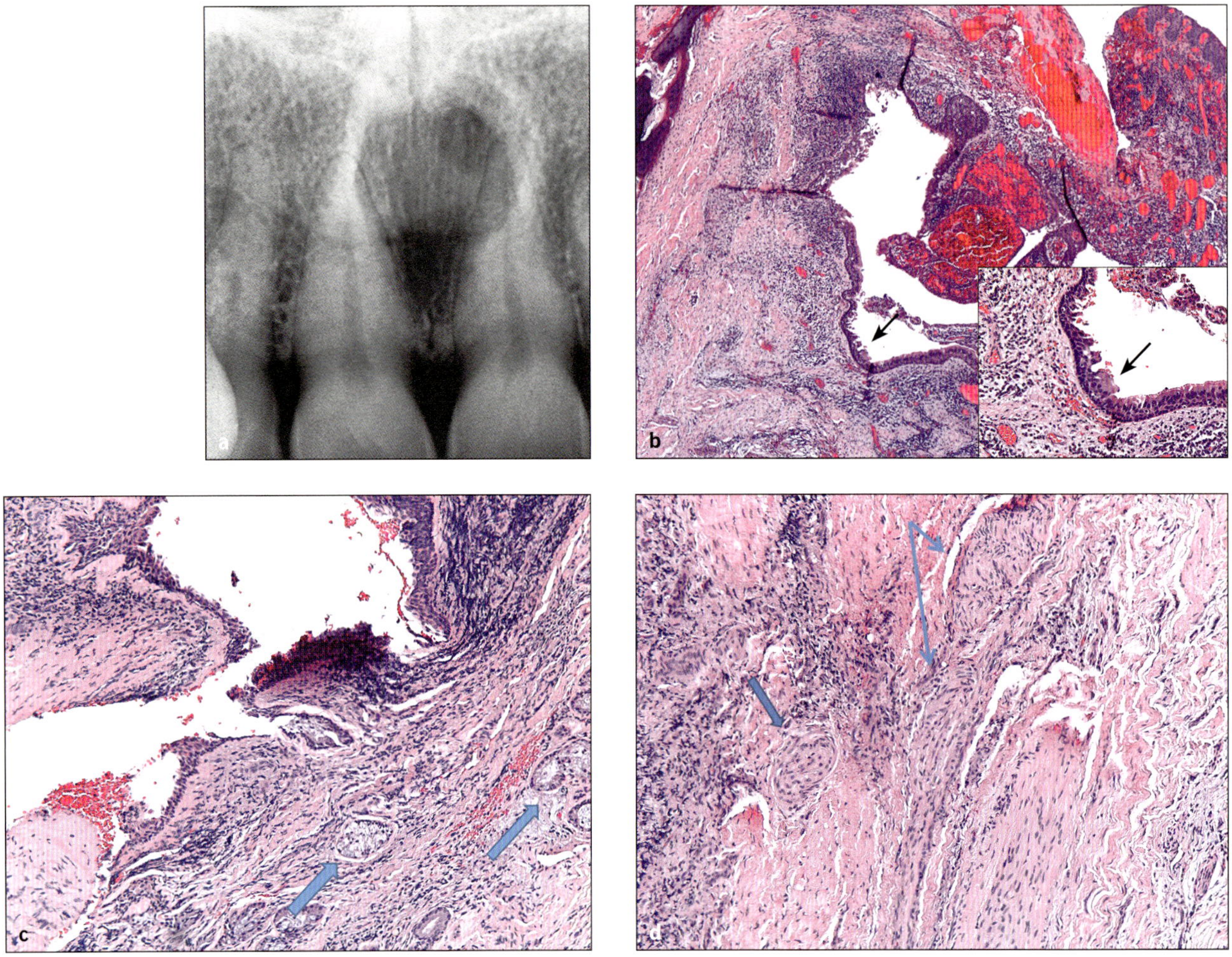

Fig 4-11 *(a)* Periapical radiograph depicting a heart-shaped radiolucency in the anterior maxilla of a 20-year-old man in association with vital teeth, characteristic of a nasopalatine duct cyst. (Courtesy of Dr Mahmoud Torabinejad, Loma Linda, California.) *(b)* Histologic examination of the enucleated cyst showing a cystic cavity lined by ciliated respiratory type epithelium *(arrow)* (h&e stain; original magnification ×60; inset ×100). *(c and d)* The cyst wall also supported minor salivary glands *(c, arrows)* and peripheral nerve bundles *(d, arrows)* (h&e stain; original magnification ×10).

radiolucency that is also associated with vital teeth (see Fig 4-11a). The radiographic presentation in addition to confirmation of tooth vitality is essential in distinguishing between nasopalatine duct cysts and radicular cysts. Further histomorphologic examination confirming the presence of respiratory-type epithelium with or without stratified squamous epithelium salivary tissue and peripheral neural tissue may further distinguish nasopalatine duct cysts from radicular cysts, which commonly display hyperplastic inflamed and edematous stratified squamous epithelial lining.

Central giant cell granuloma

Central giant cell granuloma (CGCG) is a reactive, nonneoplastic, yet also potentially expansile, aggressive, and destructive entity most commonly involving the anterior regions of the gnathic region, with a tendency to cross the midline. CGCG may present with swelling and local expansion, but there are no reliable clinical and/or pathognomonic features that can predict the lesion's behavior. Radiographically, it may present as a unilocular or multilocular radiolucency, but it may also rarely mimic periapical pathology.[122,231,232] CGCG may present with a spectrum of behavior ranging from nonaggressive to aggressive, locally destructive, and exhibiting a high incidence of postsurgical recurrence, with rapid growth, a high rate of recurrence, cortical bone perforation, root resorption, and tooth displacement.[231] Histopathologic examination reveals proliferating endothelial cells, fibroblasts, and myofibroblasts in a well-vascularized fibrocollagenous background that is packed with multinucleated, osteoclast-type giant cells. Furthermore, extravasation of

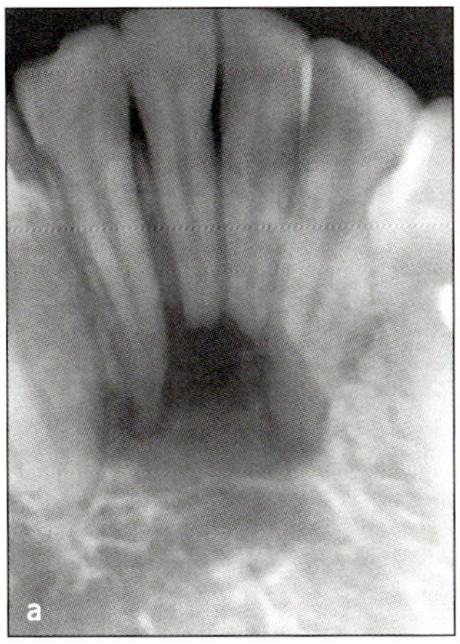

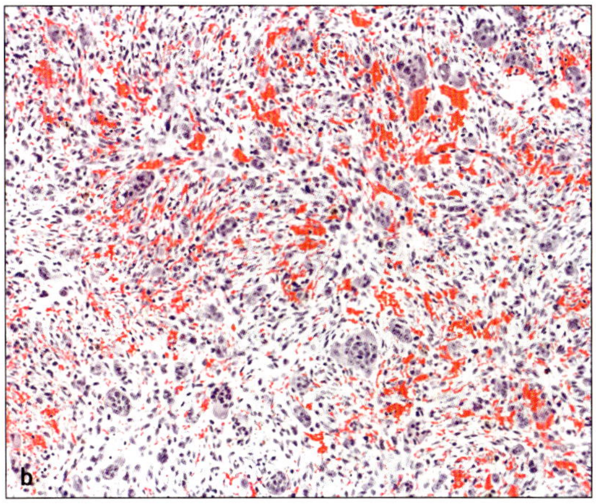

Fig 4-12 *(a)* Periapical radiograph of a CGCG identified in a periapical location. *(b)* Histomorphologic examination of the lesion demonstrating an abundance of osteoclast-type giant cells in a well-vascularized fibrocollagenous connective tissue background (h&e stain; original magnification ×60). (Courtesy of Drs Phillip Merrell and Roy Eversole, University of the Pacific.)

red blood cells and deposition of hemosiderin are commonly seen[122,231] (Fig 4-12). In 2009, Dahlkemper et al[231] reported that approximately 20% of CGCGs may present with similarities to periapical lesions and may be misdiagnosed as endodontic inflammatory lesions, and therefore root canal therapy would not be effective.[232,233] They also reported that CGCGs were less common in females, less common before age 30 years, and did not show prevalence to crossing the midline of the jaw as previously reported. The involved teeth, when seen within the context of CGCG, would respond to vitality tests. Lesions would be best managed by curettage, but radical surgery may be necessary for aggressive lesions.[122]

Intraosseous malignant tumors including metastatic carcinoma

Metastatic carcinoma is an important consideration within this category and has significant diagnostic, management, and prognostic implications.[193,234–236] The incidence of periapical pathosis representing confirmed metastatic disease ranges from 2.1% to 0.21%.[236,237] The most common region where metastatic disease is encountered is undoubtedly the posterior mandible, where lung and breast carcinomas predominate, all sites considered.[197,238–240] The identification of evidence of radiographic opacity within the metastatic disease may favor one of three sources—specifically lung, prostate, and thyroid metastasis—more than others.[122] Intraosseous malignant salivary tumors such as adenoid cystic carcinoma[241,242] and central intraosseous carcinoma (including central odontogenic carcinoma)[238,243,244] and rare malignant mesenchymal, soft tissue tumors[245] and neuroectodermal tumors[246] may also rarely masquerade as periapical pathosis. With rare exceptions where lesions may present in a periapical location, metastatic carcinoma and intraosseous malignant entities most commonly present as moth-eaten, destructive, radiolucent, radiopaque, or mixed lesions, with or without cortical perforation and/or potential jaw fracture.[122,193,234–236]

Langerhans cell disease, lymphoma, and related disorders

Langerhans cell histiocytosis (LCH) includes a group of related disorders involving the reticuloendothelial system characterized by abnormal Langerhans cell proliferation.[122,211] Of the three known subtypes of LCH—Letterer-Siwe disease, Hans Schuler Christian disease, and eosinophilic granuloma—the latter is the most common subtype and may be mistaken for periapical pathosis.[122,247] It demonstrates gnathic and extragnathic, well-demarcated, punched-out radiolucencies; tooth mobility; and a radiographic presentation that looks like teeth hanging in air. It may also be associated with focal alveolar ridge soft tissue necrosis.[122] The histomorphologic features of all types are similar, showing an abundance of mostly grooved histiocytes and eosinophils supported by a generous vascular background. Immunohistochemistry staining with CD1a and anti-S100 protein confirm the diagnosis (Fig 4-13). Electron microscopic features of the Langerhans cells known to be characteristic show tennis racket–type granules commonly referred to as *Birbeck granules*.[248,249]

Among the two well-recognized types of lymphoma—Hodgkin and non-Hodgkin lymphoma—the latter may appear in extranodal sites in up to 40% of cases.[250] Generally, non-Hodgkin lymphoma predominantly affects the lymphoid tissue of the Waldeyer's ring in the head and neck, including the tonsils, base of the tongue, and buccal mucosa, but may also rarely involve jaw bones[250–252] and may therefore mimic endodontic or periodontic space diseases, among other cystic jaw lesions[253] (Figs 4-14 and 4-15). Jaw lymphomas often present as irregular radiolucencies with well- or ill-defined outlines. When lymphomas

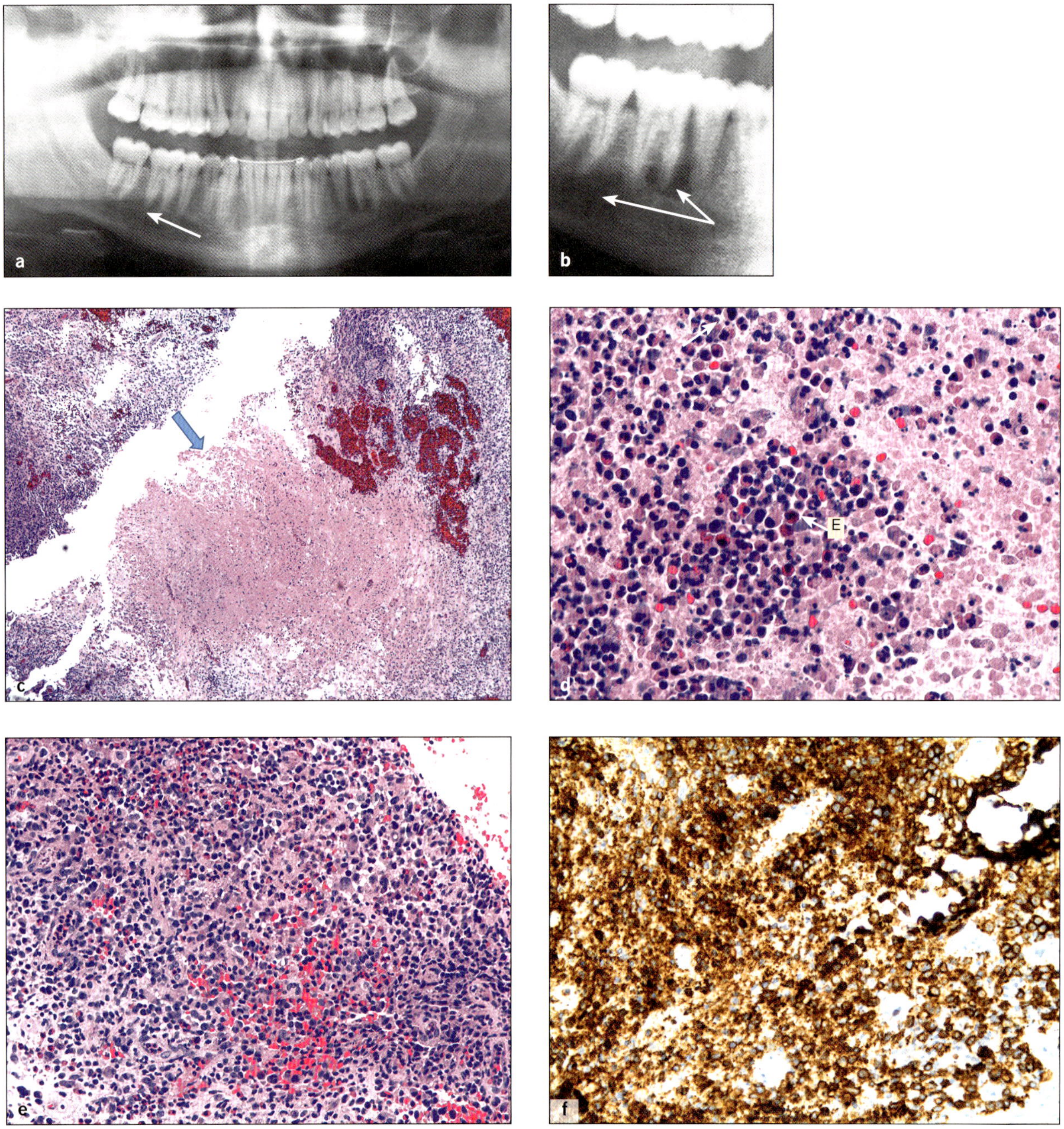

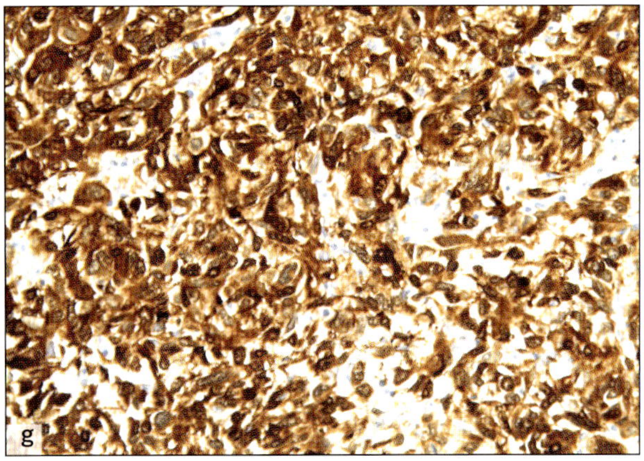

Fig 4-13 A 7-year-old boy presented with an incidental finding of a radiolucent lesion surrounding the roots of the loose mandibular right first molar. *(a)* Panoramic radiograph showing the presence of radiolucent lesions in the right mandibular body *(arrow)*. *(b)* A periapical radiograph better delineates the well-demarcated radiolucencies *(arrows)* periradicular and apical to the first and second molars, respectively. *(c)* A low-power view showing a partially necrotic tissue *(arrow)* and a dense cellular infiltrate (h&e stain; original magnification ×10). *(d)* A higher-power photomicrograph showing a dense admixture of histiocytes, many of which demonstrate grooved nuclei *(arrow)* and eosinophils (E) supported by a loose, mostly necrotic background, characteristic of LCH (h&e stain; original magnification ×60). *(e)* Parts of the cellular infiltrate showed a dense admixture of eosinophils and histiocytes (h&e stain; original magnification ×40). *(f and g)* Immunohistochemistry of LCH demonstrating intense and generalized positive labeling with CD1a and anti S-100 protein antibodies, respectively, confirming the diagnosis of LCH.

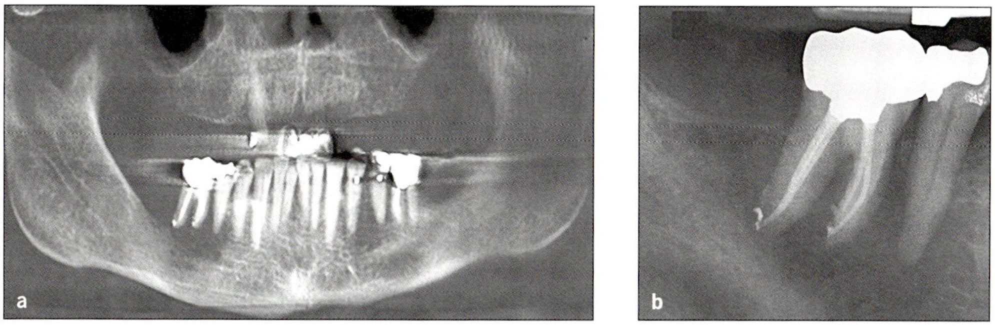

Fig 4-14 An 80-year-old man presented with a 1-month history of paresthesia and a history of endodontic treatment on the mandibular right first molar. *(a)* Panoramic radiograph demonstrates a 3-cm radiolucency apical to the endodontically treated mandibular right first molar. *(b)* A periapical radiograph of this tooth demonstrates a radiolucency apical to it. Enucleation of the lesion and histomorphologic examination demonstrated the presence of a large B-cell lymphoma, confirmed with immunohistochemistry staining and flow cytometry studies.

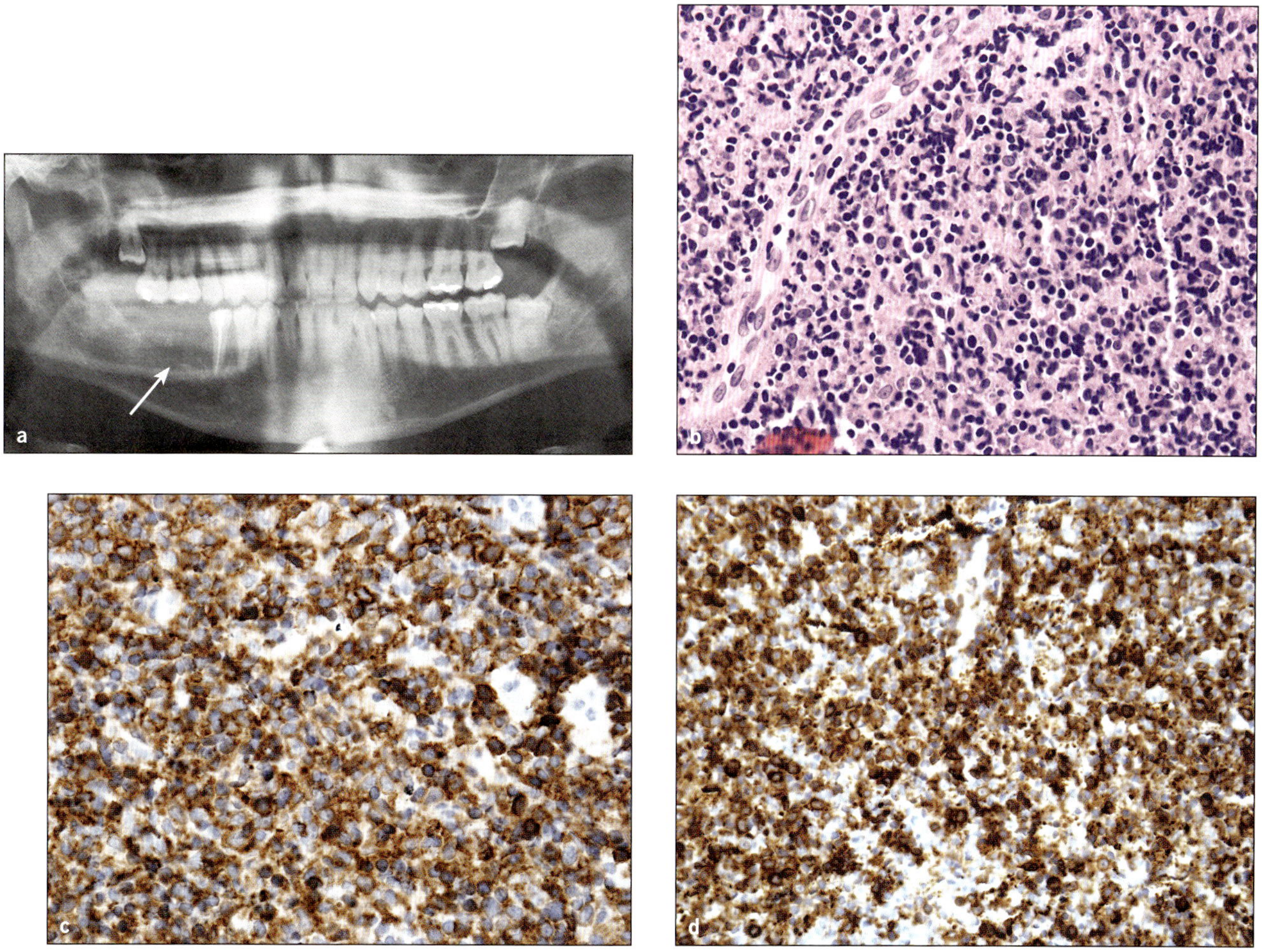

Fig 4-15 *(a)* Panoramic radiograph depicting a large radiolucency *(arrow)* in the right mandible of a 43-year-old man who presented originally to his dentist with pain and swelling, with intermittent response to antibiotics. He received three consecutive root canal treatments and several extractions within a period of 5 years. A biopsy of the persistent, refractory, painful swelling revealed the presence of a large B-cell lymphoma. *(b)* Histomorphologic examination of the lesion demonstrated a dense lymphocytic infiltrate with many large and pleomorphic cells (h&e stain; original magnification ×60). The tumor cells reacted positively with anti-CD20 *(c)* and anti-CD79a *(d)*, among several other immunohistochemistry stains, confirming the B-cell lineage of the tumor.

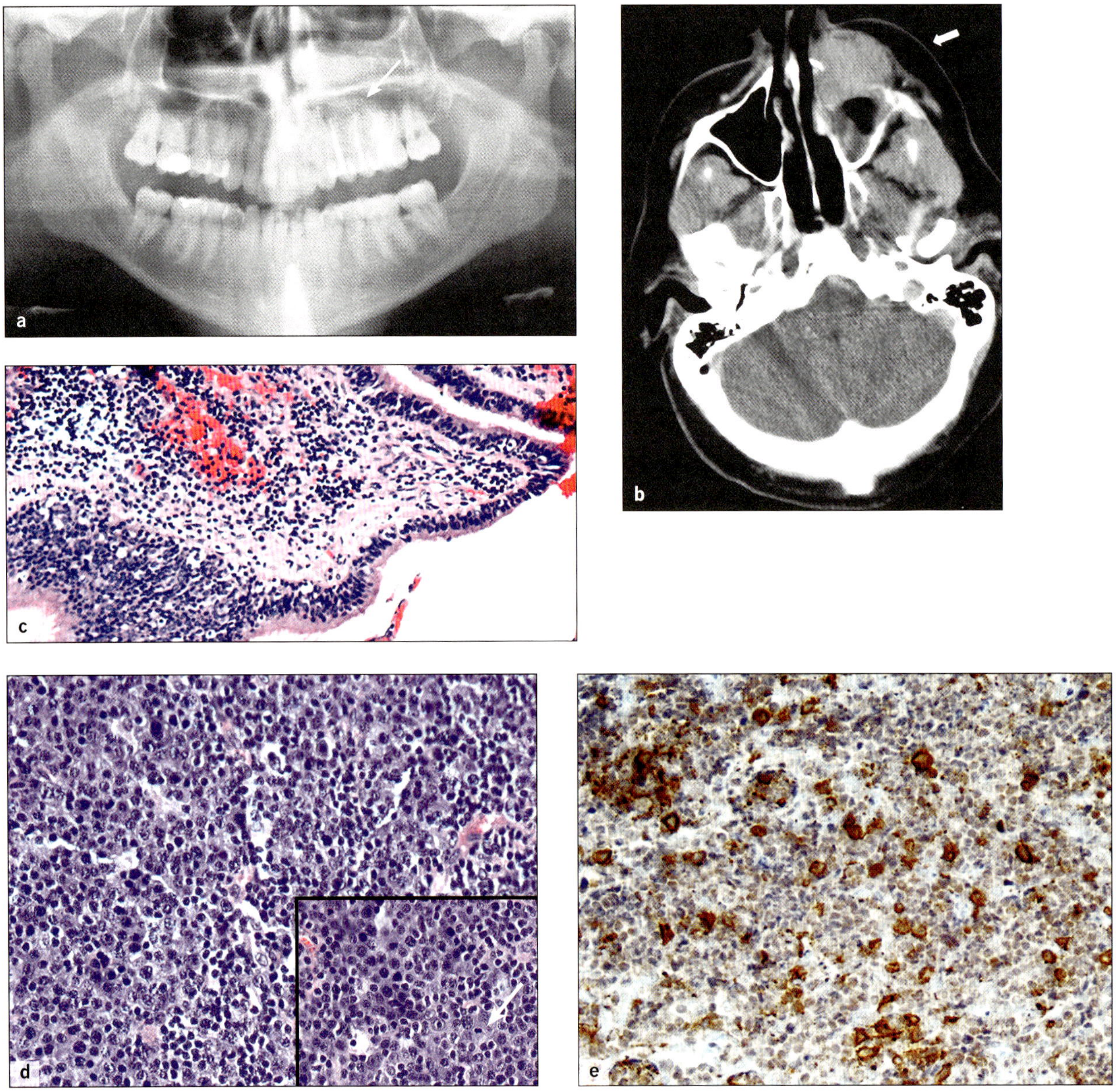

Fig 4-16 *(a)* Panoramic radiograph of a 45-year-old man who presented with a several-week history of pain and moderate swelling in the maxillary left vestibule and infraorbital area. He was diagnosed with periapical abscess *(arrow)* and accompanying cellulitis and managed with several rounds of incision and drainage, antibiotics, and consecutive root canal treatment of several left maxillary teeth after testing nonvital. *(b)* Computed tomography scan, with contrast, showing left maxillary expansion and soft tissue density within the maxillary sinus *(arrow)*. *(c)* A biopsy performed on the persistent swelling close to 6 months after his initial visit revealed inflamed sinus mucosa that supported dense, aggregated, small round blue cells (h&e stain; original magnification ×20). *(d)* Histomorphologic examination of the round blue cell population revealed the presence of an atypical pleomorphic plasma cell population, which also exhibited mitotic activity *(arrow)* (h&e stain; original magnification ×40; inset ×60). *(e)* Immunohistochemistry staining for CD138 showed diffuse positive staining, and flow cytometric analysis revealed a population of monoclonal plasma cells (approximately 41% of the total cells), expressing moderately bright CD38, CD56, and bright cytoplasmic kappa light chain. The histomorphologic features confirmed the diagnosis of solitary sinonasal plasmacytoma. (Case workup performed with the help of Dr Vishnu Reddy, University of Alabama at Birmingham.)

involve bone, biopsy material often demonstrates necrotic tissue, adding to the difficulty in reaching an accurate diagnosis.[254] This potential pitfall may be overcome via submitting the well-preserved pulpotomy (extirpated pulp) tissue for histomorphologic interpretation in suspicious cases.[255]

Plasmacytoma is a rare clonal neoplastic proliferation of plasma cells that can exist in extramedullary forms and solitary lesions of bone.[256] Lesions often appear as well-demarcated radiolucencies within the medullary cavity.[256–259] Plasmacytomas of the head and neck may partially involve bone but are often grouped under the

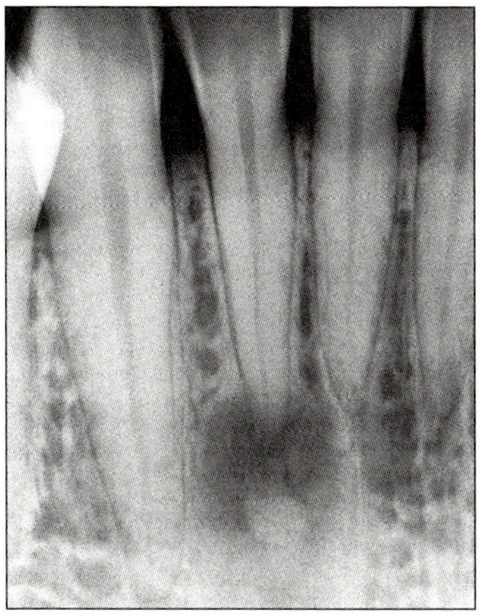

Fig 4-17 Periapical radiograph of the mandibular incisors showing periapical cemento-osseous dysplasia during the mixed lytic-blastic phase of the disease. (Courtesy of Dr Mahmoud Torabinejad, Loma Linda, California.)

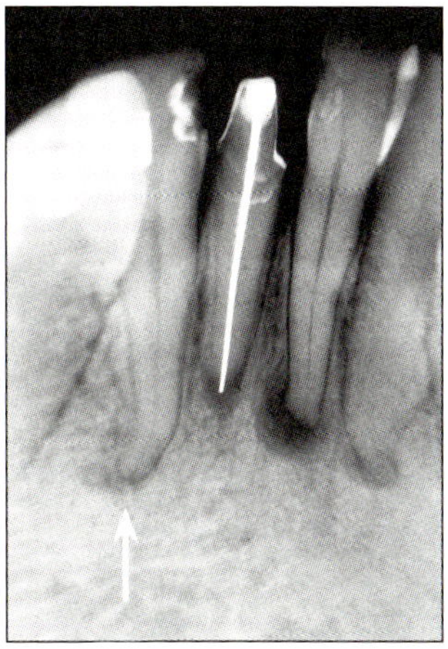

Fig 4-18 Periapical radiograph of the mandibular incisors showing the right central incisor treated with root canal therapy due to the misinterpretation of the periapical radiolucency as periapical pathology of endodontic origin. The lytic phase of cemento-osseous dysplasia is seen involving the rest of the mandibular anterior teeth except the apical region of the left central incisor *(arrow)*, where the osteoblastic phase of the condition is evident. (Courtesy of Dr Lane Thompson, Loma Linda University, California.)

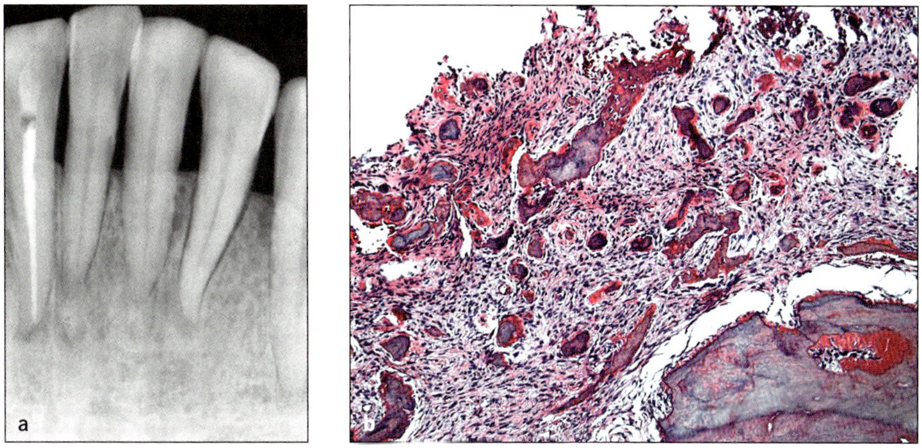

Fig 4-19 *(a)* Periapical radiograph of the mandibular incisors showing periapical cemento-osseous dysplasia involving the left lateral incisor, which has been treated with root canal therapy due to the misinterpretation of the periapical radiolucency as periapical pathology of endodontic origin. The osteoblastic phase of the condition is more evident apical to the rest of the incisors. *(b)* Histomorphologic examination of the tissue curetted from the apical region of the mandibular central incisors showing fragments of osteoid/woven bone, some of which exhibit resting lines and the majority of which demonstrate well-preserved evidence of osteoblastic rimming. The bone is supported by dense fibrocollagenous connective tissue (h&e stain; original magnification ×20).

extramedullary form with a well-documented predilection for the head and neck area.[256–258] Plasmacytoma may rarely be confused with a periapical lesion of endodontic origin, but biopsy of the tissue, usually in a lesion that fails to respond positively to root canal therapy, showing a monoclonal plasma cell infiltrate confirms the diagnosis[259] (Fig 4-16). Prolonged follow-up of these patients is of extreme importance because plasmacytomas often evolve to full-blown multiple myeloma.

Bone pathology

Several entities within this category may present as periapical pathologies. Benign fibro-osseous lesions constitute a group of neoplastic, reactive, and metabolic lesions; among this group, central cementifying ossifying fibroma (COF) and osseous dysplasia (OD) are probably the most likely to be mistaken for periapical pathology. COF is a true benign tumor of bone that is usually characterized by a well-demarcated radiolucency, radiopacity, or mixed lesion, depending on the time of discovery and examination. OD encompasses a group of reactive, non-neoplastic lesions; within this group, periapical cemento-osseous dysplasia is probably the most significant, especially because the lesions, seen apical to the mandibular incisors, are known to occur initially as osteolytic and subsequently demonstrate opacity with time. Failure to confirm the vitality status of these teeth may lead to false and unjustified root canal therapy[260–266] (Fig 4-17 to 4-19). Florid cemento-osseous dysplasia is characterized by generalized radiolucencies with opacities that typically start forming at the edges of the radiolucencies and eventually become characteristically seen throughout various proportions of the maxillary and mandibular jaw quadrants. During the lytic stages, these lesions may also be confused with periapical pathosis. Isolated cases of osteoblastoma, another benign bone tumor being misdiagnosed as periapical pathosis, are also reported.[267,268] Among other entities described, periapical infection, which is often accompanied by focal widening of the PDL and pain, may rarely lead to profound delay in the diagnosis of an osteogenic sarcoma of the jaw, a serious malignant bone tumor of the jaw that is typically painful and presents with some similarity in radiographic imaging characteristics.[269]

Other rare related disorders

Other isolated reports of rare entities presenting as periapical pathosis include nonspecific granulomatous diseases and foreign body–induced[193,270–272] as well as infectious granulomatous diseases such as *Mycobacterium tuberculosis*, aspergillosis, and histoplasmosis.[193,273] Actinomycotic colonies, most often introduced intraosseously through dental procedures, may also elicit a similar granulomatous reaction.[274–276] Inflammatory sinus conditions and a rare report of respiratory epithelial adenamatoid hamartoma and Rosai-Dorfman disease of the maxillary sinus may also be mistaken for a lesion of endodontic origin.[277–279]

Acknowledgment

The author expresses sincere gratitude and appreciation for the help and support of Mrs Carmelita Metz, administrative coordinator for the Department of Pathology, Oregon Health & Science University, School of Dentistry.

References

1. Aas JA, Griffen AL, Dardis SR, et al. Bacteria of dental caries in primary and permanent teeth in children and young adults. J Clin Microbiol 2008;46:1407–1417.
2. Loesche WJ. Microbiology of dental decay and periodontal disease. In: Baron S (ed). Medical Microbiology, ed 4. Galveston, TX: University of Texas Medical Branch, Department of Microbiology, 1997:1–45.
3. Matsuguchi T, Musikacharoen T, Ogawa T, Yoshikai Y. Gene expressions of Toll-like receptor 2, but not Toll-like receptor 4, is induced by LPS and inflammatory cytokines in mouse macrophages. J Immunol 2000;165:5767–5772.
4. Almansa Ruiz JC, Bosman AM, Steenkamp G. Bacterial profile of necrotic pulps in cheetah (acinonyx jubatus) canine teeth. J Zoo Wildl Med 2016;47:98–105.
5. Bergenholtz G. Evidence for bacterial causation of adverse pulpal responses in resin-based dental restorations. Crit Rev Oral Biol Med 2000;11:467–480.
6. Bergenholtz G, Lindhe J. Effect of soluble plaque factors on inflammatory reactions in the dental pulp. Scand J Dent Res 1975;83:153–158.
7. Bergenholtz G, Warfvinge J. Migration of leukocytes in dental pulp in response to plaque bacteria. Scand J Dent Res 1982;90:354–362.
8. Warfvinge J. Dental pulp inflammation: Experimental studies in human and monkey teeth. Swed Dent J Suppl 1986;39:1–36.
9. Hahn CL, Liewehr FR. Update on the adaptive immune responses of the dental pulp. J Endod 2007;33:773–781.
10. Hahn CL, Liewehr FR. Innate immune responses of the dental pulp to caries. J Endod 2007;3:643–651.
11. Hahn CL, Liewehr FR. Relationships between caries bacteria, host responses, and clinical signs and symptoms of pulpitis. J Endod 2007;33:213–219.
12. van Houte J, Lopman J, Kent R. The final pH of bacteria comprising the predominant flora on sound and carious human root and enamel surfaces. J Dent Res 1996;75:1008–1014.
13. Loesche WJ, Syed SA. The predominant cultivable flora of carious plaque and carious dentine. Caries Res 1973;3:201–216.
14. Bowden GH, Ekstrand J, McNaughton B, Challacombe SJ. Association of selected bacteria with the lesions of root surface caries. Oral Microbiol Immunol 1990;5:346–351.
15. Love RM, McMillan MD, Jenkinson HF. Invasion of dentinal tubules by oral streptococci is associated with collagen recognition mediated by the antigen I/II family of polypeptides. Infect Immun 1997;65:5157–5164.
16. McGrady JA, Butcher WG, Beighton D, Switalski LM. Specific and charge interactions mediate collagen recognition by oral lactobacilli. J Dent Res 1995;74: 649–657.
17. Tjäderhane L, Larjava H, Sorsa T, Uitto VJ, Larmas M, Salo T. The activation and function of host matrix metalloproteinases in dentin matrix breakdown in caries lesions. J Dent Res 1998;77:1622–1629.
18. Goldberg M, Lacerda-Pinheiro S, Six N, et al. Inflammatory and immunological aspects of dental pulp repair. Pharmacol Res 2008;58:137–147.
19. Lesot H, Bègue-Kirn C, Kübler MD, Meyer JM, Smith AJ, Cassidy N. Experimental induction of odontoblast differentiation and stimulation during reparative processes. Cell Mater 1993;3:201–217.
20. Adamkiewicz VW, Pekovic DD. Experimental pulpal Arthus allergy. Oral Surg Oral Med Oral Pathol 1980;50:450–456.
21. Bergenholtz G, Ahlstedt S, Lindhe J. Experimental pulpitis in immunized monkeys. Scand J Dent Res 1977;85:396–406.
22. Trowbridge H, Daniels T. Abnormal immune response to infection of the dental pulp. Report of a case. Oral Surg Oral Med Oral Pathol 1977;43:902–909.
23. Van Hassel HJ. Physiology of the human dental pulp. Oral Surg Oral Med Oral Pathol Oral Radiol 1971;32:126–134.
24. Tønder KJ. Vascular reactions in the dental pulp during inflammation. Acta Odontol Scand 1983;41:247–256.
25. Kakehashi S, Stanley HR, Fitzgerald RJ. The effects of surgical exposures of dental pulps in germfree and conventional laboratory rats. J South Calif State Dent Assoc 1966;34:449–451.
26. Siqueira JF Jr, Fouad AF. Endodontic microbiology. In: Torabinejad M, Fouad AF, Walton RE (eds). Endodontics: Principles and Practice, ed 5. Philadelphia: Saunders, 2014:37–48.
27. Byström A, Sundqvist G. Bacteriologic evaluation of the efficacy of mechanical root canal instrumentation in endodontic therapy. Scand J Dent Res 1981; 89:321–328.
28. Siqueira JF Jr, Rôças IN. Exploiting molecular methods to explore endodontic infections: Part 2—Redefining the endodontic microbiota. J Endod 2005;31:488–498.
29. Siqueira JF Jr, Rôças IN. Diversity of endodontic microbiota revisited. J Dent Res 2009;88:969–981.
30. Ribeiro AC, Matarazzo F, Faveri M, Zezell DM, Mayer MP. Exploring bacterial diversity of endodontic microbiota by cloning and sequencing 16S rRNA. J Endod 2011;37:922–926.
31. Nair PN. Pathogenesis of apical periodontitis and the causes of endodontic failures. Crit Rev Oral Biol Med 2004;15:348–381.
32. Kettering JD, Torabinejad M. Presence of natural killer cells in human chronic periapical lesions. Int Endod J 1993;26:344–347.
33. Wallstrom JB, Torabinejad M, Kettering J, McMillan P. Role of T cells in the pathogenesis of periapical lesions. A preliminary report. Oral Surg Oral Med Oral Pathol 1993;76:213–218.
34. Torabinejad M, Kettering JD. Identification and relative concentration of B and T lymphocytes in human chronic periapical lesions. J Endod 1985;11:122–125.
35. Abbott PV. The periapical space—A dynamic interface. Aust Endod J 2002;28: 96–107.
36. Kakeshi S, Stanley HR, Fitzgerald RJ. The effects of surgical exposures of dental pulps in germ-free and conventional laboratory rats. Oral Surg Oral Med Oral Pathol 1965;20:340–349.

37. Moller AJR, Fabricius L, Dahlen G, Ohman AE, Heyden G. Influence on periapical tissues of indigenous oral bacteria and necrotic pulp tissue in monkeys. Scand J Dent Res 1981;89:475–484.
38. Sundqvist G, Johansson E, Sjögren U. Prevalence of black-pigmented *Bacteroides* species in root canal infections. J Endod 1989;15:13–19.
39. Waltimo T, Kuusinen M, Järvensivu A, et al. Examination on *Candida* spp. in refractory periapical granulomas. Int Endod J 2003;36:643–647.
40. Sen BH, Piskin B, Demirci T. Observation of bacteria and fungi in infected root canals and dentinal tubules by SEM. Endod Dent Traumatol 1995;11:6–9.
41. Glick M, Cleveland DB, Slaking LM, Alfaro-Miranda M, Fielding AF. Intraoral cytomegalovirus lesion and HIV-associated periodontitis in a patient with acquired immunodeficiency syndrome. Oral Surg Oral Med Oral Pathol 1991;72:716–720.
42. Kabak SL, Kabak YS, Anischenko SL. Light microscopic study of periapical lesions associated with asymptomatic apical periodontitis. Ann Anat 2005;187:185–194.
43. Hojo S, Komatsu M, Okuda R, Takahashi N, Yamada T. Acid profiles and pH of carious dentin in active and arrested lesions. J Dent Res 1994;73:1853–1857.
44. Panopoulos P, Mejare B, Edwall L. Effects of ammonia and organic acids on the intradental sensory nerve activity. Acta Odontol Scand 1983;41:209–215.
45. Hahn CL, Falkler WA Jr. Correlation between thermal sensitivity and microorganisms isolated from deep caries. J Endod 1993;19:26–30.
46. Hogg SD, Whiley RA, De Soet JJ. Occurrence of lipoteichoic acid in oral streptococci. Int J Syst Bacteriol 1997;47:62–66.
47. Jacques NA, Hardy L, Knox KW, Wicken AJ. Effect of growth conditions on the formation of extracellular lipoteichoic acid by streptococcus mutans BHT. Infect Immun 1979;25:75–84.
48. Hahn CL, Falkler WA Jr. Correlation between thermal sensitivity and microorganisms isolated from deep caries. J Endod 1993;19:26–30.
49. Khabbaz MG, Anastasiadis PL, Sykaras SN. Determination of endotoxins in caries: Association with pulpal pain. Int Endod J 2000;33:132–137.
50. Bjornson HS. Activation of Hageman factor by lipopolysaccharides of *Bacteroides fragilis, Bacteroides vulgatus* and *Fusobacterium mortiferum.* Rev Infect Dis 1984;6:30–33.
51. Miller RL, Webster ME, Melmon KL. Interaction of leukocytes and endotoxin with the plasmin and kinin systems. Eur J Pharmacol 1975;33:53–60.
52. Yoshimura A, Lien E, Ingalls RR, Tuomanen E, Dziarski R, Golenbock D. Cutting edge: Recognition of gram-positive bacterial cell wall components by the innate immune system occurs via Toll-like receptor 2. J Immunol 1999;163:1–5.
53. Dziarski R, Tapping RI, Tobias PS. Binding of bacterial peptidoglycan to CD14. J Biol Chem 1998;273:8680–8690.
54. Henderson B, Wilson M. Cytokine induction by bacteria: Beyond lipopolysaccharide. Cytokine 1996;8:269–282.
55. Ginsburg I. Role of lipoteichoic acid in infection and inflammation. Lancet Infect Dis 2002;2:171–179.
56. Nair PNR. Apical periodontitis: A dynamic encounter between root canal infection and host response. Periodontol 2000 1997;13:121–148.
57. World Health Organization. Application of the International Classification of Diseases to Dentistry and Stomatology, ed 3. Geneva: World Health Organization, 1995;66–67.
58. Torabinejad M, Shabahang S. Pulp and periapical pathosis. In: Torabinejad M, Fouad A, Walton RE (eds). Endodontics: Principles and Practice, ed 5. Philadelphia: Saunders, 2014.
59. Morse DR, Seltzer S, Sinai I, Biron G. Classification. J Am Dent Assoc 1977; 94:685–689.
60. Eriksen HM. Endodontology—Epidemiologic considerations. Endod Dent Traumatol 1991;7:189–195.
61. Sullivan M, Gallagher G, Noonan V. The root of the problem: Occurrence of typical and atypical periapical pathoses. J Am Dent Assoc 2016;147:646–649.
62. Koivisto T, Bowles WR, Rohrer M. Frequency and distribution of radiolucent jaw lesions: A retrospective analysis of 9,723 cases. J Endod 2012;38:729–732.
63. Scheinfeld MH, Shifteh K, Avery LL, Dym H, Dym RJ. Teeth: What radiologists should know. Radiographics 2012;32:1927–1944.
64. Trowbridge HO. Pathogenesis of pulpitis resulting from dental caries. J Endod 1981;7:52–60.
65. Siqueira JF Jr, Rôças IN. Microbiology and treatment of acute apical abscesses. Clin Microbiol Rev 2013;26:255–273.
66. Sasaki H, Stashenko P. Interrelationship of the pulp and apical periodontitis. In: Hargreaves KM, Goodis HE, Tay FR (eds). Seltzer and Bender's Dental Pulp, ed 2. Chicago, IL: Quintessence, 2012:277–299.
67. Baumgartner JC, Siqueira JF Jr, Sedgley CM, Kishen A. Microbiology of endodontic disease. In: Ingle JI, Bakland LK, Baumgartner JC (eds). Ingle's Endodontics, ed 6. Hamilton, ON: BC Decker, 2008:221–308.
68. Marcus BJ, Kaplan J, Collins KA. A case of Ludwig angina: A case report and review of the literature. Am J Forensic Med Pathol 2008;29:255–259.
69. Boscolo-Rizzo P, Da Mosto MC. Submandibular space infection: A potentially lethal infection. Int J Infect Dis 2009;13:327–333.
70. Larawin V, Naipao J, Dubey SP. Head and neck space infections. Otolaryngol Head Neck Surg 2006;135:889–893.
71. Ogundiya DA, Keith DA, Mirowski J. Cavernous sinus thrombosis and blindness as complications of an odontogenic infection: Report of a case and review of literature. J Oral Maxillofac Surg 1989;47:1317–1321.
72. Corson MA, Postlethwaite KP, Seymour RA. Are dental infections a cause of brain abscess? Case report and review of the literature. Oral Dis 2001;7:61–65.
73. Marques DA, Silva R, Caugant DA, Josefsen R, Tronstad L, Olsen I. Characterization of streptococcus constellatus strains recovered from a brain abscess and periodontal pockets in an immunocompromised patient. J Periodontol 2004; 75:1720–1723.
74. Daramola OO, Flanagan CE, Maisel RH, Odland RM. Diagnosis and treatment of deep neck space abscesses. Otolaryngol Head Neck Surg 2009;141:123–130.
75. Huang TT, Tseng FY, Liu TC, Hsu CJ, Chen YS. Deep neck infection in diabetic patients: Comparison of clinical picture and outcomes with nondiabetic patients. Otolaryngol Head Neck Surg 2005;132:943–947.
76. Stoykewych AA, Beecroft WA, Cogan AG. Fatal necrotizing fasciitis of dental origin. J Can Dent Assoc 1992;58:59–62.
77. Tung-Yiu W, Jehn-Shyun H, Ching-Hung C, Hung-An C. Cervical necrotizing fasciitis of odontogenic origin: A report of 11 cases. J Oral Maxillofac Surg 2000; 58:1347–1352.
78. Umeda M, Minamikawa T, Komatsubara H, Shibuya Y, Yokoo S, Komori T. Necrotizing fasciitis caused by dental infection: A retrospective analysis of 9 cases and a review of the literature. Oral Surg Oral Med Oral Pathol Oral Radiol Endod 2003; 95:283–290.
79. Udaondo P, Garcia-Delpech S, Diaz-Llopis M, Salom D, Garcia-Pous M, Strottmann JM. Bilateral intraorbital abscesses and cavernous sinus thromboses secondary to streptococcus milleri with a favorable outcome. Ophthal Plast Reconstr Surg 2008;24:408–410.
80. Kim IK, Kim JR, Jang KS, Moon YS, Park SW. Orbital abscess from an odontogenic infection. Oral Surg Oral Med Oral Pathol Oral Radiol Endod 2007;103:e1–e6.
81. Koch F, Breil P, Marroquin BB, Gawehn J, Kunkel M. Abscess of the orbit arising 48 h after root canal treatment of a maxillary first molar. Int Endod J 2006;39: 657–664.
82. Stashenko P, Teles R, D'Souza R. Periapical inflammatory responses and their modulation. Crit Rev Oral Biol Med 1998;9:498–521.
83. Torabinejad M, Clagget J, Engel D. A cat model for evaluation of mechanism of bone resorption: Induction of bone loss by stimulated immune complexes and inhibition by indomethacin. Calcif Tissue Int 1979;29:207–214.
84. Torabinejad M, Kriger RD. Experimentally induced alterations in periapical tissues of the cat. J Dent Res 1980;59:87–96.
85. Torabinejad M, Eby WC, Naidorf IJ. Inflammatory and immunological aspects of the pathogenesis of human periapical lesions. J Endod 1985;11:479–488.
86. McFarland LV, Clarridge JE, Beneda HW, Raugi GJ. Fluoroquinolone use and risk factors for clostridium difficile-associated disease within a veterans administration health care system. Clin Infect Dis 2007;45;1141–151.
87. Williams BL, McCann GF, Schoenknecht FD. Bacteriology of dental abscesses of endodontic origin. J Clin Microbiol 1983;18:770–774.
88. Brook I, Frazier EH, Gher ME. Aerobic and anaerobic microbiology of periapical abscess. Oral Microbiol Immunol 1991;6:123–125.
89. Heimdahl A, Josefsson K, von Konow L, Nord CE. Detection of anaerobic bacteria in blood cultures by lysis filtration. Eur J Clin Microbiol 1985;4:404–407.
90. Lewis MA, MacFarlane TW, McGowan DA. Quantitative bacteriology of acute dento-alveolar abscesses. J Med Microbiol 1986;21:101–104.
91. Ferreira LGV, Rosin FCP, Corrêa L. Analysis of Interleukin 17A in periapical abscess and granuloma lesions [published online 28 March 2016]. Braz Oral Res 2016;30:e34.
92. Jäger A, Kuchroo VK. Effector and regulatory T-cell subsets in autoimmunity and tissue inflammation. Scand J Immunol 2010;72:173–184.
93. Oseko F, Yamamoto T, Akamatsu Y, Kanamura N, Iwakura Y, Imanishi J, Kita M. IL-17 is involved in bone resorption in mouse periapical lesions. Microbiol Immunol 2009;53:287–294.
94. Colić M, Vasilijić S, Gazivoda D, Vucević D, Marjanović M, Lukić A. Interleukin-17 plays a role in exacerbation of inflammation within chronic periapical lesions. Eur J Oral Sci 2007;115:315–320.
95. Marçal JR, Samuel RO, Fernandes D, et al. T-helper cell type 7/regulatory T-cell immunoregulatory balance in human radicular cysts and periapical granulomas. J Endod 2010;36:995–999.

96. Lewis MA, Carmichael F, MacFarlane TW, Milligan SG. A randomised trial of co-amoxiclav (augmentin) versus penicillin V in the treatment of acute dentoalveolar abscess. Br Dent J 1993;175:169–174.
97. Kuriyama T, Absi EG, Williams DW, Lewis MA. An outcome audit of the treatment of acute dentoalveolar infection: Impact of penicillin resistance. Br Dent J 2005;25:759–763.
98. Khemaleelakul S, Baumgartner JC, Pruksakorn S. Identification of bacteria in acute endodontic infections and their antimicrobial susceptibility. Oral Surg Oral Med Oral Pathol Oral Radiol Endod 2002;94:746–755.
99. Baumgartner JC, Xia T. Antibiotic susceptibility of bacteria associated with endodontic abscesses. J Endod 2003;29:44–47.
100. Jacinto RC, Gomes BP, Ferraz CC, Zaia AA, Filho FJ. Microbiological analysis of infected root canals from symptomatic and asymptomatic teeth with periapical periodontitis and the antimicrobial susceptibility of some isolated anaerobic bacteria. Oral Microbiol Immunol 2003;18:285–292.
101. Kuriyama T, Williams DW, Yanagisawa M, et al. Antimicrobial susceptibility of 800 anaerobic isolates from patients with dentoalveolar infection to 13 oral antibiotics. Oral Microbiol Immunol 2007;22:285–288.
102. Flynn TR. What are the antibiotics of choice for odontogenic infections, and how long should the treatment course last? Oral Maxillofac Surg Clin North Am 2011;23:519–536.
103. Lakhssassi N, Elhajoui N, Lodter JP, Pineill JL, Sixou M. Antimicrobial susceptibility variation of 50 anaerobic periopathogens in aggressive periodontitis: An interindividual variability study. Oral Microbiol Immunol 2005;20:244–252.
104. Gilmore WC, Jacobus NV, Gorbach SL, Doku HC, Tally FP. A prospective double-blind evaluation of penicillin versus clindamycin in the treatment of odontogenic infections. J Oral Maxillofac Surg 1988;46:1065–1070.
105. von Konow L, Kondell PA, Nord CE, Heimdahl A. Clindamycin versus phenoxymethylpenicillin in the treatment of acute orofacial infections. Eur J Clin Microbiol Infect Dis 1992;11:1129–1135.
106. Takahashi K. Microbiological, pathological, inflammatory, immunological and molecular biological aspects of periradicular disease. Int Endod J 1998;31:311–325.
107. Škaljac-Staudt G, Galić N, Katunarić M, Ciglar I, Katanec D. Immunonopathogenesis of chronic periapical lesions. Acta Stomat Croat 2001;35:127–131.
108. Torabinejad M, Bakland LK. Immunopathogenesis of chronic periapical lesions. A review. Oral Surg Oral Med Oral Pathol 1978;46:685–699.
109. de Jong EC, Smits HH, Kapsenberg ML. Dendritic cell-mediated T cell polarization. Springer Semin Immunopathol 2005;26:289–307.
110. McGeachy MJ, Cua DJ. Th17 cell differentiation: The long and winding road. Immunity 2008;28:445–453.
111. Akamine A, Anan H, Hamachi T, Maeda K. A histochemical study of the behavior of macrophages during experimental apical periodontitis in rats. J Endod 1994; 20:474–478.
112. Kawashima N, Stashenko P. Expression of bone-resorptive and regulatory cytokines in murine periapical inflammation. Arch Oral Biol 1999;44:55–66.
113. Nijweide PJ, De Grooth R. Ontogeny of the osteoclast. In: Rifkin BR, Gay CV (eds). Biology and Physiology of the Osteoclast. Boca Raton, FL: CRC, 1992;81–104.
114. Artese L, Piattelli A, Quaranta M, Colasante A, Musiani P. Immunoreactivity for interleukin 1-beta and tumor necrosis factor-alpha and ultrastructural features of monocytes/macrophages in periapical granulomas. J Endod 1991;17:483–487.
115. Safavi KE, Rossomando ER. Tumor necrosis factor identified in periapical tissue exudates of teeth with apical periodontitis. J Endod 1991;17:12–14
116. Ataoğlu T, Ungör M, Serpek B, Haliloğlu S, Ataoğlu H, Ari H. Interleukin-1beta and tumour necrosis factor-alpha levels in periapical exudates. Int Endod J 2002; 35:181–185.
117. Barkhordar RA, Hussain MZ, Hayashi C. Detection of interleukin-1 beta in human periapical lesions. Oral Surg Oral Med Oral Pathol 1992;73:334–336.
118. Lim CG, Torabinejad M, Kettering J, Linkhardt TA, Finkelman RD. Interleukin 1-beta in symptomatic and asymptomatic human periradicular lesions. J Endod 1994;20:225–227.
119. Matsuo T, Ebisu S, Nakanishi T, Yonemura K, Harada Y, Okada H. Interleukin-1 alpha and interleukin-1 beta periapical exudates of infected root canals: Correlations with the clinical findings of the involved teeth. J Endod 1994;20:432–435.
120. Čolić M, Gazivoda D, Vučević D, Vasilijić S, Rudolf R, Lukić A. Proinflammatory and immunoregulatory mechanisms in periapical lesions. Mol Immunol 2009;47: 101–113.
121. Eversole LR. Clinical Outline of Oral Pathology: Diagnosis and Treatment, ed 4. Shelton, CT: People's Medical, 2011:173.
122. Neville BW, Damm DD, Allen CM, Chi AC. Pulpal and Periapical Disease. In: Neville BW, Damm DD, Allen CM, Chi AC. Oral and Maxillofacial Pathology, ed 4. Philadelphia: Saunders, 2015:111–136.
123. Gill Y, Scully C. Orofacial odontogenic infections: Review of microbiology and current treatment. Oral Surg Oral Med Oral Pathol 1990;70:155–158.
124. Gemmell E, Carter CL, Hart DN, Drysdale KE, Seymour GJ. Antigen-presenting cells in human periodontal disease tissues. Oral Microbiol Immunol 2002;17:388–393.
125. Muglali M, Komerik N, Bulut E, Yarim GF, Celebi N, Sumer M. Cytokine and chemokine levels in radicular and residual cyst fluids. J Oral Pathol Med 2008; 37:185–189.
126. Nonaka CF, Maia AP, Nascimento GJ, de Almeida Freitas R, Batista de Souza L, Galvão HC. Immunoexpression of vascular endothelial growth factor in periapical granulomas, radicular cysts, and residual radicular cysts. Oral Surg Oral Med Oral Pathol Oral Radiol Endod 2008;106;896–902.
127. Costa Neto H, de Andrade ALDL, Gordon-Nunez MA, de Freitas RA, Galvao HC. Immunoexpression of tryptasepositive mast cells in periapical granulomas and radicular cysts. Int Endod J 2015;48:729–735.
128. Andrade AL, Nonaka CF, Gordón-Núñez MA, Freitas Rde A, Galvão HC. Immunoexpression of interleukin 17, transforming growth factor β1, and forkhead box P3 in periapical granulomas, radicular cysts, and residual radicular cysts. J Endod 2013;39:990–994.
129. Gruber BL, Kew RR, Jelaska A, et al. Human mast cells activate fibroblasts: Tryptase is a fibrogenic factor stimulating collagen messenger ribonucleic acid synthesis and fibroblast chemotaxis. J Immunol 1997;158:2310–2317.
130. Thomas VA, Wheeless CJ, Stack MS, Johnson DA. Human mast cell tryptase fibrinogenolysis: Kinetics, anticoagulation.mechanism, and cell adhesion disruption. Biochemistry 1998;37:2291–2298.
131. Santos PP, Nonaka CF, Pinto LP, de Souza LB. Immunohistochemical expression of mast cell tryptase in giant cell fibroma and inflammatory fibrous hyperplasia of the oral mucosa. Arch Oral Biol 2011;56:231–237.
132. Rodini CO, Batista AC, Lara VS. Comparative immunohistochemical study of the presence of mast cells in apical granulomas and periapical cysts: Possible role of mast cells in the course of human periapical lesions. Oral Surg Oral Med Oral Pathol Oral Radiol Endod 2004;97:59–63.
133. Teronen O, Hietanen J, Lindqvist C, et al. Mast cell-derived tryptase in odontogenic cysts. J Oral Pathol Med 1996;25:376–381.
134. Sciuba J, Fantasia J, Kahn L, Armed Forces Institute of Pathology (US), Universities Associated for Research and Education in Pathology. Tumors and Cysts of the Jaws, series 3, Atlas of Tumors Pathology. Washington, DC: Armed Forces Institute of Pathology, 2001:15–47.
135. Matthews JB, Browne RM. An immunocytochemical study of the inflammatory cell infiltrate and epithelial expression of HLA-DR in odontogenic cysts. J Oral Pathol 1987;16:112–117.
136. Rushton MA. Hyaline bodies in the epithelium of dental cysts. Proc R Soc Med 1955;48:407–409.
137. Nair PN. On the causes of persistent apical periodontitis: A review. Int Endod J 2006;39:249–281.
138. Nair PNR, Pajarola G, Luder HU. Ciliated epithelium-lined radicular cysts. Oral Surg Oral Med Oral Pathol Oral Radiol Endod 2002;94:485–493.
139. Nair PNR, Sjögren U, Figdor D, Sundqvist G. Persistent periapical radiolucencies of root-filled human teeth, failed endodontic treatments, and periapical scars. Oral Surg Oral Med Oral Pathol Oral Radiol Endod 1999;87:617–627.
140. Nair PNR. New perspectives on radicular cysts: Do they heal? Int Endod J 1998; 31:155–160.
141. Nair PNR. Pathology of apical periodontitis. In: Ørstavik D, Pitt FTR (eds). Essential Endodontology: Prevention and Treatment of Apical Periodontitis. Oxford: Blackwell, 1998:68–105.
142. Simon JHS. Incidence of periapical cysts in relation to the root canal. J Endod 1990;6:845–848.
143. Simon JHS, Chimenti Z, Mintz G. Clinical significance of the pulse granuloma. J Endod 1982;8:116–119.
144. Sonnabend E, Oh CS. Zur frage des epithels im apikalen. Granulationsgewebe (granulom) menschlicher zähne. Dtsch Zahnärztl Z 1996;21:627–643.
145. Shear M, Seward GR. Cysts of the Oral Regions, ed 3. London: Butterworth-Heinemann, 1992.
146. Daley TD, Wysocki GP, Pringle GA. Relative incidence of odontogenic tumors and oral and jaw cysts in a Canadian population. Oral Surg Oral Med Oral Pathol 1994;77:276–280.
147. Thoma KH (ed). Oral Roentgenology: A Roentgen Study of the Anatomy and Pathology of the Oral Cavity. Boston: Ritter, 1917:136–137.
148. Gardner DG. Residual cysts. Oral Surg Oral Med Oral Pathol Oral Radiol Endod 1997;84:114–115.
149. Gardner DG, Sapp JP, Wysocki GP. Odontogenic and "fissural" cysts of the jaws. Pathol Annu 1978;13:177–200.

150. Shear M. Cholesterol in dental cysts. Oral Surg Oral Med Oral Pathol 1963; 16:1465–1473.
151. Shear M. Cysts of the jaws: Recent advances. J Oral Pathol 1985;14:43–59.
152. Shear M, Altini M. Odontogenic and non-odontogenic cysts of the jaws. J Dent Assoc S Afr 1983;38:555–564.
153. Main DM. Epithelial jaw cysts: A clinicopathological reappraisal. Br J Oral Surg 1970;8:114–125.
154. Ten Cate AR. The epithelial cell rests of Malassez and the genesis of the dental cyst. Oral Surg Oral Med Oral Pathol 1972;34:956–964.
155. Torabinejad M, Theofilopoulos AN, Ketering JD, Bakland LK. Quantitation of circulating immune complexes, immunoglobulins G and M, and C3 complement component in patients with large periapical lesions. Oral Surg Oral Med Oral Pathol 1983;55:186–190.
156. Torabinejad M. The role of immunological reactions in apical cyst formation and the fate of epithelial cells after root canal therapy: A theory. Int J Oral Surg 1983;12:14–22.
157. Malassez I. Noe sur la pathologie des kystes dentaires dites periostiques. J Conn Med Prat (Paris) 1884;7:98–16.
158. Thesleff I. Epithelial cell rests of Malassez bind epidermal growth factor intensely. J Periodontal Res 1987;22:419–421.
159. Gao Z, Flaitz CM, Mackenzie IC. Expression of keratinocyte growth factor in periapical lesions. J Dent Res 1996;75:1658–1663.
160. Lin LM, Wang SL, Wu-Wang C, Chang KM, Leung C. Detection of epidermal growth factor in inflammatory periapical lesions. Int Endod J 1996;29:179–84.
161. James WW. Do epithelial odontomes increase in size by their own tension? Proc R Soc Med 1926;19:73–77.
162. Toller PA. Experimental investigations into factors concerning the growth of cysts of the jaw. Proc R Soc Med 1948;41:681–688.
163. Toller PA. The osmolarity of fluids from cysts of the jaws. Br Dent J 1970;29:275–278.
164. Harris M, Goldhaber P. The production of a bone resorbing factor by dental cysts in vitro. Br J Oral Surg 1973;10:334–338.
165. Harris M, Jenkins MV, Bennett A, Wills MR. Prostaglandin production and bone resorption by dental cysts. Nature 1973;145:213–215.
166. Brunette DM, Heersche JN, Purdon AD, Sodek J, Moe HK, Assuras JN. In vitro cultural parameters and protein and prostaglandin secretion of epithelial cells derived from porcine rests of Malassez. Arch Oral Biol 1979;24:199–203.
167. Birek C, Heersche D, Jez D, Brunette DM. Secretion of bone resorbing factor by epithelial cells cultured from porcine rests of Malassez. J Periodontal Res 1983;18:75–81.
168. Teronen O, Salo T, Laitinen J, et al. Characterization of interstitial collagenases in jaw cyst wall. Eur J Oral Sci 1995;103:141–147.
169. Bernardi L, Visioli F, Nör C, Rados PV. Radicular cyst: An update of the biological factors related to lining epithelium. J Endod 2015;41:1951–1961.
170. Güler N, Comunoğlu N, Cabbar F. Ki-67 and MCM-2 in dental follicle and odontogenic cysts: The effects of inflammation on proliferative markers. ScientificWorldJournal 2012;2012:946060.
171. Gadbail AR, Chaudhary M, Patil S, Gawande M. Actual proliferating index and p53 protein expression as prognostic marker in odontogenic cysts. Oral Dis 2009;15: 490–498.
172. Shahela T, Aesha S, Ranganathan K, et al. Immunohistochemical expression of PCNA in epithelial linings of selected odontogenic lesions. J Clin Diagn Res 2013;7:2615–2618.
173. Tekkesin MS, Mutlu S, Olgac V. Expressions of bax, bcl-2 and Ki-67 in odontogenic keratocysts (keratocystic odontogenic tumor) in comparison with ameloblastomas and radicular cysts. Turk Patoloji Derg 2012;28:49–55.
174. Singh HP, Shetty DC, Wadhwan V, Aggarwal P. A quantitative and qualitative comparative analysis of collagen fibers to determine the role of connective tissue stroma on biological behavior of odontogenic cysts: A histochemical study. Natl J Maxillofac Surg 2012;3:15–20.
175. Vij R, Vij H, Rao NN. Evaluation of collagen in connective tissue walls of odontogenic cysts—A histochemical study. J Oral Pathol Med 2011;40:257–262.
176. Tsuneki M, Cheng J, Maruyama S, Ida-Yonemochi H, Nakajima M, Saku T. Perlecan-rich epithelial linings as a background of proliferative potentials of keratocystic odontogenic tumor. J Oral Pathol Med 2008;37:287–293.
177. Lima AC, Fregnani ER, Silva-Sousa YT, da Cruz Perez DE. Parathyroid hormone/parathyroid hormone-related peptide receptor 1 expression in odontogenic cystic lesions. Int Endod J 2012;45:209–214.
178. de Moraes M, de Lucena HF, de Azevedo PR, Queiroz LM, Costa Ade L. Comparative immunohistochemical expression of RANK, RANKL and OPG in radicular and dentigerous cysts. Arch Oral Biol 2011;56:1256–1263.
179. Tekkesin MS, Mutlu S, Olgac V. The role of RANK/RANKL/OPG signalling pathways in osteoclastogenesis in odontogenic keratocysts, radicular cysts, and ameloblastomas. Head Neck Pathol 2011;5:248–253.
180. Kusafuka K, Sasaguri K, Sato S, Takemura T, Kameya T. Runx2 expression is associated with pathologic new bone formation around radicular cysts: An immunohistochemical demonstration. J Oral Pathol Med 2006;35:492–499.
181. Bando Y, Henderson B, Meghji S, Poole S, Harris M. Immunocytochemical localization of inflammatory cytokines and vascular adhesion receptors in radicular cysts. J Oral Pathol Med 1993;22:221–227.
182. Kubota Y, Ninomiya T, Oka S, Takenoshita Y, Shirasuna K. Interleukin-1alpha-dependent regulation of matrix metalloproteinase-9 (MMP-9) secretion and activation in the epithelial cells of odontogenic jaw cysts. J Dent Res 2000;79:1423–1330.
183. Honma M, Hayakawa Y, Kosugi H, Koizumi F. Localization of mRNA for inflammatory cytokines in radicular cyst tissue by in situ hybridization, and induction of inflammatory cytokines by human gingival fibroblasts in response to radicular cyst contents. J Oral Pathol Med 1998;27:399–404.
184. Bhaskar SN. Oral surgery–oral pathology conference No. 17, Walter Reed Army Medical Center. Periapical lesions—Types, incidence, and clinical features. Oral Surg Oral Med Oral Pathol 1966;21:657–671.
185. Seltzer S, Bender IB, Smith J, Freedman I, Nazimov H. Endodontic failures—An analysis based on clinical, roentgenographic, and histologic findings. Oral Surg Oral Med Oral Pathol 1967;23:517–530.
186. Nair PN. Cholesterol as an aetiological agent in endodontic failures—A review. Aust Endod J 1999;25:19-26.
187. Nair PN, Sjögren U, Figdor D, Sundqvist G. Persistent periapical radiolucencies of root-filled human teeth, failed endodontic treatments, and periapical scars. Oral Surg Oral Med Oral Pathol Oral Radiol Endod 1999;87:617–627.
188. García CC, Sempere FV, Diago MP, Bowen EM. The post-endodontic periapical lesion: Histologic and etiopathogenic aspects. Med Oral Patol Oral Cir Bucal 2007;1:585–590.
189. Nobuhara WK, del Rio CE. Incidence of periradicular pathoses in endodontic treatment failures. J Endod 1993;19:315–318.
190. Liapatas S, Nakou M, Rontogianni D. Inflammatory infiltrate of chronic periradicular lesions: An immunohistochemical study. Int Endod J 2003;36:464–471.
191. Dahl EC. Diagnosing inflammatory and non-inflammatory periapical disease. J Indiana Dent Assoc 1991:22–26.
192. Abbot PV. The periapical space—A dynamic interface. Aust Endod J 2002;28: 96-107.
193. Peters E, Lau M. Histopathologic examination to confirm diagnosis of periapical lesions: A review. J Can Dent Assoc 2003;69:598–600.
194. Faitaroni LA, Bueno MR, De Carvalhosa AA, Bruehmueller Ale KA, Estrela C. Ameloblastoma suggesting large apical periodontitis. J Endod 2008;34:216–219.
195. Schwartz S, Cohen S. The difficult differential diagnosis. Dent Clin North Am 1992;36:279–292.
196. Shelley AM, Rushton VE, Horner K. Canalis sinuosus mimicking a periapical inflammatory lesion. Br Dent J 1999;24:186;378–379.
197. Kontogiannis TG, Tosios KI, Kerezoudis NP, Krithinakis S, Christopoulos P, Sklavounou A. Periapical lesions are not always a sequelae of pulpal necrosis: A retrospective study of 1521 biopsies. Int Endod J 2015;48:68–73.
198. Hutchison IL, Hopper C, Coonar HS. Neoplasia masquerading as periapical infection. Br Dent J 1990;168:288–294.
199. Schlagel E, Seltzer RJ, Newman JI. Apicoectomy as an adjunct to diagnosis. N Y State Dent J 1973;29:156–158.
200. Sirotheau Corrêa Pontes F, Paiva Fonseca F, Souza de Jesus A, et al. Nonendodontic lesions misdiagnosed as apical periodontitis lesions: Series of case reports and review of literature. J Endod 2014;40:16–27.
201. de Moraes Ramos-Perez FM, Soares UN, Silva-Sousa YT, da Cruz Perez DE. Ossifying fibroma misdiagnosed as chronic apical periodontitis. J Endod 2010; 36:546–548.
202. Weisleder R, Yamauchi S, Caplan DJ, Trope M, Teixeira FB. The validity of pulp testing: A clinical study. J Am Dent Assoc 2009;140:1013–1017.
203. Oginni AO, Adekoya-Sofowora CA, Kolawole KA. Evaluation of radiographs, clinical signs and symptoms associated with pulp canal obliteration: An aid to treatment decision. Dent Traumatol 2009;25:620–625.
204. Faitaroni LA, Bueno MR, Carvalhosa AA, Mendonça EF, Estrela C. Differential diagnosis of apical periodontitis and nasopalatine duct cyst. J Endod 2011; 37:403–410.
205. Gutmann JL, Baumgartner JC, Gluskin AH, Hartwell GR, Walton RE. Identify and define all diagnostic terms for periapical/periradicular health and disease states. J Endod 2009;35:1658–1674.

206. Garlock JA, Pringle GA, Hicks ML. The odontogenic keratocyst: A potential endodontic misdiagnosis. Oral Surg Oral Med Oral Pathol Oral Radiol Endod 1998;85:452–456.
207. Cunha JF, Gomes CC, de Mesquita RA, Andrade Goulart EM, de Castro WH, Gomez RS. Clinicopathologic features associated with recurrence of the odontogenic keratocyst: A cohort retrospective analysis. Oral Surg Oral Med Oral Pathol Oral Radiol 2016;121:629–635.
208. Ortega A, Fariña V, Gallardo A, Espinoza I, Acosta S. Nonendodontic periapical lesions: A retrospective study in Chile. Int Endod J 2007;40:386–390.
209. Omoregie OF, Saheeb BD, Odukoya O, Ojo MA. A clinicopathologic correlation in the diagnosis of periradicular lesions of extracted teeth. J Oral Maxillofac Surg 2009;67:1387–1391.
210. Becconsall-Ryan K, Tong D, Love RM. Radiolucent inflammatory jaw lesions: A twenty-year analysis. Int Endod J 2010;43:859–865.
211. Neville BW, Damm DD, Allen CM, Bouquot JE. Oral Maxillofacial Pathology, ed 3. Philadelphia: Saunders, 2009.
212. Rajalakshmi R, Sreeja C, Vijayalakshmi D, Leelarani V. Orthokeratinised odontogenic cyst mimicking periapical cyst [published online 7 October 2013]. BMJ Case Rep doi:10.1136/bcr-2013-200883.
213. Said-Al-Naief N. Odontogenic tumors for general pathologists. Adv Exp Med Biol 2005;563:148–164.
214. de Carvalhosa AA, de Araújo Estrela CR, Borges AH, Guedes OA, Estrela C. 10-year follow-up of calcifying odontogenic cyst in the periapical region of vital maxillary central incisor. J Endod 2014;40:1695–1697.
215. Estrela C, Decurcio DA, Silva JA, Mendonça EF, Estrela CR. Persistent apical periodontitis associated with a calcifying odontogenic cyst. Int Endod J 2009; 42:539–545.
216. Gorlin RJ, Pinborg JJ, Clausen FP, Vickers RA. The calcifying odontogenic cyst—A possible analogue of the cutaneous calcifying epithelioma of Malherbe. Oral Surg Oral Med Oral Pathol 1962;15:1235–1243.
217. Buchner A, Merrell PW, Carpenter WM. Relative frequency of central odontogenic tumors: A study of 1,088 cases from northern California and comparison to studies from other parts of the world. J Oral Maxillofac Surg 2006;64:1343–1352.
218. Carvalhosa AA, Nunes FD, Pinto DDS Jr, Jorge WA, Cavalcanti MGP. Calcifying epithelial odontogenic cyst (Gorlin cyst): Report of a case. Histopathological and radiological correlation [in Portuguese]. RPG J Postgrad Dent Sch University São Paulo 2004;11:257–263.
219. Praetorius F, Ledesma-Montes C. Calcifying cystic odontogenic tumor. In: Barnes L, Evenson JW, Reichart P, Sidransky D (eds). World Health Organization Classification of Tumours: Pathology and Genetics—Head and Neck Tumours. Lyon, France: International Agency for Research on Cancer (IARC), 2005:313.
220. Chapelle KA, Stoelinga PJ, de Wilde PC, Brouns JJ, Voorsmit RA. Rational approach to diagnosis and treatment of ameloblastomas and odontogenic keratocysts. Br J Oral Maxillofac Surg 2004;42:381–390.
221. Faitaroni LA, Bueno MR, De Carvalhosa AA, Bruehmueller Ale KA, Estrela C. Ameloblastoma suggesting large apical periodontitis. J Endod 2008;34:216–219.
222. Kashyap B, Reddy PS, Desai RS. Plexiform ameloblastoma mimicking a periapical lesion: A diagnostic dilemma. J Conserv Dent 2012;15:84–86.
223. Sullivan M, Gallagher G, Noonan V. The root of the problem: Occurrence of typical and atypical periapical pathoses. J Am Dent Assoc 2016;147:646–649.
224. Gondak RO, Rocha AC, Neves Campos JG, et al. Unicystic ameloblastoma mimicking apical periodontitis: A case series. J Endod 2013;39:145–148.
225. Motamedi MH. Periapical ameloblastoma—A case report. Br Dent J 2002; 193:443–445.
226. Philipsen HP, Srisuwan T, Reichart PA, Philipsen HP, Srisuwan T, Reichart PA. Adenomatoid odontogenic tumor mimicking a periapical (radicular) cyst: A case report. Oral Surg Oral Med Oral Pathol Oral Radiol Endod 2002;94:246–248.
227. Batista AC, Filho HN, Rippert ET. Periapical radiolucency in the mandibular molar region. J Oral Maxillofac Surg 2002;60:186–189.
228. Cundiff EJ. Developing cementoblastoma: Case report and update of differential diagnosis. Quintessence Int 2000;31:191–195.
229. Hollows P, Fasanmade A, Hayter JP. Ameloblastoma—A diagnostic problem. Br Dent J 2000;188:243–244.
230. Curran AE, Miller EJ, Murrah VA. Adenomatoid odontogenic tumor presenting as periapical disease. Oral Surg Oral Med Oral Pathol Oral Radiol Endod 1997; 84:557–560.
231. Dahlkemper P, Wolcott JF, Pringle GA, Hicks ML. Periapical central giant cell granuloma: A potential endodontic misdiagnosis. Oral Surg Oral Med Oral Pathol Oral Radiol Endod 2000;90:739–745.
232. Nary Filho H, Matsumoto MA, Fraga SC, Gonçales ES, Sérvulo F. Periapical radiolucency mimicking an odontogenic cyst. Int Endod J 2004;37:337–344.
233. Movahedian B, Razavi SM, Hasheminia D, Rezaei M. Simultaneous maxillary and mandibular brown tumors in secondary hyperparathyroidism: A case report. Dent Res J 2008;5:41–45.
234. Spatafore CM, Griffin JA Jr, Keyes GG, Wearden S, Skidmore AE. Periapical biopsy report: An analysis of over a 10-year period. J Endod 1990;16:239–241.
235. Lee KJ, Cheng SJ, Lin SK, Chiang CP, Yu CH, Kok SH. Gingival squamous cell carcinoma mimicking a dentoalveolar abscess: Report of a case. J Endod 2007;33:177–180.
236. McClure SA, Movahed R, Salama A, Ord RA. Maxillofacial metastases: A retrospective review of one institution's 15-year experience. J Oral Maxillofac Surg 2009;71:178–188.
237. Shen ML, Kang J, Wen YL, et al. Metastatic tumors to the oral and maxillofacial region: A retrospective study of 19 cases in West China and review of the Chinese and English literature. J Oral Maxillofac Surg 2009;67:718–737.
238. Copeland RR. Carcinoma of the antrum mimicking periapical pathology of pulpal origin: A case report. J Endod 1980;6:655–656.
239. Block RM, Mark HI, Bushell A. Metastatic carcinoma of the breast mimicking periapical disease in the mandible. J Endod 1977;3:197–199.
240. Khalili M, Mahboobi N, Shams J. Metastatic breast carcinoma initially diagnosed as pulpal/periapical disease: A case report. J Endod 2010;36:922–925.
241. Burkes EJ Jr. Adenoid cystic carcinoma of the mandible masquerading as periapical inflammation. J Endod 1975;1:76–78.
242. Favia G, Maiorano E, Orsini G, Piattelli A. Central (intraosseous) adenoid cystic carcinoma of the mandible: Report of a case with periapical involvement. J Endod 2000;26:760–763.
243. Coonar HS. Primary intraosseous carcinoma of maxilla. Br Dent J 1979;17:47–48.
244. Ruskin JD, Cohen DM, Davis LF. Primary intraosseous carcinoma: Report of two cases. J Oral Maxillofac Surg 1988;46:425–432.
245. Jee A, Domboski M, Milobsky SA. Malignant fibrohistocytoma of the maxilla presenting with endodotically involved teeth. Oral Surg Oral Med Oral Pathol 1978; 45:464–469.
246. Davido N, Rigolet A, Kerner S, Gruffaz F, Boucher Y. Case of Ewing's sarcoma misdiagnosed as a periapical lesion of maxillary incisor. J Endod 2011;37:259–264.
247. Madrigal-Martınez-Pereda C, Guerrero-Rodriguez V, Guisado-Moya B, Meniz-Garcia C. Langerhans cell histiocytosis: Literature review and descriptive analysis of oral manifestations. Medicina Oral Patologia Oral Cirugia Bucal 2009;14: 222–228.
248. Ghadially FN, Erlandson RA. Case for the panel. Intranuclear Birbeck granules in Langerhans cell histiocytosis. Ultrastruct Pathol 1997;21:597–600.
249. Mierau GW. Intranuclear Birbeck granules in Langerhans cell histiocytosis. Pediatr Pathol 1994;14:1051–1054.
250. Pereira MI, Medeiros JA. Role of *Helicobacter pylori* in gastric mucosa-associated lymphoid tissue lymphomas. World J Gastroenterol 2014;20:684–698.
251. Djavanmardi L, Oprean N, Alantar A, Bousetta K, Princ G. Malignant non-Hodgkin's lymphoma (NHL) of the jaws: A review of 16 cases. J Craniomaxillofac Surg 2008; 36:410–414.
252. Epstein JB, Epstein JD, Le ND, Gorsky M. Characteristics of oral and paraoral malignant lymphoma: A population-based review of 361 cases. Oral Surg Oral Med Oral Pathol Oral Radiol Endod 2001;92:519–525.
253. Fischer DJ, Klasser GD, Kaufmann R. Intraoral swelling and periapical radiolucency. J Am Dent Assoc 2012;143:985–988.
254. Mopsik ER, Milobsky SA. Malignant lymphoma presenting as periapical pathology: A report of two cases. MSDA J 1995;38:175–199.
255. Melrose RJ, Cooperman HH, Abrams AM. Clinical Pathologic Conference. Odontogenic cysts. J South Calif Dent Assoc 1969;37:186–190.
256. Bataille R, Chevalier J, Rossi M, Sany J. Bone scintigraphy in plasma-cell myeloma. A prospective study of 70 patients. Radiology 1982;145:801–804.
257. Kapadia SB, Desai U, Cheng VS. Extramedullary plasmacytoma of the head and neck. A clinicopathologic study of 20 cases. Medicine (Baltimore) 1982;61:317–329.
258. Woodruff RK, Malpas JS, White FE. Solitary plasmacytoma II: Solitary plasmacytoma of bone. Cancer 1979;43:2344–2347.
259. Shah N, Sarkar C. Plasmacytoma of anterior maxilla mimicking periapical cyst. Endod Dent Traumatol 1992;8:39–41.
260. Islam MN, Cohen DM, Kanter KG, Stewart CM, Katz J, Bhattacharyya I. Florid cemento-osseous dysplasia mimicking multiple periapical pathology—An endodontic dilemma. Gen Dent 2008;56:559–562.
261. Perez-Garcia S, Berini-Aytes L, Gay-Escoda C. Ossifying fibroma of the upper jaw: Report of a case and review of the literature. Med Oral 2004;9:333–339.

262. Wilcox LR, Walton RE. Case of mistaken identity: Periapical cemental dysplasia in an endodontically treated tooth. Endod Dent Traumatol 1989;5:298–301.
263. Childers EL, Johnson JD, Warnock GR, Kratochvil FJ. Asymptomatic periapical radiolucent lesion found in an area of previous trauma. J Am Dent Assoc 1990; 121:759–760.
264. Knutsen BM, Larheim TA, Johannessen S, Hillestad J, Solheim T, Koppang HS. Recurrent conventional cemento-ossifying fibroma of the mandible. Dentomaxillofac Radiol 2002;1:65–58.
265. Drazić R, Minić AJ. Focal cemento-osseous dysplasia in the maxilla mimicking periapical granuloma. Oral Surg Oral Med Oral Pathol Oral Radiol Endod 1999; 88:87–89.
266. Smith S, Patel K, Hoskinson AE. Periapical cemental dysplasia: A case of misdiagnosis. Br Dent J 1998;185:122–123.
267. Ribera MJ. Osteoblastoma in the anterior maxilla mimicking periapical pathosis of odontogenic origin. J Endod 1996;22:142–146.
268. Hutchison IL, Hopper C, Coonar HS. Neoplasia masquerading as periapical infection. Br Dent J 1990;168:288–294.
269. Bhadage CJ, Vaishampayan S, Kolhe S, Umarji H. Osteosarcoma of the mandible mimicking an odontogenic abscess: A case report and review of the literature. Dent Update 2013;40:216–221.
270. Koppang HS, Koppang R, Solheim T, Aarnes H, Stolen SO. Cellulose fibers from endodontic paper points as an etiological factor in postendodontic periapical granulomas and cysts. J Endod 1989;15:369–372.
271. Nair PN, Sjogren U, Krey G, Sundqvist G. Therapy-resistant foreign body giant cell granuloma at the periapex of a root-filled human tooth. J Endod 1990;16:589–595.
272. Talacko AA, Radden BG. Oral pulse granuloma: Clinical and histopathological features. A review of 62 cases. Int J Oral Maxillofac Surg 1988;17:343–346.
273. Khongkhunthian P, Reichart PA. Aspergillosis of the maxillary sinuses, a complication of overfilling root canal material into the sinus: Report of two cases. J Endod 2001;27:476–478.
274. Kalnins V. Actinomycotic granuloma. Oral Surg Oral Med Oral Pathol 1971;32: 276–277.
275. Hamner JE, Schaefer ME. Anterior maxillary actinomycosis: Report of case. J Oral Surg 1965;23:60–63.
276. Martinelli C, Rulli MA. Periapical cyst associated with actinomycosis. Oral Surg Oral Med Oral Pathol 1967;24:817–820.
277. Omnell KA, Rohlin M. Case challenge. Chronic maxillary inflammation. J Contemp Dent Pract 2000;1:100–105.
278. Kessler HP, Unterman B. Respiratory epithelial adenomatoid hamartoma of the maxillary sinus presenting as a periapical radiolucency: A case report and review of the literature. Oral Surg Oral Med Oral Pathol Oral Radiol Endod 2004;97: 607–612.
279. Ojha J, McIlwain R, Said-Al Naief N. A large radiolucent lesion of the posterior maxilla. Oral Surg Oral Med Oral Pathol Oral Radiol Endod 2010;110:423–429.

Chapter Five

Diagnosis and Treatment Planning

Mahmoud Torabinejad

The major etiologic factors for tooth loss are periodontal disease, decay, and traumatic injuries. For centuries, dentists have provided information to the public regarding the value of natural dentition as well as methods and materials to prevent and treat periodontal disease, decay, and traumatic injuries. Despite these efforts, many teeth still develop periodontal disease or pulpal disease as a result of decay formation or traumatic injuries. Traditionally, the treatments for the affected teeth were periodontal procedures or root canal treatment. When these treatments were deemed inadequate, the teeth were subsequently extracted and either not replaced at all or replaced with fixed or removable prostheses. A significant improvement in the survival rates of implants in the latter part of the 20th century added another treatment option for teeth that could not be retained periodontally or endodontically (Fig 5-1). The purpose of this chapter is to discuss treatment options for teeth with periodontal or pulpal diseases.

For teeth with periodontal disease, treatment options include periodontal treatment, extraction with no replacement, and extraction with placement of a fixed partial denture (FPD) or single implant. For teeth with pulpal and periapical diseases, depending on the extent of the pulpal involvement and closure of the apices, treatment options include vital pulp therapy, apexification, regenerative endodontics, root canal treatment or extraction with no replacement, and extraction with placement of an FPD or single implant (Fig 5-2).

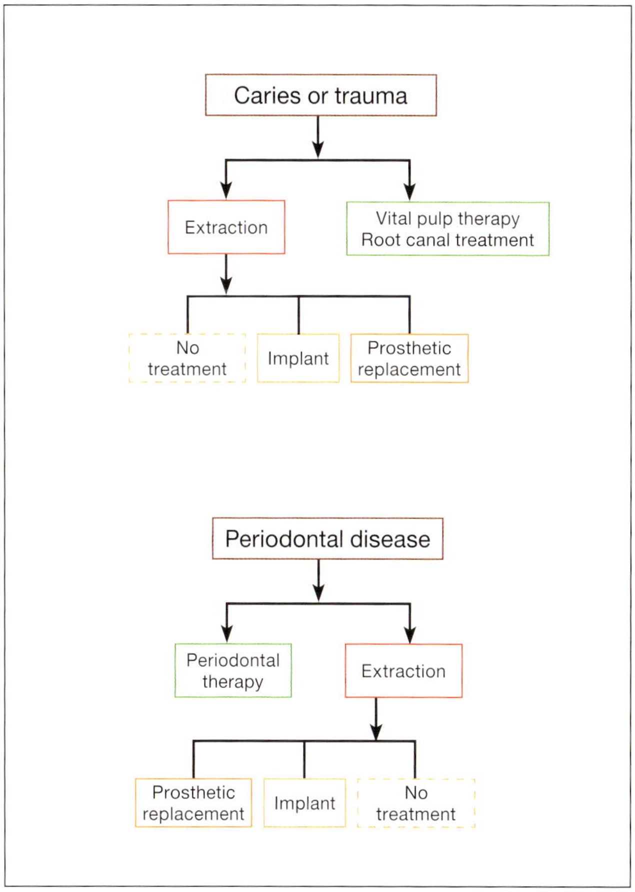

Fig 5-1 Etiologies of tooth loss and treatment options.

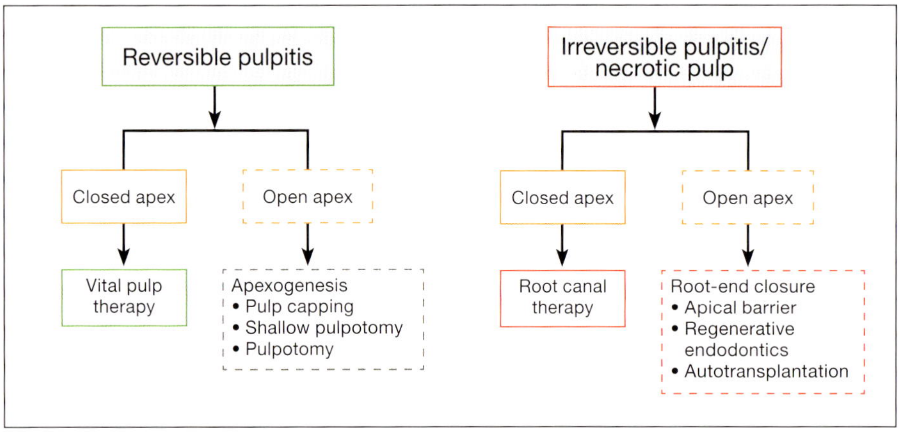

Fig 5-2 Treatment options for teeth with open and closed apices and various pulpal conditions.

Treatment Options for Teeth with Periodontal Disease

The treatment of choice for teeth with periodontal disease is periodontal therapy and preservation of the natural dentition (Fig 5-3). The main benefits of successful treatment of teeth with periodontal disease include conservation of the crown and root structure, preservation of alveolar bone and accompanying papillae, preservation of pressure perception, and lack of movement of the surrounding teeth. Several studies have shown excellent long-term prognoses for treated teeth with periodontal disease and a survival rate over 90%.[1–3]

When teeth with periodontal disease are difficult to maintain or the patient is not willing to keep his or her natural dentition for various reasons, these teeth need to be extracted (Fig 5-4). The harmful effects of extraction of these teeth are bone resorption,[4] shifting of adjacent teeth,[5–7] and reduced esthetics and chewing ability.[8] Ideally, these teeth should be replaced with FPDs or a single implant (Figs 5-5 and 5-6). The benefits of extraction and replacement of a missing tooth with an FPD include the prevention of shifting of the adjacent teeth and improved chewing ability and esthetics.[9] Studies have shown no adverse effects on the surrounding alveolar bone[10]; no difference in the attachment level between teeth supporting FPDs and a homologous tooth[11]; and no difference in plaque index, gingival index, or probing depths.[12] It has also been found that if hygiene is maintained to a high degree, no inflammation of the mucosa should be observed under the pontic, regardless of the pontic material used.[13]

Implants are indicated when natural teeth cannot be saved due to severe periodontal disease or decay or traumatic injuries.[14] Other indications for the use of implants include edentulous sites adjacent to teeth without restorations or with a need for restoration (Fig 5-7), abutment teeth with large pulp chambers, abutment teeth with a history of avulsion or luxation, teeth with infractions or vertical root fractures or an inadequate crown-to-root ratio, and teeth that cannot be prepared with adequate retention and resistance form. Other factors that affect treatment planning for single implants include the patient's systemic and local health conditions, the patient's comfort and perception, biologic factors, tooth color, soft and hard tissue biotypes, procedural complications, and adjunctive treatments.[14]

Currently, there is no study comparing the survival of periodontally treated teeth with single implant–supported crowns. In a systematic review, Torabinejad et al[15] compared the outcomes of single implant–supported crowns, FPDs, and extractions without further treatment. Survival data in this systematic review showed superior results for single implants compared with fixed prosthodontic treatment.

Treatment Options for Teeth with Pulpal and Periapical Diseases

The major factors affecting treatment planning for teeth with decay include pulpal condition and closure of the apex (see Fig 5-2). When a tooth has reversible pulpitis and an open apex, the treatment of choice is vital pulp therapy through pulp capping and partial or complete pulpotomy (Fig 5-8). When a tooth has reversible pulpitis and a closed apex, the treatment of choice is vital pulp therapy (Fig 5-9). When a tooth has irreversible pulpitis or necrotic pulp and an open apex, the treatment

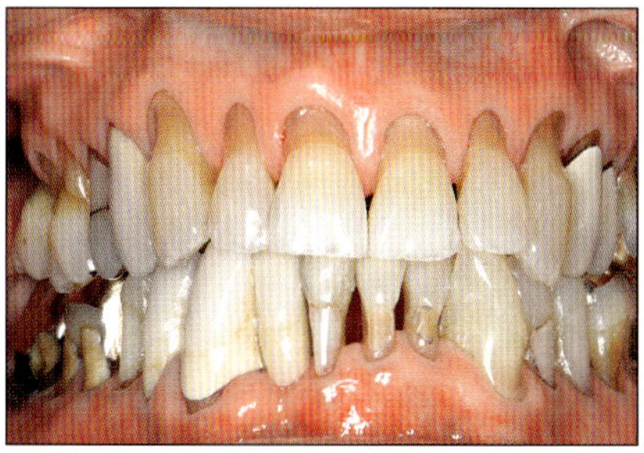

Fig 5-3 This patient was affected by severe periodontal disease and referred for multiple extractions. Periodontal treatment was performed instead, and the patient still retains all of his teeth 47 years later. (Courtesy of Dr Hessam Nowzari, Los Angeles, California.)

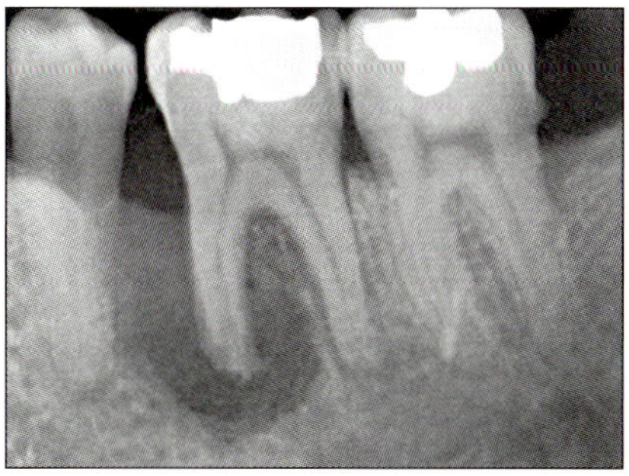

Fig 5-4 A mandibular first molar with severe periodontal disease that cannot be treated with periodontal treatment and had to be extracted.

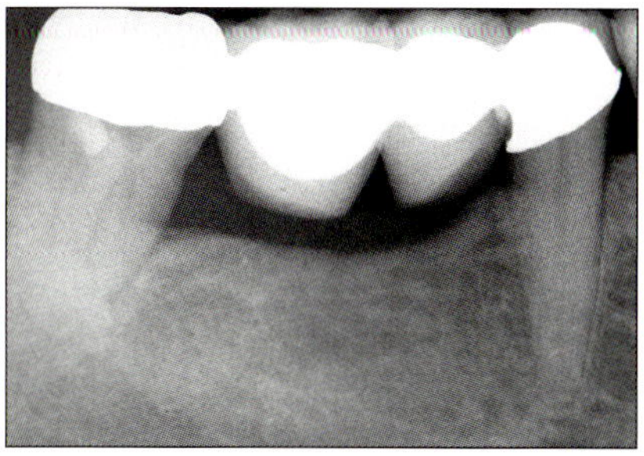

Fig 5-5 Extracted teeth are replaced with an FPD.

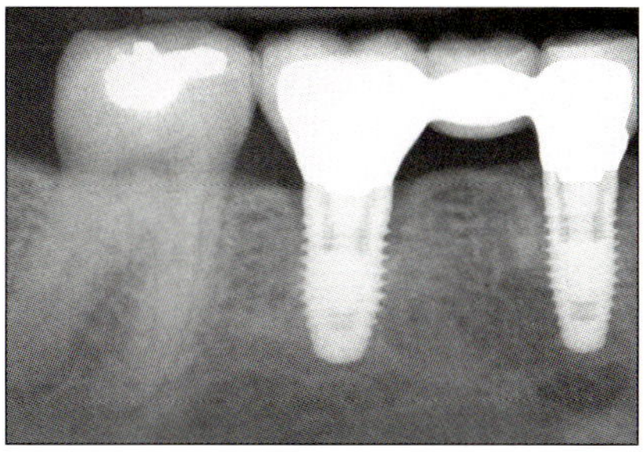

Fig 5-6 Extracted teeth are replaced with implants.

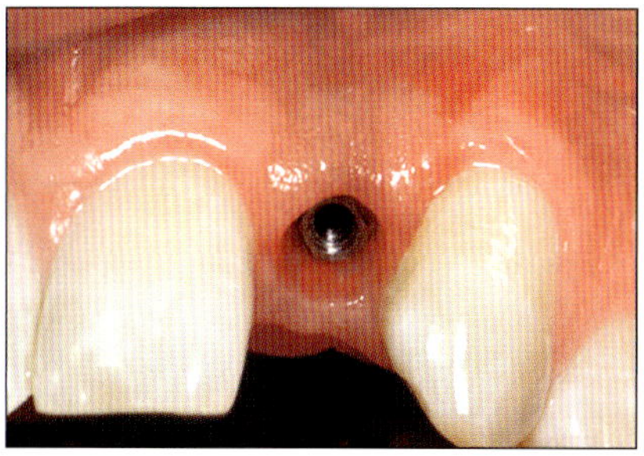

Fig 5-7 An implant is placed in an edentulous site adjacent to teeth without restorations.

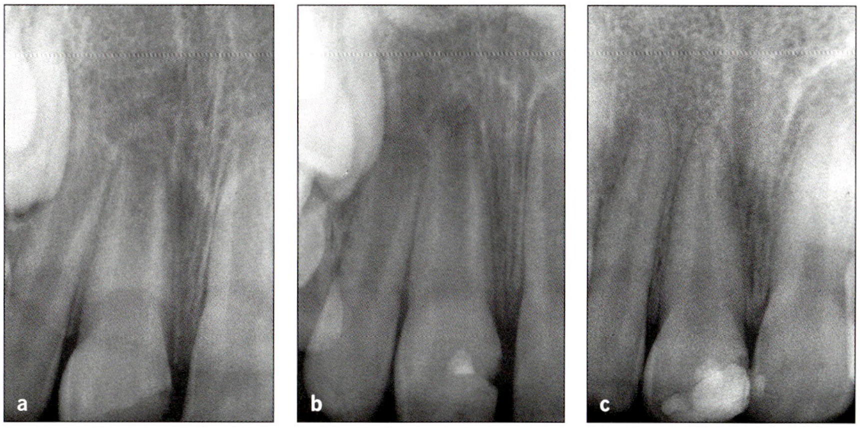

Fig 5-8 *(a)* Preoperative radiograph of a central incisor with vital pulp and an open apex. *(b)* Postoperative radiograph of the tooth after pulp capping with mineral trioxide aggregate (MTA). *(c)* Postoperative radiograph 9 years after treatment showing complete closure of the apex. The tooth had no clinical symptoms and responded within normal limits to pulp tests.

of choice is apexification (Fig 5-10) or regenerative endodontics (Fig 5-11). When a tooth has irreversible pulpitis or necrotic pulp and a closed apex, the treatment of choice is root canal treatment (Fig 5-12).

For patients who have been affected by pulpal and periapical diseases caused by decay or trauma, the main objectives of root canal treatment are to provide long-term comfort, function, and esthetics and save the natural dentition. These objectives are achieved by complete cleaning, shaping, and obturation of the canals; restoration of the affected teeth; and prevention of recontamination.[16–18]

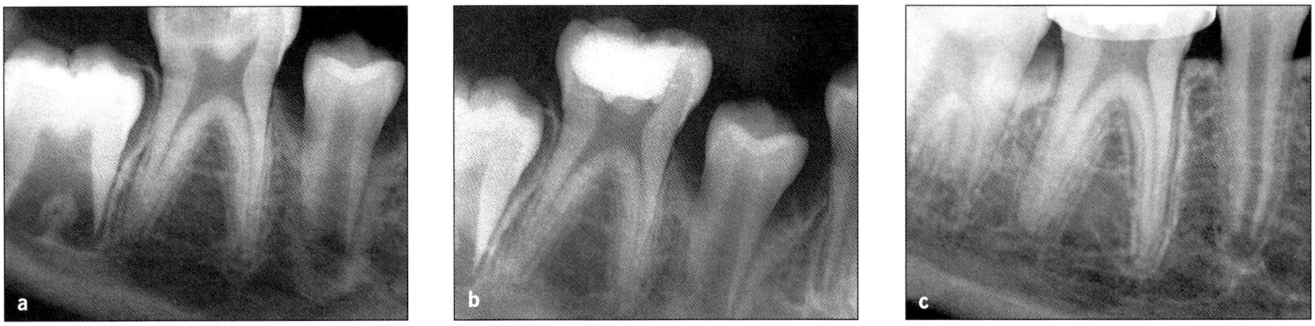

Fig 5-9 *(a)* Preoperative radiograph of a mandibular molar with vital pulp and closed apices in an 8-year-old boy. *(b)* Postoperative radiograph of the tooth after pulp capping with MTA. *(c)* Postoperative radiograph 2 years after treatment. The tooth had no clinical symptoms and responded within normal limits to pulp tests.

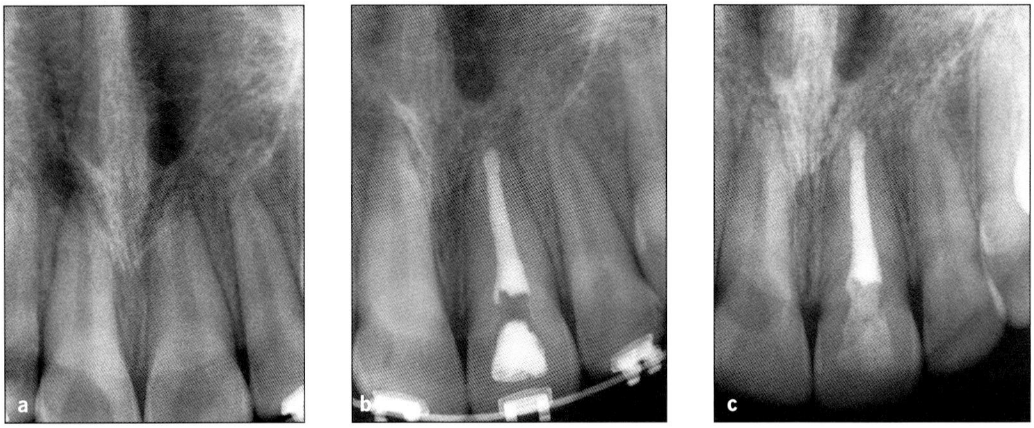

Fig 5-10 *(a)* Preoperative radiograph of a central incisor with necrotic pulp and an open apex. *(b)* Postoperative radiograph of the tooth after placement of an MTA plug and filling the rest of the canal with gutta-percha and sealer. *(c)* Postoperative radiograph 3 years after treatment showing complete closure of the apex. The tooth had no clinical symptoms.

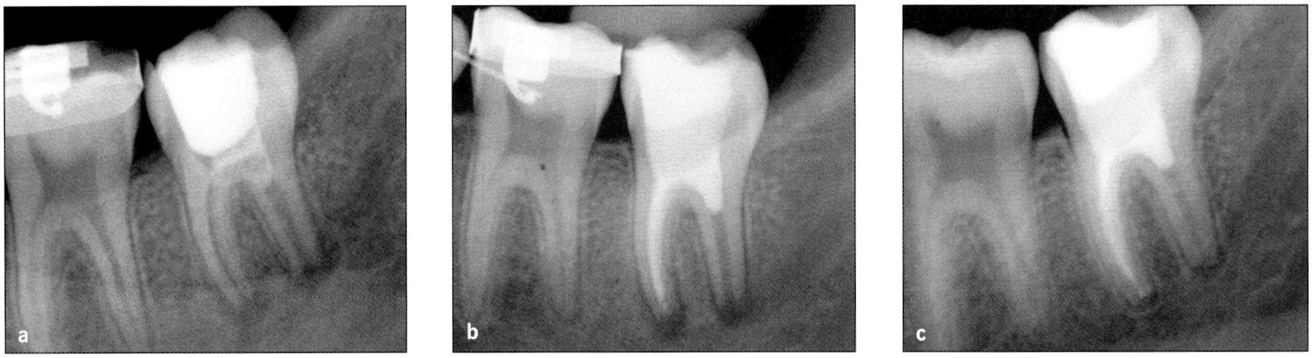

Fig 5-11 *(a)* Preoperative radiograph of a mandibular molar with necrotic pulp, closed apices in the mesial canals, and an open apex in the distal root in a 12-year-old boy. *(b)* Postoperative radiograph of the tooth after root canal treatment for the mesial roots and regenerative endodontics for the distal root. *(c)* Postoperative radiograph 1 year later showing resolution of the lesion for the mesial roots and thickening of the walls in the distal root. The tooth had no clinical symptoms.

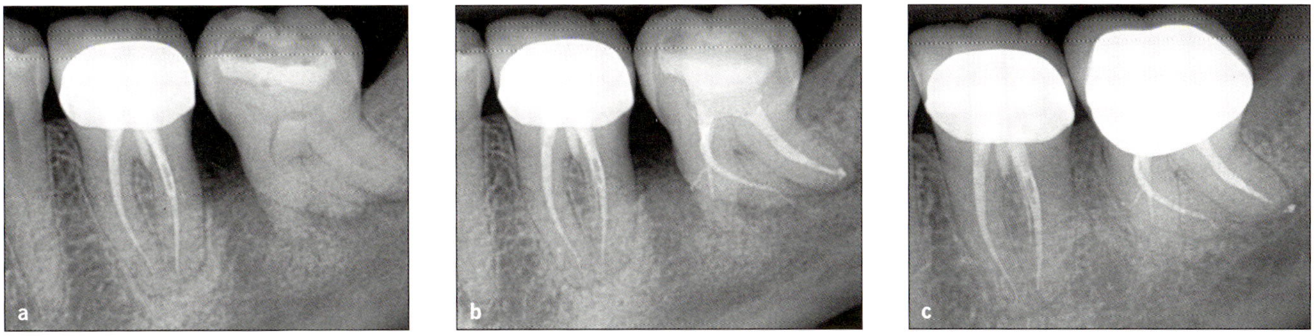

Fig 5-12 *(a)* Preoperative radiograph of a mandibular second molar with a periapical lesion and large periodontal defect. *(b)* Postoperative radiograph after initial root canal treatment and filling the main and lateral canals. *(c)* Postoperative radiograph 3 years later showing complete resolution of the periapical and periodontal lesions. (Courtesy of Dr Shahrokh Shabahang, Redlands, California.)

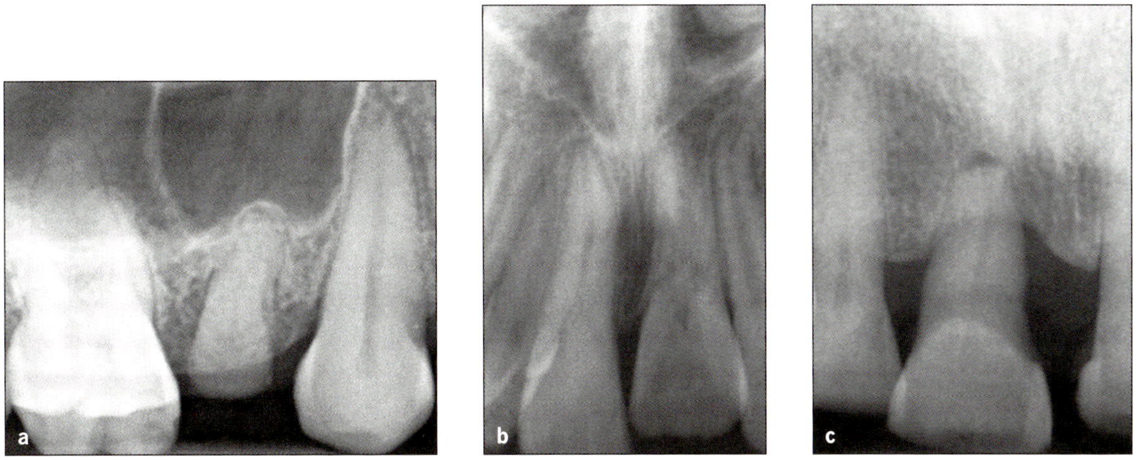

Fig 5-13 *(a)* A maxillary premolar without a restorable crown. *(b)* A central incisor with a nonsalvageable resorptive defect. *(c)* A central incisor with an inadequate crown-to-root ratio. These are all contraindications for root canal treatment.

Indications and Contraindications for Initial Root Canal Treatment

Indications for root canal treatment include teeth with irreversible pulpitis, necrotic pulps, treatable periodontal conditions, salvageable resorptive defects, favorable crown-to-root ratios, as well as teeth with or without periapical lesions that have restorable crowns.[19] Any tooth with pulpal and periapical pathosis that has a restorable crown, sound periodontal structures, an adequate crown-to-root ratio, and no major tooth resorption must be saved by root canal treatment.

Root canal treatment is contraindicated in teeth without restorable crowns or teeth with untreatable periodontal conditions, nonsalvageable resorptive defects, and inadequate crown-to-root ratios (Fig 5-13). Nonsurgical root canal treatment is a predictable procedure when it is performed properly.

Outcomes of Initial Root Canal Treatment

Nonsurgical initial root canal treatment is a highly successful procedure when diagnosis and technical aspects are carefully performed (see Fig 5-12). Several studies with large sample sizes have reported that nonsurgical root canal therapy (NSRCT) has a survival rate of more than 90% when adequately performed.[20–22] Lazarski et al[20] evaluated 44,613 NSRCT cases in the United States. They reported that 94% of the teeth that had been restored were in function and had survived at an average follow-up time of 3.5 years. Salehrabi and Rotstein[21] evaluated 1,462,935 teeth in 1,126,288 patients in the United States. They reported that at 8 years after initial NSRCT, 97% of teeth had survived without intervention. Chen et al[22] evaluated 1,557,547 teeth receiving NSRCT in Taiwan. At 5 years, they reported that 93% survived without intervention. Raedel et al[23] evaluated 556,067 teeth receiving NSRCT in Germany and reported a survival rate of 84% without intervention after 3 years.

Bernstein et al[24] examined the outcomes of NSRCT in general practice using a practice-based research network (PBRN) in the United States. At 3 to 5 years after treatment, 95% of the cases had survived without intervention. Another smaller PBRN study of 174 teeth reported an 82% survival rate with a mean follow-up time of 8.6 years.[25]

Systematic reviews of outcomes of NSRCT reveal the same results. Iqbal and Kim[26] report a six-year survival rate of 97%.[26] Torabinejad et al[15] report a similar survival rate after 6-plus years. Another systematic review, restricted to far fewer source articles, provided estimated pooled proportions of 8 to 10 years with a survival rate of 87%.[27] These results point to excellent performance of teeth treated with NSRCT over time. However, like other complex disciplines of dentistry and medicine, root canal treatment can also have some unsuccessful outcomes.

Causes of Nonhealing of Initial NSRCT

Because of the complexity of root canal systems and inadequate chemomechanical instrumentation, elimination of bacteria from the root canal systems is not always possible.[28–31] The presence of bacteria in the root canal system before obturation negatively affects the prognosis of this procedure.[32] The use of calcium hydroxide as an intracanal medicament decreases the bacterial population and improves the prognosis.[33,34] Studies have shown that inaccurate obturation lengths as well as inadequate obturation lead to worse outcomes.[35–47]

Reinfection of the root canal system after root canal treatment through coronal microleakage is a major factor for nonhealing after initial root canal treatment.[28,29,32] Other causes of nonhealing after initial root canal treatment may be related to procedural accidents and mishaps.[28,31] They include perforations, canal transportation, separated instruments, or ledge formations. Long-term delay of placement of definitive restorations after initial root canal treatment can also affect the treatment outcome.[46,48–50] Another cause of nonhealing following root canal treatment is the presence of vertical fracture that occurs after root canal treatment.[51–53] In a review paper, Nair[54] describes six main biologic factors that lead to asymptomatic radiolucencies persisting following initial root canal treatment.

Steps in Diagnosis of Nonhealing Following Initial Root Canal Treatment

When initial NSRCT is unsuccessful, the first step in solving the patient's problem is to determine the cause(s) of the nonhealing. As with initial nonsurgical treatment, diagnosis is the first and the most important phase of treatment planning. Diagnosis is a detective process and therefore must be performed carefully and systematically. A competent dentist or specialist must have adequate training in the art and science of alternative treatment options, and he or she should perform diagnostic tests, interpret the test results, psychologically manage the patient, and finally formulate an appropriate diagnosis and treatment plan. Treatment planning should address the expectations of the patient, insurance company, and dentist. An ideal treatment plan addresses the chief complaint of the patient and provides a cost-effective treatment based on patient and dentist expectations and abilities. The treatment planning should be a patient-centered process based on scientific evidence, preserving or restoring esthetics, comfort, and function for the patient.

Similar to diagnosis and treatment planning for initial NSRCT, a step-by-step systematic approach to diagnosis and treatment planning must be followed for patients who have had previous root canal treatment and may need further treatment. These steps include:

1. Ascertaining the chief complaint of the patient
2. Recording pertinent information related to the patient's medical and dental history
3. Conducting thorough subjective, objective, and radiographic examinations
4. Analyzing the obtained data
5. Formulating an appropriate diagnosis and treatment plan for the patient

A shortcut taken in these steps can result in misdiagnosis, incorrect treatment planning, and the creation of a misunderstanding between the clinician and the patient.

Chief complaint

Obtaining the chief complaint is the first step in communication between the clinician and the patient. The clinician should allow the patient to express his or her problem(s) in his or her own words. When the patient is unaware of any problem and has been referred for diagnosis or treatment, the chief complaint should be recorded as "no chief complaint" for future reference.

Health history

It is imperative to take a complete health history for new patients and to review and update the information for patients who have been treated in the office before. A comprehensive health history for a patient includes demographic data, medical history, and dental history. The written medical history form should always be supplemented with a verbal review of medical conditions and medications. Patients may forget to report a medical condition or may intentionally omit certain information due to privacy concerns or a lack of understanding that the condition or medication could be relevant to dental treatment.[55,56] Patients often fail to see the connection between their medical problems and dental treatment.[57] In one study, almost two-thirds of adult dental patients (average age 52 years) were taking prescription medications and/or over-the-counter drugs. The most common were antihypertensive medications (35%), anticoagulants (12%), psychiatric medications (10%), hypoglycemic medications (9%), and gastric ulcer medications (8%).[58]

A particular concern in treatment planning for endodontic microsurgery is the growing use of herbs, dietary supplements, and various over-the-counter medications that may cause increased bleeding during surgery.[59] For example, ginkgo, ginger, garlic, ginseng, feverfew, fish oil, and vitamin E can all increase the risk of excessive bleeding during surgery.[60] This information may change the treatment planning and treatment options for the patient.

Medical history

Medical history should include the patient's present and past physical and psychologic conditions in regards to cardiovascular system, blood disorders, metabolic profile, respiratory system, central nervous system, endocrine system, immunologic disorders, and medications taken by the patient. Advances in medicine have led to treatment being rendered not only for young individuals or patients without medical problems; the age of the patient population with pulpal or periapical pathosis is on the rise.[61] Older individuals usually have more medical problems compared with young ones. Consequently, these patients may have systemic diseases or may be taking medications that interfere with treatment options. A medically complex patient usually requires modification in treatment procedures.

A thorough medical history provides information regarding the general health of a patient as well as his or her susceptibility to infection and tendency to bleeding. Analysis of the patient's list of prescribed medications, herbs, dietary supplements, vitamins, and other over-the-counter medications is usually indicative of the medical condition of a patient and severity of his or her systemic diseases.[62] Gathering this information provides an indication of the possible complications as a result of the use of these medications as well as the emotional status of the patient. If there is any medical evidence related to the physical or psychologic disease status of the patient that might interfere with treatment, consultation with the patient's physician is indicated before starting any treatment. The consultation should be in writing and should be included in the patient's file. The American Society of Anesthesiologists' (ASA) Health Classification System is currently used for assessing the physical status of a patient. ASA I and ASA II do not usually require significant treatment modification. Patients in the ASA III category or above usually require medical consultation.[62] However, ASA category alone is only part of the risk assessment for endodontic microsurgery. The anticipated procedural stress and patient's self-reported dental anxiety must also be considered. It has been demonstrated that, compared with NSRCT, surgical endodontic therapy induces more significant physiologic changes, including increased heart rate and systolic blood pressure. Patients with above-average dental anxiety are also more likely to experience significant physiologic changes.[63]

Conditions that may affect treatment planning include cardiovascular diseases, hypertension, use of vasoconstrictors in local anesthetics, ischemic heart disease, heart murmurs and valvular disease, anticoagulant therapy including aspirin and other non-steroidal anti-inflammatory medications, bleeding disorders, arrhythmias and cardiac pacemakers, and heart failure. Certain conditions are more relevant to treatment planning for endodontic microsurgery compared with NSRCT. For example, the patient's tolerance for epinephrine must be considered, and any bleeding disorders and anticoagulant therapy or immunosuppressive conditions that may result in delayed healing or treatment failure require special attention.

Patients with valvular heart disease present two primary considerations for dental treatment: *(1)* a potential risk for infective endocarditis and *(2)* a risk of excessive bleeding in patients on anticoagulant therapy. Management considerations for patients on anticoagulant therapy are discussed in greater detail in chapter 8. Current guidelines for prevention of infective endocarditis were revised in 2007 and represent a significant change from previous American Heart Association guidelines.[64] For example, antibiotic prophylaxis is no longer recommended for patients with a history of mitral valve prolapse (with or without regurgitation), rheumatic heart disease, bicuspid valve disease, aortic stenosis, and certain congenital heart conditions. Antibiotic prophylaxis is now only recommended for patients with valvular disease associated with the highest risk of adverse outcomes from infective endocarditis. These higher-risk conditions include prosthetic heart valve, previous infective endocarditis, certain types of congenital heart disease (consult with

Box 5-1 Suggested antibiotic prophylaxis regimens

Patients not allergic to penicillin (taken orally 1 hour before procedure)
Amoxicillin
Adults: 2.0 g
Children: 50 mg/kg

Patients allergic to penicillin (taken orally 1 hour before procedure)
Clindamycin
Adults: 600 mg
Children: 20 mg/kg
or
Cephalexin
Adults: 2.0 g
Children: 50 mg/kg
or
Azithromycin or clarithromycin
Adults: 500 mg
Children: 15 mg/kg

Patients unable to take medications orally (taken intramuscularly or intravenously)
Adults: 2.0 g ampicillin or 1.0 g cefazolin or ceftriaxone
Children: 50 mg/kg ampicillin, cefazolin, or ceftriaxone

Patients allergic to penicillin who are unable to take medications orally (taken intramuscularly or intravenously)
Adults: 1.0 g cefazolin or ceftriaxone or 600 mg clindamycin
Children: 50 mg/kg cefazolin or ceftriaxone or 20 mg/kg clindamycin 30 minutes before the procedure

the patient's physician), and cardiac transplant with valvulopathy. For patients in the highest risk category, antibiotic prophylaxis is recommended for dental procedures that involve manipulation of gingival tissues or the periapical region of teeth or perforation of the oral mucosa; obviously, this includes endodontic microsurgery. For all other patients with valvular disease, the risks associated with routine antibiotic prophylaxis are greater than potential benefits.[64]

These guidelines should be considered the current best available evidence to guide clinical practice decisions; however, it is interesting to note that a recent study in England demonstrated an increase in cases of infective endocarditis following the widespread adoption of the new standards in 2008.[65] The increase in cases was found in individuals both at high risk and at lower risk of infective endocarditis. Although the increase was statistically significant, the absolute number of cases was still very low, and the authors caution that a causal relationship has not been established. The regimen for prophylactic antibiotic coverage is shown in Box 5-1.

Other conditions that affect treatment planning are diabetes, pulmonary diseases, central nervous disorders, renal disease and dialysis, a history of bisphosphonate use, bone marrow and solid organ transplantation, prosthetic joints and other prosthetic devices, pregnancy, HIV, sickle cell anemia, liver disease, adrenal suppression and long-term steroid use, and allergies to antibiotics and dental materials[62] (see chapter 16).

Dental history

A good dental history provides valuable information about the patient's attitudes toward oral health and saving the natural dentition. This information has valuable diagnostic importance and may provide clues for selecting a specific test or treatment modality. After listening with keen interest, the clinician should ask about previous dental experiences; the type of pain or discomfort; the severity, spontaneity, and duration of pain (if present); and/or the stimuli that induce or relieve pain. Obtaining this information provides clues regarding the previous adverse effect of treatment related to the tooth that has had root canal treatment or another tooth that has nothing to do with the root canal–treated tooth. Medications taken for relief of pain or discomfort also provide tips regarding the source of the patient's concern. Root canal–treated teeth usually have no sensitivity to cold or heat and are not associated with severe and spontaneous pain. Pain or discomfort related to a root canal–treated tooth usually comes after application of pressure, which indicates the presence of periradicular pathosis.

Tentative diagnosis

After careful review of the medical and dental histories of a patient and identification of the main subjective signs and symptoms of the patient's present illness, the clini-

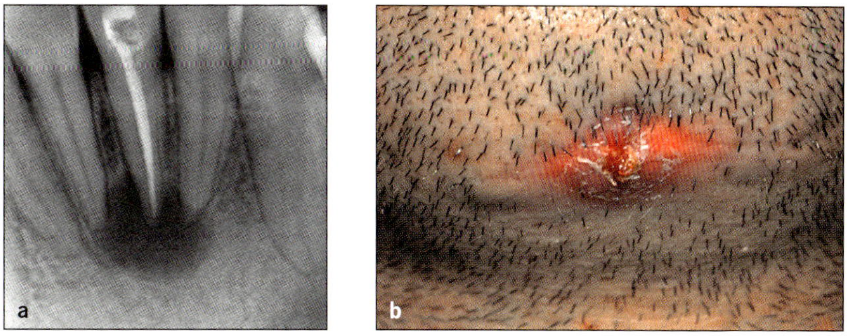

Fig 5-14 *(a)* Preoperative radiograph of a mandibular central incisor with inadequate root canal treatment with a large periapical lesion. *(b)* A large extraoral fistula on the patient's chin related to this inadequate treatment.

cian often arrives at a tentative diagnosis. The tentative diagnosis is then confirmed or modified by extra- and intraoral examinations, as well as clinical tests.

Extraoral examination

Extraoral examination consists of an evaluation of the general appearance of the face, facial asymmetry, and the presence or absence of swelling, discoloration, and skin redness. In addition, the presence or absence of extraoral scars or sinus tracts and tender and/or enlarged lymph nodes should be examined. A careful and thorough extraoral examination may provide the cause of the patient's complaint and the extent of the disease process (Fig 5-14).

Intraoral examination

Intraoral examination includes the soft and hard tissues of the oral cavity.

Soft tissues

Soft tissue examination consists of a visual and digital test of the lips, oral mucosa, cheeks, tongue, palate, and muscles of mastication. The size and shape of the oral cavity and the patient's mouth opening should be determined during intraoral examination. The color, texture, and health of marginal gingiva should be carefully evaluated. These factors affect treatment planning. The same evaluations should be performed for attached gingiva. The attached gingiva is evaluated for color, texture, and vertical dimension. Alveolar mucosa should be examined for the presence of inflammation, ulceration, discoloration, and the sinus tract stoma. Presence of a sinus tract stoma usually indicates presence of a necrotic pulp and/or chronic apical abscess and sometimes a periodontal abscess. Placement of gutta-percha into the sinus tract can aid in localizing the source of the infection (Fig 5-15). Soft tissue examination should also include identification of the gingival biotype (Fig 5-16). This biotype (thick versus thin) affects treatment planning and the type of flaps used in surgery should endodontic surgery be indicated (see chapter 9). The location, size, and texture of any muscle attachments and frena should be examined. These also affect the types of treatment and flap designs indicated for surgery.

Hard tissues

Examination of the hard tissues consists of evaluation of the dentition as well as the bones of the jaws. The number of teeth and their condition are usually indicative of the patient's interest in oral health. Patients who have poor oral health and have lost many teeth are not good candidates for retreatment surgically or nonsurgically (Fig 5-17). A mirror and an explorer should be used to determine the presence or absence of gross or recurrent marginal caries, crown fractures, defective restorations, and coronal leakage in teeth with previous root canal treatment. The thickness of the bones surrounding the teeth should be carefully examined during hard tissue examinations. The nasal spine should be palpated to determine its contour and sharpness. A delicate elevation is required to avoid tearing of the soft tissue if surgery is indicated. The location and extent of the external oblique ridge should also be noted. The depth of the vestibule should be noted during this examination. Like the gingival biotype, the depth of the vestibule also affects the types of treatment and the flap designs indicated if surgical endodontics is contemplated (Fig 5-18). The depth and height of the palate should be noted during examination of the maxillary soft and hard tissues. These factors affect the buccal or palatal surgical approach if surgery is contemplated (see chapter 12).

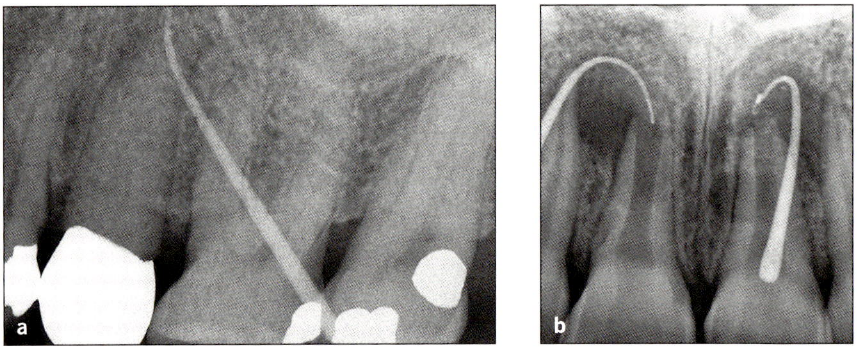

Fig 5-15 *(a)* Tracing the sinus tract stoma with a gutta-percha point shows that the source of infection is far away from the stoma. *(b)* Two sinus tract stomas are traced to the central incisors with necrotic pulps and open apices.

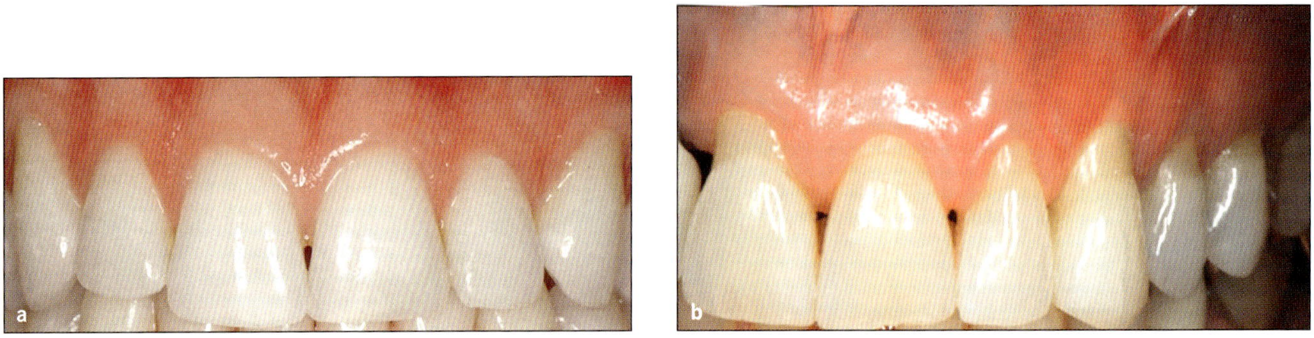

Fig 5-16 *(a)* Thin biotype. *(b)* Thick biotype.

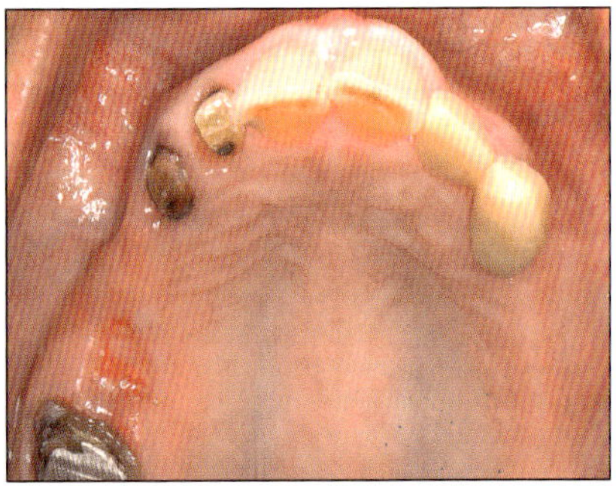

Fig 5-17 The loss of many teeth should be considered as a factor during treatment planning.

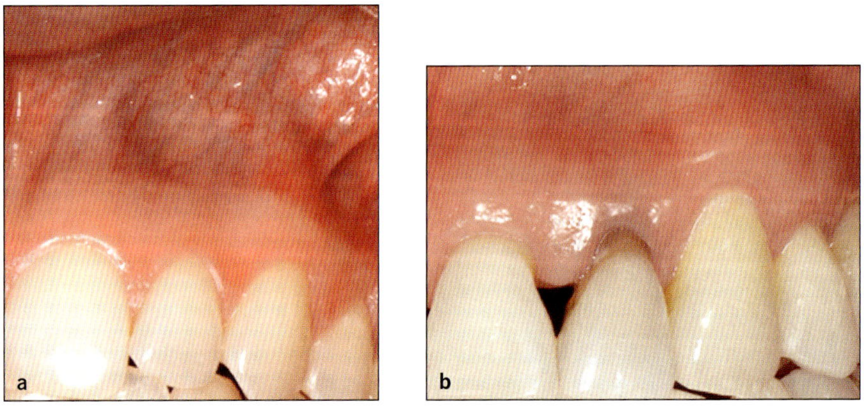

Fig 5-18 *(a)* A deep vestibule in the anterior maxilla. *(b)* A shallow vestibule in the anterior maxilla.

Clinical tests

Percussion

Percussion tests determine the presence of inflammation anywhere in the periodontal ligament caused by either pulpal or periodontal disease. In general, the percussion pain related to periodontal inflammation is milder than that related to periapical inflammation of pulpal origin. This test is performed by tapping on the incisal or occlusal surface with the end of a mirror handle held parallel or perpendicular to the crown (Fig 5-19). In teeth with severe percussion sensitivity, this test should be performed by gentle apical pressure with digital manipulation of the tooth. Another way to evaluate percussion sensitivity is to have the patient bite hard on an object such as a cotton swab or mirror handle.

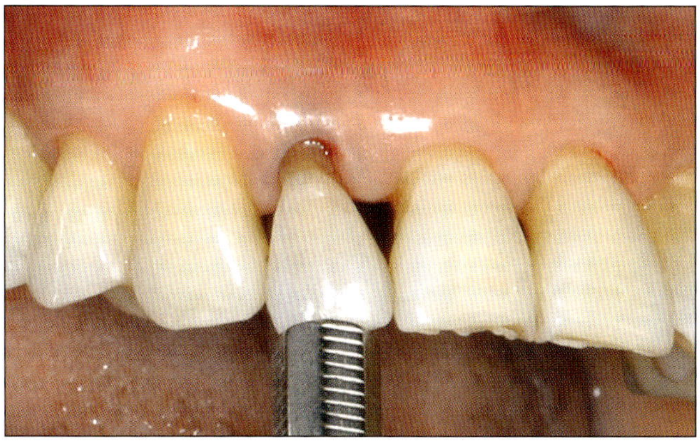

Fig 5-19 Percussion testing is performed by tapping on the incisal surface of the suspected tooth with the end of a mirror handle held parallel or perpendicular to the crown.

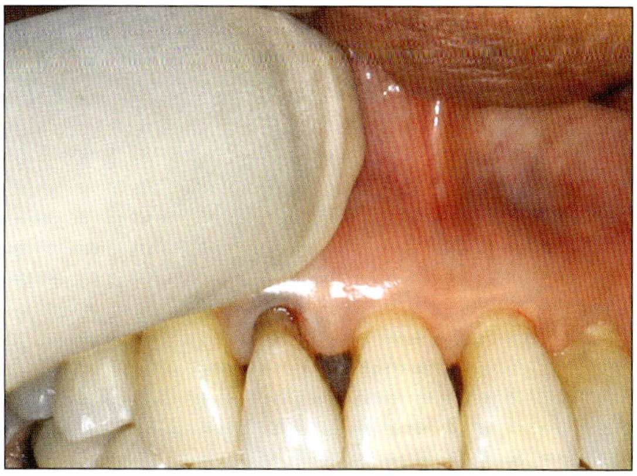

Fig 5-20 Palpation testing is performed by applying firm pressure on the mucosa overlying the hard tissues of the teeth.

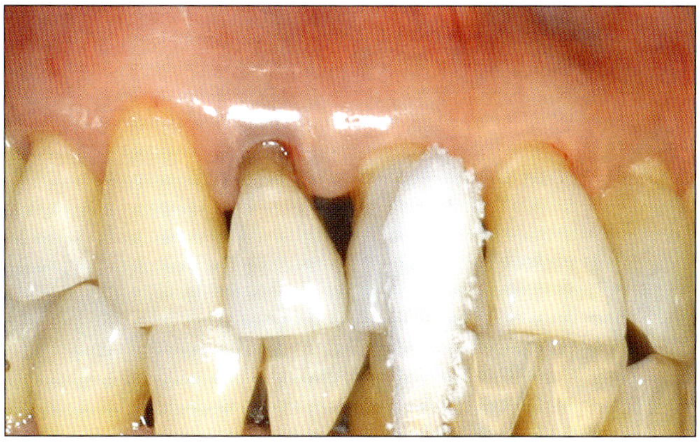

Fig 5-21 Vitality testing with cold or electricity is performed on the suspected tooth and the adjacent teeth during diagnosis and treatment planning.

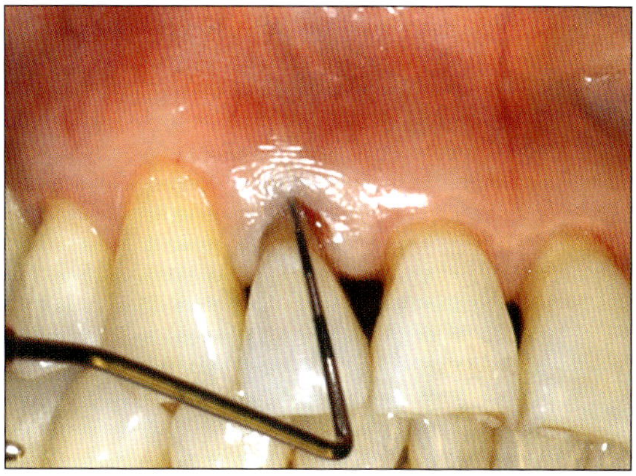

Fig 5-22 Periodontal probing is performed on the suspected tooth and the adjacent teeth during diagnosis and treatment planning. This test not only determines the source of the periodontal defect, but it also affects the flap designs if surgery is indicated.

Palpation

Like percussion sensitivity tests, palpation tests also determine the extent of inflammatory processes in the soft and hard tissues of the oral cavity. Palpation tests are performed by applying firm pressure on the mucosa overlying the hard tissues (Fig 5-20). The presence of palpation sensitivity around attached gingiva indicates periodontal disease. In contrast, the presence of palpation sensitivity in mucosa near the apices of teeth indicates periradicular disease.

Pulp vitality tests

Similar to vitality tests performed for initial root canal treatment, cold, heat, and electric pulp testing should be performed when a patient is considered for further nonsurgical or surgical treatment (Fig 5-21). The information gathered from these tests rules out other teeth and can identify the cause(s) of the patient's complaint. It is not uncommon that, after performing these tests, the clinician finds the source of the patient's complaint to be another tooth or some other cause.

Periodontal probing

Evaluation of the periodontal health of the tooth in question is an important step for diagnosis and treatment planning. Periodontal probing is an important clinical test that is often overlooked. Periapical and periodontal lesions may mimic each other and therefore require differentiation.[66] Periodontal probing not only determines the source of the periodontal defect, but it also affects flap designs and the outcome of the endodontic surgery if this treatment is indicated (Fig 5-22). Like nonrestorable teeth, teeth with severe periodontal disease involvement are poor candidates for any type of endodontic procedure including surgical or nonsurgical retreatment.

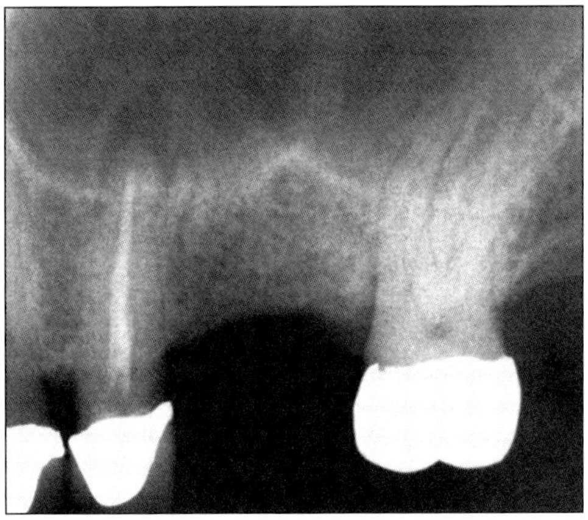

Fig 5-23 Radiographic examination shows the presence of caries lesions, defective and leaky restorations, periradicular lesions, and periodontal disease; the location of anatomical landmarks such as the maxillary sinus; the relationship of these anatomical landmarks to the apices of teeth; and the quality of root canal treatment. Careful examination of these features affects treatment planning.

Mobility

The mobility test determines the periradicular support of a tooth. Teeth with extreme mobility usually have little periradicular support and are poor candidates for surgical or nonsurgical retreatment. Occasionally, mobility decreases after successful surgical or nonsurgical retreatment if the source of the periradicular tissue loss is eliminated.

Radiographic examination

Radiographs allow evaluation of mineralized tissues such as teeth and bone. They reveal general information regarding teeth, their roots, their crowns and crown-root ratios, as well as the bone levels of surrounding teeth. Radiographs also show the presence of caries lesions, defective and leaky restorations, periradicular lesions, and periodontal disease; the location of anatomical landmarks such as the maxillary sinus, incisive and mental foramina, and the mandibular canal and its relationship with the apices of teeth; and the quality of root canal treatment (Fig 5-23). In addition, they show the presence of radiolucencies as well as radiopaque structures such as a buccal oblique ridge or exostosis. The data gathered during radiographic examination provides valuable information that affects treatment planning.

Unfortunately, clinicians have a tendency to rely on radiographs too much and come to their final diagnostic decision based on a single radiograph. Radiographs are a useful tool and have diagnostic value, but they have many limitations. Inflammatory changes in the pulp tissue are not visible, and periradicular lesions cannot be detected in their early stages. Periradicular pathosis is detected when the inflammatory process erodes the cortical plates.[67,68] Radiographs are only two-dimensional and may not show the third dimension of objects in the oral cavity. Recent advances in radiology have resulted in development of cone beam computed tomography (CBCT) and visualization of the third dimension of objects in the oral cavity. This technology is useful for diagnosis and treatment planning for surgical and/or nonsurgical retreatment (see chapter 6).

After conducting the above examinations and tests, the clinician should be able to arrive at a final diagnosis and prepare a proper treatment plan. The gathered information should be discussed with the patient in clear, precise, and understandable language. The presentation to the patient should include the scientific aspects of the treatment options and the reasons, features, and benefits of the proposed treatments. The American Association of Endodontists has published material that is designed to assist patients in understanding various treatment options. These resources (in print and electronic formats) answer the most frequently asked questions about treatment procedures, problems, and prognosis (www.aae.org).

Patient consent

Informed consent is an important part of treatment planning for any proposed procedure. The treatment and its alternatives should be discussed in layman's terms and must include a candid assessment of benefits, risks, and costs involved. To document the understanding and acceptance or rejection of the treatment options, a consent form should be signed by the patient or guardian and witnessed by a third party. This form is an agreement between the patient and the practitioner and becomes a part of the patient's permanent record. If changes are made in the treatment plan, they must be discussed and added to the document, along with the date and the patient's and dentist's signatures.

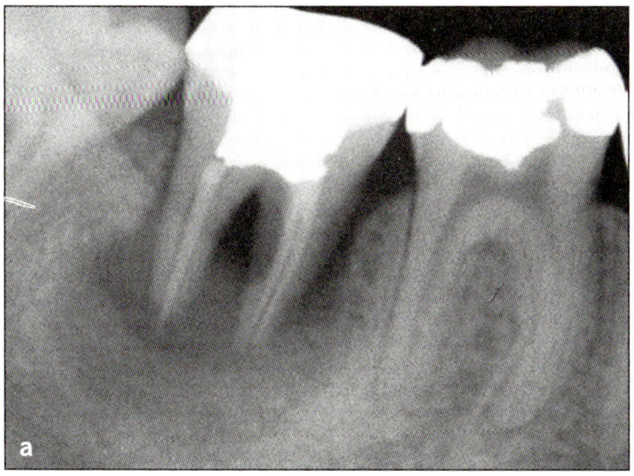

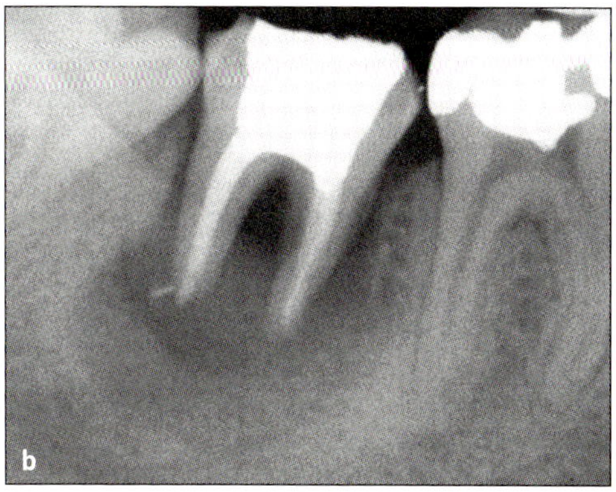

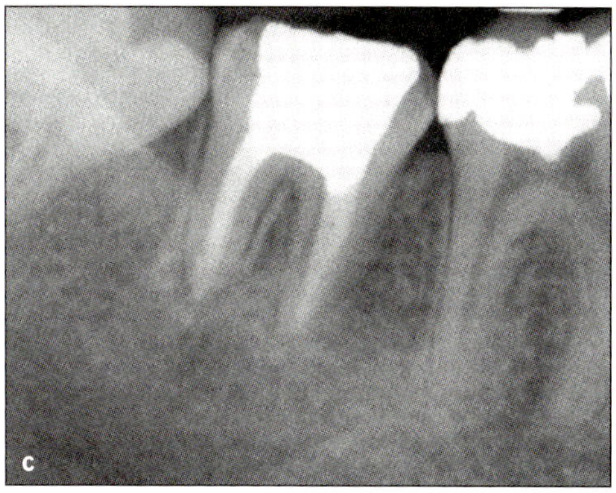

Fig 5-24 *(a)* Preoperative radiograph of a mandibular second molar with inadequate root canal treatment and a large periapical lesion. *(b)* Postoperative radiograph after retreating the root canals and filling them with MTA. *(c)* Postoperative radiograph 9 months later showing complete resolution of the periapical pathosis. (Courtesy of Dr H. J. Kang, Westlake Village, California.)

It must be remembered that the vast majority of teeth with initial root canal treatment heal without any further intervention. But like other procedures in medicine or dentistry, some cases do not heal and need further treatment.

Treatment Options Following Nonhealing of Initial Root Canal Treatment

Clinical examinations of teeth that have not healed following initial root canal treatment may show the presence of palpation and percussion sensitivity, localized swelling, leaky or missing coronal restorations, and recurrent caries. Radiographic examinations of these teeth may reveal the presence of untreated canals, poor obturation, separated instruments, and recurrent caries. The main cause of nonhealing is the presence of bacteria in the root canal system.[54] When initial root canal treatment fails to promote healing, the goals of further treatment are to eliminate infection, improve the quality of obturation, and save the natural dentition. The treatment options are currently nonsurgical retreatment, endodontic surgery, replantation, transplantation, or extraction.

Nonsurgical Retreatment

Indications

If the quality of previous root canal treatment can be improved, nonsurgical retreatment is usually the first treatment of choice (Fig 5-24). Nonsurgical retreatment is indicated in motivated patients with teeth that are restorable, have sound periodontal conditions, possess favorable crown-to-root ratios, and are accessible nonsurgically. The nonsurgical retreatment option allows the clinician to improve the quality of disinfection and obturation compared with the initial treatment and addresses possible coronal leakage with placement of a better coronal restoration. Nonsurgical retreatment prior to surgical treatment has been shown to improve the outcome of surgical endodontics.[30,69] Retreatment procedures usually require special skills, instruments, and advanced training.[31,70]

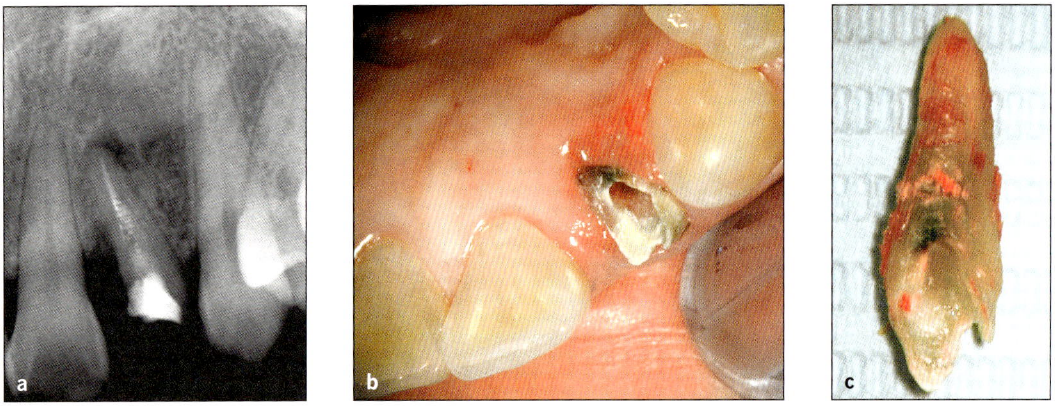

Fig 5-25 *(a)* Preoperative radiograph of a maxillary lateral incisor with inadequate root canal treatment and a periapical lesion. *(b)* A clinical image of the area shows the presence of inadequate tooth structure for placement of a crown and two adjacent teeth without restorations. *(c)* The tooth was extracted and replaced with a single implant.

Contraindications

An unmotivated patient, nonrestorable teeth, teeth with inadequate periodontal support, teeth with an unfavorable crown-to-root ratio, and teeth that are inaccessible nonsurgically are the main contraindications for nonsurgical retreatment of teeth with nonhealing conditions (Fig 5-25). In addition, single-rooted teeth with vertical root fractures are not suitable candidates for nonsurgical retreatment.

Benefits and risks

The main benefits of nonsurgical retreatment are retention of the patient's natural dentition and avoiding extraction. The main risks include damage to the existing crown during access preparation, root fracture during post removal, and accidental procedures such as ledge formation, root perforations, and separation of instruments. Furthermore, nonsurgical retreatment may result in extensive removal of tooth structure and weaken the tooth, which may impact the retreatment outcome and lead to the necessity for extraction training.[70]

Outcomes

Studies have shown that a high percentage of nonsurgically retreated cases are successful after retreatment.[71–74] Based on these reports, it appears that if a nonhealing case is retreated by conventional nonsurgical means, the success rate is high, especially in teeth without periapical lesions and when the cause of failure is identified and corrected.[75]

Surgical Endodontics

When nonsurgical retreatment is not possible or does not succeed, surgical treatment (surgical endodontics) is needed to retain a tooth that would otherwise be extracted (Fig 5-26). Surgical endodontics does not involve simply resecting the apex of a root, preparing a root-end cavity, and placing a root-end filling material. The goals of this procedure are sealing of all portals of communication between the root canal system and periradicular tissues, eliminating contaminants from the periradicular tissues, providing an environment for complete regeneration of periradicular tissues, and saving the natural dentition. During the past 20 years, the art and science of surgical endodontics have significantly changed. With the use of the operating microscope, microsurgery instruments, and new root-end filling materials, surgical endodontics has saved numerous teeth that might otherwise have been extracted.[76]

History of surgical endodontics

Surgical endodontics is not a new procedure; it has a long history (Table 5-1). The first modern endodontic textbook on surgical endodontics was published by Arens, Adams, and DeCastro,[77] followed by other textbooks in 1998.[76] The results from scientific investigations and the clinical techniques and concepts developed during the second half of the 20th century have formed the foundation of what is known and is being practiced in the 21st century. However, surgical endodontics is continually evaluated and modified to improve its long-term clinical outcomes.[76]

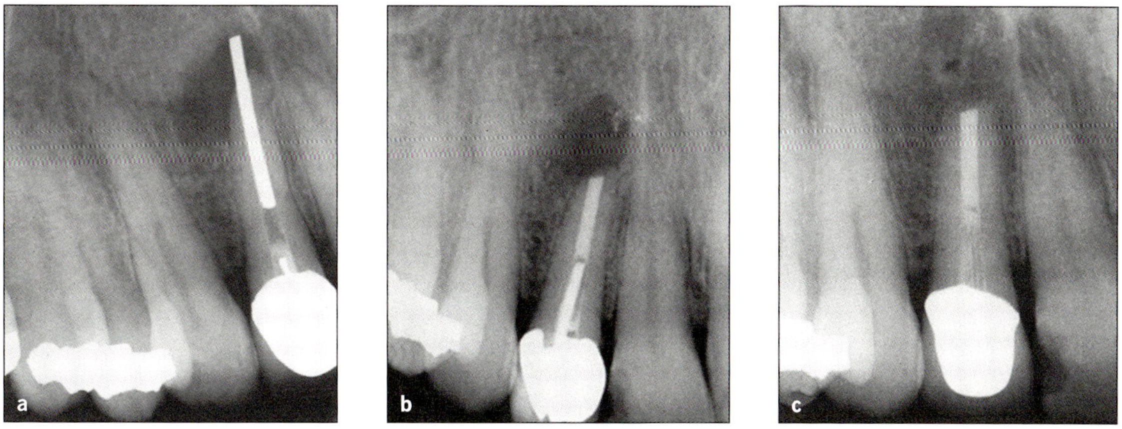

Fig 5-26 *(a)* Periapical radiograph showing an extensive radiolucency around the apex of the maxillary right incisor with an overextended silver point and an inadequate coronal seal. *(b)* The root canal was retreated nonsurgically and surgically using MTA as a root canal filling material. *(c)* Radiograph 3 years later showing complete resolution of the periapical lesion. (Courtesy of Dr Christopher Sechrist, Redlands, California.)

Table 5-1 Examples of historical reports related to endodontic surgery (1884–1998)

Authors	Year	Described techniques
Farrar	1884	Root amputation
Black	1886	Apicoectomy
Rhein	1890	Root amputation
Schamberg	1906	Flap design
Koch	1909	Fistulation
Buckley	1914	Flap design
Lucas	1916	Amalgam as a root-end filling
Fawn	1927	Causes of surgical endodontic failures
Coolidge	1930	Cementum formation over resected roots
Hill	1931	Cementum formation over resected roots
Maxmen	1959	Scope of periapical surgery
Luebke et al	1964	Indications for endodontic surgery
Arens et al	1981	Endodontic surgery
Gutmann and Harrison	1991	Endodontic surgery
Bellizzi and Loushine	1991	Endodontic surgery
Arens et al	1998	Endodontic surgery

Surgical endodontic procedures consist of incision and drainage, periapical surgery, and adjunctive surgery procedures like perforation repair, root resection, hemisection, bicuspidization, as well as tooth replantation and tooth transplantation.

Incision and drainage

The objective of incision and drainage is to evacuate exudates and purulence from a soft tissue swelling. This procedure not only results in patient comfort, but it also speeds healing and recovery.[76]

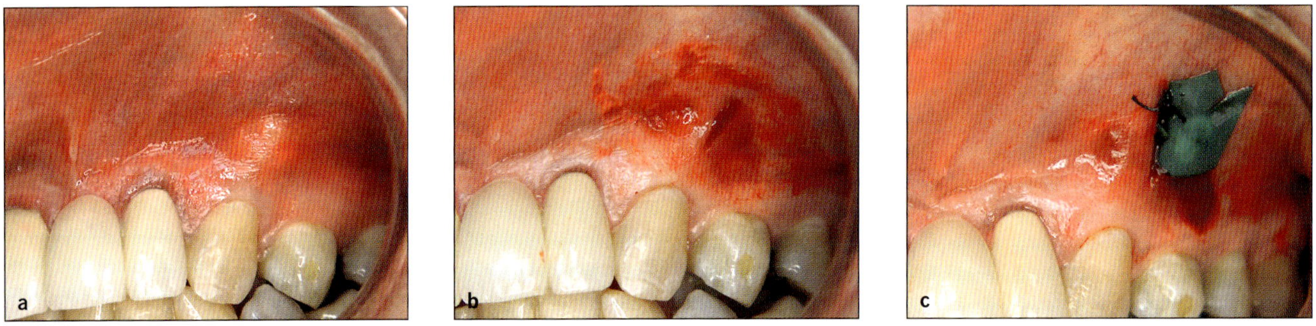

Fig 5-27 *(a)* A fluctuant swelling associated with the maxillary left canine with pulpal necrosis and an acute abscess. *(b)* A vertical incision is placed over the abscess. *(c)* A rubber drain is sutured in place for continued drainage for a few days.

Indications

Drainage through the soft tissue is accomplished most effectively when the swelling is fluctuant[76] (Fig 5-27). If the swelling is nonfluctuant or firm, incision for drainage often results in drainage of only blood and serous fluids. Incision and drainage sometimes is performed before endodontic surgery. Endodontic surgery should be performed when the incision has completely healed.

Contraindications

There are very few contraindications for the use of incision and drainage. Patients with bleeding disorders must be approached with caution. Hematologic screening is indicated for these patients. Anatomical landmarks such as the mental foramen, maxillary sinus, incisive foramen, and an inferior alveolar canal near the apical abscess should be approached carefully during incision and drainage.[77]

Procedures

Anesthesia

Obtaining profound anesthesia is essential to performing incision and drainage. Because of the presence of severe inflammation, accomplishing this task with routine anesthetic techniques might be difficult. In some cases, regional block anesthetic techniques such as mandibular blocks for posterior areas, including Gow-Gates (Video 5-1) and Vazirani-Akinosi (Video 5-2) blocks, bilateral mental blocks for the anterior mandible, posterior superior alveolar blocks for the posterior maxilla, and second division block (Video 5-3) or infraorbital block (Video 5-4) for the anterior maxilla are needed to obtain profound anesthesia. In addition, in cases of severe percussion sensitivity, intraosseous and intraligamental injections are extremely helpful to provide effective anesthesia (Videos 5-5 and 5-6). If none of these procedures work, nitrous oxide/oxygen sedation or intravenous sedation can be used to perform incision and drainage with less pain and discomfort (see chapters 8 and 16).

Incision

After obtaining anesthesia, the incision is made vertically with a No. 11 scalpel. The advantage of vertical incisions is that they are parallel with the major blood vessels and nerves and leave very little scarring. The incision should be made firmly through the soft tissue into the periosteum and bone.

Drainage

After making the initial incision, a small closed hemostat can be placed in the incision line to obtain more drainage. To maintain a path for drainage, a drain cut from rubber dam can be placed and sutured to the edge of the envisioned tissue. The drain should be removed within 2 to 3 days (Video 5-7).

Periapical surgery

The purpose of performing periapical surgery is to stop egress of irritants from the root canal system into the periradicular tissues. This is accomplished by gaining access to the root end, or any part of it, and sealing the portals of exit with a biocompatible material that allows complete regeneration of periradicular tissues.

Indications

The indications for periapical surgery have undergone dramatic changes in the last two decades.[76] These changes are evident especially when dealing with the treatment

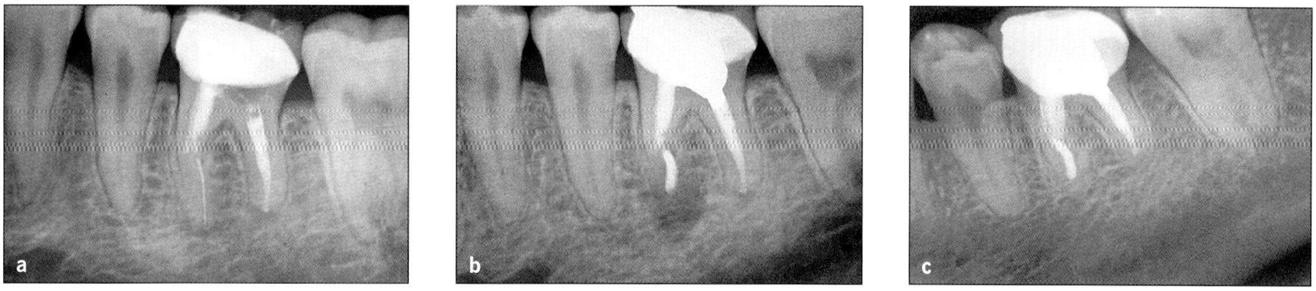

Fig 5-28 *(a)* A nickel-titanium file is separated inside the mesiobuccal canal of the mandibular first molar. *(b)* Because of patient discomfort, surgery was performed to remove this instrument. MTA was used as a root-end filling material. *(c)* Periapical radiograph 32 months later showing complete healing.

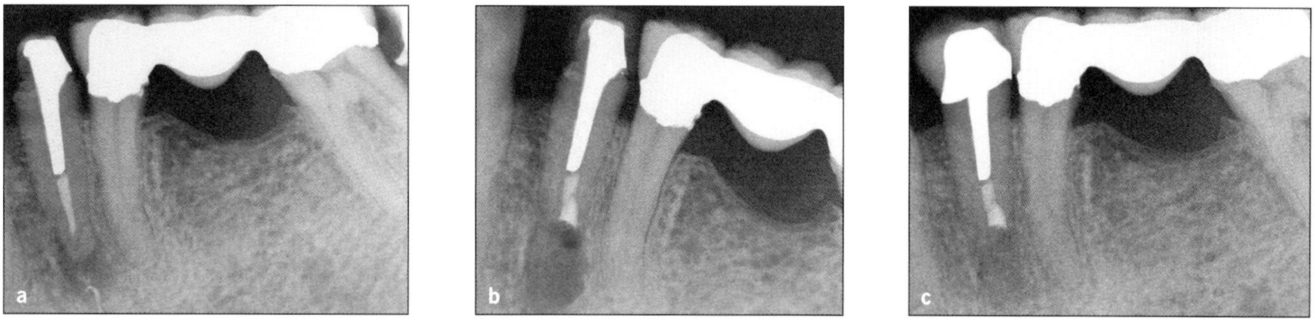

Fig 5-29 *(a)* Inadequate root canal treatment, a large post, extrusion of filling materials into the periapical tissues, and patient discomfort led to a decision to perform periapical surgery on the mandibular first premolar. *(b)* Postoperative radiograph after endodontic surgery. MTA was used as a root-end filling material. *(c)* Periapical radiograph 4½ years later showing complete healing and a functional tooth.

of failed nonsurgical endodontic treatments. The most important principle of endodontic diagnosis and treatment planning is that the primary treatment option for failed endodontic treatment should be nonsurgical endodontic retreatment whenever possible. The importance of thorough and meticulous presurgical planning cannot be overemphasized. Not only must the practitioner and staff be thoroughly trained, but also all necessary instruments, equipment, and supplies must be readily available in the treatment room. This requires that every step of the procedure be carefully planned and analyzed. The potential for possible complications must be anticipated and incorporated into the presurgical planning. Good patient communication is essential for thorough surgical preparation. It is important that the patient understands the reason surgery is needed as well as other treatment options available. The patient must be informed of the prognosis for a successful outcome and the risks involved in the surgical procedure in addition to the benefits. It is also important that the patient is informed of the possible short-term effects of the surgery, such as pain, swelling, discoloration, and infection.[76]

The main indications for periapical surgery are failing root canal treatments; procedural accidents; irretrievable materials in the root canal or periapical tissues; anatomical complexity of the root canal system that prevents complete cleaning, shaping, and obturation of the root canal system through the coronal access; symptomatic cases; adjunctive surgeries; and exploratory surgery.

Failing root canal treatments. When previous NSRCT cannot be improved or performed because regaining access to the canal or removing posts would carry a risk of perforation or root fracture and/or create a restorative problem, surgical endodontics is indicated.

Procedural accidents. As with other disciplines in dentistry, performing root canal treatment can result in mishaps and procedural accidents. These include ledge formation, root perforation, separated instruments, and underfilled or overfilled canals. Most of these accidents can be corrected nonsurgically. However, when nonsurgical correction of these accidents is not feasible or practical, periapical surgery is indicated to save these teeth (Fig 5-28).

Irretrievable filling materials. Root canal filling materials within the root canals can usually be removed from the roots by an orthograde approach. However, when obturation materials cannot be removed nonsurgically (Video 5-8) or are beyond the root canal space, surgical endodontics is indicated to save the tooth (Fig 5-29). See Videos 5-9 and 5-10.

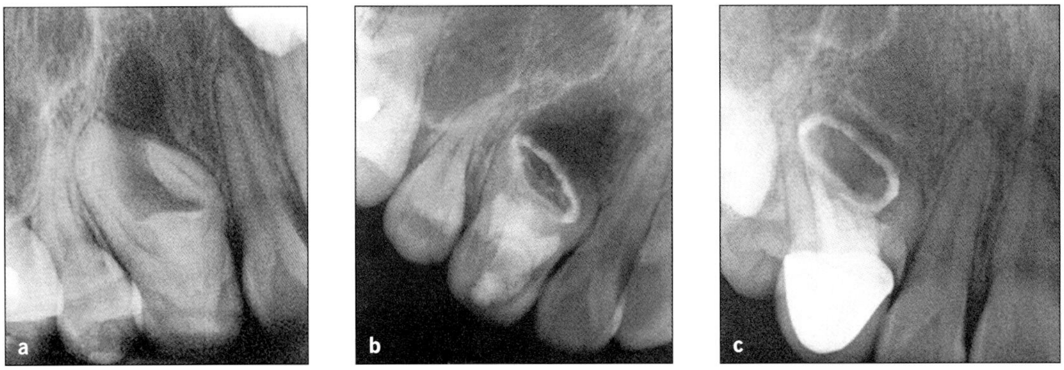

Fig 5-30 *(a)* Preoperative radiograph of the right anterior maxilla shows the presence of dens invaginatus in the canine. *(b)* Because of the presence of this anomaly in the tooth, the large lesion, and the inability to perform NSRCT, periapical surgery was performed. *(c)* Postoperative radiograph 20 months later showing complete resolution of the lesion associated with the canine.

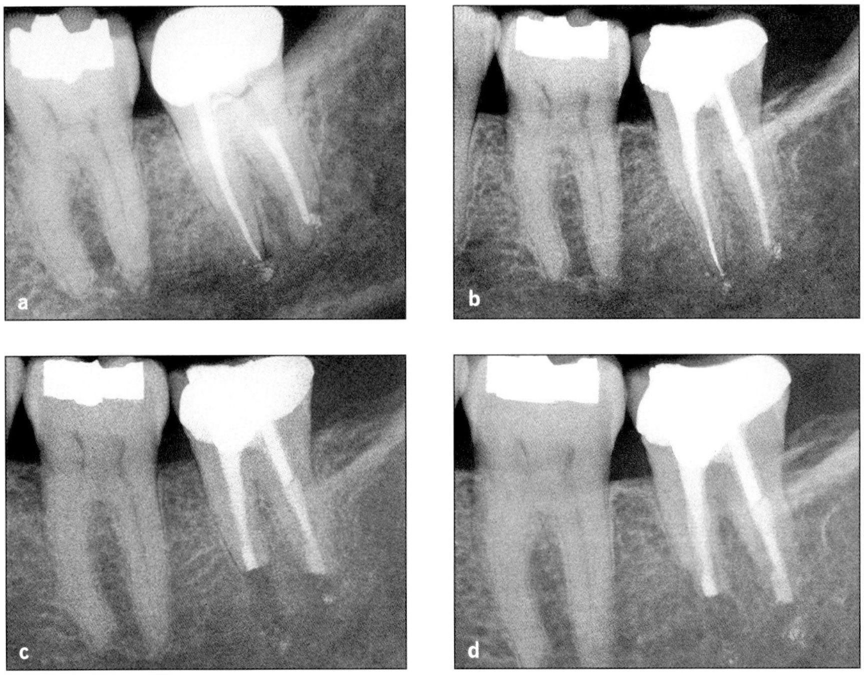

Fig 5-31 *(a)* Preoperative radiograph of a mandibular second molar with completed root canal treatment. The tooth stayed symptomatic after treatment. *(b)* Postoperative radiograph of the tooth after nonsurgical retreatment. The tooth stayed symptomatic again after retreatment. A tooth replantation was planned for the patient. *(c)* Immediate postoperative radiograph after tooth replantation. *(d)* Postoperative radiograph 2 years later showing complete healing.

Anatomical complexity of the root canal system. Complex anatomy, severe curvature, and canal calcifications that cannot be handled nonsurgically are indications for surgical endodontics (Fig 5-30).

Symptomatic cases. Nonsurgical retreatment usually results in relief of pain and discomfort for most patients. However, when nonsurgical retreatment is not possible and symptoms persist during (Video 5-11) or following (Video 5-12) initial treatment or retreatment, surgical endodontics should be considered to relieve pressure and reduce pain and discomfort for the patient[76] (Fig 5-31).

Adjunctive surgeries. Adjunctive surgical procedures are those that are required to repair defects that occur as a result of either procedural accidents or pathologic

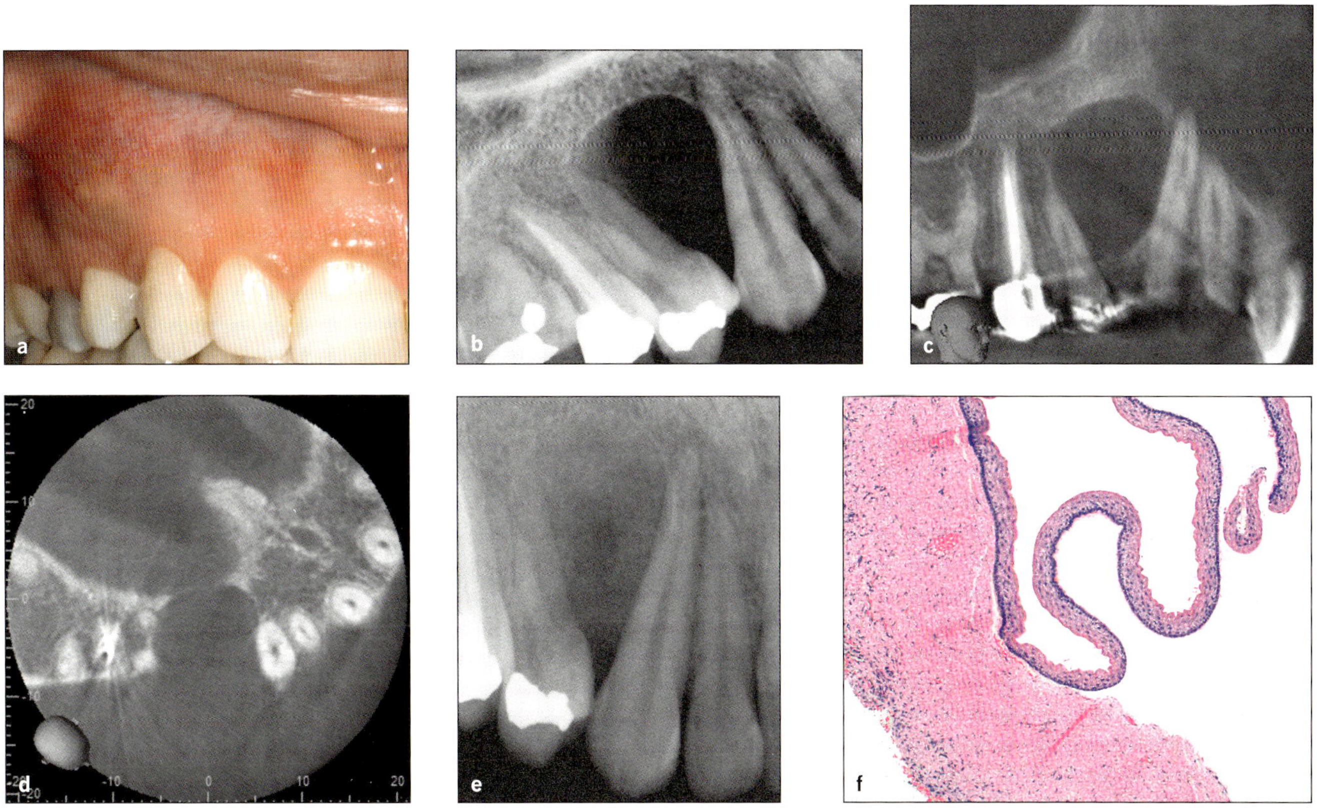

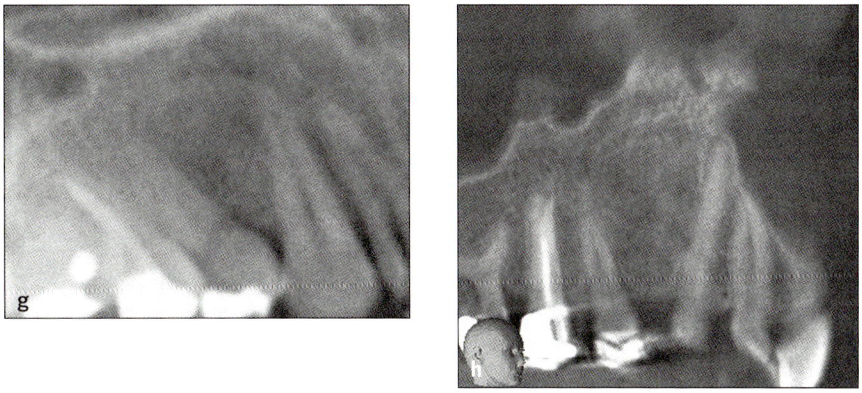

Fig 5-32 *(a)* Clinical view of the maxillary right region showing the presence of swelling between the canine and first premolar in a 25-year-old woman. *(b)* Periapical radiograph showing the presence of a large lesion between the canine and maxillary first premolar. *(c)* A sagittal view of the region with CBCT showing the extent of the lesion. *(d)* An axial view of the region with CBCT showing that the lesion has almost perforated the maxillary sinus. *(e)* Because the teeth in this region responded within normal limits, a biopsy was performed. A postoperative radiograph was taken after removal of the lesion. The detect was filled with freeze-dried bone, and a resorbable membrane was placed over the bone graft material. *(f)* Histologic examination of the tissue specimens removed during exploratory surgery revealed the presence of an odontogenic keratocyst between the canine and first premolar. *(g)* Postoperative radiograph 1 year later showing complete resolution of the lesion. *(h)* A sagittal view of the region with CBCT 1 year after surgery showing complete healing.

processes. They include repair of perforations, repair of resorptive defects, root resection, hemisection, crown lengthening, tooth replantation, and transplantation (see chapter 15).

Exploratory surgery. A majority of periapical lesions are caused by infection of root canal systems. However, there are some radiolucencies that are not caused by root canal infection and may mimic periapical lesions of endodontic origin (see chapter 4). Suspicious and nonhealing lesions require exploratory surgery including a biopsy for histologic examination (Fig 5-32 and Video 5-13).

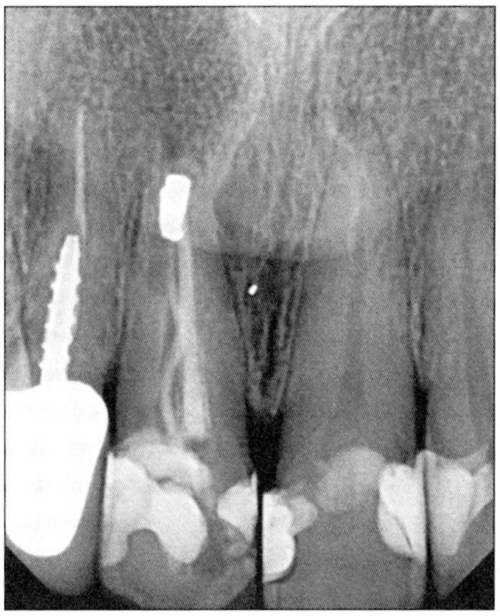

Fig 5-33 Performing periapical surgery on a tooth with inadequate root canal treatment that can be retreated nonsurgically is an indiscriminate act and a contraindication for endodontic surgery.

Contraindications

There are few contraindications for periapical surgery. They include medical or systemic complications, indiscriminate use of periapical surgery, anatomical factors, and an unidentified cause of treatment failure.[76]

Medical or systemic complications. Serious systemic diseases in patients with blood disorders, terminal diseases, uncontrolled diabetes, severe heart diseases, and compromised immune systems are examples of contraindications for periapical surgery. Consultation with the patient's physician is indicated.

Indiscriminate use of surgery. Indiscriminate use of periapical surgery for those cases that can be handled nonsurgically is unethical and should not be practiced (Fig 5-33). Periapical surgery is contraindicated when nonsurgical treatment is feasible and could probably result in successful outcomes. Torabinejad et al[72] performed a systematic review to compare the clinical and radiographic outcomes of nonsurgical retreatment with those of endodontic surgery. They found that although endodontic surgery offered more favorable initial success rates, nonsurgical retreatment offered more favorable long-term outcomes.[72] This finding supports the concept that nonsurgical retreatment should be the first choice before attempting periapical surgery.

Benefits and risks of surgical endodontics

The main benefits of surgical endodontics are retention of the patient's natural dentition and avoiding extraction. The main risks of surgical endodontics include damage to the gingival tissue and scar tissue formation after surgery, as well as postoperative complications such as bruising and paresthesia.

Outcomes of surgical endodontics

Examination of the outcomes of traditional endodontic surgery has shown a relatively high success rate for this procedure.[72] Recent advances in the art and science of endodontic surgery have improved significantly because of the use of the microscope, angled ultrasonic surgical instruments, and new root-end filling materials[78] (see chapter 17).

Adjunctive procedures

Adjunctive surgery procedures include perforation repair, root resection, hemisection, and bicuspidization, as well as tooth replantation and transplantation. The indications, contraindications, and techniques involved with these procedures are described in chapter 15.

References

1. Hirschfeld L, Wasserman B. A long-term survey of tooth loss in 600 treated periodontal patients. J Periodontol 1978;49:225–237.
2. McFall WT Jr. Tooth loss in 100 treated patients with periodontal disease. A long-term study. J Periodontol 1982;53:539–549.
3. Becker W, Berg L, Becker BE. The long term evaluation of periodontal treatment and maintenance in 95 patients. Int J Periodontics Restorative Dent 1984;4(2):54–71.
4. Johnson K. A study of the dimensional changes occurring in the maxilla following tooth extraction. Aust Dent J 1969;14:241–244.
5. Love WD, Adams RL. Tooth movement into edentulous areas. J Prosthet Dent 1971;25:271–278.
6. Shugars DA, Bader JD, White BA, Scurria MS, Hayden WJ Jr, Garcia RI. Survival rates of teeth adjacent to treated and untreated posterior bounded edentulous spaces. J Am Dent Assoc 1998;129:1089–1095.
7. Aquilino SA, Shugars DA, Bader JD, White BA. Ten-year survival rates of teeth adjacent to treated and untreated posterior bounded edentulous spaces. J Prosthet Dent 2001;85:455–460.
8. Oosterhaven SP, Westert GP, Schaub RM, van der Bilt A. Social and psychologic implications of missing teeth for chewing ability. Community Dent Oral Epidemiol 1988;16:79–82.
9. Torabinejad M. Effects of dental implants on treatment planning for prosthodontics, periodontics and endodontics. In: Ingle JI, Bakland LK, Baumgartner JC (eds). Endodontics, ed 6. Hamilton, Ontario: BC Decker, 2008:105–117.
10. Wyatt CC. The effect of prosthodontic treatment on alveolar bone loss: A review of the literature. J Prosthet Dent 1998;80:362–366.
11. Ericsson SG, Marken KE. Effect of fixed partial dentures on surrounding tissues. J Prosthet Dent 1968;20:517–525.
12. Silness J, Gustavsen F. Alveolar bone loss in bridge recipients after six and twelve years. Int Dent J 1985;35:297–300.
13. Tolboe H, Isidor F, Budtz-Jorgensen E, Kaaber S. Influence of pontic material on alveolar mucosal conditions. Scand J Dent Res 1988;96:442–447.
14. Torabinejad M, Goodacre CJ. Endodontic or dental implant therapy: The factors affecting treatment planning. J Am Dent Assoc 2006;137:973–977.
15. Torabinejad M, Anderson P, Bader J, et al. The outcomes of endodontic treatment, single implant, fixed partial denture and no tooth replacement: A systematic review. J Prosthet Dent 2007;98:285–311.
16. Sundqvist G. Bacteriological studies of necrotic dental pulps [thesis]. Umeå, Sweden: University of Umeå, 1976.
17. Bergenholtz G. Micro-organisms from necrotic pulp of traumatized teeth. Odontol Revy 1974;25:347–358.
18. Kantz WE, Henry CA. Isolation and classification of anaerobic bacteria from intact pulp chambers of non-vital teeth in man. Arch Oral Biol 1974;19:91–96.
19. Walton RE, Torabinejad M. Diagnosis and treatment planning. In: Walton RE, Torabinejad M (eds). Principles and Practice of Endodontics, ed 3. Philadelphia: Saunders, 2002:49–70.
20. Lazarski MP, Walker WA 3rd, Flores CM, Schindler WG, Hargreaves KM. Epidemiological evaluation of the outcomes of nonsurgical root canal treatment in a large cohort of insured dental patients. J Endod 2001;27:791–796.
21. Salehrabi R, Rotstein I. Endodontic treatment outcomes in a large patient population in the USA: An epidemiological study. J Endod 2004;30:846–850.
22. Chen S, Chueh L, Hsiao CK, Tsai MY, Ho SC, Chiang CP. An epidemiologic study of tooth retention after nonsurgical endodontic treatment in a large population in Taiwan. J Endod 2007;33:226–229.
23. Raedel M, Hartmann A, Bohm S, Walter MH. Three-year outcomes of root canal treatment: Mining an insurance database. J Dent 2015;43:412–417.
24. Bernstein SD, Horowitz AJ, Man M, et al; Practitioners Engaged in Applied Research and Learning (PEARL) Network Group. Outcomes of endodontic therapy in general practice: A study by the Practitioners Engaged in Applied Research and Learning Network. J Am Dent Assoc 2012;143:478–487.
25. Gilbert GH, Tilashalski KR, Litaker MS, McNeal SF, Boykin MJ, Kessler AW; DPBRN Collaborative Group. Outcomes of root canal treatment in Dental Practice-Based Research Network practices. Gen Dent 2010;58:28–36
26. Iqbal MK, Kim S. For teeth requiring endodontic therapy, what are the differences in the outcomes of restored endodontically treated teeth compared to implant-supported restorations? Int J Oral Maxillofac Implants 2007;22(suppl 1):96–116 [erratum 2008;23:56].
27. Ng YL, Mann V, Gulabivala K. Tooth survival following non-surgical root canal treatment: A systematic review of the literature. Int Endod J 2010;43:171–189.
28. Allen RK, Newton CW, Brown CE Jr. A statistical analysis of surgical and nonsurgical endodontic retreatment cases. J Endod 1989;15:261–266.
29. Hoen MM, Pink FE. Contemporary endodontic retreatments: An analysis based on clinical treatment findings. J Endod 2002;28:834–836.
30. Friedman S, Stabholz A. Endodontic retreatment—Case selection and technique. Part 1: Criteria for case selection. J Endod 1986;12:28–33.
31. Ruddle CJ. Nonsurgical retreatment. J Endod 2004;30:827–845.
32. Sjögren U, Figdor D, Persson S, Sundqvist G. Influence of infection at the time of root filling on the outcome of endodontic treatment of teeth with apical periodontitis. Int Endod J 1997;30:297–306.
33. Weiger R, Rosendahl R, Lost C. Influence of calcium hydroxide intracanal dressings on the prognosis of teeth with endodontically induced periapical lesion. Int Endod J 2000;33:219–226.
34. Kim D, Kim E. Antimicrobial effect of calcium hydroxide as an intracanal medicament in root canal treatment: A literature review—Part II. In vivo studies. Restor Dent Endod 2015;40:97–103.
35. Pirani C, Chersoni S, Montebugnoli L, Prati C. Long-term outcome of non-surgical root canal treatment: A retrospective analysis. Odontology 2015;103:185–193.
36. Ng YL, Mann V, Gulabivala K. A prospective study of the factors affecting outcomes of non-surgical root canal treatment: Part 2: Tooth survival. Int Endod J 2011;44:610–625.
37. Kojima K, Inamoto K, Nagamatsu K, et al. Success rate of endodontic treatment of teeth with vital and nonvital pulps. A meta-analysis. Oral Surg Oral Med Oral Pathol Oral Radiol Endod 2004;97:95–99.
38. Hamedy R, Shakiba B, Pak JG, Barbizam JV, Ogawa RS, White SN. Prevalence of root canal treatment and periapical radiolucency in elders: A systematic review. Gerodontology 2016;33:116–127.
39. Stoll R, Betke K, Stachniss V. The influence of different factors on the survival of root canal fillings: A 10-year retrospective study. J Endod 2005;31:783–790.
40. Kirkevang LL, Orstavik D, Horsted-Bindslev P, Wenzel A. Periapical status and quality of root canal fillings and coronal restorations in a Danish population. Int Endod J 2000;33:509–515.
41. De Moor RJ, Hommez GM, De Boever JG, Delme KI, Martens GE. Periapical health related to the quality of root canal treatment in a Belgian population. Int Endod J 2000; 33:113–120.
42. Segura-Egea JJ, Jiménez-Pinzón A, Poyato-Ferrera M, Velasco-Ortega E, Ríos-Santos JV. Periapical status and quality of root fillings and coronal restorations in an adult Spanish population. Int Endod J 2004;37:525–530.
43. Siqueira JF Jr. Aetiology of root canal treatment failure: Why well-treated teeth can fail. Int Endod J 2001;34:1–10.
44. Frisk F. Epidemiological aspects on apical periodontitis. Studies based on the Prospective Population Study of Women in Göteborg and the Population Study on Oral Health in Jönköping, Sweden. Swed Dent J Suppl 2007;189:11–78.
45. Gillen BM, Looney SW, Gu LS, Loushine BA, et al. Impact of the quality of coronal restoration versus the quality of root canal fillings on success of root canal treatment: A systematic review and meta-analysis. J Endod 2011;37:895–902.
46. Liang Y, Li G, Shemesh H, Wesselink PR, Wu M. The association between complete absence of post-treatment periapical lesion and quality of root canal filling. Clin Oral Investig 2012;16:1619–1626.
47. Bergenholtz G, Lekholm U, Milthon R, Engstrom B. Influence of apical overinstrumentation and overfilling on re-treated root canals. J Endod 1979;5:310–314.
48. Chong BS. Coronal leakage and treatment failure. J Endod 1995;21:159–160.
49. Begotka BA, Hartwell GR. The importance of the coronal seal following root canal treatment. Va Dent J 1996;73(4):8–10.
50. Hartwell GR, Loucks CA, Reavley BA. Bacterial leakage of provisional restorative materials used in endodontics. Quintessence Int 2010;41:335–339.
51. Tamse A. Iatrogenic vertical root fractures in endodontically treated teeth. Endod Dent Traumatol 1988;4:190–196.
52. Sedgley CM, Messer HH. Are endodontically treated teeth more brittle? J Endod 1992;18:332–335.
53. Fuss Z, Lustig J, Katz A, Tamse A. An evaluation of endodontically treated vertically fractured roots: Impact of operative procedures. J Endod 2001;27:46–48.
54. Nair PN. On the causes of persistent apical periodontitis: A review. Int Endod J 2006;39:249–281.
55. Fenlon MR, McCartan BE. Validity of a patient self-completed health questionnaire in a primary care dental practice. Community Dent Oral Epidemiol 1992;20:130–132.
56. McDaniel TF, Miller D, Jones R, Davis M. Assessing patient willingness to reveal health history information. J Am Dent Assoc 1995;126:375–379.
57. Smeets EC, de Jong KJ, Abraham-Inpijn L. Detecting the medically compromised patient in dentistry by means of the medical risk-related history. A survey of 29,424 dental patients in The Netherlands. Prev Med 1998;27:530–535.

58. Fitzgerald J, Epstein JB, Donaldson M, Schwartz O, Jones C, Fung K. Outpatient medication use and implications for dental care: Guidance for contemporary dental practice. J Can Dent Assoc 2015;81:f10.
59. Norred CL, Brinker F. Potential coagulation effects of preoperative complementary and alternative medicines. Altern Ther Health Med 2001;7:58–67.
60. Chang LK, Whitaker DC. The impact of herbal medicines on dermatologic surgery. Dermatol Surg 2001;27:759–763.
61. Eriksen H. Endodontology—Epidemiologic considerations. Endod Dent Traumatol 1991;7:189–195.
62. Johnson BR, Epstein JB. Management considerations for the medically complex endodontic patient. In: Rotstein I, Ingle JI (eds). Ingle's Endodontics, ed 7. Shelton, CT: People's Medical, 2017 [in press].
63. Georgelin-Gurgel M, Diemer F, Nicolas E, Hennequin M. Surgical and nonsurgical endodontic treatment-induced stress. J Endod 2009;35:19–22.
64. Wilson W, Taubert KA, Gewitz M, et al; American Heart Association Rheumatic Fever, Endocarditis and Kawasaki Disease Committee, Council on Cardiovascular Disease in the Young; Council on Clinical Cardiology; Council on Cardiovascular Surgery and Anesthesia; Quality of Care and Outcomes Research Interdisciplinary Working Group; American Dental Association. Prevention of infective endocarditis: Guidelines from the American Heart Association: a guideline from the American Heart Association Rheumatic Fever, Endocarditis and Kawasaki Disease Committee, Council on Cardiovascular Disease in the Young, and the Council on Clinical Cardiology, Council on Cardiovascular Surgery and Anesthesia, and the Quality of Care and Outcomes Research Interdisciplinary Working Group. J Am Dent Assoc 2007;138:739–760.
65. Dayer MJ, Jones S, Prendergast B, Baddour LM, Lockhardt PB, Thornhill MH. Incidence of infective endocarditis in England, 2000–13: A secular trend, interrupted time-series analysis. Lancet 2015;385(9974):1219–1228.
66. Torabinejad M, Rotstein I. Endodontic-periodontic interrelationship. In: Torabinejad M, Fouad A, Walton RE (eds). Endodontic Principles and Practice, ed 5. Philadelphia: Saunders, 2015:106–120.
67. Bender IB. Factors influencing the radiographic appearance of bony lesions. J Endod 1982;8:161–170.
68. Lee SJ, Messer HH. Radiographic appearance of artificially prepared periapical lesions confined to cancellous bone. Int Endod J 1986;19:64–72.
69. Taschieri S, Machtou P, Rosano G, Weinstein T, Del Fabbro M. The influence of previous non-surgical re-treatment on the outcome of endodontic surgery. Minerva Stomatol 2010;59:625–632.
70. Bogen G, Handysides R. Retreatment. In: Torabinejad M, Fouad A, Walton RE (eds). Endodontic Principles and Practice, ed 5. Philadelphia: Saunders, 2015:355–375.
71. Farzaneh M, Abitbol S, Friedman S. Treatment outcome in endodontics: The Toronto study. Phases I and II: Orthograde retreatment. J Endod 2004;30:627–633.
72. Torabinejad M, Corr R, Handysides R, Shabahang S. Outcomes of nonsurgical retreatment and endodontic surgery: A systematic review. J Endod 2009;35:930–937.
73. Ng YL, Mann V, Gulabivala K. Outcome of secondary root canal treatment: A systematic review of the literature. Int Endod J 2008;41:1026–1046.
74. Salehrabi R, Rotstein I. Epidemiological evaluation of the outcomes of orthograde endodontic retreatment. J Endod 2010;36:790–792.
75. Bergenholtz G, Lekholm U, Milthon R, Heden G, Odesjö B, Engström B. Retreatment of endodontic fillings. Scand J Dent Res 1979;87:217–224.
76. Torabinejad M, Sabeti M, Glickman G. Surgical endodontics. In: Rotstein I, Ingle JI (eds). Ingle's Endodontics, ed 7. Shelton, CT: People's Medical, 2017 [in press].
77. Arens DE, Adams WR, DeCastro RA. Endodontic Surgery. Philadelphia: Harper & Row, 1981.
78. Torabinejad M, White S. Endodontic treatment options following unsuccessful initial root canal treatment: Alternatives to single implants. J Am Dent Assoc 2016;147:214–220.

Chapter Six

Cone Beam Computed Tomography in Treatment Planning of Periapical Surgery

Mohamed I. Fayad, Bruno C. Azevedo, Richard Rubinstein

Cone beam computed tomography (CBCT) is a diagnostic imaging modality that provides high-quality, accurate three-dimensional (3D) representations of the osseous elements of the maxillofacial skeleton. CBCT has great potential to become a valuable tool in modern endodontic microsurgical procedures. The different applications of CBCT in diagnosis, treatment planning, and long-term outcome evaluation of periapical surgery are reviewed in this chapter. Cases are presented to demonstrate the benefit of CBCT information in presurgical assessment, case selection, and treatment planning in endodontic microsurgery. The chapter also discusses how to use CBCT to identify and manage cases involving vital structures (maxillary sinus, inferior alveolar nerve [IAN], mental nerve, and nasopalatine bundle) and to evaluate the outcome of periapical microsurgery.

Intraoral and extraoral imaging modalities are invaluable tools to the overall assessment of the oral maxillofacial complex. Periapical (PA), bitewing (BW), and panoramic radiographs allow for two-dimensional (2D) imaging examination of teeth and tooth-bearing areas. PA radiographs play a major role in the endodontic imaging diagnosis and, according to the joint statement between the American Association of Endodontists (AAE) and the American Academy of Oral and Maxillofacial Radiology (AAOMR) published in 2015, "should be considered the imaging modality of choice in the evaluation of the endodontic patient."[1]

Interpretation of 2D radiographs in dentistry is limited due to the complex anatomy associated with the oral cavity and the imaging projection restrictions, such as flattening 3D structures into 2D images.[2] Historically, 2D images have been known to have significant problems because of vertical and horizontal imaging projection errors such as elongation, foreshortening, magnification, and overlapping of anatomical structures.[3] These problems made precise diagnosis and surgical planning of endodontic surgical cases a challenge, and until recently, access to 3D imaging such as CT was limited.[3]

However, in 1997, Dr Yoshinori Arai from Nihon University in Japan announced the development of the first high-resolution, small-volume CT scanner dedicated to the oral and maxillofacial complex. Another technologic breakthrough was the ability to process and reconstruct 3D images in ordinary desktop computers.[4,5] This new imaging modality was originally termed *ortho-CT*.[5] Dr Arai's work led to a 3D revolution in dentistry and the endodontic specialty, allowing dentists to acquire small, high-resolution 3D volumes of the maxilla and mandible in office. This small-volume scanner also involved reduced radiation dose and cost compared with medical CT. In the early 2000s, the term *ortho-CT* evolved to *cone beam volumetric tomography* (CBVT) and later to *cone beam computed tomography* (CBCT).[3]

CBCT imaging has proven to be better than conventional radiographs for visualization of the maxillofacial complex, including root canal anatomy, and accurate detection of apical pathologies and root fractures.[3,6] CBCT quickly became an important tool for endodontic surgical cases. The ability to observe tooth and bony anatomy in three dimensions without superimposition and sliced into submillimeter layers delivers invaluable information to surgeons before, during, and after surgical procedures.

According to the AAE/AAOMR 2015 statement, small-volume high-resolution CBCT should be considered as the imaging modality of choice when evaluating the nonhealing of previous endodontic treatment to help determine the need for further treatment—nonsurgical, surgical, or extraction—and for presurgical treatment planning to localize the root apex/apices and to evaluate the proximity to adjacent anatomical structures.[1]

CBCT Hardware

CBCT scanners can be divided into two categories: dedicated and multifunction. Dedicated CBCT scanners can only acquire 3D volumes and have no other imaging capabilities. They typically have larger footprints due to wider air gap (distance between the area sensor and the x-ray emitter) and offer multiple fields of view, ranging from small to full head scan capabilities.[3] The patient may be positioned as standing, sitting, or in a supine position depending on the manufacturer. Multifunction CBCT scanners can acquire multiple 2D/3D imaging modalities, including panoramic radiographs, lateral and frontal cephalograms, open and closed 2D temporomandibular joint (TMJ) views, and CBCT volumes. These units have small footprints, and their designs are based on 2D digital panoramic units.

Different types of sensors such as image intensifier screens (IIS) and flat-panel displays (FPD) are currently used on multifunction units.[7,8] There are significant differences between them. IIS sensors are much bigger and bulkier than FPD sensors and are sensitive to magnetic fields, which typically translates to a shorter life span and regular calibration sessions. During image acquisition, photons are converted into an optical signal by the input phosphor screen, and this signal is in turn converted to electrons by the photocathode screen. The electric field inside the image intensifier will accelerate the electrons and convert them back to an optical signal at the output phosphor screen. The intensity of the optical signal is adjusted by the optical iris, and the signal is then detected by the charge-coupled device.[7,8]

This complex image formation generates a volume in the shape of a sphere and can lead to geometric distortions at the edges of the volume. New reconstruction software can reduce such artifacts, but noise is still part of the volume. This distortion could potentially reduce the measurement accuracy of CBCT units and their resolution. One advantage, however, is a reduced radiation dose to the patient. Flat-panel images are produced in a thin film of amorphous silicon with a large area sensor.[8] The photons are read by a scintillator that converts x-rays into an electric signal, which is read directly on the flat panel. This allows for a distortion-free image and better dynamic range, maximized performance, and longer sensor life span when compared with IIS.[7,8]

Image acquisition on both scanners relies on the same imaging acquisition principles: a C-arm with an area sensor (IIS or FPD) and an x-ray source rotating around the patient's head or region of interest. Multiple images/frames, referred to as *base images*, are captured by the sensors. The number of base images acquired depends on the rotation angle (180 degrees vs 360 degrees), sensor frame capture per second, resolution protocol, and exposure protocols (continuous or pulsating). In general, the larger the number of base images, the better the image quality/resolution, fewer reconstruction imaging artifacts, and higher radiation dose.[3,4,7,8]

After acquisition is finished, all base images or raw data are transferred to a computer for reconstruction. CBCT data is typically incomplete because only part of the anatomy is acquired during image capture, and a reconstruction filter is used to improve the data quality. The Feldkamp algorithm is the most popular filter used in CBCT reconstruction.

CBCT Volume

The CBCT volume is made of 3D pixels called *voxels*.[9–11] CBCT voxels are small cubes that are isometrics and isomorphs. Their size is an important factor when determining the spatial resolution of a CBCT scan/scanner. In theory, the smaller the voxel, the better the scanner's ability to display detail. However, because CBCT is a complex imaging system, final resolution needs to take into consideration more than just voxel size. It also depends on the type of sensor (FPD has higher resolution than IIS), number of base images acquired, air gap distance, quality of the sensor, acquisition time, use of patient stabilization devices, and software filters.

After images are reconstructed by the acquisition software, the volume is available for visualization. Multiplanar reconstruction (MPR) allows the clinician to visualize the volume in three different planes of space: axial, sagittal, and coronal. The axial plane allows the clinician to evaluate the volume from bottom to top to bottom. This plane allows for visualization of perforation or expansion of cortical plates. The coronal plane runs from anterior to posterior to anterior. This plane is important when interpreting the maxillary sinuses and buccal-palatal or lingual cortication of the posterior teeth. The sagittal plane slides from lateral to medial to lateral (following the midsagittal plane). This plane is preferable during the investigation of anterior teeth and TMJ pathologies. Volume-rendering reconstruction is also visualized; 3D rendering of the anatomy is important to better visualize key anatomical structures and to improve perception of key anatomical features.[10,11]

Users can also control the slice thickness and slice interval of the navigation. Slice thickness controls thickness of the 3D planes. As a general rule, the smaller the voxel size display, the more noise is shown within the volume. Slice interval controls how much the cursors will move from image to image. In the MPR view, slice interval and slice thickness are linked together and are typically 1 mm. If more detail is needed, they can be changed to submillimeter values consistent with the smaller acquisition voxel at the expense of adding more noise to the volume. Surgical case navigation through a volume should strike a balance between those values in order to maximize resolution and minimize noise.[9–11]

CBCT Applications in Endodontics

As a new imaging modality in dentistry, CBCT is increasing its importance in the modern dental practice. The benefit of CBCT scans in the fields of endodontics, surgery, orthodontics, periodontics, implants, and pathology is vastly described in the scientific literature; however, there are nuances and limitations to this imaging modality. Medicolegal issues, cost, imaging artifacts, and increased patient radiation dose are important topics to be considered before the adoption of this technology. From a medicolegal standpoint, it is important to remember that doctors are required to interpret the full volume and not only the region of interest. In general, small-volume CBCT scans cover the same anatomy as 2D images, and minimal competency on their interpretation is required. In addition, it is also important to stress that oral and maxillofacial radiology is a recognized specialty in dentistry; in case of doubt during interpretation, referral of the patient volume to a dental radiologist is encouraged.

There are approximately 75 different dental CBCT scanners on the world market, and competition between companies has significantly reduced the cost of the scanners. As they become more affordable and more available to practitioners, their price will continue to fall. CBCT billing is currently being addressed by the American Dental Association (ADA) and the AAE, and insurance reimbursement is expected to be resolved at some time in the near future.

CBCT scans are associated with multiple types of artifacts such as noise and poor soft tissue display. Artifacts can compromise the final image quality and should be minimized at all costs. The most common artifacts in CBCT scanning are movement and beam hardening. Patient movement is typically associated with longer acquisition times and/or poor patient stabilization. Movement artifact will generate blurred images and double cortication throughout the anatomy. Those artifacts reduce image quality and could potentially mask key anatomical and pathologic findings. Beam hardening and scatter artifacts are produced in areas of metal restorations, dental implants, root canal–treated teeth,[3] and orthodontic braces. The dark band surrounding those metals and the scatter white lines associated with metal and high density are associated with polychromatic photons generated from the tube head. Because the energy levels of those photons are not consistent, high-density structures such as metal attenuate the photons in the diagnostic spectrum, therefore hardening the beam of radiation and generating those types of artifacts.

The increased radiation dose to the patient is a controversial topic in dentistry and medicine. Several national and international initiatives are aimed to bring awareness to increased radiation dose associated with imaging examinations. When discussing the issue, it is important to stress that dentistry uses relatively low levels of radiation and that no current studies can prove beyond any doubt a link between the radiation dose levels used in dentistry and cancer. CBCT scans should be used when the benefit of the information provided outweighs potential risks. The radiation dose associated with CBCT scans used in endodontics varies from 20 to 100 microsieverts. The American Association of Physicists in Medicine state that doses below 50,000 carry such a low risk that it may be nonexistent. Furthermore, hypothetical cancer risk in patient populations exposed to such low doses is highly speculative and should be discouraged.[12]

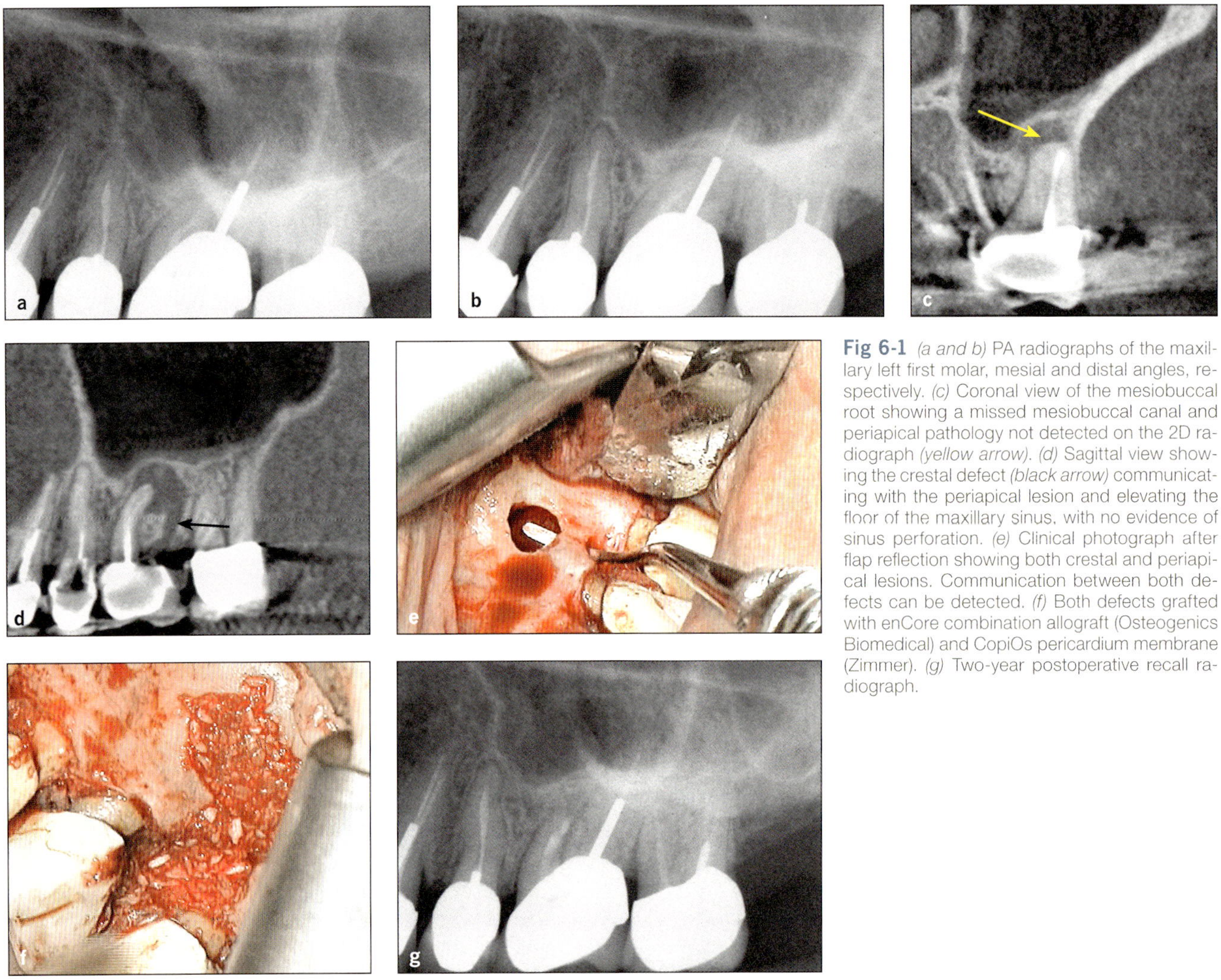

Fig 6-1 *(a and b)* PA radiographs of the maxillary left first molar, mesial and distal angles, respectively. *(c)* Coronal view of the mesiobuccal root showing a missed mesiobuccal canal and periapical pathology not detected on the 2D radiograph *(yellow arrow)*. *(d)* Sagittal view showing the crestal defect *(black arrow)* communicating with the periapical lesion and elevating the floor of the maxillary sinus, with no evidence of sinus perforation. *(e)* Clinical photograph after flap reflection showing both crestal and periapical lesions. Communication between both defects can be detected. *(f)* Both defects grafted with enCore combination allograft (Osteogenics Biomedical) and CopiOs pericardium membrane (Zimmer). *(g)* Two-year postoperative recall radiograph.

Potential Applications of CBCT in Treatment Planning of Endodontic Microsurgery

CBCT is a radiographic method that allows the clinician to visualize an individual tooth or teeth in relation to the surrounding structures and to create 3D images of the area of study. Traditional radiographic examinations are usually limited to 2D views captured using radiographic film or digital sensors. Because 2D methods reproduce the 3D anatomy as a 2D image, essential information of the 3D anatomy of the tooth/teeth and adjacent structures is frequently obscured, and even with paralleling techniques, distortion and superimposition of dental structures in PA views is unavoidable (Fig 6-1).

The role of CBCT in planning for periapical microsurgery has been well documented.[13–16] A major advantage of CBCT that has been reported is the 3D geometric accuracy compared with conventional radiographs. Compared with PA films, CBCT has been reported to be a more sensitive means to detect changes in density of the bony structures[17] and for the presence of periapical rarefaction. CBCT enables periapical disease evidenced by radiolucent changes at the root apex to be detected earlier than conventional radiographs.[1] CBCT scans resulted in 62% more periapical radiolucent areas being detected on individual roots of posterior mandibular and maxillary teeth when compared with two angled PA radiographs. In situations where patients have poorly localized symptoms associated with an untreated or previously root-filled tooth and clinical and PA radiographic examination show no evidence of disease, CBCT may be indicated to detect the presence of previously undiagnosed periapical disease. 3D visualization of any lesions and the increased accuracy for the diagnosis of the periapical status has been reported.[18,19] Axial, coronal, and sagittal views of CBCT images also eliminate the superimposition of anatomical structures.

Apical surgery in maxillary and mandibular molars is often associated with difficulties. These difficulties include the close proximity of the apices or periapical lesions to vital structures. In the posterior maxilla, the roots of maxillary teeth overlap with anatomical structures such as the maxillary sinus and the zygomatic buttress. The roots of maxillary posterior teeth and their periapical tissues can be visualized separately and in all three orthogonal planes without superimposition of the overlying zygomatic buttress, alveolar bone, and adjacent roots. In the posterior mandible, the roots of the mandibular premolars and molars can be located in close proximity to the mental foramen and the mandibular canal.

Both medical CT and CBCT have been used for the planning of periradicular endodontic surgery.[20,21] 3D imaging allows the anatomical relationship of the root apices to important neighboring anatomical structures to be clearly identified.

CBCT for surgical treatment planning when roots are in close proximity to the mental bundle and IAN

Communication between the root apices of mandibular posterior teeth and the mandibular canal is not rare and has to be taken into consideration when performing apical microsurgery to avoid iatrogenic nerve damage.[22]

The mean distance between the mandibular canal and the apices of the adjacent teeth was evaluated in a recent study.[23] A total of 821 mandibular second premolars and 597 first, 508 second, and 48 third molars were included in this study. The mean distances were 4.2, 4.9, 3.1, and 2.6 mm, respectively. The occurrence of a direct relationship between the root tips and the mandibular canal was noted in 3.2%, 2.9%, 15.2%, and 31.3% of the involved teeth, respectively. Women were affected almost twice as often as men. No significant differences were found concerning the location (right/left) of the teeth ($P > .05$). Significantly shorter distances from the mandibular canal to the root apices were found in patients younger than 35 years of age compared with those who were older.

Velvart et al[20] found that the relationship of the mandibular canal to the root apices could be determined in every case when using medical CT but in less than 40% of cases when using conventional radiography. Similar results could most likely be achieved with CBCT using considerably less radiation.

Figures 6-2 to 6-4 demonstrate a series of surgical cases in which CBCT was a valuable aid in accurate treatment planning for periapical surgery for teeth with roots in close proximity to the mental bundle and IAN.

CBCT for surgical treatment planning when roots are in close proximity to the maxillary sinus

When surgical treatment planning the posterior maxilla, one should evaluate the maxillary sinus for the presence of mucosal thickening near the affected root and the proximity of the root end and lesion to the sinus and sinus membrane. This preoperative 3D evaluation makes presurgical treatment planning easier and allows the operator to predict potential complications in advance, such as a sinus perforation. Rigolone et al[21] concluded that CBCT may play an important role in periapical microsurgery of palatal roots of maxillary first molars. The distance between the cortical plate and the palatal root apex can be measured, and the presence or absence of the maxillary sinus between the roots can be assessed. In addition, the thickness of the cortical plate, the cancellous bone pattern, fenestrations, the shape of the maxilla, and the inclination of the roots of teeth planned for periapical surgery should be able to be determined before initiating treatment. Root morphology can be visualized in three dimensions, as can the number of root canals and whether they converge or diverge from each other. Unidentified (and untreated) root canals in root-filled teeth may be identified using axial slices; these canals may not be readily identifiable with PA radiographs even if taken at different angles. In two recent studies, the thickness and the anatomical characteristics of the sinus membrane and cortical bone were evaluated using CBCT in patients treatment planned for periapical microsurgery in the maxillary molar region.[24,25] The sinus membrane in the vicinity of roots with apical lesions tends to be significantly thicker when compared with the roots of teeth without apical pathosis.[21]

Roots of maxillary posterior teeth can also frequently extend into the maxillary sinus. Pagin et al[26] found on a random sample of CBCT scans that 35.9% of maxillary posterior tooth roots abutted the sinus wall while 14.3% of the roots protruded into the sinus.

Depending on the lesion and sinus perforation size, guided tissue regeneration (GTR) could be indicated (for further discussion of GTR, see chapter 15). If GTR is indicated, CBCT imaging provides 3D information of the maxillary sinus septa. Even though Underwood[27] published a detailed description of maxillary sinus anatomy in 1910, for decades these septa were considered clinically insignificant anatomical variations. Now, however, we

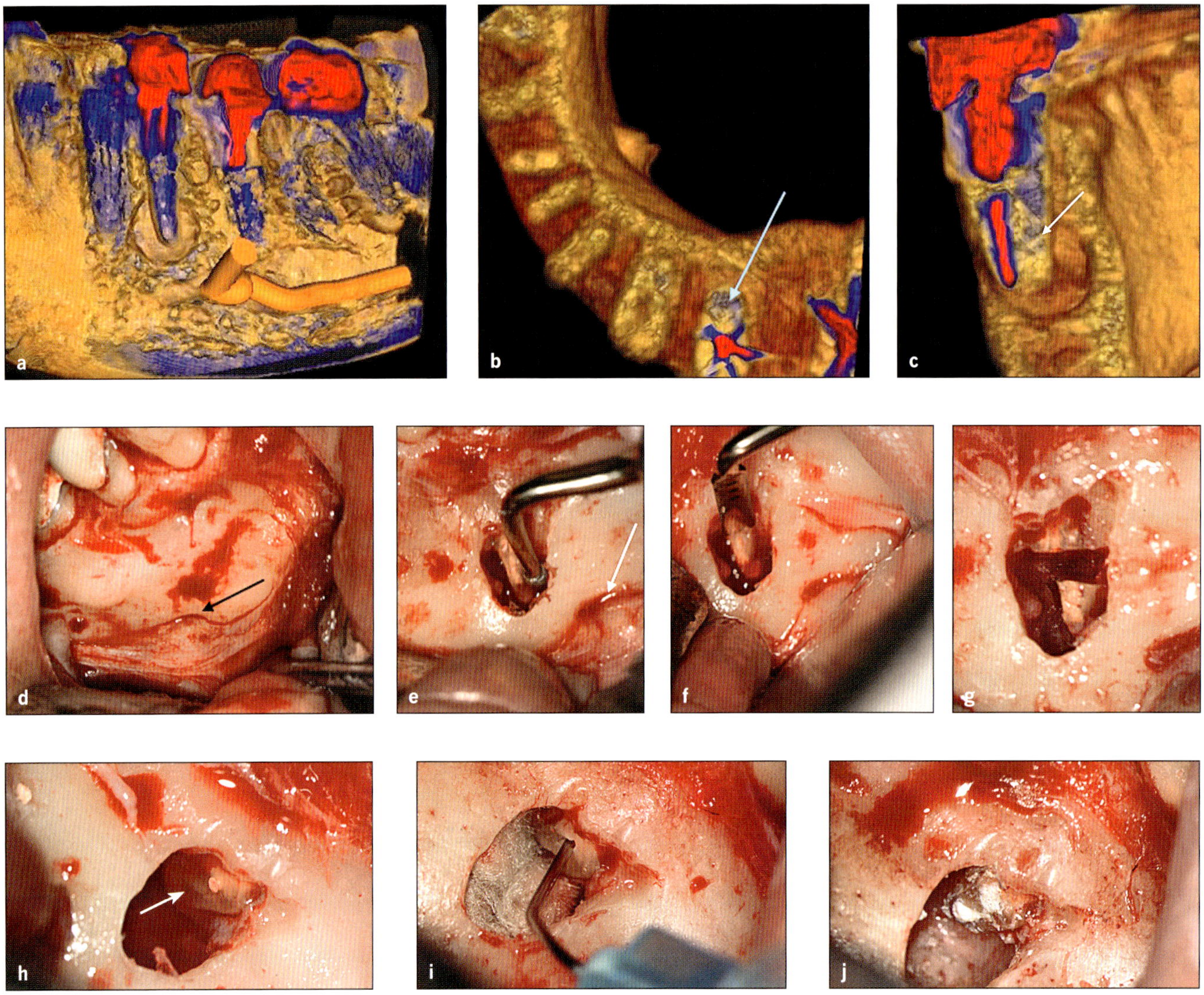

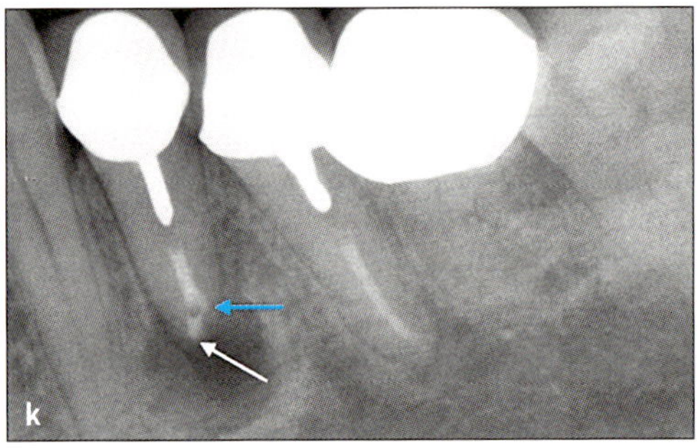

Fig 6-2 *(a)* 3D rendering of the mandibular left first premolar showing the periapical lesion and its relationship to the mental bundle. *(b and c)* Axial and coronal 3D renderings showing the untreated lingual canal *(blue and white arrows)*. Treatment options were discussed with the patient, and the patient preferred the surgical approach due to the presence of the cast post and core. The extent of the lesion buccolingually as well as the relationship of the root to the buccal and lingual cortical plates can be evaluated from the coronal view *(c)*. *(d)* Clinical image after flap reflection and identification of the mental bundle *(black arrow)*. *(e)* Because of the close proximity of the root to the mental bundle *(white arrow)*, a piezoelectric surgery insert OT5 (Mectron) was used for the osteotomy. *(f)* Root resection performed with OT7S-3 insert (Mectron). *(g)* Resected apical third with the OT7S-3 insert. *(h)* Clinical image demonstrating the untreated lingual canal *(white arrow)* and isthmus. *(i)* Application of Endo-Sequence BC Sealer (Brasseler USA) into the apical preparation prior to placement of the Root Repair Material (RRM) (Brasseler USA). *(j)* RRM material filling in the buccal and lingual canals. *(k)* Postoperative radiograph demonstrating the RRM filling in the lingual canal *(white arrow)* and buccal canal *(blue arrow)*.

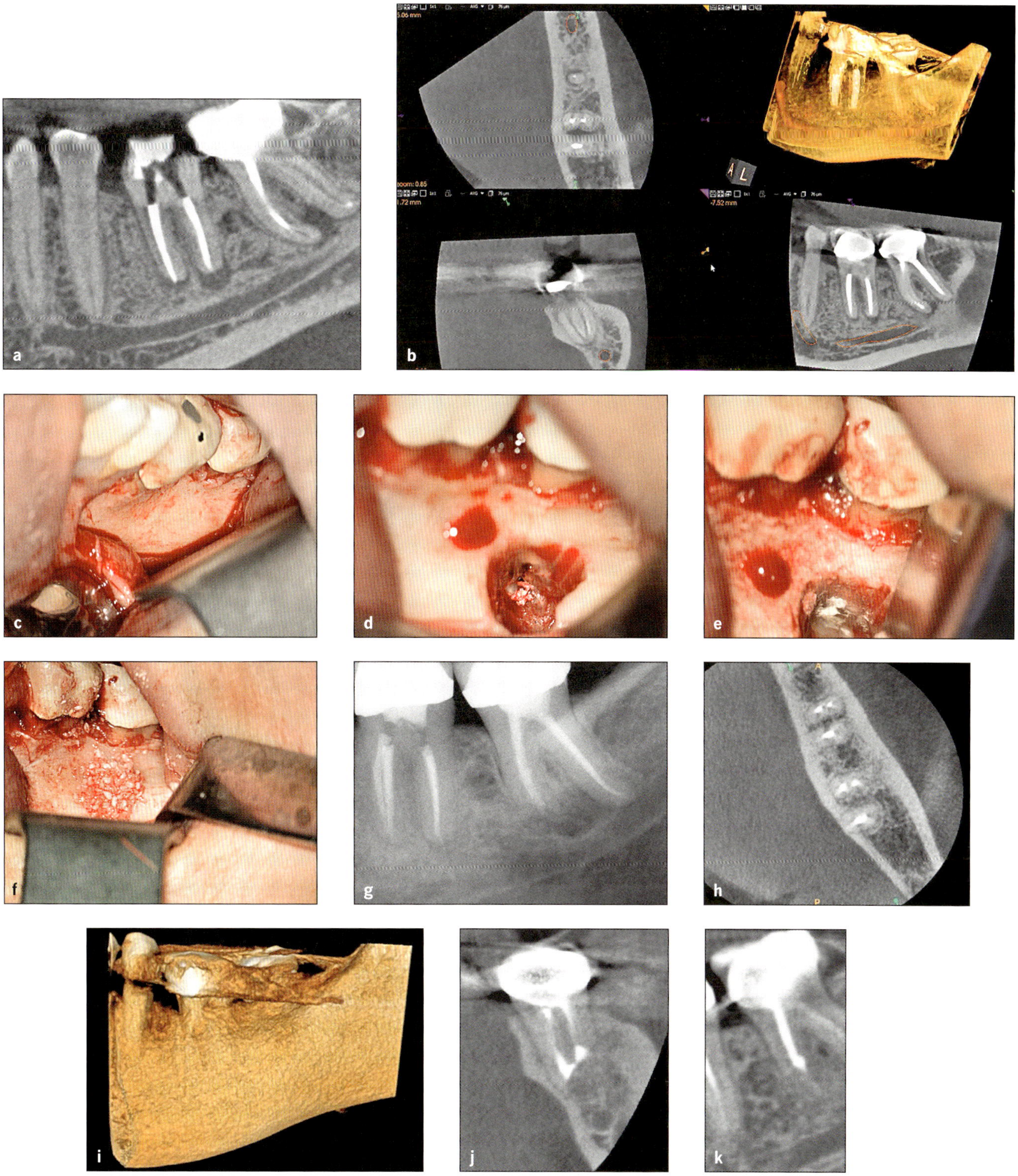

Fig 6-3 *(a)* CBCT sagittal view of a mandibular left second molar that was referred for periapical microsurgery. The first molar was retreated nonsurgically. *(b)* CBCT of the axial, coronal, and sagittal views and a 3D rendering demonstrating the proximity of the IAN to the mesial root of the second molar. *(c)* Clinical photograph after surgical flap reflection showing the buccal cortical plate. *(d)* Osteotomy and resection of the mesial root. *(e)* Clinical photograph demonstrating the mineral trioxide aggregate (MTA) root-end filling. *(f)* Periapical defect grafted with Puros allograft material (Zimmer) before placement of CopiOs membrane. *(g)* Immediate postsurgical radiograph. *(h to k)* Eighteen-month postoperative CBCT images demonstrating complete remodeling of the defect and the buccal cortical plate.

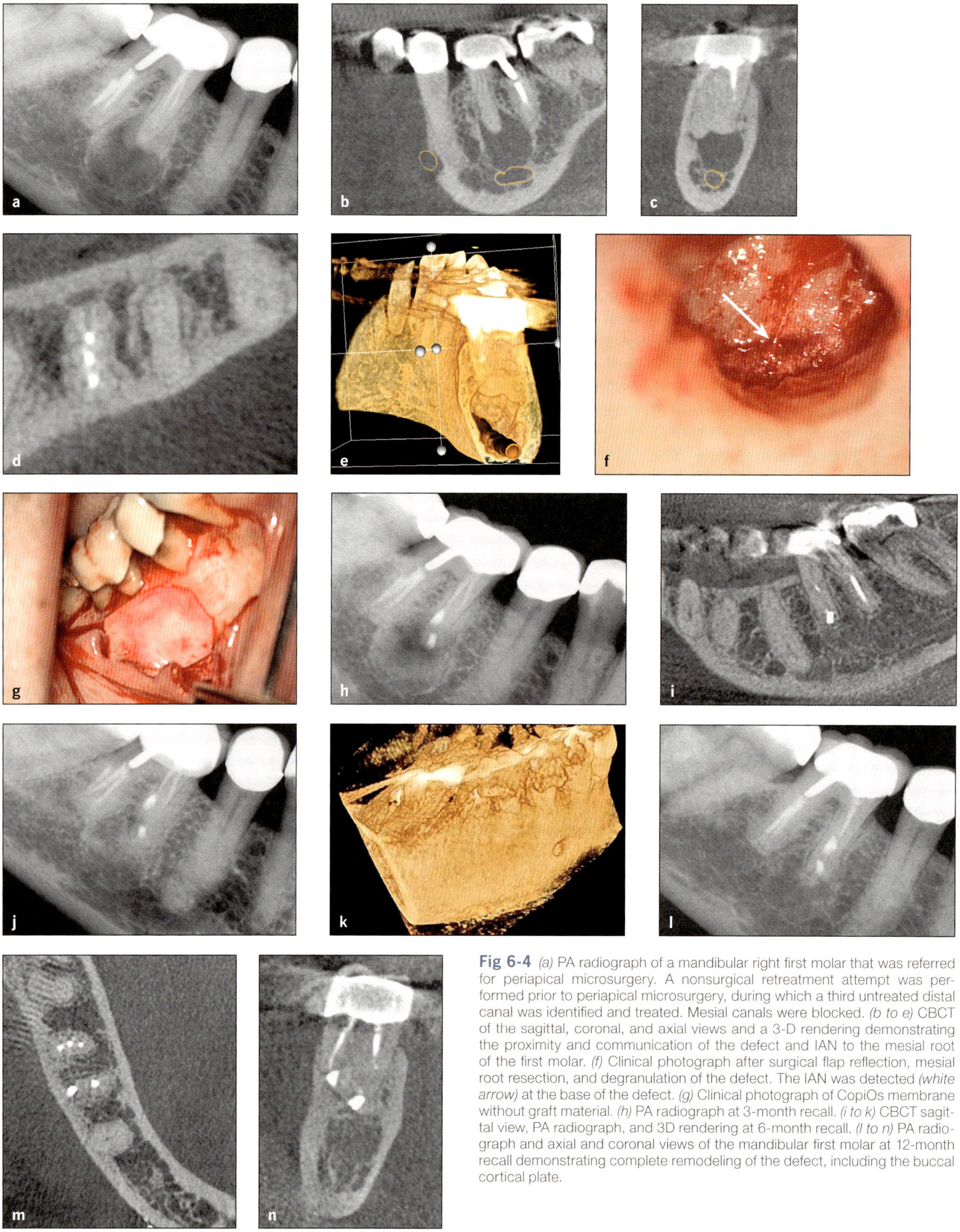

Fig 6-4 *(a)* PA radiograph of a mandibular right first molar that was referred for periapical microsurgery. A nonsurgical retreatment attempt was performed prior to periapical microsurgery, during which a third untreated distal canal was identified and treated. Mesial canals were blocked. *(b to e)* CBCT of the sagittal, coronal, and axial views and a 3-D rendering demonstrating the proximity and communication of the defect and IAN to the mesial root of the first molar. *(f)* Clinical photograph after surgical flap reflection, mesial root resection, and degranulation of the defect. The IAN was detected *(white arrow)* at the base of the defect. *(g)* Clinical photograph of CopiOs membrane without graft material. *(h)* PA radiograph at 3-month recall. *(i to k)* CBCT sagittal view, PA radiograph, and 3D rendering at 6-month recall. *(l to n)* PA radiograph and axial and coronal views of the mandibular first molar at 12-month recall demonstrating complete remodeling of the defect, including the buccal cortical plate.

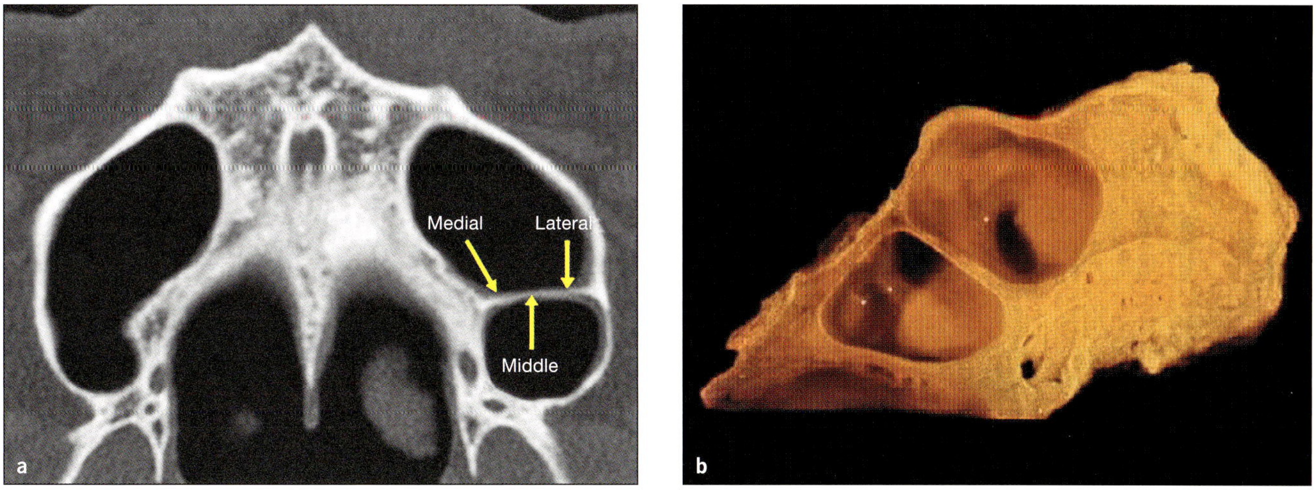

Fig 6-5 *(a)* CBCT axial view demonstrating maxillary sinus septa. *(b)* 3D CBCT rendering demonstrating maxillary sinus septa.

must understand the normal anatomy of the maxillary sinus and any anatomical variations because the sinus elevation is a complicated procedure and the membrane is susceptible to perforation during apical surgery in the presence of a septum.[28] Therefore, only when the prevalence, location, and morphology of the sinus septa are understood can a precise surgical plan be made and complications from sinus surgery be prevented.

The prevalence of sinus septa varies from 16% to 58%. The location and the shape of the septa are important because they provide support for the absorbable membranes (Fig 6-5). Sinus septa can be divided into primary septa and secondary septa. The primary septa arise from the development of the maxilla, whereas the secondary septa are said to arise from the irregular pneumatization of the sinus floor following tooth loss. In other words, primary septa are congenital, and secondary septa are acquired. The septa above the apical area of an edentulous ridge cannot be distinguished into primary or secondary septa without previous radiographic records. Therefore, it can be said that septa above teeth are primary while septa above an edentulous ridge are primary or secondary. The location of reported septa demonstrated a greater prevalence in the middle region (from the distal aspect of the second premolar to the distal aspect of the second molar; 50%). This was followed by the anterior region (from the mesial to distal aspect of the second premolar; 24%) and the posterior region (the distal aspect of the second molar region; 22.7%).[29] We can assume that secondary septa develop more frequently in the area above lost molars because of earlier extraction of molars than premolars.

Figures 6-6 and 6-7 demonstrate two surgical cases in which CBCT was a valuable aid in accurate treatment planning for periapical surgery for teeth with roots in close proximity to the maxillary sinus.

CBCT for surgical treatment planning for teeth with large periapical lesions

The true size, location, and extent of periapical disease should finally be appreciated, and the actual root to which the lesion is associated should be able to be identified with confidence. Accurate analysis of the volume of bone defects is an important step for clinical evaluation before performing endodontic surgery as well as for monitoring the outcomes of therapy (increased/decreased volume after treatment).

The outcome of periapical surgery can be affected by several factors, among which the size and location of the periapical bone loss and the presence of bacteria are thought to be among the most important. Knowledge of the lesion size is important when a decision is to be made for the use of GTR techniques (for further discussion of GTR techniques, refer to chapter 15). In large periapical defects, lesions will often be filled with fibrous connective tissue referred to as *scar tissue*. The ingrowth of non-osteogenic tissues and the downgrowth of the epithelial tissue along the root surface can result in incomplete repair.

Several software packages already provide clinicians with a dedicated tool for assessing the volumes of regions

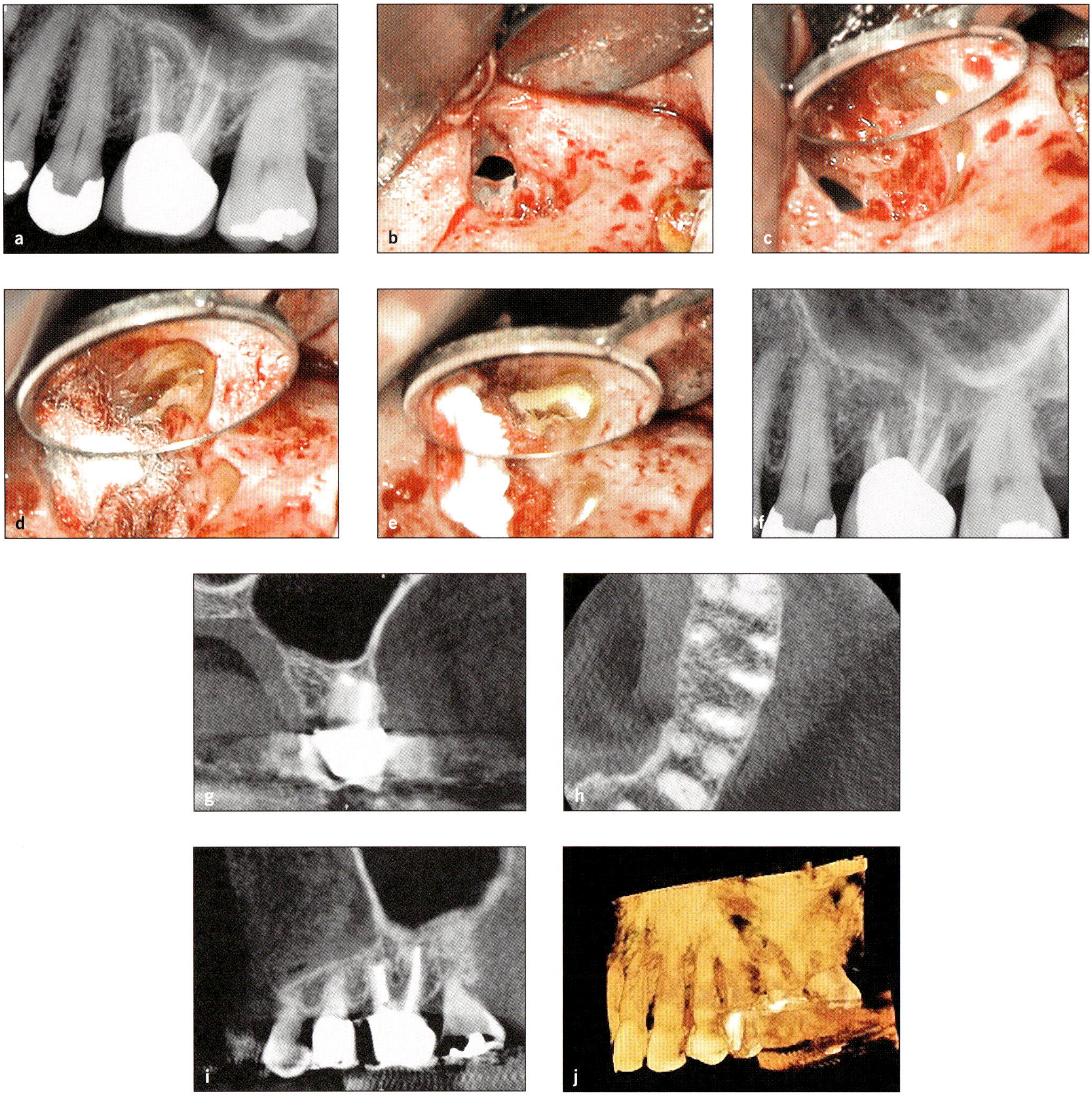

Fig 6-6 *(a)* PA radiograph of a maxillary left first molar referred for periapical surgery. *(b and c)* Clinical photograph demonstrating sinus communication after degranulation of the defect. *(d)* Clinical photograph demonstrating the protection of the sinus communication with CollaCote (Zimmer) and methylene blue staining of the mesiobuccal root resection to confirm complete resection and location of the untreated mesiolingual canal prior to ultrasonic root-end preparation. *(e)* Root-end filling with MTA. *(f)* Postoperative radiograph. *(g to j)* Eight-year recall CBCT images demonstrating the coronal *(g)*, axial *(h)*, and sagittal *(i)* views and a 3D rendering *(j)*. Complete bone regeneration of the buccal plate as well as the floor of the sinus can be visualized.

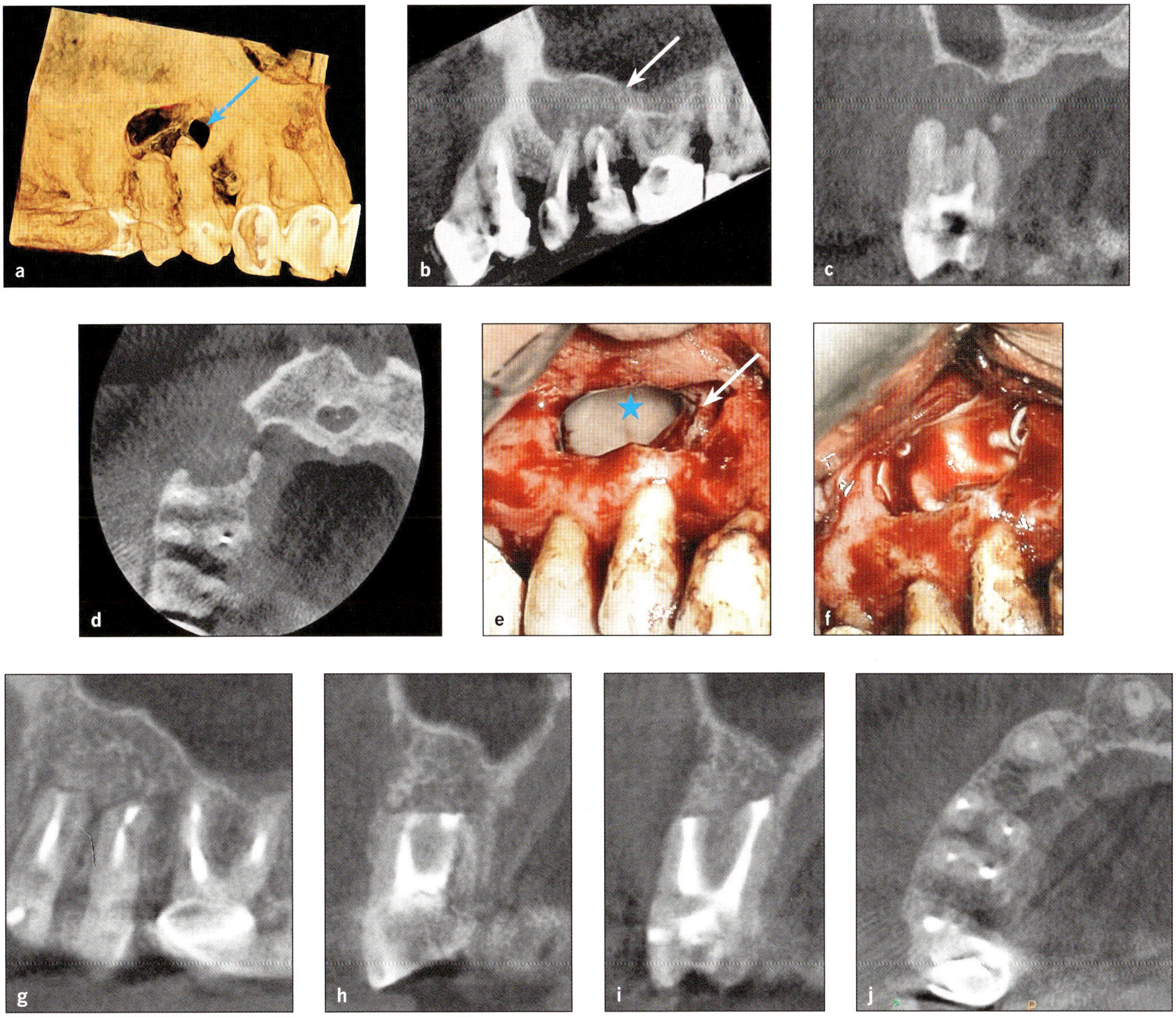

Fig 6-7 *(a)* CBCT 3D rendering of maxillary right premolars referred for periapical microsurgery. Perforation of the maxillary sinus can be visualized *(blue arrow)*. *(b)* Sagittal view of the premolars. Perforation of the maxillary sinus is noted *(white arrow)*. *(c)* Coronal view of the first premolar demonstrating the through-and-through nature of the periapical defect. *(d)* Axial view demonstrating the mesiodistal extent of the periapical defect. *(e)* Clinical image demonstrating the large maxillary sinus communication, vasculature *(blue star)*, and the maxillary sinus septa *(white arrow)* that will be utilized to hold the absorbable membrane. *(f)* CopiOs membrane placed prior to the placement of Infuse bone morphogenetic proteins (Medtronic) and bone grafting with an enCore combination. *(g to j)* Two-year postoperative CBCT images of the premolars demonstrating bone remodeling observed in the sagittal view *(g)*, coronal view of the first premolar *(h)*, coronal view of the second premolar *(i)*, and axial CBCT view *(j)*. Both buccal and palatal cortical plate remodeling can be observed.

of interest in cubic millimeters. However, to obtain an accurate volume estimation, it is necessary to obtain linear measurements across all of the slices that encompass the region of interest, which makes volume estimation very time-consuming. Dedicated software packages solve this issue by allowing for interpolation between several separated slices. Furthermore, volume analysis can be performed on the axial, sagittal, or coronal plane using software packages such as the XoranCAT (version 3.1.62, Xoran Technologies), which is used regularly to work with i-CAT images. OnDemand3D (version 1.0, CyberMed) and KDIS 3D (version 2.1.11, Kodak Dental Systems) are examples of software that are able to assess DICOM (Digital Imaging and Communications in Medicine) images.

The use of high-resolution images derived from CBCT data sets enables the linear measurement of lesions in the maxilla and mandible in three planes of space. Measurements on different planes make it possible to obtain real volumetric assessments. Esposito et al[30] evaluated the accuracy and reliability of volumes measured on CBCT images as compared with physical measurements. Twenty-seven bone defects were created around the apices of eight teeth in a single young bovine mandible to simulate periapical lesions of different sizes and shapes. The volume of each defect was determined by taking an impression of the defect using a silicone material. The samples were scanned using an Accuitomo 170 CBCT unit (J. Morita), and the data were uploaded into a newly developed dedicated software tool. Two endodontists acted as independent and calibrated observers. They analyzed each bone defect for volume size. The differences between the direct volumetric measurements and the measurements obtained with the CBCT images were statistically assessed using a lack-of-fit test. A correlation study was undertaken using the Pearson product-moment correlation coefficient. Intra- and interobserver agreement was also evaluated.

Statistical analysis showed no significant differences between the reference values and the software-based volume measurements, proving that this software is accurate. Intra- and interobserver agreement was excellent, showing a strong correlation between the two variables. The authors concluded that CBCT proved to be a reliable method in vitro for the estimation of endodontic lesion volumes in bovine jaws. Therefore, this may constitute a new, validated technique for the accurate evaluation and follow-up of apical periodontitis. Figure 6-8 illustrates the use of CBCT to determine the size of the periapical lesion as well as treatment planning prior to the surgical procedure.

CBCT for surgical outcome evaluation

Perhaps the most exciting area in which CBCT may be applied in endodontics is in determining the outcome of treatment.[31,32] Detailed CBCT scans should result in a more objective and therefore more accurate determination of the outcome of endodontic treatment. The CBCT images are geometrically accurate, and there is no distortion of the teeth being assessed or superimposition of overlying anatomy as often seen with conventional film and digitally captured PA radiographs. Recently, clinical studies have compared the diagnostic value of 2D and 3D radiography for the postsurgical assessment of periapical healing following periapical microsurgery.[33–35] There was a higher agreement when evaluating healing in the 3D evaluation when compared with the 2D method. The results of these studies demonstrated that the percentage of repair was different for both methods. More remaining defects were detected after periapical microsurgery on CBCT images than on PA radiographs. The lower rate of healing observed on 3D radiographs could be attributed to the type of the bony defect, which may require regenerative procedures or longer observation periods for healing assessment.

Traditionally, the criteria for healing assessment of apical surgery are based on the work by Rud et al[36] and Molven et al.[37] However, a recent study has shown that these 2D criteria may not be valid for the evaluation of 3D.

Simon et al[38] compared the ability of CBCT and biopsy with histologic examination to differentiate between periapical cysts and granulomas in teeth with large periapical lesions. They stated that grayscale value measurements of periapical lesions on CBCT images were able to differentiate solid (granulomas) from cystic or cavity (cyst) type lesions. They further concluded that CBCT may be clinically more accurate and more useful than biopsy. If confirmed, these findings may influence the decision-making process when considering a nonsurgical or surgical approach to endodontic retreatment.

A recent study evaluated the concordance of 2D and 3D radiography and histopathology in the diagnosis of periapical lesions.[39] The final histologic diagnosis of the periapical lesions included 55 granulomas (94.8%) and 3 cysts (5.2%). Radiographic assessment overestimated cysts by 28.4% (CBCT imaging) and 20.7% (PA radiography), respectively. The authors concluded that in order to establish a final diagnosis of an apical radiolucency, the tissue specimen should be evaluated histologically and specified as a granuloma (without epithelium) or a cyst (with epithelium). Analysis of 2D or 3D radiograph-

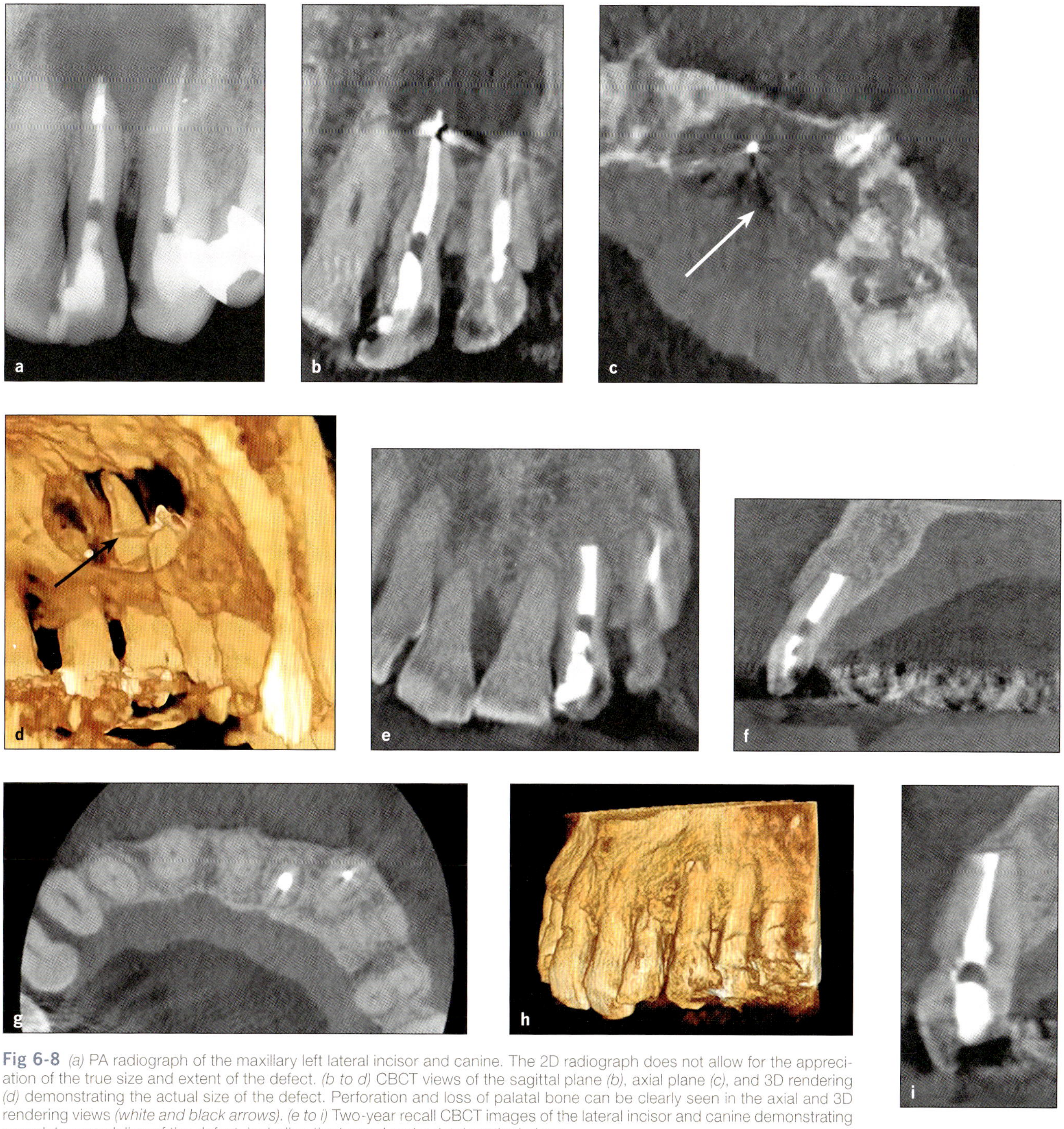

Fig 6-8 *(a)* PA radiograph of the maxillary left lateral incisor and canine. The 2D radiograph does not allow for the appreciation of the true size and extent of the defect. *(b to d)* CBCT views of the sagittal plane *(b)*, axial plane *(c)*, and 3D rendering *(d)* demonstrating the actual size of the defect. Perforation and loss of palatal bone can be clearly seen in the axial and 3D rendering views *(white and black arrows)*. *(e to i)* Two-year recall CBCT images of the lateral incisor and canine demonstrating complete remodeling of the defect, including the buccal and palatal cortical plates.

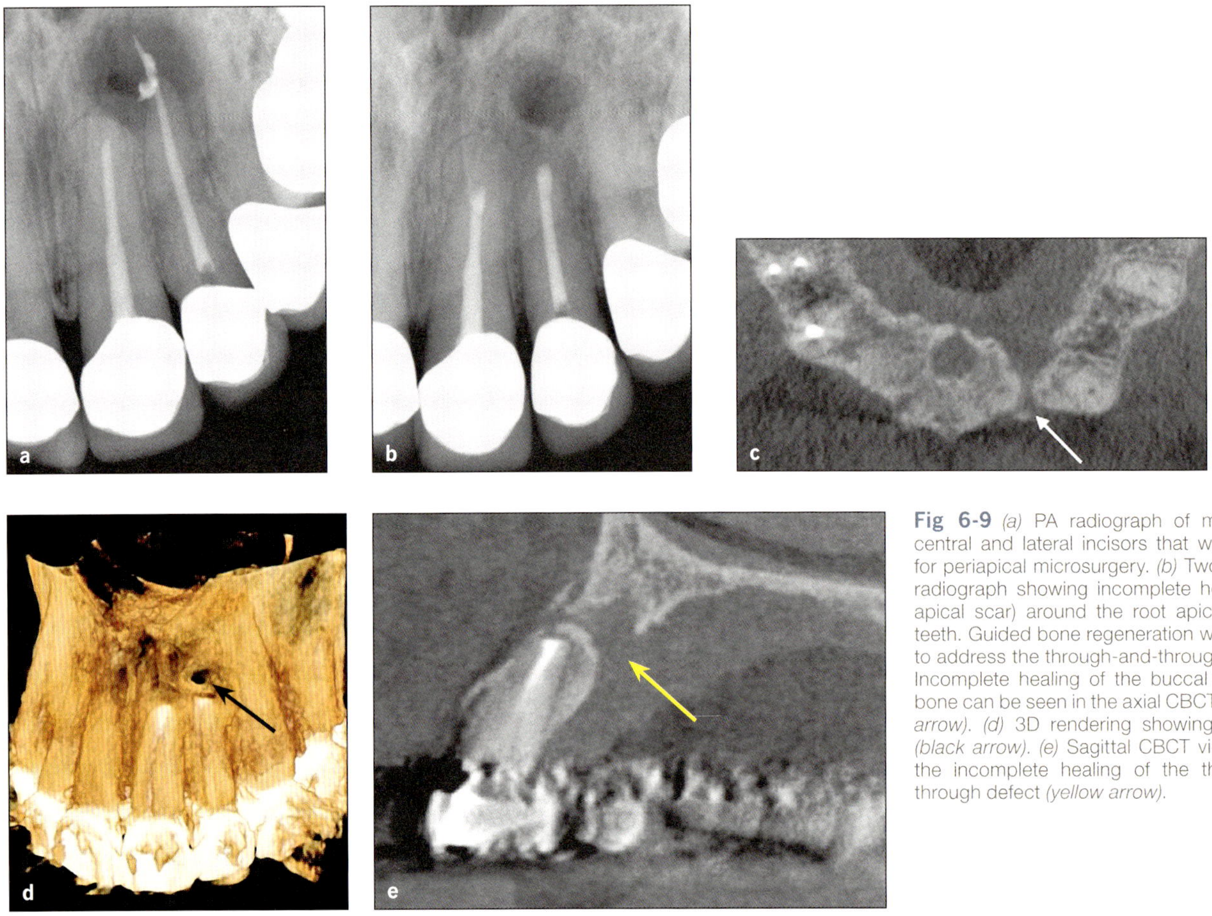

Fig 6-9 *(a)* PA radiograph of maxillary left central and lateral incisors that were referred for periapical microsurgery. *(b)* Two-year recall radiograph showing incomplete healing (periapical scar) around the root apices of these teeth. Guided bone regeneration was not used to address the through-and-through defect. *(c)* Incomplete healing of the buccal and palatal bone can be seen in the axial CBCT view *(white arrow)*. *(d)* 3D rendering showing the defect *(black arrow)*. *(e)* Sagittal CBCT view showing the incomplete healing of the through-and-through defect *(yellow arrow)*.

ic images alone results only in a tentative diagnosis that should be confirmed with biopsy.

Two recent studies evaluated the outcome of endodontic microsurgery utilizing CBCT technology.[35,40] Von Arx et al[34] evaluated a new CBCT-based criteria in a prospective clinical study for the radiographic outcome assessment 1 year after apical surgery using four different indices. Reformatted buccolingual CBCT sections through the longitudinal axis of the treated roots were analyzed. Radiographic healing was assessed at the resection plane (R index), within the apical area (A index), at the cortical plate (C index), and regarding a combined apical-cortical area (B index). All readings were performed twice to calculate the intraobserver agreement (repeatability). Second-time readings were used for analyzing the interobserver agreement (reproducibility). All study parameters showed excellent intraobserver agreement (repeatability). With regard to interobserver agreement (reproducibility), the B index (healing of apical and cortical defects combined) and the R index (healing on the resection plane) showed substantial congruence and thus are to be recommended in future studies when using buccolingual CBCT sections for radiographic outcome assessment of apical surgery.

Kim et al[40] evaluated the size, volume, and other parameters of preoperative periapical lesions measured from CBCT images as potential prognostic factors in endodontic microsurgery. The mesiodistal (Lx), apicocoronal (Ly), and buccolingual (Lz) diameter; the volume (V) of the periapical lesions; the destruction of the cortical bone; and the height of the buccal bone plate (Lb) were measured independently by two examiners. The outcome was classified as a success or failure based on the clinical and radiographic evaluation at least 1 year after the surgical procedures were performed. The main finding of this study was that the outcome of endodontic microsurgery was influenced by the volume of the preoperative periapical lesion. Periapical lesions smaller than 50 mm^3 in volume were associated with significantly higher successful outcomes. The preoperative linear diameter of the lesion, destruction of the cortical bone, and height of the buccal bone plate were not found to be significant predictors. The findings from the previous studies could influence the decision-making for the utilization of GTR techniques in apical microsurgery.

Future research may show that root-filled teeth that appear to have "healed" on conventional radiographs may still have signs of periapical disease (eg, widened periodontal ligament space, periapical radiolucency) when imaged using CBCT. This in turn may have implications for decision-making and selection criteria when considering placing or replacing coronal restorations on teeth that have previously been treated with endodontics and appear to have successfully healed radiographically. There is a need to define the criteria of radiographic healing in CBCT following periapical microsurgery.

Figure 6-9 demonstrates a surgical case in which CBCT was a valuable aid in accurate outcome assessment of periapical surgery.

Clinicians must remember that CBCT still uses ionizing radiation and is not without risk. Radiation exposure to the patient must be kept as low as reasonably practicable, and evidence-based selection criteria for CBCT must be adhered to. Endodontic cases should be judged individually, and until further evidence is available, CBCT should only be considered when it has been decided that conventional radiographic view(s) are yielding limited information and that further radiographic details are required for diagnosis and treatment planning. The AAE/AAOMR position statement on the use of CBCT in endodontics is a valuable document that lists recommendations to help the clinician decide when it is appropriate to use CBCT imaging in the diagnosis, treatment planning, and execution of nonsurgical and surgical procedures.[1]

References

1. Special Committee to Revise the Joint AAE/AAOMR Position Statement on use of CBCT in Endodontics. AAE and AAOMR joint position statement: Use of cone beam computed tomography in endodontics 2015 update. Oral Surg Oral Med Oral Pathol Oral Radiol 2015;120:508–512.
2. Lofthag-Hansen S, Huumonen S, Gröndahl K, Gröndahl HG. Limited cone-beam CT and intraoral radiography for the diagnosis of periapical pathology. Oral Surg Oral Med Oral Pathol Oral Radiol Endod 2007;103:114–119.
3. Scarfe WC, Farman AG. What is cone-beam CT and how does it work? Dent Clin North Am 2008;52:707–730.
4. Arai Y, Tammisalo E, Iwai K, Hashimoto K, Shinoda K. Development of a compact computed tomographic apparatus for dental use. Dentomaxillofac Radiol 1999;28:245–248.
5. Honda K, Larheim TA, Johannessen S, Arai Y, Shinoda K, Westesson PL. Ortho cubic super-high resolution computed tomography: A new radiographic technique with application to the temporomandibular joint. Oral Surg Oral Med Oral Pathol Oral Radiol Endod 2001;91:239–243.
6. Estrela C, Bueno MR, Azevedo BC, Azevedo JR, Pécora JD. A new periapical index based on cone beam computed tomography. J Endod 2008;34:1325–1331.
7. Jaffraya DA, Siewerdsen JH. Cone-beam computed tomography with a flat-panel imager: Initial performance characterization. Med Phys 2000;27:1311–1323.
8. Baba R, Ueda K, Okabe M. Using a flat-panel detector in high resolution cone beam CT for dental imaging. Dentomaxillofac Radiol 2004;33:285–290.
9. Schulze R, Heil U, Gross D, et al. Artefacts in CBCT: A review. Dentomaxillofac Radiol 2011;40:265–273.
10. Tanimoto H, Arai Y. The effect of voxel size on image reconstruction in cone-beam computed tomography. Oral Radiol 2009;25:149–153.
11. Mah P, Reeves TE, McDavid WD. Deriving Hounsfield units using grey levels in cone beam computed tomography. Dentomaxillofac Radiol 2010;39:323–335.
12. American Association of Physicists in Medicine. AAPM Position Statement on Radiation Risks from Medical Imaging Procedures: Policy no. PP 25-A. www.aapm.org/org/policies/details.asp?id=318&type=PP. Accessed 13 January 2017.
13. Cheung G, Wei WL, McGrath C. Agreement between periapical radiographs and cone-beam computed tomography for assessment of periapical status of root filled molar teeth. Int Endod J 2013;46:889–895.
14. Esposito SA, Huybrechts B, Slagmolen P, et al. A novel method to estimate the volume of bone defects using cone-beam computed tomography: An in vitro study. J Endod 2013;39:1111–1115.
15. Bornstein MM, Lauber R, Sendi P, von Arx T. Comparison of periapical radiography and limited cone-beam computed tomography in mandibular molars for analysis of anatomical landmarks before apical surgery. J Endod 2011;37:151–157.
16. Low KM, Dula KD, Bürgin W, von Arx T. Comparison of periapical radiography and limited cone-beam tomography in posterior maxillary teeth referred for apical surgery. J Endod 2008;34:557–562.
17. Tsai P, Torabinejad M, Rice D, Azevedo B. Accuracy of cone-beam computed tomography and periapical radiography in detecting small periapical lesions. J Endod 2012;38:965–970.
18. Tyndall DA, Rathore S. Cone-beam diagnostic applications: Caries, periodontal bone assessment, and endodontic applications. Dent Clin North Am 2008;52: 825–841.
19. Cotton TP, Geisler TM, Holden DT, Schwartz SA, Schindler WG. Endodontic applications of cone-beam volumetric tomography. J Endod 2007;33:1121–1132.
20. Velvart P, Hecker H, Tillinger G. Detection of the apical lesion and the mandibular canal in conventional radiography and computed tomography. Oral Surg Oral Med Oral Pathol Oral Radiol Endod 2001;92:682–628.
21. Rigolone M, Pasqualini D, Bianchi L, Berutti E, Bianchi SD. Vestibular surgical access to the palatine root of the superior first molar: "Low-dose cone-beam" CT analysis of the pathway and its anatomic variations. J Endod 2003;29:773–775.
22. Kovisto T, Mansur Ahmad M, Bowles W. Proximity of the mandibular canal to the tooth apex. J Endod 2011;37:311–315.
23. Bürklein S, Grund C, Schäfer E. Relationship between root apices and the mandibular canal: A cone-beam computed tomographic analysis in a German population. J Endod 2015;41:1696–1700.
24. Maillet M, Bowles WR, McClanahan SL, John MT, Ahmad M. Cone-beam computed tomography evaluation of maxillary sinusitis. J Endod 2011;37:753–757.
25. Bornstein MM, Wasmer J, Sendi P, Janner SF, Buser D, von Arx T. Characteristics and dimensions of the Schneiderian membrane and apical bone in maxillary molars referred for apical surgery: A comparative radiographic analysis using limited cone beam computed tomography. J Endod 2012;38:51–57.
26. Pagin O, Centurion BS, Rubira-Bullen IR, Alvares Capelozza AL. Maxillary sinus and posterior teeth: Accessing close relationship by cone-beam computed tomographic scanning in a brazilian population. J Endod 2013;39:748–751.
27. Underwood AS. An inquiry into the anatomy and pathology of the maxillary sinus. J Anat Physiol 1910;44:354–369.
28. Boyne PJ, James RA. Grafting of the maxillary sinus floor with autogenous marrow and bone. J Oral Surg 1980;38:613–616.
29. Lee WJ, Lee SJ, Kim HS. Analysis of the location and prevalence of maxillary sinus septa. J Periodontal Implant Sci 2010;40:56–60.
30. Esposito SA, Huybrechts B, Slagmolen P, et al. A novel method to estimate the volume of bone defects using cone-beam computed tomography: An in vitro study. J Endod 2013;39:1111–1115.
31. De Paula-Silva FW, Junior MS, Leonardo MR, Consolaro A, da Silva LA. Cone-beam computerized tomographic, radiographic, and histologic evaluation of periapical repair in dogs' post-endodontic treatment. Oral Surg Oral Med Oral Pathol Oral Radiol Endod 2009;108:796–805.
32. Kourkouta S, Bailey G. Periradicular regenerative surgery in a maxillary central incisor: 7-year results including cone-beam computed tomography. J Endod 2014;40:1013–1019.
33. Christiansen R, Kirkevang LL, Gotfredsen E, Wenzel A. Periapical radiography and cone beam computed tomography for assessment of the periapical bone defect 1 week and 12 months after root-end resection. Dentomaxillofac Radiol 2009;38:531–536.
34. Von Arx T, Janner SF, Hänni S, Bornstein MM. Agreement between 2D and 3D radiographic outcome assessment one year after periapical surgery. Int Endod J 2016;49:915–925.

35. Tanomaru-Filho M, Jorge ÉG, Guerreiro-Tanomaru JM, Reis JM, Spin-Neto R, Gonçalves M. Two- and tridimensional analysis of periapical repair after endodontic surgery. Clin Oral Investig 2015;19:17–25.
36. Rud J, Andreasen JO, Jensen JE. Radiographic criteria for the assessment of healing after endodontic surgery. Int J Oral Surg 1972;1:195–214.
37. Molven O, Halse A, Grung B. Observer strategy and the radiographic classification of healing after endodontic surgery. Int J Oral Maxillofac Surg 1987;16:432–439.
38. Simon JH, Enciso R, Malfaz JM, Roges R, Bailey-Perry M, Patel A. Differential diagnosis of large periapical lesions using cone-beam computed tomography measurements and biopsy. J Endod 2006;32:833–837.
39. Bornstein MM, Bingisser AC, Reichart PA, Sendi P, Bosshardt DD, von Arx T. Comparison between radiographic (2-dimensional and 3-dimensional) and histologic findings of periapical lesions treated with apical surgery. J Endod 2015;41:804–811.
40. Kim D, Ku H, Nam T, Yoon TC, Lee CY, Kim E. Influence of size and volume of periapical lesions on the outcome of endodontic microsurgery: 3-dimensional analysis using cone-beam computed tomography. J Endod 2016;42:1196–1201.

Chapter Seven

Magnification and Illumination in Apical Surgery

Richard Rubinstein

One of the most important developments in surgical endodontics in recent years has been the introduction of the surgical operating microscope. In the late 1980s and early 1990s, a handful of endodontists throughout the world began experimenting with the operating microscope to see if there were any applications that could be used in apical surgery. They felt that they could provide better treatment if they could further magnify and illuminate the surgical field beyond what was available with conventional loupes and surgical headlamps. The results were overwhelming. Cases that once seemed impossible became easy and exciting to operate on, and teeth that might otherwise have been extracted had a predictable chance for retention.

Several Paths Cross

The separate pursuits of intention, knowledge, and technology on occasion overlap and over time result in clinical solutions that benefit patients. The development of apical microsurgery is such an example. The desire to eliminate disease at the root end, the need to obtain a clearer understanding of the complexities of pulpal anatomy, and the utilization of enhanced magnification and illumination have fathered contemporary apical surgery, more accurately described as apical microsurgery.

Elimination of Disease at the Root End

While the origins of apical surgery can be traced to pre-Columbian times,[1,2] contemporary endodontic surgery began its journey in the early 1960s along with the recognition of endodontics as a specialty in the United States in 1964. Emphasis was placed on root-end filling materials and their sealing ability. As apical surgical procedures evolved, much controversy existed, and personal choices evolved with little biologic basis. Surgery at this time, and until recently, was often performed with inadequate lighting, no magnification, and a limited ar-

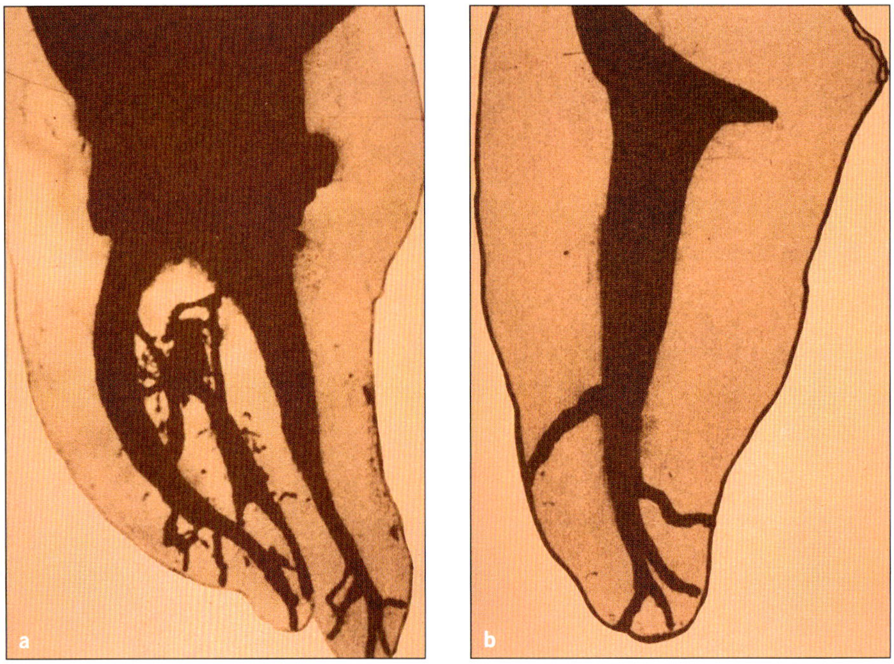

Fig 7-1 *(a)* Hess model of a mandibular molar showing anatomical complexities throughout the root canal system. *(b)* Hess model of a mandibular premolar showing anatomical complexities in the apical terminus.

mamentarium. Frank et al[3] reported that the success rate in apical surgeries sealed with amalgam, which had been considered a successful procedure, dropped to 57.7% after 10 years. Guttmann and Harrison identified the task of modern-day endodontics as striving to "eliminate the art and craft otherwise inherent in surgical endodontics—the heuristic—and encourage a relentless, honest pursuit of the contemporary challenges of endodontic surgery."[4] Shabahang recently described apical surgery as endodontic therapy through a surgical flap. The main purpose of apical surgery is to remove a portion of a root with anatomical complexities laden with tissue debris and microorganisms or to seal the canal when a complete seal cannot be accomplished through nonsurgical means.[5] The complexity of these root canal spaces has only recently been appreciated.

Anatomical Complexities

Walter Hess, a Swiss dentist, first published his landmark anatomical studies in the early 1920s.[6] When his work was first published, many clinicians felt that the anatomical complexities reported were artifacts created by injecting vulcanite rubber under too much pressure (Fig 7-1). However, more progressive thinkers of that time believed that the results had merit and sought more effective ways to clean, shape, and obturate root canal systems. More recently, Takahashi and Kishi, using a dye infusion process, also studied anatomical complexities.[7] These models clearly show the majesty and grace of the human dental pulp (Fig 7-2). Weller et al[8] studied the incidence and location of the isthmus in the mesiobuccal root of the maxillary first molar and found a partial or complete isthmus 100% of the time at the 4-mm level of resection. West looked at the relationship between failed endodontics and unfilled or underfilled portals of exit (POEs).[9] Using a centrifuged dye, he identified that 100% of the failed specimens studied had at least one underfilled or unfilled POE.[9] Because 93% of the canal ramifications occur in the apical 3 mm, logically the clinician should attempt to treat the root canal system to the full extent of the anatomy.[7] Failure to address these anatomical concerns will leave the etiology of failure unremoved, and reinfection, even after the removal of a periapical lesion, may reoccur. Clearly, root canal systems are more complex than previously thought. Significant pulpal anatomy such as accessory canals and isthmi has to be considered when performing both surgical and nonsurgical endodontic treatment. The acceptance of the significance of these anatomical complexities and the need to eliminate them may in fact have been the genesis of modern apical surgery, which could further be appreciated with the introduction of magnification.

Fig 7-2 Takahashi models. *(a)* Mesial view of the mesial root of a mandibular molar. Note the midroot isthmus and the apical bifidity of the buccal canal. Also note the multiple apical termini. *(b)* Mandibular second premolar. Note how the single canal bifurcates, rejoins, and then splits once more at the canal terminus. *(c)* Maxillary central incisor. Note the multiple portals of exit in the apical third of the root. *(d)* Mandibular molar. Note the anatomical complexities present in both roots.

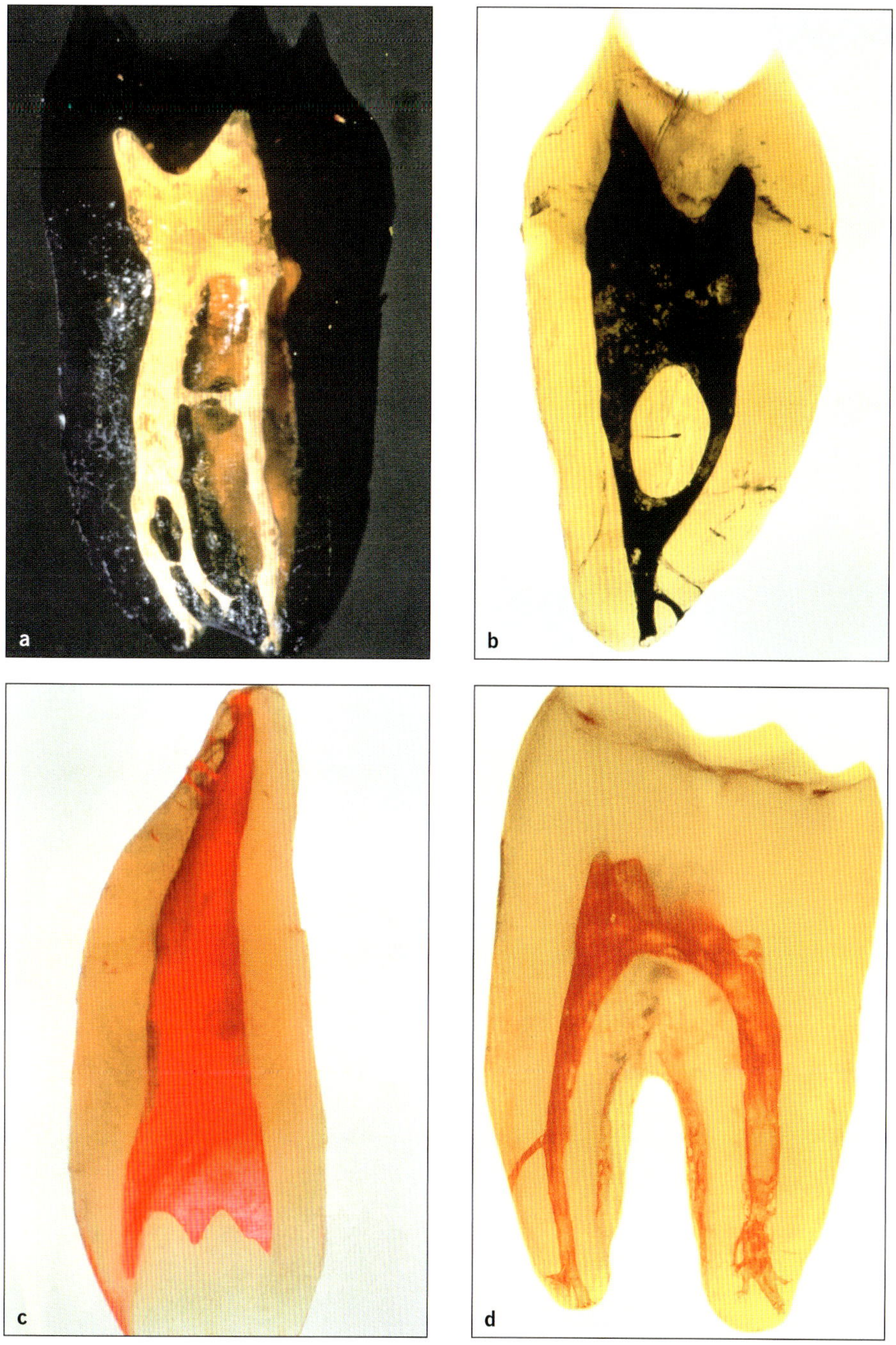

A Brief History of Magnification

Although the first accurate lenses were not made until about the year 1300, credit for the first microscope is usually given to Hans and Zacharias Jansen, a father and son who operated a Dutch lens-grinding business, around 1595.[10] They produced both simple (single lens) and compound (two lenses) microscopes.

Using a compound microscope, in 1665 Robert Hooke coined the word *cell* while describing features of plant tissue.[10] Another pioneer of microscopy, Antonie van Leeuwenhoek produced single lenses powerful enough to enable him to observe bacteria 2 to 3 microns in diameter in 1674.[10]

Little was done to improve the microscope until the middle of the 19th century when Carl Zeiss, Ernst Abbe, and Otto Schott devoted significant time to develop the microscope as we know it today. While Zeiss concentrated on the manufacturing process, Abbe and Schoot concentrated their time on the theoretical study of optical principles and conducted research on glass.[11] Their product was the genesis of the surgical operating microscope (SOM) that ultimately found its way into the practice of medicine.

The Evolution of Magnification and Illumination in Medicine

In 1921, Dr Carl Nylen of Germany reported the use of a monocular microscope for operations to correct chronic otitis of the ear.[12] The unit had two magnifications of ×10 and ×15 and a 10-mm-diameter view of the field. This microscope had no illumination.

In 1922, the Zeiss Company (Germany), working with Dr Gunnar Holmgren of Sweden, introduced a binocular microscope for treating otosclerosis of the middle ear. This unit had magnifications of ×8 to ×25 with field-of-view diameters of 6 to 12 mm.

In the United States, ophthalmologists were using the slit lamp for examination of the anterior structures of the eye before World War II, but it was the otologists who introduced the SOM to the medical community. In the late 1940s, Dr Jules Lempert, a leading mastoid surgeon from New York, had been using loupes to perform his surgery. Dr Lempert realized the limitations of loupes; he needed more magnification and illumination and was in search of a microscope. While attending a show of industrial equipment in Germany, he found a microscope that he felt he could adapt. This was the Zeiss epi-teknoscope. Zeiss sold three of these units to the Storz Instrument Company in St Louis, Missouri, one of which went to the Lempert Institute of Otology. The epi-teknoscope was based on Galilean optics. Galilean optics are those optics that focus at infinity. This is markedly different from Greenough optics (convergent optics), which are found in dissecting or laboratory microscopes. Greenough-type microscopes necessitate observation with convergent eyes, resulting in accommodation of the observer and eye fatigue. The advantage of Galilean optics is that the light beams going to each eye are parallel. With parallel light instead of converging light, the operator's eyes are at rest as if he or she were looking off into the distance. Therefore, operations that use the SOM and take several hours can be performed without eye fatigue (Haper M, personal communication, 2005).

Dr Samuel Rosen, an otologist from Philadelphia, learned of the microscope that Dr Lempert had obtained. He also purchased one and developed a procedure to replace the stapes mobilization technique with one that could restore permanent hearing after the tiny bones of the middle ear had ossified (Lowrence B, personal communication, 1989).

The formal introduction of the binocular operating microscope was in 1953 when Zeiss introduced the Opton ear microscope. This was the forerunner of the OPMI 1 (the first modern microscope). The Opton had a five-step magnification changer that could produce magnifications from ×1.2 to ×40 and field-of-view diameters from 4.8 to 154 mm. Working distances were a remarkable 200 to 400 mm. The Opton had built-in coaxial illumination, which added immensely to visual acuity (Haper M, personal communication, 2005).

The use of the SOM in ophthalmology developed at a much slower rate. Many ophthalmic procedures could be performed without the microscope. Initially, loupes seemed adequate, and emphasis was placed on developing better loupes. Light amplification was not a particular problem because side illumination was available. The need for a coaxial illumination light source (found in an SOM) did not become important to the ophthalmologists until they started performing extracapsular cataract extraction. In order to see the posterior capsule, a red reflex from the retina was needed. This reflex is produced by coaxial illumination. Many ophthalmologists during the early 1970s felt that the SOM made simple and highly successful operations complicated and drawn out. However, a few clinicians began to use the "ear scope," as it was called, to perform cataract removal. They soon recognized the advantages of the wide field, better depth of focus, better illumination, and variable magnification when using the SOM instead of loupes (Lowrence B, personal communication, 1989).

The development of the SOM in neurosurgery was similar to that in ophthalmology. In 1966, while performing cranial nerve dissections at the University of California, Los Angeles on closed-circuit television for dental students, Dr Peter Jannetta, a neurosurgeon, made an anatomical discovery. The trigeminal nerve is generally described as emerging in the cerebellopontine angle in two bundles: sensory (portio major) and motor (portio minor). Jannetta noted a portio intermedius, which he theorized needed to be preserved when cutting the portio major in order to preserve light touch perception after surgery for trigeminal neuralgia. Using the SOM, he further developed a microvascular decompression procedure to visualize and free up small blood vessels wrapped around the trigeminal nerve root, thereby relieving compression on the nerve and eliminating the symptoms of trigeminal neuralgia.[13]

In the mid 1970s, Contraves AG of Zurich, in conjunction with Dr M Gazi Yasargil (Switzerland) and Dr Leonard Malis (USA), introduced a neurosurgical floor stand that combined a perfectly balanced suspension of the microscope with electromagnetic locking of each pri-

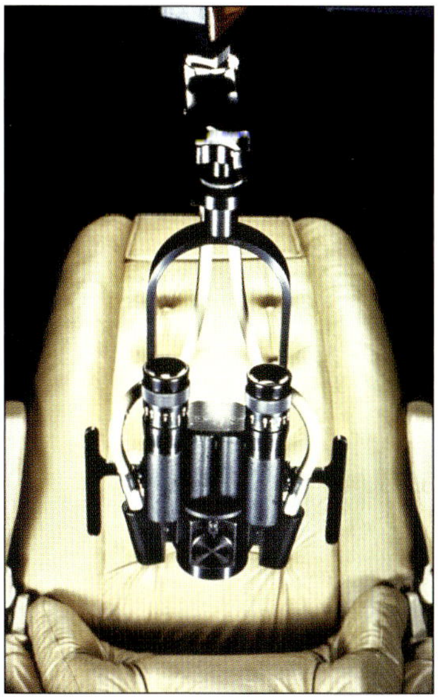

Fig 7-3 The original DentiScope. (Courtesy of Dr Noah Chivian, West Orange, New Jersey.)

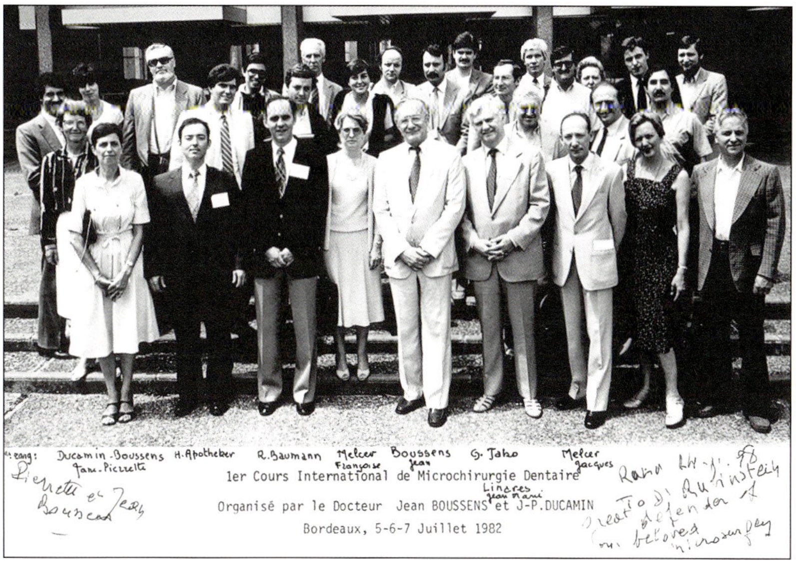

Fig 7-4 Attendees at the First International Congress in Microsurgical Dentistry. (Courtesy of Dr Jean Boussens, Bordeaux, France.)

mary axis of the various floor stand elements (Haper M, personal communication, 2005). Advancements of this nature made the SOM a mainstay in the modern hospital operating room for all medical disciplines.

The Evolution of Magnification and Illumination in Dentistry and Endodontics

The use of magnification to enhance visualization in dentistry dates back over a century. In 1876, Dr Edwin Saemisch, a German ophthalmologist, introduced simple binocular loupes to surgery.[14] Soon after, dentists began experimenting with loupes to assist in the performance of precision dentistry, and this continued to be standard practice until the late 1970s.

In 1962, Dr Geza Jako, an otolaryngologist, used the SOM in oral surgical procedures.[15] Dr Robert Baumann, an otolaryngologist and practicing dentist, described the use of the otologic microscope in dentistry in 1977.[16] He predicted that the SOM would find a place in the armamentarium of the modern dentist as it did in otorhinolaryngology, neurosurgery, vascular medicine, and gynecology.

In 1978, Dr Harvey Apotheker, a dentist from Massachusetts, and Dr Jako began the development of a microscope specifically designed for dentistry. In 1980, Dr Apotheker coined the term *microdentistry*.[17,18] The DentiScope (Fig 7-3) was manufactured by Chayes-Virginia and was marketed by Johnson & Johnson. The DentiScope had a single magnification of ×8 and dual fiberoptic lights that were directed toward the surgical field. The unit could be mounted on a mobile stand or could be permanently mounted to a wall. Unfortunately, due to lack of initial interest in the product, the DentiScope was dropped from production. Despite this setback, there was still interest in using the SOM in dentistry.

In July 1982, the First International Congress in Microsurgical Dentistry was held in Bordeaux, France (Fig 7-4). Drs Jean Boussens and Ducamin-Boussens chaired the meeting. In attendance were many of the early pioneers, including Drs Baumann, Jako, and Apotheker (Boussens J, personal communication, 1997). Dr Apotheker continued to work with and perform research on the operating microscope. In 1984, along with Dr Howard Reuben, they reported its use for the first time in apical surgery.[19] Two years later, Dr Howard Selden reported his experience with the SOM.[20]

Interest surged again among endodontists in 1989 when Drs Noah Chivian and Sandy Baer formed a company called Microdontics and sold the remaining DentiScopes. All of these microscopes found their way into endodontic offices throughout the United States by the end of the decade.

Dr Gabriele Pecora gave the first presentation on the use of the SOM in surgical endodontics at the 1990 annual session of the American Association of Endodontists in Las Vegas, Nevada. He used the Zeiss OPMI I SOM. Dr Richard Rubinstein and Dr Gary Carr began using medical-grade microscopes for apical surgery in 1990 and reported on their experience.[21–24] Shortly thereafter, Dr

Carr founded the Pacific Endodontic Research Foundation, which was dedicated to teaching microendodontics.

In March 1993, 11 years after the introduction of the DentiScope, the first symposium on microscopic endodontic surgery was held at the University of Pennsylvania School of Dental Medicine. The first university-based training program was founded at that university shortly thereafter.

By 1995, there was considerable increase in the use of the SOM. Microscope companies such as Zeiss, Global, and JEDMED offered microscopes with a variety of features that could accommodate virtually any practitioner and office environment. Improved lighting systems, variable adjustable binoculars, and improved ergonomics created opportunities for visual acuity that were far superior to what was available just a decade earlier.

In the summer of 1995, a workshop was held for endodontic department chairmen and program directors to address the need for enhanced magnification and its role in advanced specialty education programs. The American Association of Endodontists sponsored the workshop. Drs Carr, Rubinstein, Ruddle, West, Kim, Arens, and Chivian, all early pioneers in endodontic microscopy, taught the course that was both lecture and hands-on. At the end of the 2-day workshop, there was a unanimous decision among the teachers to recommend to the Commission on Dental Accreditation of the American Dental Association that proficiency in the use of the microscope in both surgical and nonsurgical treatment be included in postgraduate endodontic education programs. The Commission met in January 1996, and the mandatory teaching of microscopy was passed and included in the new Accreditation Standards for Advanced Specialty Education Programs in Endodontics. The new standards went into effect in January 1997. Later the term *microscopy* was amended to *magnification* to include the use of loupes, headlamps, and endoscopy. As in medicine, the incorporation of the SOM moved slowly, but it has ultimately changed the fields of both surgical and nonsurgical endodontics and the way they are practiced.

In 1999, Mines et al[25] reported the frequency of use of the microscope, as a function of years since completing advanced endodontic training, as follows: < 5 years, 71%; 6 to 10 years, 51%; and > 10 years, 44%. The average rate of utilization was 52%. The most frequent use of the microscope in apical surgery was in root-end preparations and in placing root-end fillings. In 2008, Kersten et al[26] repeated the study and reported the results as follows: < 10 years, 95%; 10 to 14 years, 90%; 16 to 20 years, 82%; and > 20 years, 78%. The average utilization had increased to 90%.[26] Since this study was reported, more residents have completed programs and are now in practice, and more nonusers have retired. One can assume that the frequency of utilization has increased and will continue to increase in time.

As an alternative to the SOM, some practitioners use loupes, loupes in conjunction with headlamps, and the recently introduced endoscope for apical surgery. A review of each of these choices of magnification and illumination will point out their benefits and limitations as surgical adjuncts.

Loupes

Historically, dental loupes have been the most common form of magnification used in apical surgery (Fig 7-5). Loupes are essentially two monocular microscopes with lenses mounted side by side and angled inward (convergent optics) to focus on an object. The disadvantage of this arrangement is that the eyes must converge to view an image. This convergence over time will create eye strain and fatigue, and as such, loupes were never intended for lengthy procedures. Most dental loupes used today are compound in design and contain multiple lenses with intervening air spaces. This is a significant improvement over simple magnification eyeglasses but falls short of the more expensive prism loupe design.

Prism loupes are the most optically advanced type of loupe magnification available today. They are actually low-power telescopes that use refractive prisms. Prism loupes produce better magnification, larger fields of view, wider depths of field, and longer working distances than other types of loupes. Only the SOM provides better magnification and optical characteristics than prism loupes.

The disadvantage of loupes is that ×3.5 to ×4.5 is the maximum practical magnification limit. Loupes with higher magnification are available, but they are quite heavy and, if worn for a long period of time, can produce significant head, neck, and back strain. In addition, as magnification is increased, the field of view and depth of field decrease, which limits visual opportunity.

Visual acuity is heavily influenced by illumination. An improvement to using dental loupes is obtained when a fiberoptic headlamp system is added to the visual armamentarium (Fig 7-6). Surgical headlamps can increase light levels as much as four times that of conventional dental operatory lights. Another advantage of the surgical headlamp is that because the fiberoptic light is mounted in the center of the forehead, the light path is always in the center of the visual field.

Endoscopy

Endoscopy is a surgical procedure whereby a long tube is inserted into the body, usually through a small incision. It is used for diagnostic purposes, examination, and surgical procedures in many medical fields. Goss and Bosanquet[27] reported that Ohnishi first used the endoscope in den-

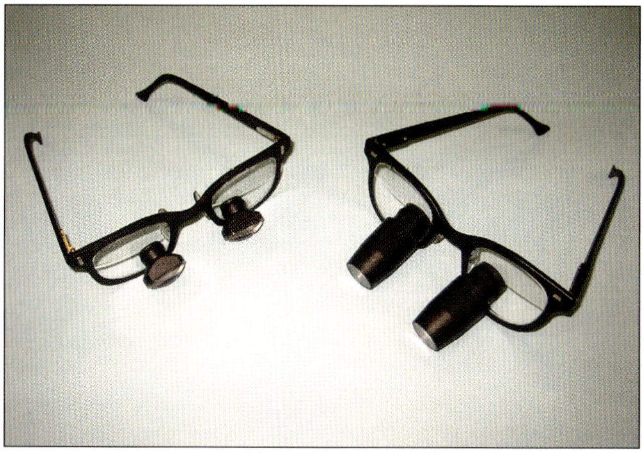

Fig 7-5 Dental loupes with ×2.5 and ×3.5 magnification (Designs for Vision).

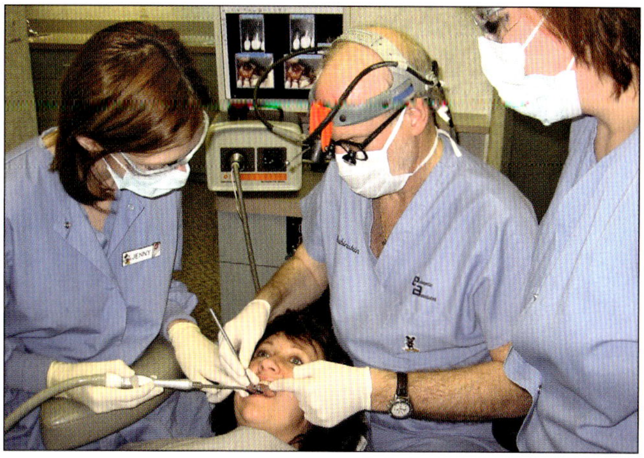

Fig 7-6 Surgeon with surgical headlamp and ×2.5 loupes (Designs for Vision).

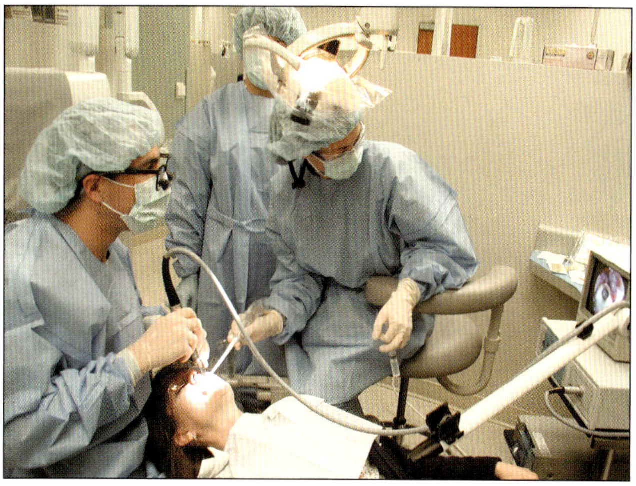

Fig 7-7 The EVS utilizes a fixed rod lens for apical surgery. (Courtesy of Dr James Bahcall, University of Illinois at Chicago.)

tistry to perform an arthroscopic procedure of the temporomandibular joint in 1975. Detsch et al[28] first used the endoscope in endodontics to diagnosis dental fractures in 1979. Held et al[29] and Shulman and Leung[30] reported the first use of the endoscope in surgical and nonsurgical endodontics in 1996. Bahcall et al[31] presented an endoscopic technique for endodontic surgery in 1999.

The endoscopic system consists of a telescope with a camera head, a light source, and a monitor for viewing. The traditional endoscope used in medical procedures consists of rigid glass rods and can be used in apical surgery and nonsurgical endodontics. A 2.7-mm lens diameter, 70-degree angulation, 3-cm-long rod lens is recommended for surgical endodontic visualization, and a 4-mm lens diameter, 30-degree angulation, and 4-cm-long rod lens is recommended for nonsurgical visualization through an occlusal access opening.[32] The recently introduced flexible fiberoptic orascope is recommended for intracanal visualization and has a 0.8-mm tip diameter, 0-degree lens, and working portion that is 15 mm in length.

The term *orascopy* describes the use of either the rigid rod lens endoscope or the flexible orascope in the oral cavity. One of the first units introduced, the EVS (Endodontic Visualization System, JEDMED) incorporates both endoscopy and orascopy in one unit (Fig 7-7). The EVS allows for two methods of documentation. The camera head used in the EVS is an S-video camera, and as such, documentation is usually accomplished by recording streaming video onto tape or a digitized format. Digital stills can be obtained by using the JEDMED Medicapture system, which can work with any existing video system. Images are captured on a USB flash drive in either JPEG or BMP format, with a resolution of up to 1024 × 768 pixels, and transferred to a computer for editing and placement into case reports or presentations. Updated versions are now available with the Medicapture system incorporated into the camera head.

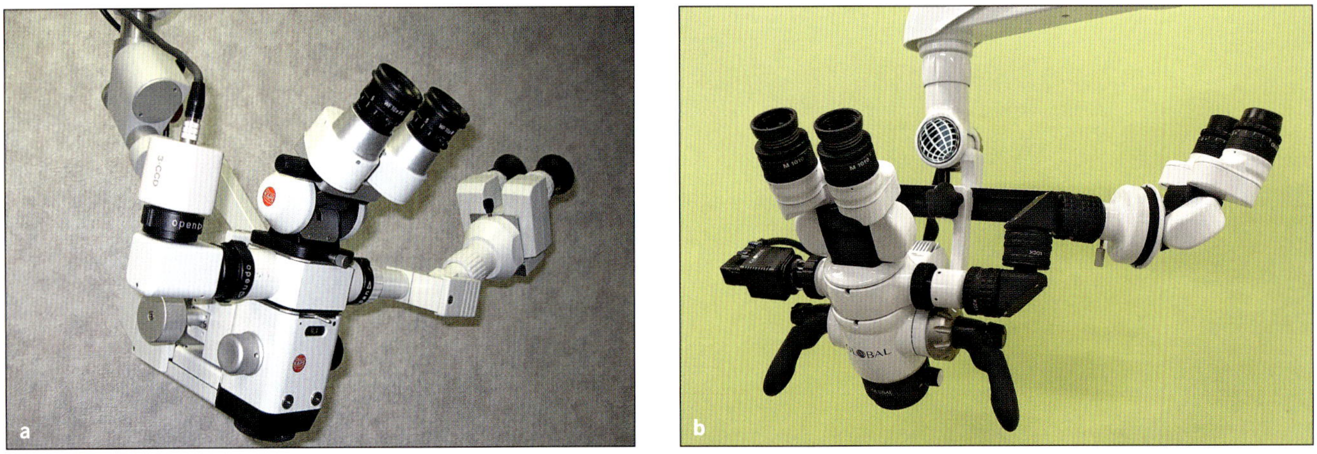

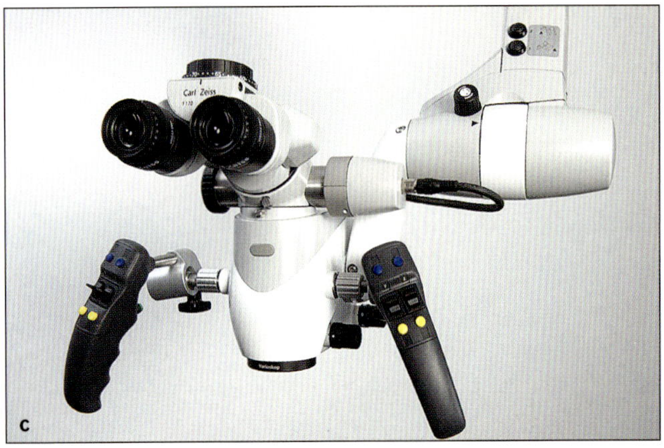

Fig 7-8 *(a)* JEDMED V-Series SOM with assistant binoculars, three-chip video camera, and counterbalanced arms. *(b)* Global A-6 SOM with assistant observation scope, high-definition digital camera, and 100,000-lux illumination. *(c)* Zeiss OPMI PROergo SOM with magnetic clutches, power zoom, and power focus on the handgrips.

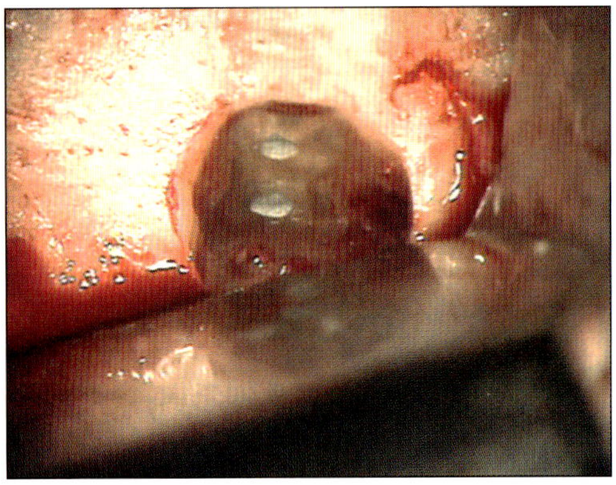

Fig 7-9 Micromirror view of Grey MTA Plus retrofill (Avalon Biomed) at ×16.

Clinicians who use orascopic technology appreciate the fact that it has a nonfixed field of focus, which allows visualization of the treatment field at various angles and distances without losing focus and depth of field.[33] Unlike when loupes or a microscope is used, the endoscope and orascope are in much closer proximity to the field of treatment. Moving the lens closer to the point of observation creates various levels of magnification. This equates to greater clarity at higher magnification, often in the range of ×30 to ×40. Because of this close proximity to the point of observation, factors like condensation and blood can affect the clarity of the image, and the use of antifog solutions are recommended. Furthermore, endoscopes and orascopes will not provide a discernible image when placed in blood, dictating the need for excellent hemostasis in the operating field. Observation of the surgical field for both the operator and the assistant is through a monitor (see Fig 7-7). Critics of this form of magnification point out that the images viewed are two-dimensional (2D) and too restrictive to be useful when compared with the stereoscopic images provided with loupes or microscopes.

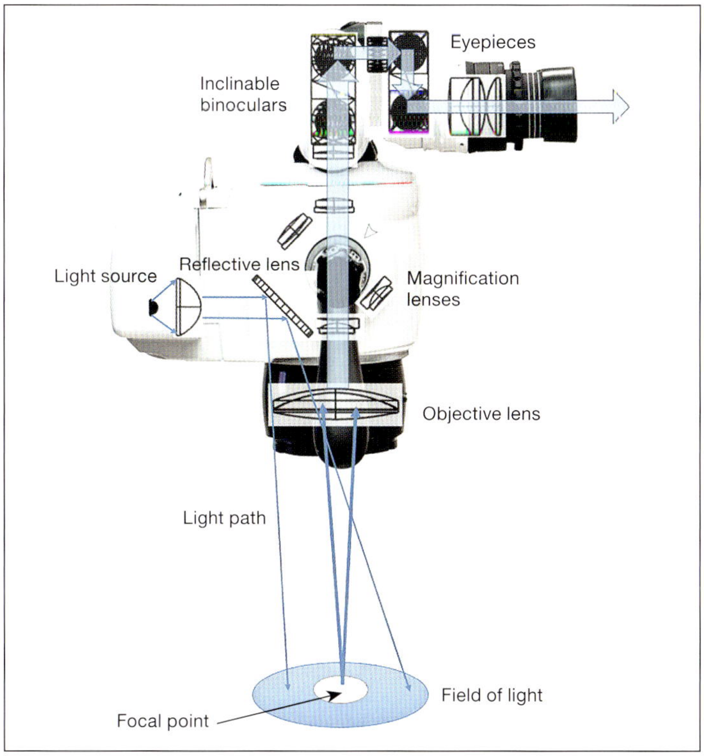

Fig 7-10 Cross-sectional diagram of a typical five-step SOM head showing the turret ring, magnification lenses, and light path in the body of the microscope.

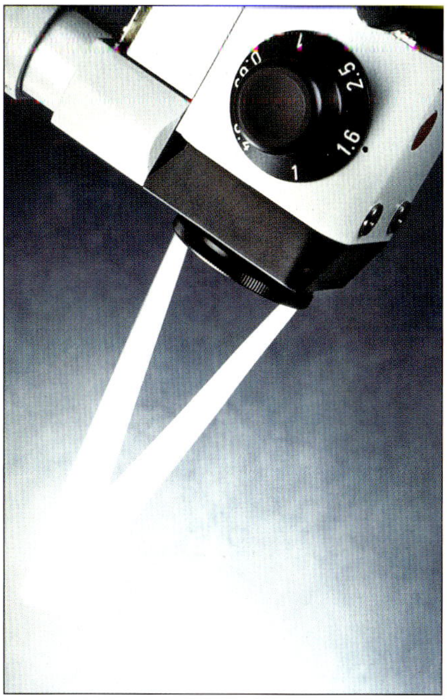

Fig 7-11 Turning the dial rotates the turret ring inside the body of the SOM and creates five magnification factors.

Orascopy was never intended to replace loupes or the microscope but rather to complement these other forms of magnification when specific magnification is needed.[34] Bahcall and Barss recommend using ×2 to ×2.5 loupes for visualization in conjunction with the use of the endoscope in apical surgery to reflect gingival tissue, remove cortical and medullary bone, and isolate the root end. They further recommend that the endodontist hold the endoscope with a comfortable pen grasp while the assistant retracts the gingival tissue and suctions during surgical treatment.[32]

Surgical operating microscope

Most microscopes can be configured to magnifications up to ×40 and beyond (Fig 7-8), but limitations in depth of field and field of view make it impractical. The lower-range magnifications (×2.5 to ×8) are used for orientation to the surgical field and allow for a wide field of view. Mid-range magnifications (×10 to ×16) are used for operating. Higher-range magnifications (×20 to ×30) are used for observing fine detail. The most significant advantages of using the SOM are in visualizing the surgical field and in evaluating surgical technique (Fig 7-9). Clearly, if a task can be seen better, it can be performed better. Fractures, POEs, and canal isthmi can be readily seen and dealt with accordingly.

Magnification fundamentals

The magnification possibilities of a microscope are determined by the power of the eyepiece (available as ×10, ×12.5, ×16, and ×20), the focal length of the binoculars, the magnification changer factor, and the focal length of the objective lens. Diopter settings on the eyepieces adjust for accommodation and refractive error of the operator. *Accommodation* is the ability to focus the lens of our eyes, which decreases as we age, and *refractive error* is the degree to which we need to wear corrective glasses. As in a typical pair of field binoculars, adjusting the distance between the two binocular tubes sets the interpupillary distance. Binoculars are now available with variable inclinable tubes and can rotate from 0 to 220 degrees and beyond to accommodate virtually any head position.

Magnification changers are available in three-, five-, or six-step manual changers, with manual zoom or power zoom changers. Manual step changers consist of lenses that are mounted on a turret (Fig 7-10). The turret is connected to a dial that is located on the side of the microscope housing (Fig 7-11). The dial positions one lens in front of the other within the changer to produce a fixed

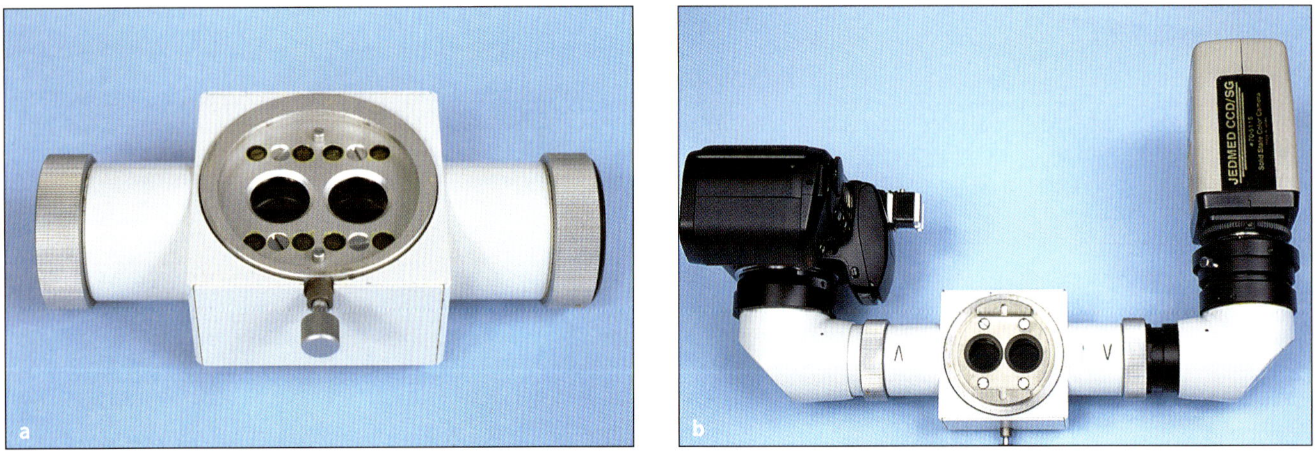

Fig 7-12 *(a)* A 50:50 beam splitter. *(b)* A 50:50 beam splitter with 35-mm digital camera and video camera.

magnification factor. Rotating the dial reverses the lens positions and produces a second magnification factor. A typical five-step changer has two sets of lenses and a blank space on the turret without a lens. When you factor in the power of the eyepiece, the focal lengths of the binoculars, and the objective lens with the magnification changer lenses, five fixed powers of magnification are obtained: two from each lens combination and one from the blank space.

A manual zoom changer is merely a series of lenses that move back and forth on a focusing ring to give a wide range of magnification factors. A power zoom changer is a mechanized version of the manual zoom changer. Power and manual zoom changers avoid the momentary visual disruption or jump that is observed with manual step changers as you rotate the turret and progress up or down in magnification.

The SOM is focused much like a laboratory microscope. The manual focusing control knob is located on the side of the microscope housing and changes the distance between the microscope and the surgical field. As the control knob is turned, the microscope is brought into focus. Some microscopes are fine focused by turning a focusing ring mounted on the objective lens housing.

Some microscopes have power zoom and power focus features. These features are often combined and located in foot controls, which allow for hands-free operation. The Zeiss OPMI PROergo has its power zoom and power focus adjustments located on both sides of the handgrips of the microscope (see Fig 7-8c). This microscope also features magnetic clutches, which keep the microscope head in a locked and stable position.

The focal length of the objective lens determines the operating distance between the lens and the surgical field. With the objective lens removed, the microscope focuses at infinity and performs as a pair of field binoculars. A variety of objective lenses are available with focal lengths ranging from 100 to 400 mm. A 175-mm lens focuses at about 7 inches, a 200-mm lens focuses at about 8 inches, and a 400-mm lens focuses at about 16 inches. Many endodontic surgeons use a 200-mm lens; this allows adequate room to place surgical instruments and still be comfortably close to the patient.

As mentioned earlier, as the magnification is increased, the depth of field and field of view both decrease. While this is a limitation for fixed-magnification loupes, it is not a limiting factor with the SOM because of the variable ranges of magnification. If the depth of field or field of view is too narrow, the operator merely needs to back off on the magnification as necessary to view the desired field.

Illumination fundamentals

The light provided in an SOM is two to three times more powerful than that in surgical headlamps and, in many endodontists' offices, has replaced standard overhead operatory lighting.

As can be seen in Fig 7-10, the illumination pathway of the microscope starts at its source and is reflected through a condensing lens to a series of prisms and then through the objective lens to the surgical field. After the light reaches the surgical field, it is then reflected back through the objective lens, through the magnification changer lenses, through the binoculars, and then exits to the eyes as two separate beams of light. The separation of the light beams is what produces the stereoscope effect that allows us to see depth.

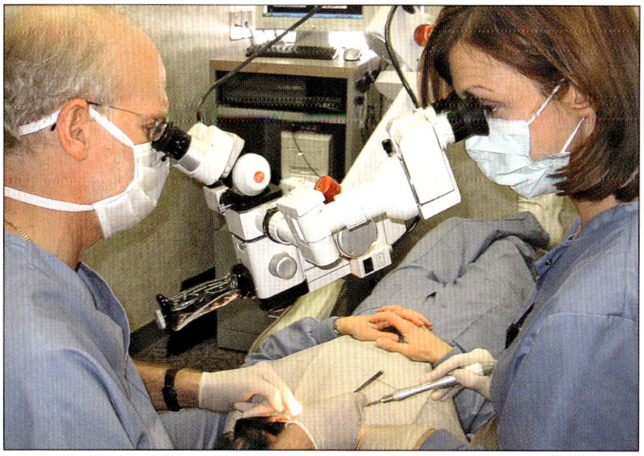

Fig 7-13 Doctor and assistant at the SOM.

Illumination with the SOM is coaxial with the line of sight. This means that light is focused between the eyes in such a fashion that you can look into the surgical site without seeing any shadows. Elimination of shadows is made possible because the SOM utilizes Galilean optics. As stated earlier, Galilean optics focus at infinity and send parallel beams of light to each eye. With parallel light, the operator's eyes are at rest, and therefore lengthy operations can be performed without eye fatigue.

Accessories

A beam splitter (Fig 7-12) can be inserted in the pathway of light as it returns to the operator's eyes. The function of the beam splitter is to supply light to an accessory such as a video camera or a digital still camera. With a 50:50 beam splitter, half of the light is available to the operator, and the remaining light can be equally split between a digital still camera and a video camera. Other configurations are also available. In addition, an assistant articulating binocular can be added to the microscope array (see Fig 7-8a) and substituted for one of the cameras. The advantages of adding assistant articulating binoculars are numerous. The assistant becomes optically important to the surgical team and develops a keener understanding not only of what is expected in the surgery but also of why it is expected (Fig 7-13). He or she sees stereoscopically exactly what the operator sees. Placement of a surgical suction becomes accurate, and the assistant can visually anticipate the surgeon's next step in the procedure. Most clinicians have found that bringing the assistant into the visual sphere increases job satisfaction significantly.

An eyepiece with a reticule field can be substituted for a traditional eyepiece. The reticule field helps the operator center the surgical field and assists with surgical photography.

Parfocusing the microscope

Before the microscope can be used, it must be made parfocal. This means that it is in focus throughout the entire range of magnification. In addition, when the microscope is parfocused, accessories such as cameras and auxiliary binoculars are also in focus. The necessary process is detailed below.

1. If you wear glasses, fold the rubber cups on the eyepieces to their downward position.
2. Set the interpupillary distance as you would a pair of field binoculars.
3. Set any fine focus device (which will vary depending on the manufacturer) so that it is in the center position.
4. Set the diopter settings of both eyepieces to zero.
5. With the microscope set at the highest magnification factor, focus the microscope on a fixed object.
6. When the object is in focus, set the microscope to the lowest magnification factor.
7. Close the left eye and turn the diopter setting of the right eyepiece either + or – until the object is in focus in the right eye.
8. Close the right eye and turn the diopter setting of the left eyepiece either + or – until the object is in focus in the left eye.
9. The microscope is now parfocused and will not need to be changed unless it is to be used by an operator who has different optical requirements.

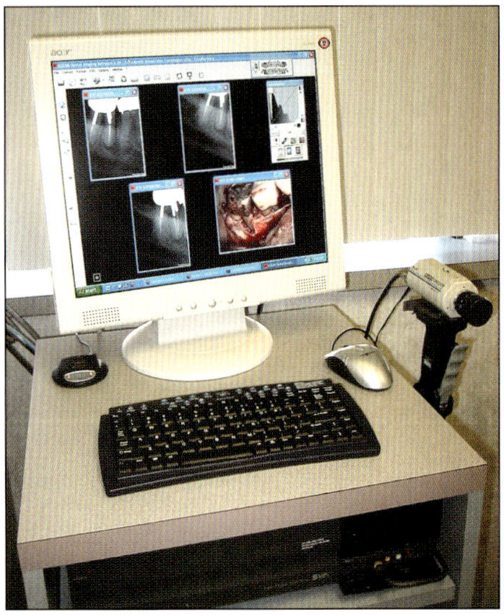

Fig 7-14 Digital radiographs and clinical images on a 19-inch flat-panel LCD screen.

Determining magnification

A frequently asked question is "how do I know what power I'm working at?" While charts are available from the various manufacturers, there is a simple formula that can help the operator calculate the working magnification.

$$\text{Total magnification} = \frac{\text{Focal length of binoculars}}{\text{Focal length of objective lens}} \times \text{Magnification factor} \times \text{Power of eyepieces}$$

For example, if the magnification factors are 0.5, 0.66, 1.0, 1.5, and 2.0; the focal length of the binoculars is 160 mm; the power of the eyepieces is ×10; and the focal length of the objective lens is 200 mm, then the total magnifications are as follows:

$$\frac{160}{200} \times 0.5 \times 10 = \times 4$$

$$\frac{160}{200} \times 0.66 \times 10 = \times 5.3$$

$$\frac{160}{200} \times 1.0 \times 10 = \times 8$$

$$\frac{160}{200} \times 1.5 \times 10 = \times 12$$

$$\frac{160}{200} \times 2.0 \times 10 = \times 16$$

Documentation

Historically, there have been a number of ways to incorporate documentation while using the microscope. Among them have been 35-mm photography, sublimation dye prints, and videotaping. With the introduction of digital radiography systems, clinical images can now be captured on a video capture card installed on the operatory computer. The video camera mounted on the microscope's beam splitter sends a real-time video signal, and an unlimited number of images can be captured or recorded during the procedure. These images can then be saved along with radiographic images and reviewed with the patient after the surgery (Fig 7-14). Digitally created clinical and radiographic images can then be exported to a Microsoft Word document for case reporting or placed into PowerPoint presentations for teaching purposes.

Using the microscope and digital radiographic systems in this way provides opportunities for unsurpassed doctor-patient communication. Furthermore, communication with referring dentists and teaching possibilities are also enhanced.

Care and maintenance of the microscope

An SOM is a costly item and should last a long time if properly maintained and cared for. Dust is the greatest enemy of a microscope, and as such the microscope should be covered when not in use. The SOM lenses should be treated like a fine pair of glasses and frequently cleaned with lens-cleaning solution. Prior to the use of such solutions, observable dust particles should be removed from all lens surfaces by using a camel hair brush or compressed air. After applying the lens-cleaning solution, use a cotton-tipped applicator and, starting at the center of the lens, move the applicator in increasing circu-

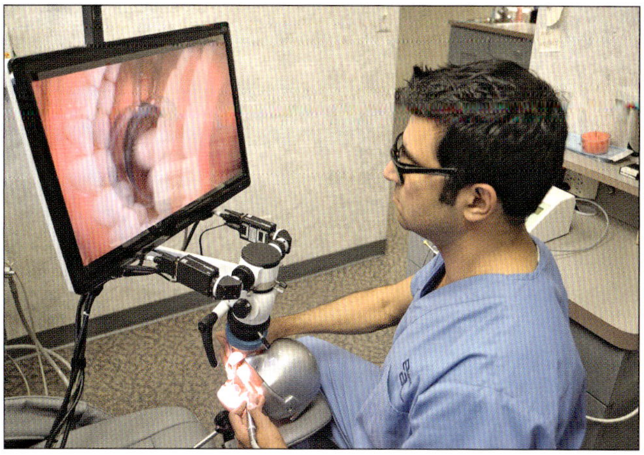

Fig 7-15 Operator demonstrating the use of a 3D imaging system.

lar motions until you reach the outer rim of the lens. Then lift the applicator off the lens surface. The objective lens should be completely removed and cleaned on both sides. Dust can also be removed by using lens-cleaning paper or ultrafine fiber cloths that trap dust and dirt, which is then squeegeed away.

Residual Oil Remover (V-Vax Products) is considered by many to be the best and safest optical cleaning formula available. Dirt particles are emulsified, and light transmission is increased by ½ an f-stop. It was originally made for Zeiss and is currently used in the space program. The product is sprayed on and removed with lens paper or a microfiber cloth.

While it is very important to clean all the lens surfaces, it is important not to attempt to clean the internal parts of any lenses. If you feel that there is dirt or dust on the inside of a sealed component, it should be returned to the manufacturer for professional cleaning. Avoid using any abrasive disinfection solutions on lens surfaces, because they will remove the antireflective coating over time. Disinfection of exposed surfaces should be limited to the body of the microscope and not the lenses. Products such as Sani-Cloth (PDI), a dual-chain quaternary/alcohol disinfectant, can be used to disinfect the surfaces of the SOM.

A variety of surgical barriers are available for use with the SOM. Elaborate disposable and autoclavable sterile drapes can be used in an operating room environment. Adhesive coverings such as Allrap and Cover-All are available from most dental supply companies and provide an adequate surface barrier. These products can be cut to size and placed on most contact surfaces of the microscope. Sterilizable rubber knobs can be purchased from the various microscope companies and fit over magnification and focusing knobs to provide a sterile barrier.

3D Imaging: 3D Vision Systems

Three-dimensional (3D) imaging systems such as the one produced by 3D Vision Systems are designed from the ground up for dentistry. The third-generation prototype (Fig 7-15) has a passive 3D imaging system with 720p resolution and a latency of 50 msec. The microscope head magnifies the image, which is captured by two 3D cameras. The signal is then processed and sent to a 22-inch 3D monitor. The depth of field is 100 mm. There is an HDMI outlet for 2D recording. Whether or not it could replace the SOM in apical surgery is unknown. However, it may ultimately replace the use of the endoscope and orascope as it is hands free, puts the monitor directly in front of the operator, and allows the operator to work in a heads-up position.

Another 3D imaging system is the MoraVision 3D clinical operating camera system designed by Dr Assad Mora, a practicing prosthodontist. This 3D system (Fig 7-16a) consists of a 4-inch cube housing two high-definition video cameras, a light source, a microphone, and a 3D video microprocessor, all suspended by a relatively small articulation arm mounted on a pole. A foot control allows for hands-free focusing and zoom magnification. When an HDMI cable is connected to a 3D monitor, the magnified 3D image is viewed in real time with passive 3D glasses. The glasses use two polarizing filters set on either side of the frame at 90 degrees to one another. The degree of magnification varies with the size of the viewing monitor. On average, a 42-inch monitor provides a range between ×10 and ×13. The depth of field is 25 to 75 mm at ×8. A second monitor can be added so that the assistant can view the same 3D field as the operator. Options to record video in either 2D or 3D or capture still photos in 2D are available. Some clinicians have already

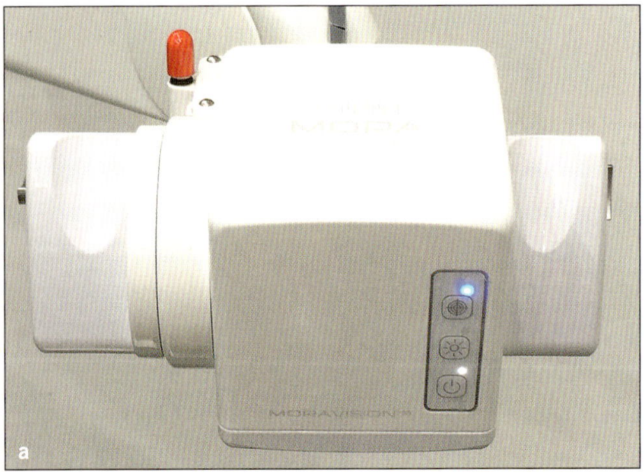

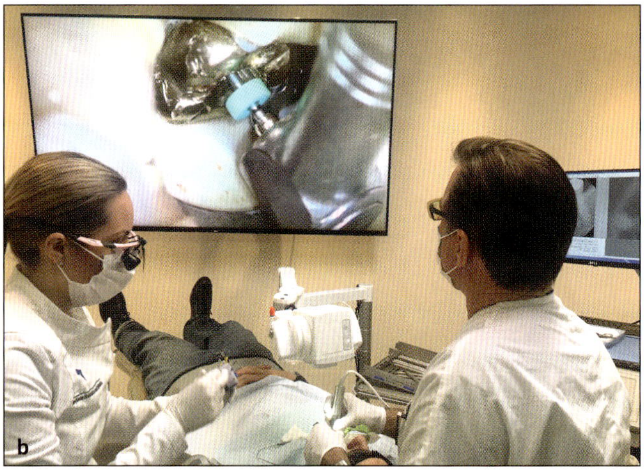

Fig 7-16 *(a)* MoraVision 3D housing. *(b)* Operator working with MoraVision 3D. (Courtesy of MoraVision.)

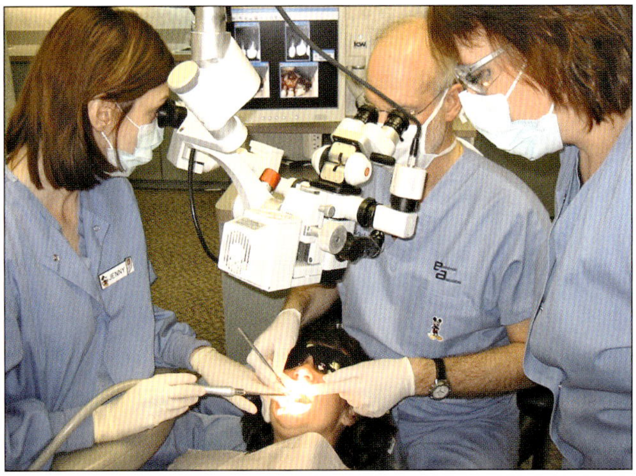

Fig 7-17 Left-handed doctor utilizing two assistants during apical surgery.

replaced their microscopes with this camera system (Fig 7-16b) and report that the 180-degree hemispheric range of motion over the patient's head allows for significant postural freedom not afforded by the SOM.

Ergonomics

As stated earlier, the binoculars on many SOMs have variable inclination. This means that the operator's head can develop and maintain a comfortable position. All stooping and bending is eliminated, thereby forcing the operator to sit up straight, tilting the pelvis forward, and aligning the spine in proper position. Proper positioning is further enhanced when the operator uses a surgical operating stool with arm supports and can have his or her thighs parallel to the floor. In addition, both feet should be placed flat on the floor. This upright positioning should create a double S-curvature of the spine, with lordosis in the neck, kyphosis in the mid-back, and lordosis again in the lower spine. Such posturing is not possible when the clinician is wearing a headlamp and loupes or using an endoscope. With these devices, there is still the tendency to bend over the patient, creating poor ergonomics and leading to head, neck, and shoulder strain. Constant bending over the patient collapses the diaphragm and may inhibit oxygen exchange, causing fatigue later in the workday. This is eliminated with the upright positioning achieved while using the SOM.

While performing apical surgery, the clinician should utilize two assistants (Fig 7-17). The primary assistant or suctioning assistant is seated so that he or she can observe the doctor's perspective through the assistant articulating microscope. The secondary assistant stands to the doctor's dominant side and is responsible for placing instruments into the doctor's hand. If desired, the secondary assistant can view the surgery in real time on either of two monitors placed in the operatory that display digital radiographs and real-time video. Positioned this way, the doctor should never have to take his or her eyes away from the SOM and the surgical field and should be able to maintain appropriate and beneficial posture throughout the entire procedure.

Operating positions must be comfortable for the doctor, the assistants, and the patient. Proper operating position is determined by six factors: the patient's head position, the dental chair position, the microscope position, the doctor's position, the assistants' positions, and the position of any assistant observation devices such as an assistant articulating binocular. All of these components are capable of moving in 3D space. There must be good communication throughout the surgery as slight adjustments in any of the six factors may significantly improve the comfort level, allowing lengthy procedures to be performed with little or no fatigue.

Misconceptions About Surgical Microscopes

Magnification

A frequently asked question is "how powerful is your microscope"? The question really addresses the issue of useable power. Useable power is the maximum object magnification that can be used in a given clinical situation relative to the depth of field and field of view. The question then becomes "how usable is the maximum power"? While magnification in excess of ×30 is attainable, it is of little value while performing apical surgery. Working at higher magnification is extremely difficult because slight movements by the patient continually throw the field out of view and out of focus. The operator is then constantly recentering and refocusing the microscope. This wastes a considerable amount of time and creates unnecessary eye fatigue. Those clinicians who use the endoscope for apical surgery would also agree that higher magnifications are for critical evaluation only and not for operating.

Illumination

There is a limit to the amount of illumination that an SOM can provide. As you increase magnification, you decrease the effective aperture of the microscope and therefore limit the amount of light that can reach the surgeon's eyes. This means that as higher magnifications are selected, the surgical field will appear darker. In addition, if a beam splitter is attached to the microscope, less light will be available for the photo adapters and auxiliary assistant binoculars. This decrease in illumination at higher magnification is not a problem while using the endoscope because the light source of the endoscope is at the tip of the endoscope and the camera compensates for any light loss. Furthermore, depth-of-field concerns while using the endoscope are not an issue because the aperture of the endoscope is quite small and, as in photography, as you decrease aperture or f-stop you increase depth of field.

Depth perception

Before apical surgery can be performed with an SOM, the clinician must feel comfortable receiving an instrument from his assistant and placing it between the microscope and the surgical field. As stated earlier, the operating space between the objective lens and the surgical field is determined by the focal length of the objective lens, which should be large enough to accommodate the clinician's hand and surgical instruments. Learning depth perception and orientation to the microscope takes time and patience. There is a learning curve, and it will vary among operators. As a general rule, it is suggested that each clinician reorient himself or herself to the SOM prior to beginning each procedure and practice various surgical scenarios with the assistants prior to each case. If the clinician is not a recent graduate of an advanced specialty training program in endodontics, it is strongly suggested that he or she enroll in a university-based microsurgical training program or take a continuing education course prior to purchasing a microscope to avoid making costly mistakes.

Access

One of the problems encountered in conventional apical surgery is gaining physical access to the sight of infection. The SOM will not improve access to the surgical field. If access is limited for traditional surgical approaches, it will be even more limited when the microscope is placed between the surgeon and the surgical field. Use of the SOM, however, will create a much better view of the surgical field. This is particularly true in diagnosing craze lines and cracks along the beveled surface of a root or when the surgeon is preparing a tiny isthmus between two canals ultrasonically. Because vision is enhanced so dramatically, apical surgery can now be performed with a higher degree of confidence and accuracy. Repeated use of the microscope and concurrent stereoscopic visualization will help the clinician develop visual imagery of the various stages of apical surgery, which is necessary in learning sophisticated surgical skills.

Flap design and suturing

Incising and reflecting soft tissue flaps are not high-magnification procedures. In many cases, they can be performed with the naked eye or with low-power loupes. Basic single interrupted stitch suturing can also be performed with little to no magnification. While the microscope could be used at low magnification, little is gained from its use in these applications. However, with the introduction of the delicate papilla base incisional flap design, which requires the use of 7-0 sutures and a minimum of two sutures per papilla, microscopic magnification with a minimum of ×4.3 is suggested.[35] The SOM is used at its best advantage for osteotomy, apicoectomy, apical preparation, retrofilling, and documentation.

References

1. Saville MH. Pre-Columbian decoration of teeth in Ecuador with some account of the occurrence of the custom in other parts of North and South America. Am Anthropol 1913;15:377–394.
2. Andrews RR. Evidence of Prehistoric dentistry in Central America. Trans Pan Am Med Cong 1893;2:1872–1873.
3. Frank AL, Glick DH, Patterson SS, Weine FS. Long-term evaluation of surgically placed amalgam fillings. J Endod 1992;18:391–398.
4. Gutmann JL, Harrison JW. Surgical Endodontics. Boston: Blackwell, 1991.
5. Shabahang S; American Association of Endodontics Research and Scientific Affairs Committee. State of the art and science of endodontics. J Am Dent Assoc 2005;136:41–52.
6. Hess W, Zürcher E, Dolamore WH. The anatomy of the root-canals of the teeth of the permanent dentition. New York: William Wood, 1925.
7. Kim S, Pecora G, Rubinstein R. Color Atlas of Microsurgery in Endodontics. Philadelphia: Saunders, 2001.
8. Weller RN, Niemczyk SP, Kim S. Incidence and position of the canal isthmus. Part 1. Mesiobuccal root of the maxillary first molar. J Endod 1995;21:380–383.
9. West JD. The relationship between the three-dimensional endodontic seal and endodontic failures [thesis]. Boston: Boston University, 1975.
10. Stevenson JR. Founding fathers of microscopy. Department of Microbiology, Miami University. https://www.cas.miamioh.edu/mbiws/microscopes/fathers.html. Accessed 8 December 2016.
11. Vision Engineering. About: Technology. http://www.visioneng.com/about/technology/microscope_history. Accessed 8 December 2016.
12. Nylen C. The microscope in aural surgery: Its first use and later development. Acta Otolaryngol 1921;116:226–240.
13. Shelton M. Working in a Very Small Place: The Making of a Neurosurgeon. New York: Vintage, 1990.
14. Shanelec DA. Optical principles of loupes. J Calif Dent Assoc 1992;20(11):25–32.
15. Apotheker H. Letter to the editor. Dent Today 1997;16:2.
16. Baumann R. How may the dentist benefit from the operating microscope? Quintessence Int 1977;5:17–18.
17. Apotheker H, Jako G. A microscope for use in dentistry. J Microsurg 1981;3:7–10.
18. Apotheker H, Jako G. The applications of the dental microscope: Preliminary report. J Microsurg 1981;3:103–106.
19. Reuben HL, Apotheker H. Apical surgery with the dental microscope. Oral Surg Oral Med Oral Pathol 1984;57:433–435.
20. Selden HS. The role of the dental operating microscope in endodontics. Pa Dent J (Harrisb) 1986;53(3):36–37.
21. Rubinstein R. New horizons in endodontic surgery. Part I. The operating microscope. Oak County (MI) Dent Rev 1991;30:7.
22. Rubinstein R. New horizons in endodontic surgery. Part II. Periapical ultrasonics and more. Oak County (MI) Dent Rev 1992;30:9.
23. Carr G. Microscopes in endodontics. J Calif Dent Assoc 1992;11:55–61.
24. Pecora G, Andreana S. Use of dental operating microscope in endodontic surgery. Oral Surg Oral Med Oral Pathol 1993;75:751–758.
25. Mines P, Loushine RJ, West LA, Liewehr FR, Zadinsky JR. Use of the microscope in endodontics: A report based on a questionnaire. J Endod 1999;25:755–758.
26. Kersten DD, Mines P, Sweet M. Use of the microscope in endodontics: Results of a questionnaire. J Endod 2008;34:804–807.
27. Goss AN, Bosanquet AG. Temporomandibular joint arthroscopy. J Oral Maxillofac Surg 1986;44:614–617.
28. Detsch SG, Cunningham WT, Langloss JM. Endoscopy as an aid to endodontic diagnosis. J Endod 1979;5:60–62.
29. Held SA, Kao YH, Wells DW. Endoscope—An endodontic application. J Endod 1996;22:327–329.
30. Shulman BB, Leung A. Endoscopic surgery: An alternative technique. Dent Today 1996;15(9):42–45.
31. Bahcall JK, DiFiore PM, Poulakidas TK. An endoscopic technique for endodontic surgery. J Endod 1999;25:132–135.
32. Bahcall J, Barss J. Orascopic visualization technique for conventional and surgical endodontics. Int Endod J 2003;36:441–447.
33. Bahcall JK, Barss JT. Orascopy: A vision for the new millennium, Part 2. Dent Today 1999;18(9):82–85.
34. Bahcall JK, Barss JT. Orascopic endodontics: Changing the way we "think" about endodontics in the 21st century. Dent Today 2000;19(5):50–55.
35. Velvart P. Papilla base incision: A new approach to recession-free healing of the interdental papilla after endodontic surgery. Int Endod J 2002;35:453–460.

Chapter Eight

Local Anesthesia and Hemostasis

Bradford R. Johnson, Hamid Abedi

The ability to predictably achieve profound anesthesia is one of the foundational skills for clinicians who perform endodontic microsurgery. Fear of pain is a primary reason that patients avoid dental treatment,[1] and considering that the majority of endodontists are not equipped or trained to provide deep sedation or general anesthesia, endodontic surgeons must be able to provide a pain-free experience using only local anesthesia, with the possible addition of anxiolytic medications and/or nitrous oxide/oxygen sedation. It is not the intention of this chapter to replicate the content of the excellent textbooks already available on local anesthesia; rather, it provides an overview of general principles and will focus primarily on the aspects of local anesthesia that are specifically relevant to surgical endodontics.

Hemostasis during endodontic microsurgery is inextricably tied to local anesthesia because the epinephrine component of dental local anesthetics provides the first, and arguably the most important, ingredient for successful hemostasis. Therefore, this chapter also focuses on the most clinically relevant aspects of surgical hemostasis. The authors invite interested readers to pursue more in-depth exposure to the basic science underlying hemostasis from one of the many excellent sources available on this topic.

Mechanism of Action of Local Anesthesia

At a fundamental level, local anesthetics function by preventing the generation and conduction of a nerve impulse. The neuron is the basic unit of the nervous system and allows for transmission of noxious stimuli from peripheral oral structures to the central nervous system via sensory afferent neurons. The action of local anesthetics is most closely tied to structural aspects of the axon. The axon is encased in a thin nerve membrane (axolemma), and some nerve fibers are covered by an additional lipid layer of myelin. Constrictions of the nerve sheath are called *nodes of Ranvier*, and it is this area of the axon that is exposed to the extracellular environment. At rest, there is a difference in electrical charge between the inside and outside of the membrane, with the interior negatively charged in relation to the exterior. This polarization of the nerve is maintained by sodium (Na^+) and potassium (K^+) pumps. When a stimulus is applied, there is a rapid increase in permeability to Na^+ ions. This decreases the interior negative charge, and a firing threshold is reached, which generates an action potential and subsequent transmission of a nerve impulse. At the most basic level, local anesthetics work primarily by binding to Na^+ ion channels in the neuronal membrane and inhibiting depolarization, thereby blocking conduction of a nerve impulse.[2]

Duration of action, potency, and time of onset

Duration of action is an especially important factor in endodontic microsurgery for several reasons. First, unlike nonsurgical root canal treatment, if anesthesia wears off before completion of a surgical procedure, it can be difficult to reinject in areas where a mucoperiosteal flap has been reflected. Second, longer-acting local anesthesia can also enhance postoperative analgesia. Finally, the duration of anesthesia is closely related to the duration of hemostatic control in the surgical area. The protein-binding ability of the cationic hydrophilic part of the local anesthetic is related to the duration of action. For example, bupivacaine has very strong protein-binding abilities, which allows it to be effective for many hours when given as a regional block.

Potency is related to lipid solubility. Greater lipid solubility enhances the diffusion through the nerve sheet as well as the neural membranes of the axon. Bupivacaine is more lipid soluble than lidocaine, and therefore it is more potent and can be prepared as a 0.5% concentration rather than a 2% to 4% concentration.[3]

Local anesthetics are weak bases, and for them to be stable in solution they are formulated as hydrochloride salts. As such, the molecules exist in a quaternary, water-soluble state at the time of injection. This form will not penetrate the neuron. The time of onset of local anesthesia is therefore predicated on the ionization constant (pKa) of the anesthetic, which predicts the proportion of molecules that exist in the cationic and lipid-soluble base form in equal amounts.

Types of local anesthesia

Ester anesthetics

Ester local anesthetics (eg, procaine) are of interest primarily from a historical perspective. First introduced in the early 1900s, they were largely replaced with amide-type local anesthetics in the 1940s. Procaine was associated with a higher incidence of allergic reactions and fell out of common use for dental procedures after the introduction of lidocaine and other amide-type local anesthetics.[4]

Topical benzocaine is the only widely used ester-type anesthetic in dentistry and is not available in injectable form. Both 5% lidocaine and 20% benzocaine have shown some effectiveness in specific situations when used as a topical anesthetic prior to injection. Application for at least one minute to dry mucosa is important and has been demonstrated in some studies to be moderately effective for reducing injection pain when giving an infiltration injection in the buccal vestibular mucosa, although the value for palatal injections is more limited, and no benefit was found for use in deeper regional block injections, such as an inferior alveolar nerve block.[5–7]

Amide anesthetics

Lidocaine hydrochloride. Lidocaine is an amide anesthetic, originally introduced by Nils Lofgren in 1943 and cleared for use in the United States in 1948. Compared with procaine, lidocaine is more potent, with a longer duration of action and faster onset. This, together with the fact that the drug has an excellent safety record and few drug-drug interactions, makes it a very useful anesthetic.[8–10] The most common formulation is 2% with 1:100,000 epinephrine. In endodontic microsurgery, 2% lidocaine with 1:50,000 epinephrine is also used and has specific benefits and limitations, as discussed later in this chapter.

Mepivacaine hydrochloride. Mepivacaine is an important drug as it produces only mild vasodilation and is one of the few commercially available local anesthetics that is marketed as a 3% solution without a vasoconstrictor, which can be very useful for patients with limited tolerance for epinephrine or other vasoconstrictors. However, local anesthetics without a vasoconstrictor are generally not recommended for primary anesthesia of the surgical site due to decreased duration of action and no vasoconstriction to assist with surgical hemostasis. Therefore, 3% mepivacaine is often recommended for intraosseous anesthesia to avoid the transient tachycardia routinely seen when using local anesthetics with a vasoconstrictor.

Bupivacaine hydrochloride. Bupivacaine has a pKa of 8.1, which means it has a longer onset of action compared with other local anesthetics discussed in this chapter. Bupivacaine is available as a 0.5% solution with 1:200,000 epinephrine, and its primary attribute in surgery is its long duration of action when used in regional block anesthesia. Studies have shown that bupivacaine does not appear to be more effective than 2% lidocaine with 1:80,000 epinephrine for the inferior alveolar nerve block,[11] but it can be effective for postoperative pain control, especially if combined with pretreatment use of a nonsteroidal anti-inflammatory drug (NSAID).[12] The patient may also require fewer opioid analgesics when bupivacaine is used for local anesthesia.[13] The slower onset of action often necessitates first using a faster-acting local anesthetic, such as lidocaine, to allow rapid onset of anesthesia followed by bupivacaine for prolonged anesthesia.

Because of the long duration of action, it is usually not recommended for children due to the risk of postoperative, self-inflicted soft tissue injury.

Articaine hydrochloride. Articaine is an amide/ester anesthetic available as a 4% solution with either 1:100,000 or 1:200,000 epinephrine and has been claimed by some to be more effective than other local anesthetics.[14,15] Articaine is unique among amide anesthetics in that it has a thiophene ring instead of the benzene ring found in other amide anesthetics. This ester group means that articaine gets metabolized in both the blood plasma and the liver. Since its introduction, articaine has been popular with dentists because of its reputation for superior diffusion through bone and better anesthetic efficacy. According to some reports, articaine has garnered the majority of the dental market in many of the countries in which it is available.[16,17] Reported risks of articaine include potential for methemoglobinemia and possible increased incidence of paresthesia following regional nerve block injection, although this latter claim is somewhat controversial.[18,19] Gaffen and Haas[20] looked at all cases of nonsurgical paresthesia reported during a 10-year period (1999–2008) by a professional liability insurance provider in Canada. According to their calculations, the occurrence of paresthesia was 1 in 609,000 injections. About 80% involved paresthesia of the tongue, while altered sensation in the lip and chin accounted for most of the other cases. Of the 182 cases of paresthesia reported, almost 60% were associated with articaine, 16% with prilocaine, and 13% with lidocaine. For the two local anesthetic drugs commonly available for dental use as 4% solutions (ie, articaine and prilocaine), the frequency of reported paresthesia was significantly greater than expected. A review of the literature is inconclusive with respect to its efficacy compared with other anesthetics, with some suggesting significantly more success[21–25] and others showing no significant difference.[26–34]

Vasoconstrictors

All injectable local anesthetics are vasodilators. This leads to lower efficacy because the local anesthetic is more rapidly transported away from the surgical site into the systemic circulation. This may also lead to increased bleeding, which is particularly relevant during surgery. Vasoconstrictors constrict the blood vessels and control the tissue perfusion. Their addition is important because they allow local anesthetics to be effective longer[35,36]; produce lower blood levels of anesthetic, thereby decreasing the potential for systemic toxicity; and decrease bleeding during surgery.

The most common type of vasoconstrictor used in local anesthetics, and the most appropriate for endodontic surgery, is epinephrine. Epinephrine works on the alpha and beta adrenergic receptors.[37] The primary action of epinephrine is on smaller arterioles and precapillary sphincters. During surgery, local anesthetic with 1:50,000 epinephrine is an effective aid in obtaining adequate hemostasis. Of note is the fact that as the levels of epinephrine decrease with time, its effect on the beta receptors is predominant, and this can cause a rebound effect whereby vasodilation and bleeding result. This is often seen hours after surgery.[38]

Considerations unique to endodontic microsurgery

Because endodontic surgery requires both soft tissue and hard tissue anesthesia, as well as hemostasis provided by the epinephrine component, it is recommended to wait at least 10 minutes after local anesthetic injection to allow for adequate anesthesia and hemostasis, even though the usual soft tissue signs of anesthesia may appear more rapidly.

Mandibular arch

A standard inferior alveolar and long buccal nerve block is usually indicated as the starting point for surgery in the mandibular arch. Two alternatives to the standard inferior alveolar block are the Gow-Gates block (see Video 5-1) and the Vazirani-Akinosi block (see Video 5-2). Although neither of these injection techniques has been proven superior to the standard inferior alveolar nerve block, they may be preferred by some clinicians. In patients with limited opening or trismus, the Vazirani-Akinosi block may be useful because this injection is performed with the patient's mouth closed. The usual anesthetic of choice for mandibular nerve block anesthesia is 2% lidocaine with 1:100,000 epinephrine, which is supplemented by a buccal vestibular injection of one or two cartridges of 2% lidocaine with 1:50,000 epinephrine for enhanced anesthesia and hemostasis. Long-acting local anesthetics such as 0.5% bupivacaine with 1:200,000 epinephrine have a soft tissue duration of action of 6 to 10 hours when used as a mandibular block injection, but the relatively low epinephrine concentration can result in increased intraoperative bleeding.[39,40] A useful strategy to provide increased postoperative analgesia is to administer a long-acting local anesthetic at the end of a surgical procedure, prior to dismissing the patient.[41,42]

Maxillary arch

The approach to local anesthesia for endodontic surgery in the maxillary arch is similar to that used for nonsurgical endodontic therapy, with a few differences. First, buccal vestibular infiltration over the tooth requiring surgery is performed using one cartridge of 2% lidocaine with 1:50,000 epinephrine. To maximize the hemostatic properties of epinephrine, it is important to inject in the vestibular fold, not the more apically positioned muscle attachments, which can result in vasodilation instead of vasoconstriction. Adjacent teeth are then anesthetized with solutions containing 1:100,000 epinephrine, extending at least one tooth beyond the area of the planned incisions. Next, approximately 1 mL of local anesthetic solution is slowly injected in the palatal tissues adjacent to the root apex. To reduce patient discomfort associated with palatal injections, place topical anesthetic with firm pressure for 1 minute prior to initiating the injection; start by injecting a small amount of local anesthetic, wait 2 minutes, then complete the injection. Regional nerve blocks such as posterior superior alveolar, second division (see Video 5-3), and infraorbital (see Video 5-4) may also be used in the maxillary arch for a greater field of anesthesia, but at the expense of somewhat diminished localized vasoconstriction activity.

Adjunctive therapy

Nitrous oxide/oxygen analgesia

Nitrous oxide/oxygen sedation can be used as a safe adjunct to local anesthesia to help reduce anxiety and provide analgesia. Nitrous oxide is a colorless, odorless gas and is an effective analgesic/anxiolytic agent causing central nervous system depression and euphoria with little respiratory depression.[43] Nitrous oxide requires special equipment and may be particularly useful in children during dental and medical surgical procedures.[44,45]

Analgesic properties of nitrous oxide are thought to be achieved by releasing endogenous opiate peptides, and activation of opioid receptors and its anxiolytic effect involve the activation of gamma-aminobutyric acid (GABA) receptors through the binding site for benzodiazepines.[46]

Oral conscious sedation

A significant number of patients defer or avoid dental treatment due to fear. Dionne et al[47] found that 18% of patients who typically avoid dental treatment would be willing to see the dentist if a drug was available to make them less nervous. Oral sedation has been used in dental offices for over 100 years and, with proper training and monitoring, can be a safe and reliable method to relax patients and enhance the surgical experience. The clinician must receive proper training for conscious sedation and must comply with all local regulatory requirements.

Benzodiazepines are the preferred drugs for conscious sedation. They act by facilitating the physiologic inhibitory effects of GABA, the major inhibitory neurotransmitter in the brain.[48] Triazolam, diazepam, and lorazepam are the most common benzodiazepines. Of the three, triazolam has the shortest half-life, approximately 1.5 to 5.5 hours, and is well-suited for dental procedures. A typical dosing schedule for an average, healthy adult is 0.25 mg triazolam at bedtime the night before surgery, followed by 0.25 mg 1 hour before surgery. As with all medications, the dose should be adjusted based on age, weight, and medical conditions. The patient should also be advised that he or she must be accompanied and driven to and from the appointment by an adult. As an alternative to oral dosing, triazolam can be effective in about 15 minutes when crushed and administered sublingually.[49]

Management of anesthetic failure and discontinuous anesthesia

In general, the same regional block and infiltration techniques used for nonsurgical endodontic treatment are used for surgical treatment. Perhaps the most significant difference in the local anesthetic protocol between nonsurgical and surgical endodontic therapy is the benefit gained from judicious use of anesthetic solutions containing 1:50,000 epinephrine. As previously noted, managing discontinuous anesthesia or a duration of action that is shorter than the procedure is more of a challenge after a surgical flap has been reflected.

Intraosseous anesthesia can be used either prior to surgery to enhance depth of anesthesia and possibly improve hemostasis or during surgery to manage discontinuous anesthesia. Examples of intraosseous systems are depicted in Figs 8-1 and 8-2 (see also Video 5-5). Although there are minor differences between intraosseous anesthesia systems, the general concept is the same. First, a single-use, disposable perforator tip placed in a low-speed or electric handpiece is used to create a small opening through the attached gingiva (unless a soft tissue flap has already been reflected) and buccal cortical plate, dropping into the cancellous bone space. Light pressure should be used so as to not overheat the bone. Initial resistance will be felt as the perforator tip engages the buccal bone, followed by a distinct decrease in resistance as the tip drops into the less dense cancellous bone. Next, local anesthetic is delivered directly into the cancellous bone surrounding the tooth using an ultrashort needle sized to match the perforator tip. Systemic effects of epinephrine are more pronounced with intraosseous injections, so it is important to limit the quantity of anesthetic with epinephrine. Transient tachycardia, usually lasting less than 4 or 5 minutes, is almost certain following intraosseous injection with solutions containing 1:100,000 epinephrine. However, no significant change in systolic, diastolic, or mean arterial blood pressure is expected.[50] Even so, solu-

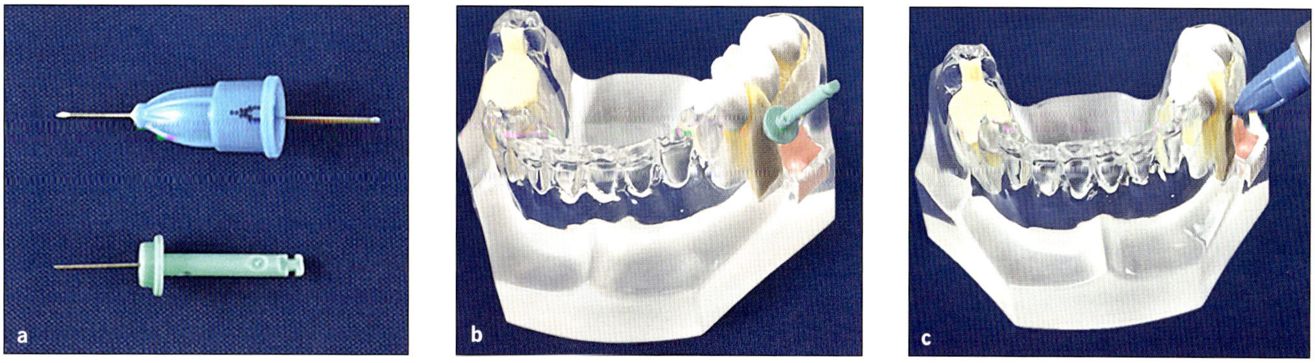

Fig 8-1 Stabident system (Fairfax Dental). *(a)* A 27-gauge ultrashort needle *(top)* and 27-gauge solid wire with beveled tip perforator *(bottom)*. *(b)* Proper angulation and interproximal position of the perforator tip after penetration into cancellous bone (the low-speed handpiece has been removed for better visualization). The perforator tip is removed prior to placement of the local anesthetic needle. *(c)* The ultrashort needle is inserted to the hub, and local anesthetic is slowly injected.

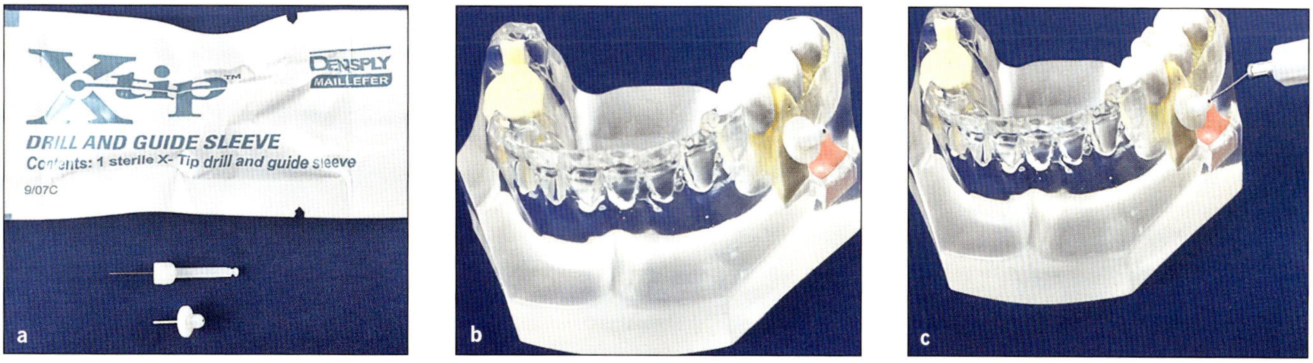

Fig 8-2 X-tip system (Dentsply). *(a)* X-tip package *(top)* and disassembled perforator tip and sleeve *(bottom)*. *(b)* The X-tip assembly is driven by a low-speed handpiece into the interproximal bone, and the tip and sleeve are then separated, leaving the sleeve in place. *(c)* An ultrashort needle is inserted completely into the X-tip sleeve, and anesthetic solution is slowly injected (image shows only initial insertion).

tions containing 1:50,000 epinephrine should not be used for intraosseous anesthesia. Local anesthetic solutions without a vasoconstrictor (eg, 3% mepivacaine) may provide sufficient short-term local anesthesia in situations of discontinuous anesthesia, but the duration of action will be less than solutions containing 1:100,000 epinephrine, and no additional hemostasis will be achieved.

Regional block injections (eg, inferior alveolar, posterior superior alveolar, or infraorbital) or reinjection can be reasonably effective when not in the immediate area of a reflected surgical flap. In the maxillary arch, a supplemental palatal injection with 1 mL of lidocaine with 1:100,000 epinephrine is often effective, at least as a short-term measure. Injection on the palate with 1 mL of local anesthetic between the first and second premolars and about midway between the marginal gingiva and the midline of the palate (anterior middle superior nerve block) can provide anesthesia from the ipsilateral central incisor to second premolar, often proving useful when a buccal flap has been reflected in this area and buccal infiltration is not possible.

Medical considerations and safety of local anesthetics

Use in pregnancy

Although endodontic surgical procedures for pregnant patients can often be deferred until after delivery, the presence of pain or recurrent infection could shift the balance in favor of surgery during pregnancy, especially if it can be scheduled during the second trimester. In fact, endodontic microsurgery is typically no more invasive than a surgical extraction and could be considered more conservative and appropriate therapy than prolonged use of analgesics and/or antibiotics during pregnancy. Of the commonly used local anesthetic agents, only lidocaine and prilocaine, with or without epinephrine, are US Food and Drug Administration (FDA) category B drugs and therefore considered safest for use during pregnancy.[51] The most commonly available local anesthetic without a vasoconstrictor is 3% mepivacaine, which is FDA category C. The use of a local anesthetic with epinephrine is recommended for the pregnant patient as it has several benefits including greater duration of anesthesia, more profound anesthesia, and decreased potential for systemic toxicity from the lidocaine due to delayed systemic uptake and metabolism of the local anesthetic.

Maximum safe dose of epinephrine in patients with cardiovascular disease

Compared with nonsurgical root canal therapy, which can often be performed with limited or no vasoconstrictor, microsurgical procedures can be very challenging without the hemostatic benefits of a local anesthetic with vasoconstrictor. Safe management of patients with moderate to severe cardiovascular disease requires careful attention to the amount of epinephrine used. Although high-quality clinical research on this topic is lacking, the use of 0.036 to 0.054 mg of epinephrine (two to three cartridges of local anesthetic with 1:100,000 epinephrine) is generally considered safe for most patients with cardiovascular disease, except those with severe disease and other specific conditions.[52–54] For practical purposes, this may preclude the use of a local anesthetic with 1:50,000 epinephrine, because the quantity of local anesthetic used would need to be reduced by 50%. A reasonable strategy for patients with advanced cardiovascular disease or reported sensitivity to epinephrine is to titrate the dose—that is, slowly inject one-half to one cartridge of local anesthetic and wait several minutes to gauge the response before proceeding with an additional injection. Vasoconstrictors should be avoided or used with extreme caution in patients with poorly controlled hypertension, arrhythmias that are refractory to treatment, myocardial infarction within the past month, coronary artery bypass graft within the past 3 months, stroke within the past 6 months, and uncontrolled congestive heart failure. When in doubt about a patient's ability to tolerate an endodontic surgical procedure, medical consultation is indicated.

The maximum safe dose of a local anesthetic is not the same for all products. For example, the maximum allowable dose for lidocaine is 7 mg/kg (up to 500 mg), which converts to approximately 13 cartridges of 2% lidocaine with 1:100,000 epinephrine for an average, healthy adult. For endodontic microsurgery, it is more appropriate to observe a typical maximum dose (TMD) that is equivalent to 8 cartridges of 2% lidocaine with 1:100,000 epinephrine. The TMD for 4% articaine with 1:100,000 epinephrine (TMD = 7 cartridges) or 3% mepivacaine without vasoconstrictor (TMD = 5.5 cartridges) are both lower than the TMD for 2% lidocaine with 1:100,000 epinephrine.[55] Pediatric and elderly patients, as well as those with significant systemic disease, are more likely to reach toxic levels of local anesthetic at a lower dose than healthy adults, so extra caution must be exercised with these patients.

Drug interactions

The vasoconstrictor in local anesthetics is more likely than the anesthetic agent itself to be responsible for a drug-drug interaction. Serious drug interactions with epinephrine and other vasoconstrictors have been associated with nonselective beta-blockers (eg, propranolol, nadolol, and timolol maleate), monoamine oxidase inhibitors (eg, isocarboxazid, phenelzine, selegiline, and tranylcypromine), and tricyclic antidepressants (eg, amitriptyline, desipramine, and nortriptyline).

Possible allergy

True allergy to an amide local anesthetic (eg, lidocaine, articaine, prilocaine, and mepivacaine) is extremely rare, but any such report should be investigated. The most common adverse reaction following local anesthetic injection is psychogenic,[56,57] characterized by a report of tachycardia, syncope, or general uneasiness. Reaction to the epinephrine component of a local anesthetic is not uncommon and can result from an inadvertent intravascular injection or a general sensitivity to catecholamines such as epinephrine. This is not a true allergic reaction. A true allergy will almost certainly have been detected during prior routine dental treatment. An allergic reaction to the sulfite preservatives used in local anesthetics containing epinephrine is also believed to be very rare but has been reported.[58–61]

Surgical Hemostasis

Value of vasoconstrictors in local anesthetic

Endodontic microsurgery is unique compared with most other oral surgical procedures in that the main reason for good hemostasis is the need for a relatively blood-free field around the apex of the root to allow for proper visualization of the area, placement of root-end filling materials, and inspection for possible root fractures.[62] In addition, adequate hemostasis during the surgical procedure minimizes surgical time, which leads to less postoperative bleeding and swelling. The first step in assuring adequate hemostasis is the use of a local anesthetic with vasoconstrictor. The vasoconstrictor of choice is epinephrine due to decreased stimulation of alpha receptors compared with alternative vasoconstrictors such as norepinephrine and levonordefrin.[63]

In a relatively small clinical study comparing blood loss during periodontal flap surgery using 2% lidocaine with either 1:50,000 or 1:100,000 epinephrine, twice as much blood loss occurred when the 1:100,000 epinephrine solution was used compared with the 1:50,000 epinephrine solution.[64] This difference could have practical implications in endodontic microsurgery and supports the position that injection of local anesthetic solutions with 1:50,000 epinephrine should allow for improved visualization and management of the surgical field. Additional discussion of the safe use of local anesthetics with epinephrine can be found in the previous section, "Medical considerations and safety of local anesthetics."

Anticoagulant therapy

Anticoagulant drug therapy is prescribed for a variety of medical conditions and includes warfarin (Coumadin, Bristol-Myers-Squibb), aspirin and other antiplatelet agents (eg, clopidogrel, ticlopidine, prasugrel, and ticagretor), novel oral anticoagulants, and novel oral antiplatelet drugs. In addition, NSAIDs and many herbal medications (eg, garlic, ginkgo, ginger, ginseng, feverfew, fish oil, and others) have anticoagulant activity. A thorough medical history is required because patients may fail to consider herbal medications as drugs. As a general statement, anticoagulant therapy usually should not be discontinued or modified prior to endodontic microsurgery because doing so can increase the risk for a thromboembolic event, and bleeding can almost always be controlled with local measures.[65–67] However, it is important to understand the specific mechanism of action of an anticoagulant drug and the appropriate method for measuring the level of anticoagulation, as well as the patient-specific indication for anticoagulant therapy. In addition, even though the risk for excessive bleeding may be minimal for most patients undergoing endodontic microsurgery,[68] medical consultation is often indicated to help assess the potential risk of a thromboembolic event if a decreased level of anticoagulation is desired because the bleeding that occurs at higher levels of anticoagulation can potentially interfere with optimal visualization of the surgical field and the placement of root-end filling materials.

The standard test for measuring warfarin activity is the International Normalized Ratio (INR), and bleeding risk should be minimal if the INR is within the normal therapeutic range of 2.0 to 3.5.[66] A recent clinical study concluded that even patients with an INR between 3.5 and 4.2 were at no greater risk for bleeding during oral surgery procedures than patients in the 2.0 to 3.5 range.[69] However, warfarin level and therefore level of anticoagulation is notoriously difficult to maintain in the desired therapeutic range. Thus, an INR test the day of surgery is recommended. If postsurgical antibiotics are given for more than 5 days, disruption of the normal gastrointestinal flora can alter vitamin K absorption and therefore increase the INR.[70]

Two newer alternatives for patients requiring anticoagulant therapy have been recently introduced and are gaining popularity. Novel oral anticoagulants (NOACs) are an alternative for most patients except those with artificial heart valves. NOACs have fewer interactions with foods and other drugs than warfarin and do not require regular monitoring. However, standardized coagulation assays are of limited value in measuring the level of anticoagulation,[71] and therefore it is more difficult to predict potential bleeding risk during surgical procedures. And, unlike warfarin, only one of the commonly prescribed NOACs currently has an FDA-cleared reversal agent. Novel oral antiplatelet drugs have been recently introduced, and little clinical guidance is available.[67]

Endodontic microsurgery is usually possible in patients on anticoagulant therapy, but considering the wide variety of drugs currently used for anticoagulation, along with indications for anticoagulation therapy that range from minimal to very serious, a medical consultation is usually advised.[67]

Inherited or acquired bleeding disorders

Any patient reporting a history of an inherited or acquired bleeding disorder requires medical consultation prior to surgical intervention. Replacement of deficient coagulation factors or a platelet transfusion prior to endodontic surgery may be required. Examples of bleeding disorders include thrombocytopenia, hemophilia, and von Willebrand disease. The potential for increased bleeding should also be considered in patients with impaired liver function.

Local hemostatic agents

Preoperative phase

As previously noted, profound local anesthesia with the use of a vasoconstrictor is not only essential to ensure patient comfort during the procedure, but also it is the first and arguably the most important step in establishing adequate hemostasis for endodontic microsurgery. Infiltration with one or two cartridges of 2% lidocaine with 1:50,000 epinephrine in the surgical field will help assure

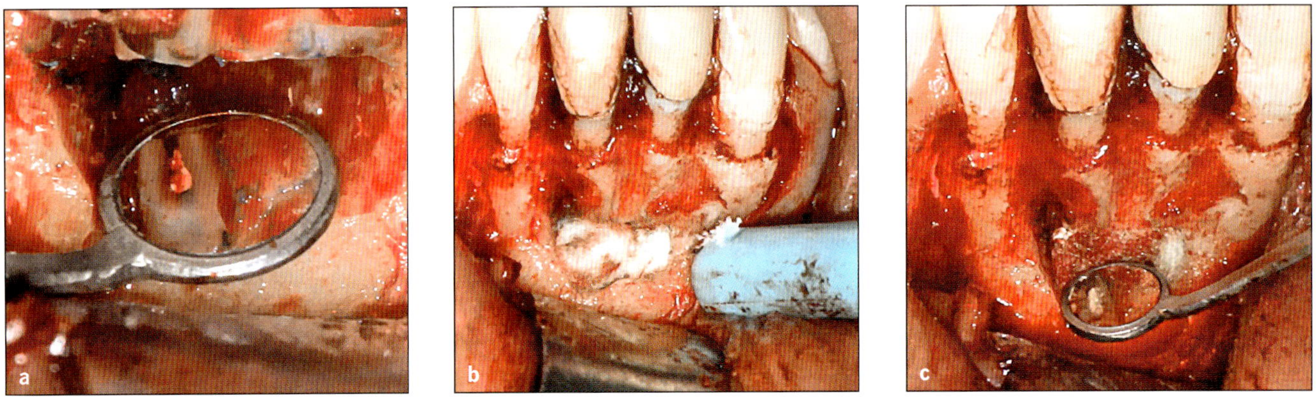

Fig 8-3 *(a)* Osteotomy and resected root end of a mandibular left central incisor viewed with a micromirror. Although the root end can be clearly visualized, oozing of blood in the surgical site would make placement of a root-end filling difficult. *(b)* Racellet pellets placed in the bony crypt for hemostasis. *(c)* View of the root end after placement of root-end filling material. Racellet pellets are still in place but must be removed prior to wound closure. (Case courtesy of Dr Jonathan Ee, Aurora, Ontario.)

hemostasis during the procedure. However, there is no or very limited value of using 1:50,000 solutions for block injections. In fact, the additional epinephrine can result in increased mean arterial blood pressure and tachycardia, which can increase patient anxiety and place some patients at greater risk of an adverse event.

Intraoperative phase

Bone wax. Bone wax is composed of beeswax and isopropyl palmitate and produces physical tamponade of small exposed blood vessels and capillaries in the bony crypt. However, the use of bone wax for microsurgical hemostasis is not recommended because it can impair healing by initiation of a foreign body reaction and decrease clearance of microorganisms.[72,73] In addition, effective and more biocompatible alternatives are readily available.[74]

Cautery. Cautery involves the application of a handheld heat source (such as most devices used for warm obturation techniques) or an electrosurgery device to a visibly bleeding or oozing vessel, but it should be limited to isolated areas due to the potential for delayed healing.[75–77] Cautery causes hemostasis by coagulation of blood and tissue proteins.

Calcium sulfate. When mixed and placed in the bony crypt, calcium sulfate provides a physical barrier to bleeding. After the material has set, it can be carved away from the root-end area, leaving a layer in contact with the bone. Unlike bone wax, calcium sulfate does not inhibit healing. After completion of root-end preparation and filling, the excess calcium sulfate can be left in place or removed.[78,79] In a small clinical study comparing calcium sulfate, cotton gauze, and ferric sulfate for hemostasis during endodontic surgery, calcium sulfate was found to be superior to the other two products.[80]

Vasoconstrictors. Racemic epinephrine cotton pellets (Racellet #2, Pascal) are often used to control bleeding during endodontic microsurgery[81] (Fig 8-3). All granulation tissue should be removed prior to placement of the cotton pellets to ensure direct contact with the bone.[81] After placing one epinephrine cotton pellet in the bony crypt, several additional plain cotton pellets are packed on top of the epinephrine pellet, and pressure is applied for several minutes. The plain cotton pellets are then removed, and the epinephrine pellet is left in place to provide a physical barrier to mild oozing of blood and to catch any debris resulting from root-end preparation and filling. If hemostasis is inadequate, the steps may be repeated.

Although the epinephrine content of these pellets is much higher than the amount contained in local anesthetic, the systemic effect appears to be minimum when used as described.[82] Epinephrine is bound to alpha-1 and alpha-2 adrenergic receptors and creates a strong and almost immediate vasoconstriction of small blood vessels and capillaries in the bony crypt, therefore limiting systemic uptake. One potential concern with using cotton pellets in the bony crypt is that cotton fibers may remain in the crypt after removal of the pellet and potentially interfere with healing. This risk can be minimized by using the surgical operating microscope to isolate and carefully remove any embedded cotton fibers prior to curetting the bony crypt and stimulating bleeding. CollaCote (Zimmer Dental) saturated with 10 drops of 2.25% racepinephrine inhalation solution may be considered as an alternative to racemic epinephrine cotton pellets.[83]

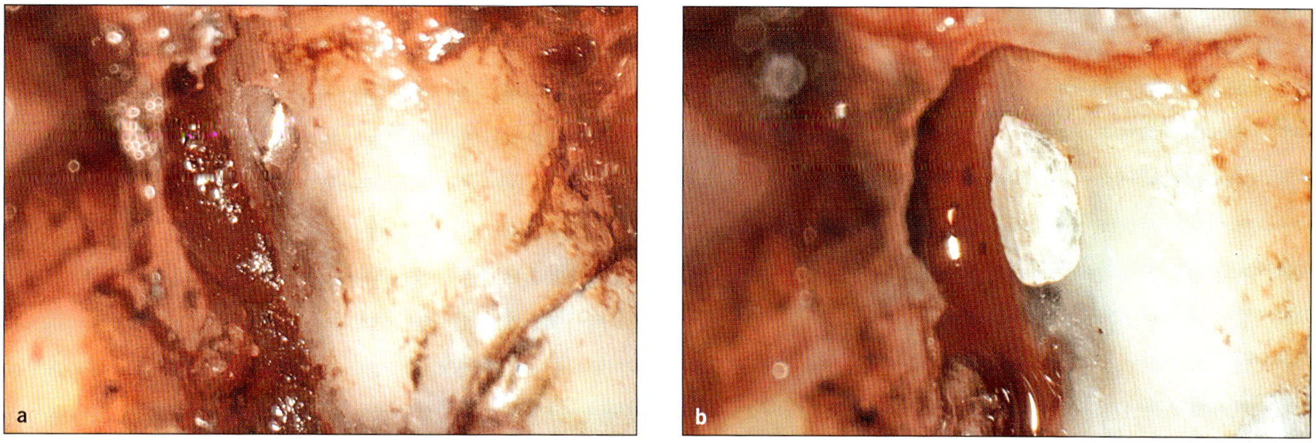

Fig 8-4 *(a)* Post perforation repair on the lateral surface of a maxillary right lateral incisor with ferric sulfate coagulum in place. *(b)* Filling material in place with the ferric sulfate coagulum removed and fresh bleeding induced. (Case courtesy of Dr Richard Rubinstein, Farmington Hills, Michigan.)

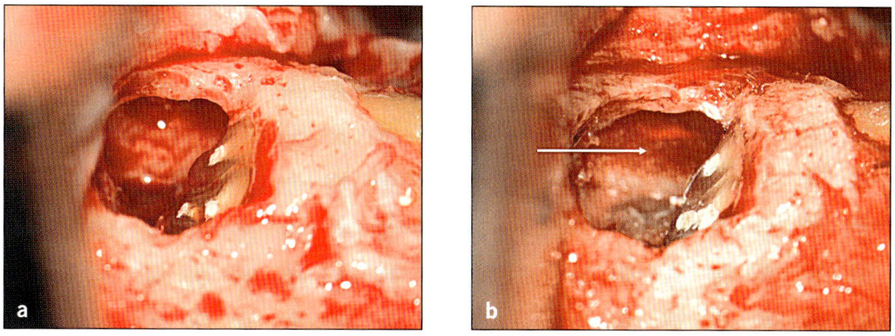

Fig 8-5 *(a)* Osteotomy and root-end resection completed on the mesiobuccal and distobuccal roots of a maxillary left second molar. *(b)* A layer of collagen is placed on the distal wall of the bony crypt *(arrow)* to control oozing and catch any excess root-end filling material. (Case courtesy of Dr Mohamed I. Fayad, Chicago, Illinois.)

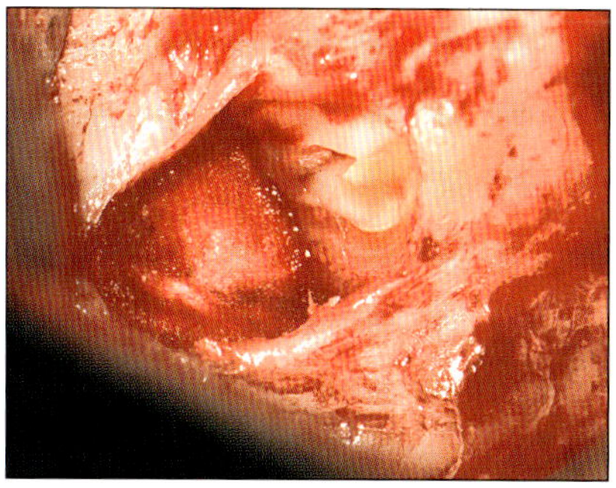

Fig 8-6 Root-end resection and preparation of a maxillary right second premolar. Collagen is packed in the bony crypt for hemostasis.

Ferric sulfate. Ferric sulfate (Cut-Trol, Ichthys) is a hemostatic necrotizing agent with a very low pH that was first introduced for use in restorative dentistry to help control bleeding from the gingival sulcus. Tissue proteins are agglutinated and then plug capillary orifices. The use of ferric sulfate as a hemostatic agent for use in endodontic surgery has been explored in animal model studies with generally favorable results, as long as the material was completely removed from the surgical site prior to wound closure.[84,85] However, failure to remove the ferric sulfate from the bony crypt resulted in a foreign body reaction and significantly impaired healing (Fig 8-4).

Thrombin. Thrombin has a long history in medicine for localized surgical hemostasis but is not commonly used for endodontic microsurgery due to handling properties and expense.[86] Thrombin is produced from bovine prothrombin and prepared as a dry powder and reacts directly with blood fibrinogen to induce clotting.

Gelfoam. Gelfoam (Pfizer) is a water-insoluble gelatin-based product prepared from purified porcine skin. The mode of action is believed to be mostly mechanical by formation of an artificial clot and partially related to alteration of the intrinsic blood clotting pathway. Although Gelfoam is absorbable, it may delay initial healing, and therefore removal prior to wound closure is advised.

Absorbable collagen. A variety of collagen-based products are available to assist with surgical hemostasis (eg, CollaCote, CollaPlug, and CollaTape [Zimmer Dental] and HeliCote [Integra]; Figs 8-5 and 8-6). The collagen is obtained from purified bovine tendon. On contact with blood, collagen causes platelet aggregation with subsequent fibrin clot formation, and hemostasis occurs in 2 to 6 minutes.

Surgicel. Surgicel (Ethicon) is an oxidized regenerated cellulose product prepared in a variety of fiber configurations. When it comes in contact with blood, it has antimicrobial properties (presumably due to its low pH) and is primarily a physical barrier to bleeding by formation of a sticky artificial coagulum.[87] Although Surgicel is absorbable over time, retention in the wound site is not recommended because it can delay healing.[88,89] ActCel (Coreva Health Sciences) is a similar soluble regenerated cellulose product. One potentially desirable attribute of cellulose products is that they are not derived from animal tissues, which may be preferred by some patients.

Chitosan products. HemCon (Tricol Biomedical) is derived from chitosan, a naturally occurring biocompatible polysaccharide from shellfish that was originally developed as a hemostatic agent for use in battlefield trauma. Cleared uses now include oral surgical procedures. A sticky mass is formed when in contact with blood, effectively sealing a wound while allowing time for the natural coagulation pathway and clotting to occur. Chitosan has natural antimicrobial activity, including activity against many microorganisms commonly associated with oral infections. In a rabbit study, HemCon was compared with ferric sulfate using the osseous wound model developed by Jeansonne et al.[85] There was no statistically significant difference in hemostasis and wound healing between the two groups, although a statistically significant increase in new bone formation was observed in the HemCon group.[90] A clinical oral surgery (extractions) study found significantly enhanced hemostasis and favorable wound healing in the HemCon group compared with the control group.[91]

Strategies to decrease the potential for postoperative bleeding and ecchymosis

Some minor postoperative bleeding and ecchymosis is not uncommon but typically is minimal. Unlike extractions, endodontic microsurgery allows for suturing and primary closure over the surgical site. Obviously, some patients, especially those on oral anticoagulant therapy or with bleeding disorders, require close postoperative monitoring. NSAIDs and some antibiotics (eg, cephalosporins, macrolides, and quinolones) can increase the potential for postoperative bleeding, although this is more of a risk for patients on anticoagulant therapy.[67]

Applying gentle pressure to the repositioned flap with a moistened sterile cotton gauze for several minutes is suggested, both before and after suturing, to displace any excess blood and allow for stabilization of the initial fibrin stage of the blood clot. If excessive bleeding from the suture puncture sites is observed, placement of medical-grade cyanoacrylate on the suture wounds may be helpful.[67] An acrylic splint, fabricated prior to surgery, is indicated for palatal root surgery and is especially important for patients for whom the potential for postoperative bleeding is a concern. The flap should be inspected after suturing to ensure close approximation of all tissue margins and control bleeding. If additional local anesthesia is desired for the immediate postoperative time period, care must be taken not to inject directly under the repositioned flap. The patient is returned to an upright position for 10 to 15 minutes, and the surgical area is inspected once more prior to dismissing the patient. A cold compress is given to the patient with instructions to apply to the face in the surgery area—on for 20 minutes, then off for 20 minutes—for the remainder of the day. The patient is given a package of sterile cotton gauze to control minor bleeding if necessary. The vast majority of situations involving postoperative oozing of blood can be self-managed by application of direct pressure with moistened cotton gauze. For further discussion of postoperative instructions, see chapter 13.

References

1. Ayers C, Abrams RA. Attitudes of consumers toward dentistry and dentists. J Dent Pract Adm 1989;6:22–28.
2. De Jong RH, Wagman IH. Physiological mechanisms of peripheral nerve block by local anesthetics. Anesthesiology 1963:24:684–722.
3. Becker DE, Reed KL. Essentials of local anesthetic pharmacology. Anesth Prog 2006;53:98–108.
4. Wilson AW, Deacock S, Downie IP, Zaki G. Allergy to local anesthetic: The importance of thorough investigation. Br Dent J 2000;188:320–322.
5. Rosivack RG, Koenigsberg SR, Maxwell KC. An analysis of the effectiveness of two topical anesthetics. Anesth Prog 1990;37:290–292.
6. Meechan JG. Effective topical anesthetic agents and techniques. Dent Clin North Am 2002;46:759–766.
7. Rosa AL, Sverzut CE, Xavier SP, Lavrador MA. Clinical effectiveness of lidocaine and benzocaine for topical anesthesia. Anesth Prog 1999;46:97–99.
8. Brown RS, Paluvoi S, Choksi S, Burgess CM, Reece ER. Evaluating a dental patient for local anesthesia allergy. Comp Contin Educ Dent 2002;23:125–134.
9. Ball IA. Allergic reactions to lignocaine. Br Dent J 1999;186:524–526.
10. Thyssen JP, Menné T, Elberling J, Plaschke P, Johansen JD. Hypersensitivity to local anaesthetics—Update and proposal of evaluation algorithm. Contact Dermatitis 2008;59:69–78.
11. Parirokh M, Yosefi MH, Nakhaee N, Abbott PV, Manochehrifar H. The success rate of bupivacaine and lidocaine as anesthetic agents in inferior alveolar nerve block in teeth with irreversible pulpitis without spontaneous pain. Restor Dent Endod 2015;40:155–160.
12. Moore PA. Bupivacaine: A long-lasting local anesthetic for dentistry. Oral Surg 1984;58:369–374.
13. Mesgarzadeh AH, Afsari H, Pourkhamne S, Shahamfar M. Efficacy of bilateral mental nerve block with bupivacaine for postoperative pain control in mandibular parasymphysis fractures. J Dent Res Dent Clin Dent Prospects 2014;8:172–175.
14. Evans G, Nusstein J, Drum M, Reader A, Beck M. A prospective, randomized, double-blind comparison of articaine and lidocaine for maxillary infiltrations. J Endod 2008;34:389–393.
15. Abdulwahab M, Boynes S, Moore P, et al. The efficacy of six local anesthetic formulations used for posterior mandibular buccal infiltration anesthesia. J Am Dent Assoc 2009;140:1018–1024.
16. Schertzer ER Jr. Articaine vs. lidocaine. J Am Dent Assoc 2000;131:1242–1243.
17. Weaver JM. Articaine, a new local anesthetic for American dentists: Will it supersede lidocaine? Anesth Prog 1999;46:111–112.
18. Becker DE, Reed KL. Local anesthetics: Review of pharmacological considerations. Anesth Prog 2012;59:90–101.

19. Sambrook PJ, Smith W, Elijah J, Goss AN. Severe adverse reactions to dental local anaesthetics: Systemic reactions. Aust Dent J 2011;56:148–153.
20. Gaffen AS, Haas DA. Retrospective review of voluntary reports of nonsurgical paresthesia in dentistry. J Can Dent Assoc 2009;75:579.
21. Kanaa MD, Whitworth JM, Corbett IP, Meechan JG. Articaine and lidocaine mandibular buccal infiltration anesthesia: A prospective randomized double-blind cross-over study. J Endod 2006;32:296–298.
22. Robertson D, Nusstein J, Reader A, Beck M, McCartney M. The anesthetic efficacy of articaine in buccal infiltration of mandibular posterior teeth. J Am Dent Assoc 2007;138:1104–1112.
23. Abdulwahab M, Boynes S, Moore P, et al. The efficacy of six local anesthetic formulations used for posterior mandibular buccal infiltration anesthesia. J Am Dent Assoc 2009;140:1018–1024.
24. Batista da Silva C, Aranha Berto L, Cristina Volpato M, et al. Anesthetic efficacy of articaine and lidocaine for incisive/mental nerve block. J Endod 2010;36:438–441.
25. Srinivasan N, Kavitha M, Loganathan CS, Padmini G. Comparison of anesthetic efficacy of 4% articaine and 2% lidocaine for maxillary buccal infiltration in patients with irreversible pulpitis. Oral Surg Oral Med Oral Pathol Oral Radiol Endod 2009;107:133–136.
26. Costa CG, Tortamano IP, Rocha RG, Francischone CE, Tortamano N. Onset and duration periods of articaine and lidocaine on maxillary infiltration. Quintessence Int 2005;36:197–201.
27. Oliveira PC, Volpato MC, Ramacciato JC, Ranali J. Articaine and lignocaine efficiency in infiltration anaesthesia: A pilot study. Br Dent J 2004;197:45–46.
28. Evans G, Nusstein J, Drum M, Reader A, Beck M. A prospective, randomized, double-blind comparison of articaine and lidocaine for maxillary infiltrations. J Endod 2008;34:389–393.
29. Donaldson D, James-Perdok L, Craig BJ, Derkson GD, Richardson AS. A comparison of Ultracaine DS (Articaine HCl) and Citanest forte (Prilocaine HCl) in maxillary infiltration and mandibular nerve block. J Can Dent Assoc 1987;53:38–42.
30. Haas DA, Harper DG, Saso MA, Young ER. Comparison of articaine and prilocaine anesthesia by infiltration in maxillary and mandibular arches. Anesth Prog 1990;37:230–237.
31. Haas DA, Harper DG, Saso MA, Young ER. Lack of differential effect by Ultracaine (articaine) and Citanest (prilocaine) in infiltration anaesthesia. J Can Dent Assoc 1991;57:217–223.
32. Claffey E, Reader A, Nusstein J, Beck M, Weaver J. Anesthetic efficacy of articaine for inferior alveolar nerve blocks in patients with irreversible pulpitis. J Endod 2004;30:568–571.
33. Tortamano IP, Siviero M, Costa CG, Buscariolo IA, Armonia PL. A comparison of the anesthetic efficacy of articaine and lidocaine in patients with irreversible pulpitis. J Endod 2009;35:165–168.
34. Maniglia-Ferreira C, Almeida-Gomes F, Carvalho-Sousa B, et al. Clinical evaluation of the use of three anesthetics in endodontics. Acta Odontol Latinoam 2009;22:21–26.
35. Brown G. The influence of adrenaline, noradrenaline vasoconstrictors on the efficacy of lidocaine. J Oral Ther Pharmacol 1968;4:398–405.
36. Cowan A. Further clinical evaluation of prilocaine (Citanest), with and without epinephrine. Oral Surg Oral Med Oral Pathol 1968;26:304–311.
37. Ahlquist RP. A study of adrenotropic receptors. Am J Physiol 1948;153:586–600.
38. Sveen K. Effect of the addition of a vasoconstrictor to local anesthetic solution on operative and postoperative bleeding, analgesia, and wound healing. Int J Oral Surg 1979;8:301–306.
39. Hiava GL, Reinhardt RA, Kalkwarf KL. Etidocaine HCl local anesthetic for periodontal flap surgery. J Periodontol 1984;55:364–367.
40. Sisk AL, Dionne RA, Wirdzek PR. Evaluation of etidocaine hydrochloride for local anesthesia and postoperative pain control in oral surgery. J Oral Maxillofac Surg 1984;42:84–88.
41. Danielsson K, Evans H, Holmlund A, Kjellman O, Nordenram A, Persson NE. Long-acting local anesthetics in oral surgery: Clinical evaluation of bupivacaine and etidocaine for mandibular nerve block. Int J Oral Maxillofac Surg 1986; 15:119–126.
42. Gordon SM, Dionne RA, Brahim J, Jabir F, Dubner R. Blockade of peripheral neuronal barrage reduces postoperative pain. Pain 1997;70:209–215.
43. Paterson SA, Tahmassebi JF. Paediatric dentistry in the new millennium: 3. Use of inhalation sedation in paediatric dentistry. Dent Update 2003;30:350–358.
44. Burnweit C, Diana-Zerpa JA, Nahmad MH, et al. Nitrous oxide analgesia for minor pediatric surgical procedures: An effective alternative to conscious sedation? J Pediatr Surg 2004;39:495–499.
45. Otley CC, Nguyen TH. Conscious sedation of pediatric patients with combination oral benzodiazepines and inhaled nitrous oxide. Dermatol Surg 2000;26:1041–1044.
46. Emmanouil DE, Quock RM. Advances in understanding the actions of nitrous oxide. Anesth Prog 2007;54:9–18.
47. Dionne RA, Yagiela JA, Coté CJ, et al. Balancing efficacy and safety in the use of oral sedation in dental outpatients. J Am Dent Assoc 2006;137:502–513.
48. Malamed SF. Sedation: A Guide to Patient Management, ed 5. St Louis: Mosby, 2009.
49. Berthold CW, Dionne RA, Corey SE. Comparison of sublingually and orally administered triazolam for premedication before oral surgery. Oral Surg Oral Med Oral Pathol Oral Radiol Endod 1997;84:119–124.
50. Reader A, Nusstein J, Drum M. Successful Local Anesthesia for Restorative Dentistry and Endodontics. Chicago: Quintessence, 2011:110–111.
51. Donaldson M, Goodchild JH. Pregnancy, breast-feeding and drugs used in dentistry. J Am Dent Assoc 2012;143:858–871[erratum 2012;143:1187].
52. Bader JD, Bonito AJ, Shugars DA. Cardiovascular effects of epinephrine on hypertensive dental patients: Summary. In: AHRQ Evidence Report Summaries. Rockville, MD: Agency for Healthcare Research and Quality (US), 1998–2005.
53. Herman WW, Konzelman JL Jr, Prisant LM; Joint National Committee on Prevention, Detection, Evaluation, and Treatment of High Blood Pressure. New national guidelines on hypertension: A summary for dentistry. J Am Dent Assoc 2004;135:576–584.
54. Yagiela JA. Injectable and topical local anesthetics. In: Ciancio SG (ed). ADA Guide to Dental Therapeutics, ed 3. Chicago: American Dental Association, 2003.
55. Patton LL. Medical emergencies. In: Patton LL, Glick M (eds). The ADA Practical Guide to Patients with Medical Conditions, ed 2. Hoboken, NJ: John Wiley & Sons, 2016:451–464.
56. Hensten A, Jacobsen N. Allergic reactions in endodontic practice. Endod Topics 2005;12:44-51.
57. Hensten-Pettersen A, Jacobsen N. Perceived side effects of biomaterials in prosthetic dentistry. J Prosthet Dent 1991;65:138–144.
58. Forman GH, Ord RA. Allergic endodontic angio-oedema in response to periapical endomethasone. Brit Dent J 1986;160:348–350.
59. Kunisada M, Adachi A, Asano H, Horikawa T. Anaphylaxis due to formaldehyde released from root-canal disinfectant. Contact Dermatitis 2002;47:215–218.
60. Haikel Y, Braun JJ, Zana H, Boukari A, de Blay F, Pauli G. Anaphylactic shock during endodontic treatment due to allergy to formaldehyde in a root canal sealant. J Endod 2000;26:529–531.
61. Braun JJ, Zana H, Purohit A, et al. Anaphylactic reactions to formaldehyde in root canal sealant after endodontic treatment: Four cases of anaphylactic shock and three of generalized urticaria. Allergy 2003;58:1210–1215.
62. Jang Y, Kim E. Cardiovascular effect of epinephrine in endodontic microsurgery: A review. Restor Dent Endod 2013;38:187–193.
63. Johnson BR, Fischer DJ, Epstein JB. The medically complex endodontic patient. In: Ingle JI, Bakland LK, Baumgartner JC (eds). Ingle's Endodontics, ed 6. Hamilton, ON: BC Decker, 2008:749–779.
64. Buckley JA, Ciancio SG, McMullen JA. Efficacy of epinephrine concentration in local anesthesia during periodontal surgery. J Periodontol 1984;54:653–657.
65. Wahl MJ. Myths of dental surgery in patients receiving anticoagulant therapy. J Am Dent Assoc 2000;131:77–81.
66. Jeske AH, Suchko GD; ADA Council on Scientific Affairs and Division of Science; Journal of the American Dental Association. Lack of a scientific basis for routine discontinuation of oral anticoagulant therapy before dental treatment. J Am Dent Assoc 2003;134:1492–1497.
67. Kämmerer PW, Frerich B, Liese J, Schiegnitz E, Al-Nawas B. Oral surgery during therapy with anticoagulants—A systematic review. Clin Oral Invest 2015;19:171–180.
68. Cho YW, Kim E. Is stopping of anticoagulant therapy really required in a minor dental surgery? How about in an endodontic microsurgery? Restor Dent Endod 2013;38:113–118.
69. Bajkin BV, Vujkov SB, Milekic BR, Vuckovic BA. Risk factors for bleeding after oral surgery in patients who continued using oral anticoagulant therapy. J Am Dent Assoc 2015;146:375–381.
70. Aldridge E, Cunningham LL Jr. Current thoughts on treatment of patients receiving anticoagulation therapy. J Oral Maxillofac Surg 2010;68:2879–2787.
71. Noll A. Coagulation assays and the new oral anticoagulants. American College of Cardiology. http://www.acc.org/latest-in-cardiology/articles/2015/06/22/12/06/coagulation-assays-and-the-new-oral-anticoagulants. Published 22 June 2015, accessed 1 July 2016.
72. Aurelio J, Chenail B, Gerstein H. Foreign-body reaction to bone wax. Report of a case. Oral Surg Oral Med Oral Pathol 1984;58:98–100.
73. Johnson P, Fromm D. Effects of bone wax on bacterial clearance. Surgery 1981; 89:206–209.
74. Witherspoon DE, Gutmann JL. Haemostasis in periradicular surgery. Int Endod J 1996;29:135–149.

75. Azzi R, Kenney EB, Tsao TF, Carranza FA Jr. The effect of electrosurgery on alveolar bone. J Periodontol 1983;54:96–100.
76. Nixon KC, Adkins KF, Keys DW. Histological evaluation of effects produced in alveolar bone following gingival incision with an electrosurgical scalpel. J Periodontol 1975;46:40–44.
77. Trent CS. Electrocautery versus epinephrine-injection tonsillectomy. Ear Nose Throat J 1993;72:520–522.
78. Walsh WR, Morberg P, Yu Y, et al. Response of a calcium sulfate bone graft substitute in a confined cancellous defect. Clin Orthop Relat Res 2003;(406):228–236.
79. Clokie CM, Moghadam H, Jackson MT, Sandor GK. Closure of critical sized defects with allogenic and alloplastic bone substitutes. J Craniofac Surg 2002;13:111–121.
80. Scarano A, Artese L, Piattelli A, Carcinci F, Mancino C, Iezzi G. Hemostasis control in endodontic surgery: A comparative study of calcium sulfate versus gauzes and versus ferric sulfate. J Endod 2012;38:20–23.
81. Kim S, Rethnam S. Hemostasis in endodontic microsurgery. Dent Clin North Am 1997;41:499–511.
82. Vickers FJ, Baumgartner JC, Marshall G. Hemostatic efficacy and cardiovascular effects of agents used during endodontic surgery. J Endod 2002;28:322–323.
83. Vy CH, Baumgartner JC, Marshall JG. Cardiovascular effects and efficacy of a hemostatic agent in periradicular surgery. J Endod 2004;30:379–383.
84. Lemon RR, Steele PJ, Jeansonne BG. Ferric sulfate hemostasis: Effect on osseous wound healing. Left in situ for maximum exposure. J Endod 1993;19:170–173.
85. Jeansonne BG, Boggs WS, Lemon RR. Ferric sulfate hemostasis: Effect on osseous wound healing. II. With curettage and irrigation. J Endod 1993;19:174–176.
86. Kim S, Kratchman S. Modern endodontic surgery concepts and practice: A review. J Endod 2006;32:601–623.
87. Keshavarzi S, MacDougall M, Lulic D, Kasasbeh A, Levy M. Clinical experience with the Surgicel family of absorbable hemostats (oxidized regenerated cellulose) in neurosurgical applications: A review. Wounds 2013;25:160–167.
88. Nappi JF, Lehman JA Jr. The effects of Surgicel on bone formation. Cleft Palate J 1980;17:291–296.
89. Petersen JK, Krogsgaard J, Nielsen KM, Nørgaard EB. A comparison between 2 absorbable hemostatic agents: Gelatin sponge (Spongostan) and oxidized regenerated cellulose (Surgicel). Int J Oral Surg 1984;13:406–410.
90. Azargoon H, Williams BJ, Solomon ES, Kessler HP, He J, Spears R. Assessment of hemostatic efficacy and osseous wound healing using HemCon dental dressing. J Endod 2011;37:607–611.
91. Malmquist JP, Clemens SC, Olen HJ, Wilson SL. Hemostasis of oral surgery wounds with the HemCon Dental Dressing. J Oral Maxillofac Surg 2008;66:1177–1183.

Chapter Nine

Soft Tissue Management

Peter Velvart, Ove A. Peters

Clinical success in endodontic surgery extends beyond the mere treatment of apical periodontitis. Surgical treatment of periapical periodontitis involves the removal of necrotic material and tissue breakdown products, treatment of the infection of the root canal system, and a fluid-tight obturation of the treated portals of exit.[1] In order to allow these procedures to take place, the soft tissues have to be mobilized. Three types of flaps dominate the possible surgical approach: sulcular, submarginal, and papilla-preserving incisions. The handling of the tissues—including incision, raising the flap, handling during the procedure, and suturing—is responsible for the ultimate outcomes, mainly the amount of gingival recession and attachment loss. Consequently, a successful outcome not only depends on endodontic aspects of the treatment but also includes all involved dentoalveolar structures. Reports regarding the impact of periodontal conditions on the overall success rate are rather scarce; however, Jansson et al[2] studied the relationship between apical and marginal healing in endodontic surgery and demonstrated the persistence of endodontic infection as a contributing factor for progression of attachment loss. On the other hand, following periodontal procedures, impaired periodontal healing in teeth with periapical lesions was observed.[3]

Esthetic consequences following any dental procedures have become a significant factor to be considered in addition to eradication of pathosis. In surgical treatment, the least traumatic approach and tissue handling have a positive effect on the esthetic result. The ultimate goal in modern dentistry is regeneration, extending the mere repair of lost tissues.

Achievement of so-called "white esthetics" refers to natural visible tooth structures with tooth-colored materials. With restorative techniques, it is possible to come very close to a natural appearance of teeth. This notion has reached a very high level of importance.[4] The term *pink esthetics*, in contrast, refers to soft tissues and underlying bone, which are both equally important for an optimal esthetic result after surgical intervention. Management of periodontal tissues with appropriate surgical techniques, followed by proper long-term oral hygiene, significantly impacts esthetics after a surgical procedure. The objective of preserving oral structures is no longer sufficient without considering the esthetics for all involved dentoalveolar components.[5]

This chapter addresses factors affecting soft tissue management in order to gain access to the underlying bone covering the roots in need of surgical intervention. Emphasis is placed on the considerations of classic and recent soft tissue management methods in reference to biologic and esthetic outcomes.

Biology of the Periodontal Tissues

While each of the dentoalveolar structures is distinct in its location and tissue architecture, they function together as a unit. They influence each other, and pathologic changes as well as treatment trauma have marked effects on repair and regeneration.

The periodontium comprises four components: gingiva, periodontal ligament, alveolar bone, and cementum. The gingiva reaches from the papilla to the mucogingival junction, where it joins the alveolar mucosa. The gingiva is divided into papillae, marginal gingiva, and attached gingiva (Fig 9-1). The gingival tissue attaches to the tooth with the junctional epithelial attachment. Further apically, the attachment consists of connective tissue and periodontal ligament between the alveolar bone and cementum on the root surface. Gargiulo and others[6] describe the biologic width as a measure to be respected; its dimension is approximately 2 mm in total and can be described as the sum of the junctional epithelial attachment width (0.97 mm) and connective tissue attachment width (1.07 mm).

The papilla has an important function, namely to fill the interproximal space between the neighboring teeth, and its presence is esthetically critical. The papilla has a buccal and lingual peak separated by the col area, forming a concave depression. The papilla is covered with keratinized oral epithelium and both nonkeratinized sulcular and squamous stratified col epithelium.[7–9] The height of the gingiva from the mucogingival junction to the gingival margin is highest on the labial aspect of the maxillary incisors and decreases in height toward distal areas.[10]

Gingival epithelium

Depending on location and composition, the gingival epithelium can be divided into oral gingival, oral sulcular, and junctional epithelium.

Oral gingival epithelium

The oral gingival epithelium extends from the mucogingival junction to the tip of the gingival crest. It is between 0.2 and 0.3 mm thick and has largely a protective function.[11] The oral gingival epithelium is a keratinized squamous stratified epithelium that forms four cell layers. Above the connective tissue, in close contact to the basement membrane, lies an active layer of cells, the stratum basale. These rather small cells multiply continuously, and as they mature into keratinized cells they become the stratum spinosum. The cells of the spinous layer make up the thickest part of the epithelium. The transformation process closer to the surface renders the cells flatter (stratum granulosum). The most superficial cell layer (stratum corneum) consists of flat cells in close contact, mostly without nuclei.

In the stratum spinosum, dendritic (Langerhans) cells may be found. They play an important role in the inflammation process. Langerhans cells bind to antigens and transmit the information to macrophages and lymphocytes.[12]

Oral sulcular epithelium

The sulcular epithelium is located between the gingival crest and the most coronal portion of the junctional epithelium, forming the lining of the gingival sulcus. In a healthy situation, the depth of the sulcus is about 0.5 mm. There are structural similarities to the oral gingival epithelium. The sulcular epithelium is less permeable and displays small infiltration of neutrophils compared with the junctional epithelium.

Junctional epithelium

The junctional epithelium extends from the base of the gingival sulcus to a level approximately 2 mm coronal from the crestal bone. In healthy conditions, without attachment loss, the junctional epithelium reaches the cementoenamel junction. It is closely adapted to the tooth surface and fulfills sealing and attachment functions.

The junctional epithelium is different from the sulcular and the oral epithelium in both its origin and structure. Triangular in form, in the most apical part it consists of few cell layers, and toward the sulcus the thickness increases gradually to 15 to 30 layers. The reproduction rate of the stratum basale cells is high, and these cells then exfoliate into the gingival sulcus. Intact junctional epithelium contains migrating neutrophils; their presence rapidly increases when an inflammatory process develops. In addition to the neutrophils, T lymphocytes are found.[13]

In contrast to other oral epithelia with little extracellular space present, junctional epithelium shows gaps between cells. This could be responsible for the increased permeability of water, nutrients, and toxic substances through the epithelium. The intercellular matrix not only helps cell adhesion but also aids the attachment to the tooth surface and base membrane separating the epithelium from the connective tissue.[14,15] Epithelial cells are metabolically active and capable of reacting to external stimuli by synthetizing cytokines, growth factors, and enzymes.[16,17]

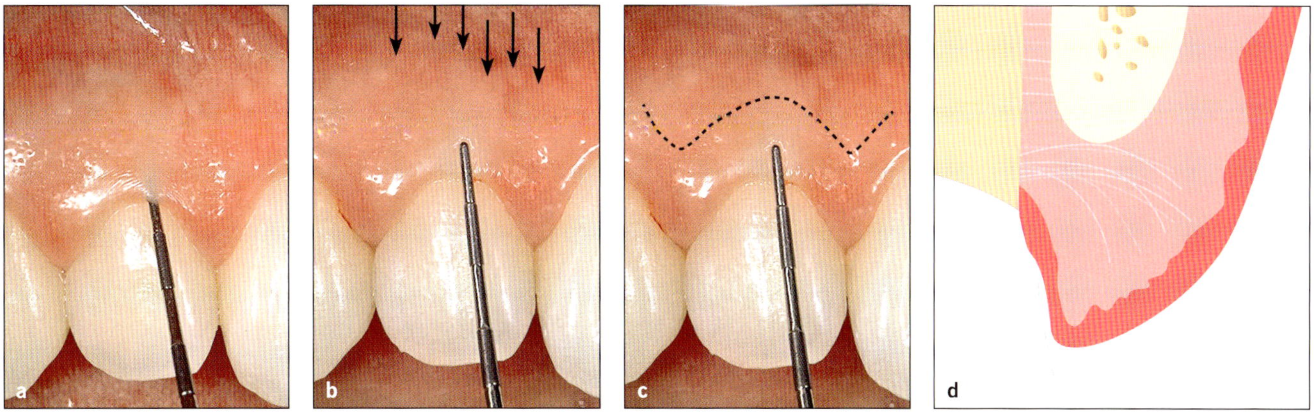

Fig 9-1 Determination of the width of the attached gingiva. *(a)* Measurement of the probing depth. The gingival tissue over the probe represents the free gingiva. *(b) Arrows* mark the mucogingival line. The distance between the tip of the probe (representing the probing depth) and the mucogingival junction is the width of the attached gingiva. *(c) Dashed line* represents the location for proper placement of a submarginal incision. *(d)* Schematic drawing of the components of the so-called biologic width. (Parts *a* to *c* reprinted from Velvart[1] with permission.)

Gingival connective tissue

Fibroblasts, a major cellular component of the connective tissue, are of mesenchymal origin. They synthesize extracellular matrix, take part in the regulatory process, and respond to a variety of stimulants. Fibroblasts produce cytokines, enzymes, enzyme inhibitors, and matrix macromolecules. The function of these enzymes is to regulate the degradation of the matrix during remodeling and turnover.[18] Fibroblasts are sensitive to changes in the extracellular matrix as well as to the presence of growth factors or cytokines. When injury occurs, fibroblasts are able to migrate and attach to various substrates that attract them.

Collagen fibers, a major component of the matrix, are organized in a distinct architectural pattern. They are classified according to their location, origin, and insertion (eg, dentoalveolar, transgingival, interseptal, or circular fibers). Supragingival fibers are responsible for the attachment of the gingiva to teeth and provide a basis for its firmness and biomechanical resistance.

Gingival changes during inflammation

Bacterial infection is the predominant cause for disease development. The epithelium acts in several ways in the presence of bacteria. Not only is it a mechanical barrier against invasion of bacteria, but it also initiates the first signals of bacterial assault to the underlying connective tissue. The increased permeability of the junctional epithelium is particularly important in initiating cellular signaling processes. Epithelial cells are also capable of producing substances that can attract neutrophils. As the bacterial accumulation continues, intercellular spaces begin to widen further, easing the passage of the inflammatory exudate to the gingival sulcus and at the same time allowing molecules from the external surface to move toward connective tissue.

As the high level of infiltration and exudation persists, ongoing tissue damage is established. Marked migration of neutrophils and activation of macrophages and lymphocytes can be observed within connective tissue. At the same time, cells of the basal layer are capable of producing collagenases, which degrade the underlying collagen fibers. The junctional epithelium starts to migrate in an apical direction, resulting in formation of a periodontal pocket.[19]

The inflammatory process is marked by an increased number and size of capillary loops in the connective tissue adjacent to the junctional epithelium. A specific feature of venules is their facilitation of neutrophil migration rather than lymphocyte migration. A variety of additional factors present in the local environment determine the activity of fibroblasts, affecting migration, adhesion, proliferation, and the matrix synthesis.[20]

Signs of tissue destruction are detectable as early as 3 to 4 days after plaque accumulation.[21] The inflammatory response remains contained within the gingival tissues for prolonged periods of time. However, should the balance between bacteria and host defense shift unfavorably, uncontrolled tissue destruction can take place, and the inflammation may expand deeper into the periodontal ligament and alveolar bone, resulting in attachment loss together with apical migration of junctional epithelium.

Functional Aspects

Interdental papilla

The tissue between two adjacent teeth, named the *papilla*, is roughly pyramidal and triangular in shape.[22] The specific contour, width, and contact point area of the neighboring crowns determine whether the papilla has one peak or, for most cases, both a lingual and a buccal peak joined by a concave col.[23] The papilla usually fills the entire interproximal space between neighboring teeth. Tarnow et al[24] studied the factors influencing papilla height and found that the presence or absence of the interdental papilla depends on the distance between the contact point and the crest of the bone. When the distance from the contact point to the bone measured 5 mm or less, the papilla was present almost 100% of the time. With a distance of 6 mm, the papilla was present 56% of the time, and when the distance measured 7 mm or more, the papilla was present 27% of the time or less.

Holmes[23] excised interdental papillae in 16 dental students: one from the anterior and one from the posterior area of each student. From 32 specimens, 22 papillae did not regenerate to their original shape and height. The regenerated papillae appeared flatter and did not fill the embrasure as completely as before excision, and the cols were less concave.

Blood supply

The blood vessels supply the alveolar mucosa and gingiva through interconnected pathways. There are subepithelial capillaries of the gingiva and alveolar mucosa, the vascular network within the periosteum, the intraseptal vessels in the bone marrow, and the plexus of the periodontium. The periosteal and periodontal networks connect directly through Volkmann canals.[25] The gingiva and periosteum receive blood supply from supraperiosteal vessels, which run roughly along the long axis of the teeth. They branch in the lamina propria of the gingiva and spread to the periosteum. Minor communications exist between intraseptal vessels penetrating the interdental bone and periodontal ligament, which fuel the gingiva with blood. These multiple interconnections between different plexus help supply blood and nutrients to tissues when surgically severed.

Access to the site of apical pathosis

Proper access to the area to be treated is one of the key factors for a successful surgical procedure. Lesions of endodontic origin are present in the bone around the root. This necessitates exposing the bone surface by a full-thickness flap consisting of periosteum and gingival and mucosal tissues. Various factors must be considered prior to placing an incision and selecting the flap design.

Regional anatomical structures

The location and path of blood vessels as well as nerves must be known so that they can be protected and preserved during the surgical procedure. Within the general anatomical framework, their precise location can vary from one patient to another. When mandibular premolars or molars are involved in a surgical procedure, the protection of the neurovascular bundle is crucial. The mental foramen is usually present between mandibular premolars, apical or adjacent to the apices of the premolars. Dental radiographs do not visualize the mental foramen and the mandibular canal predictably.[26] Klinge et al[27] assessed periapical radiographs, panoramic radiographs, as well as tomography and found none of these methods to be predictable in detecting the mandibular canal. Computed tomography (CT) not only allows for detection of neurovascular and other anatomical structures (ie, the maxillary sinus) but also shows real transverse and vertical relations between bone surface, lesion, and root. When distances measured in the scan were compared with the actual in vivo situation, 70% corresponded exactly, and 94% of the values were within ±1 mm of the real measurements.[27] Cone beam CT has replaced spiral CT scans in dental offices due to its limited radiation exposure and is now increasingly used as a tool for diagnosis and treatment planning in endodontics.[28–30]

Periodontal Conditions

Soft tissue management in surgical endodontics is heavily influenced by periodontal conditions in the region of intervention. Probing depth around all involved teeth should be measured. This involves continuous probing around the entire circumference of the tooth, noting any furcation involvement in multirooted teeth. A clear distinction should be made between histologic pocket depths and clinically measured probing depth. In a completely healthy situation, these distances correspond approximately. Gingival inflammation will increase the probing depth reading due to resorption of collagen fibers in the connective tissue (see "Biology of the Periodontal Tissues"). In the case of acute gingivitis or periodontitis, the periodontal probe will slide into the pocket and penetrate the junctional epithelium as well as connective tissue to the level of crestal bone or where collagen fibers are still intact. Consequently, the measured probing depths are

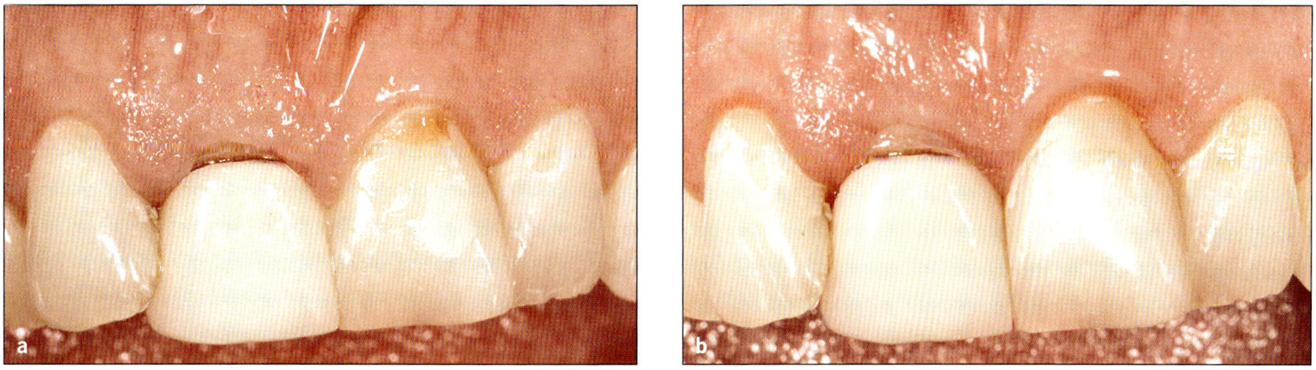

Fig 9-2 Recession following a surgical procedure on the maxillary left central incisor. *(a)* Preoperative condition. *(b)* Recall at 1 year. Note the increased retraction of the gingival margin and exposure of the root surface. (Reprinted from Velvart et al[38] with permission.)

generally larger than the actual histologic attachment level or pocket depth.[31] Further reason for overestimation of pocket depth is the presence of gingival swelling. The amount of swelling and the degree of inflammation corresponds to bleeding on probing. As the accumulation of bacteria is the main reason for inflammation, every attempt should be made to reduce the amount of plaque in the oral environment. This can be achieved in three ways: by the dental hygienist, with meticulous oral hygiene, and by rinsing with 0.2% chlorhexidine twice daily 1 week prior to and 2 weeks after the surgical intervention. Chlorhexidine has been shown to significantly reduce plaque growth,[32,33] to minimize postoperative discomfort, and to promote healing.[34,35] In general, less plaque results in reduced contamination of the surgical site and atmosphere for the surgeon and staff.[36]

The determination of the width of attached gingiva is a further factor to be considered for planning the proper placement of an incision. When a submarginal incision is considered, a minimum of 2 mm of attached gingiva is required for the survival of the nonmobilized tissue and to maintain a stable position of the gingival margin.[37] The attached gingiva is determined by subtracting the probing depth from the distance between the gingival margin and the mucogingival junction (see Fig 9-1).

Critical to the survival of the soft tissues is sufficient blood supply. As described earlier, marginal gingiva receives nutrients from crestal vessels and to a minor extent from the periodontal ligament. Insufficient blood supply and traumatic handling of the tissues, including excessive drying, can lead to necrosis of the nonreflected tissue with a deleterious esthetic result.

Coronal Restoration

The presence, type, and quality of the restorative work must be considered. Restorative work in general represents an irritation factor for the gingival tissues. Overextended restorations should be corrected during a presurgical dental hygiene phase. Special reference should be made to the position of the restoration margin in relation to the gingival margin. In visible areas, frequently subgingival margin placement is observed to avoid esthetic drawbacks of a discolored root surface or visible metal portions of the restoration. Manipulation of soft tissues will result in some degree of recession, which might expose the restoration margin (Fig 9-2). Management of this problem is discussed later in the chapter.

Patient-Related Factors

The healing process depends heavily on the biotype of gingival tissue. Patients with a thick tissue appearance tend to display coronal soft tissue regrowth to the former level in crown lengthening procedures, while patients with a thin tissue biotype show a higher degree of recession following surgical interventions.[39–41] Next to soft tissue factors, the integrity and thickness of the underlying bone plays a role in mucogingival stability.[42]

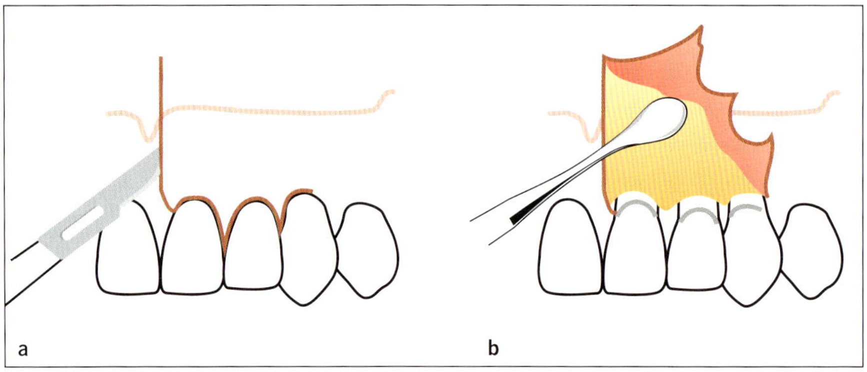

Fig 9-3 *(a)* The triangular flap requires a sulcular incision, usually with mesial placement of the vertical releasing incision. *(b)* Flap reflected. (Reprinted from Velvart[1] with permission.)

Flap design

The success of any surgical procedure depends largely on the extent to which adequate access can be obtained. Endodontic surgery first requires exposure of the bone overlying the tip of the root(s). To access the bone, a full-thickness flap or a combination of a full-thickness and a split-thickness flap must be raised. This means a soft tissue flap, which consists of gingival and mucosal tissue as well as periosteum. In order to mobilize the flap, various modes of incision can be selected, including horizontal incisions (sulcular and submarginal) and vertical releasing incisions. It is critical that incisions and flap elevations are carried out in a manner such that soft tissue healing by primary intention is facilitated. This is secured by *(1)* performing complete and sharp incision of the tissues, *(2)* avoiding severing of the tissues during flap elevation, and *(3)* preventing dehydration of tissue remnants on the root surface during the procedure.

Semilunar flap

A semilunar flap consists of a straight or curved horizontal incision in the alveolar mucosa over the apical area, placed all the way to the bone. A multitude of disadvantages have made this flap design obsolete. The semilunar flap will only provide limited access to the apical area. It will sever a maximum of blood vessels by cutting horizontally. Incisions should not be placed over existing or surgically created bone defects but rather over sound bone. Oral tissue at the apical level to a large extent consists of elastic fibers and muscle attachments, both of which exert pulling forces on reapproximated surgical wound margins. This retractive force will not only make suturing difficult but will also result in a constant tension on the flap, poor alignment of wound edges, gap formation, and impaired healing.[43]

Triangular flap

A horizontal incision extending one or two teeth distally and mesially to the involved area, combined with only one vertical releasing incision, forms the triangular flap (Fig 9-3 and Videos 9-1 and 9-2). The incision extends from a point 1 to 2 mm short of the mucobuccal fold to a point at the distal or mesiolabial line angle of the selected tooth. From there, a horizontal incision in the gingival sulcus continues to a point two to three teeth to the opposite side of the surgical site. For palatal roots that are not accessible from the buccal, a palatal triangular flap is raised. In order to prevent damage to the neurovascular bundle at the palatal foramen and avoid substantial bleeding, the releasing incision should be placed between the canine and first premolar (see Video 9-2).

The main advantage of this flap design is easy repositioning and minimal disruption of the vascular supply to the flap. The triangular flap is indicated for correction of marginally located processes such as perforations, cervical root resorptions, or apicoectomies involving teeth with short roots. If it turns out that the access is too limited, the triangular flap can be converted easily to a rectangular flap by placing an additional releasing incision at the distal end of the horizontal incision (see below). The main drawback of this flap design is a risk of recession due to the marginal line of incision.

Rectangular flap

The rectangular flap is formed by a horizontal incision with two vertical releasing incisions (Fig 9-4 and Video 9-1) and is perhaps the most frequently used flap in endodontic surgery. At the terminal point of the horizontal incision of a triangular flap, a vertical incision is made extending from the crestal tissue at the mesial or distal line angle of the last tooth to the mucobuccal fold.

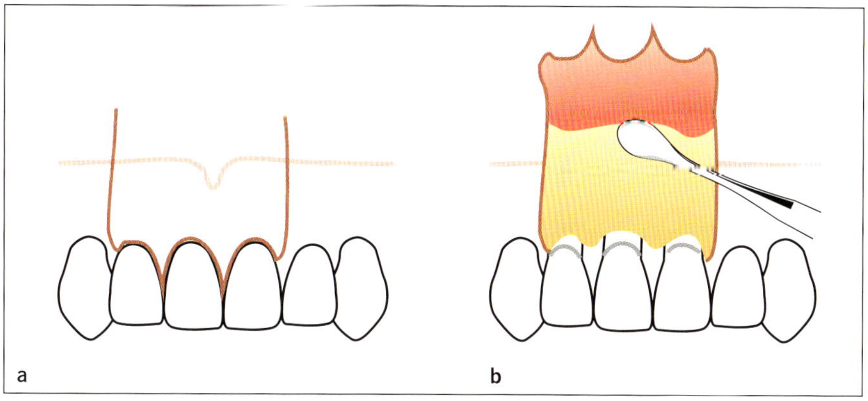

Fig 9-4 *(a)* The rectangular flap involves two vertical releasing incisions combined with a marginal sulcular incision. The releasing incisions are placed at least one tooth away from the tooth to be operated on, except in the area of the mental foramen, which should not be subjected to vertical incisions. *(b)* Flap reflected. (Reprinted from Velvart[1] with permission.)

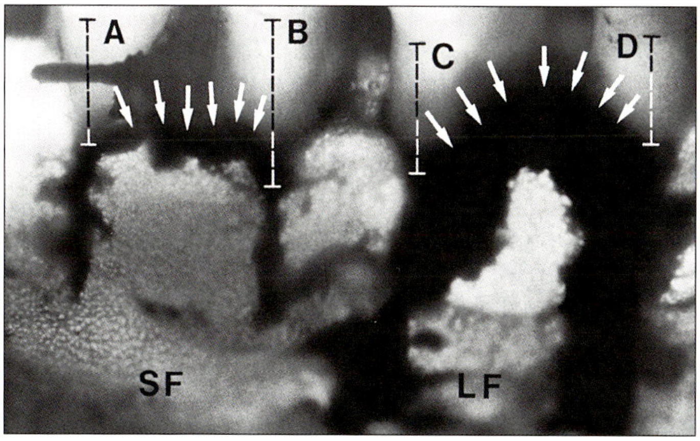

Fig 9-5 Fluorescein angiography following placement of a short (SF) versus long (LF) full-thickness flap, 24 hours after surgery. A to B and C to D indicate the distances from the cementoenamel junction to the respective flap margin. *Arrows* indicate the clinical flap outline and hypofluorescent areas of subsequent necrosis. (Reprinted from Mörmann and Ciancio[45] with permission.)

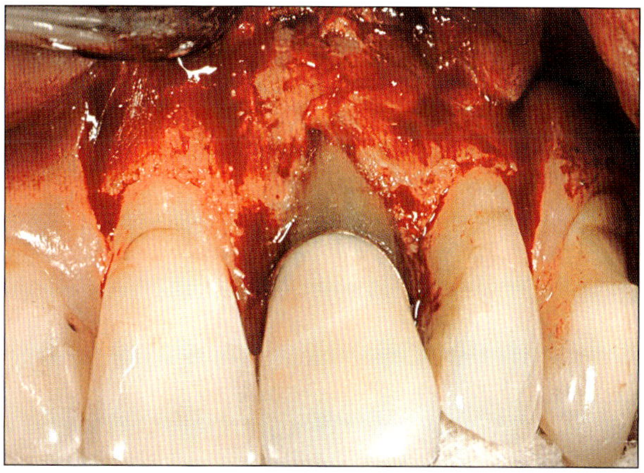

Fig 9-6 Rectangular sulcular full-thickness flap involving a tooth with a discolored root covered with a metal-ceramic crown. (Reprinted from Velvart et al[38] with permission.)

The rectangular flap will give excellent surgical access to the apical area in any region. The difference between the rectangular and trapezoidal version is the degree of divergence of the vertical incisions. Blood vessels run roughly parallel to the long axis of the teeth.

In order to disrupt the vascular supply as little as possible, the vertical incision should be placed parallel to the root. This favors the rectangular flap.[44] On the other hand, the blood supply and survival of the mobilized tissue appeared to be the best when the base was broader than the proximal end of the flap.[45] For this reason, vertical incisions should never be placed in a converging pattern; rather, the flap width should be extended one or two teeth mesially or distally to the tooth involved. Figure 9-5 shows the difference in circulation disturbance in a short full-thickness flap compared with a long full-thickness flap of comparable flap width by means of fluorescein angiography. Mörmann and Ciancio[45] studied the effect of various types of surgical procedures on the gingival capillary blood circulation. The circulation changes observed suggested that flaps receive their major blood supply from their apical aspect, but not exclusively. However, the horizontal marginal incision severed the anastomoses between the gingival and periodontal vasculature. Flap blood perfusion was maintained up to the point where the ratio of length to width of the parallel pedicle flap equaled 2:1. Several authors have confirmed this finding.[46,47] The length-to-width ratio requirement usually favors a slight trapezoidal shape of the flap, with strong preference of extending the horizontal dimension of the flap over several teeth. Repositioning the tissue and wound closure in the rectangular and trapezoidal flaps is typically straightforward because of the definite position of the papillae during reapproximation of the tissue. In esthetically critical areas with prosthetic restorations involving subgingivally placed crown margins (Fig 9-6), postoperative recession is a potential outcome, leading to an esthetically compromising exposure of the crown mar-

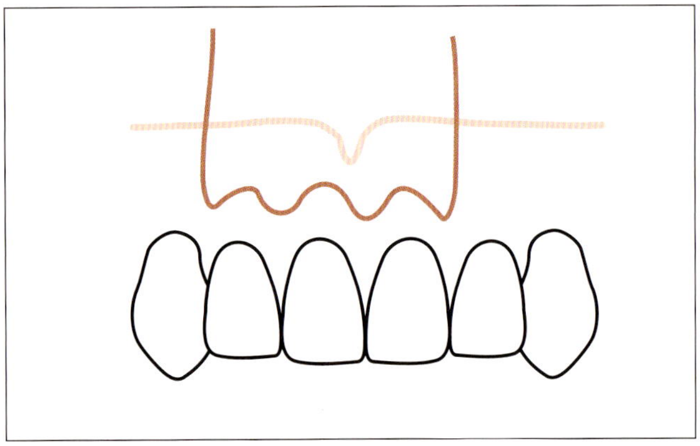

Fig 9-7 Submarginal incision consisting of two vertical incisions connected by a scalloped horizontal incision within the attached gingiva. (Reprinted from Velvart[1] with permission.)

gins (see Fig 9-2). Using a proper atraumatic and gentle surgical technique with appropriate wound management minimizes such esthetic disadvantages.

Submarginal flap

The submarginal flap, also referred to as the *Ochsenbein-Luebke flap*,[48] is formed by a scalloped horizontal submarginal incision placed within the attached gingiva, which follows roughly parallel to the contour of the gingival margin (see Figs 9-1a to 9-1c). The horizontal incision continues with two vertical releasing incisions (Fig 9-7). These vertical incisions extend from a point 1 to 2 mm short of entering the mucobuccal fold to a point on the attached gingiva approximately 3 to 5 mm above or below the marginal gingiva and the sulcus depth (Video 9-3).

The submarginal flap is only to be used when there is a broad attached gingiva and when the expected apical lesion or surgical bony access will not involve the incision margins. This flap design has the advantage of preserving the marginal gingiva and does not expose the marginal crestal bone. Pihlstrom et al[49] studied healing results when a sulcular full-thickness flap was elevated in an area with shallow pockets (1 to 3 mm). They observed loss of attachment, which was still present 6½ years postoperatively. The Ochsenbein-Luebke flap, on the other hand, is typically associated with minimal gingival recession. For example, von Arx et al[39] reported significantly less recession for the submarginal incision compared with a sulcular and papilla base incision. However, this difference was not significant at the 5-year recall appointment, indicating that the incision technique mainly affected marginal healing within the first year after apical surgery.[50]

Except for the rare risk of massive loss of marginal tissue due to a possible insufficient blood supply to the nonreflected gingival tissue (see above) or poor treatment planning, the risk of scarring is another disadvantage of submarginal flap design. As a consequence of dehydration of the tissue, the flap sometimes tends to shrink during surgery, resulting in tension and difficulty in replacing and securing it by suturing.

Papilla base flap

The papilla base flap consists of two releasing vertical incisions connected by the papilla base incision and intrasulcular incision in the cervical area of the tooth (Video 9-4). This flap was designed to prevent recession of the papilla. A microsurgical blade of a size not exceeding 2.5 mm in width should be used. Controlled and minute movement of the surgical blade within the small dimensions of the interproximal space is crucial. The papilla base incision requires two different incisions at the base of the papilla. A first shallow incision severs the epithelium and connective tissue to the depth of 1.5 mm from the surface of the gingiva (Fig 9-8, *blue line*). This guarantees sufficient thickness of the coronal end of the split-thickness flap portion. The path is a curved line connecting one side of the papilla to the other. The incision begins and ends perpendicular to the gingival margin (Fig 9-9). The scalpel is held perpendicular to the gingival surface. In the second step, the scalpel retraces the base of the previously created incision while inclined vertically, toward the crestal bone margin. The second incision results in a split-thickness flap in the apical third of the base of the papilla (see Fig 9-8). From this point on apically, a full-thickness mucoperiosteal flap is elevated (Fig 9-10). Although the papilla base flap achieves predictable healing results, this technique requires a skilled surgeon. Atraumatic handling of the soft tissues is of utmost importance in order to obtain rapid healing through primary intention. The epithelium of the partial-thickness flap has to be supported by underlying connective tissues, otherwise it will break down

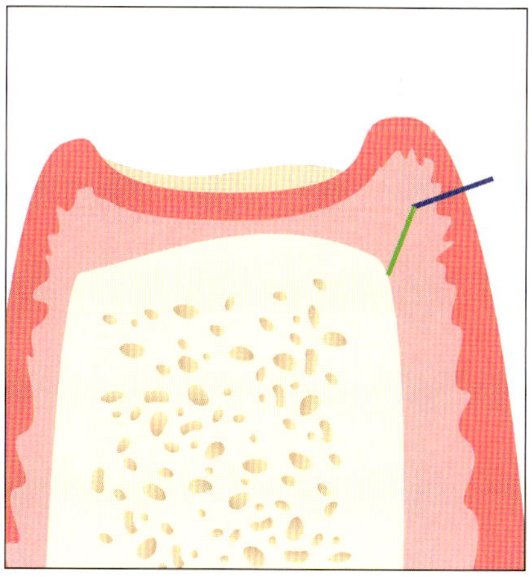

Fig 9-8 Schematic drawing of incision type for the papilla base flap. The first shallow incision is placed at the lower end of the papilla in a slightly curved line, perpendicular to the gingival margin *(blue line)*. A second incision is placed directed to the crestal bone margin from the base of the previously created incision *(green line)*. The result is a split-thickness flap on the base of the papilla.

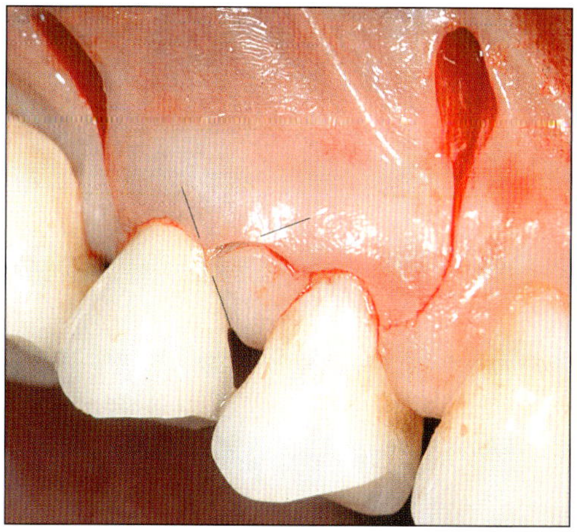

Fig 9-9 Curved incision placed perpendicular to the gingival margin *(lines)*. (Reprinted from Velvart et al[51] with permission.)

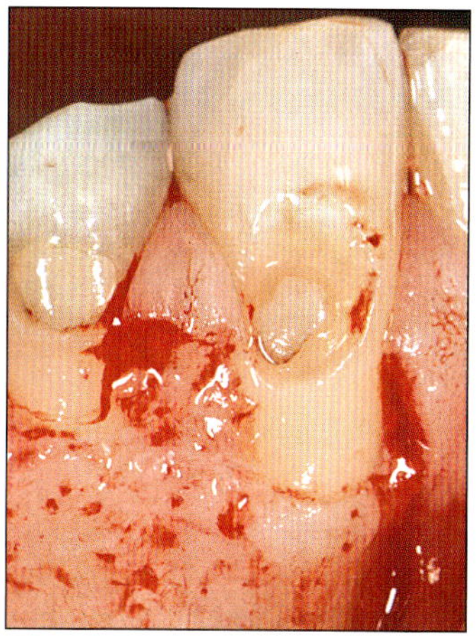

Fig 9-10 Elevated spit-thickness flap showing the papilla base incision with the major part of the papilla unaltered. (Reprinted from Velvart et al[51] with permission.)

and lead to scar formation. On the other hand, excessive thickness of the connective tissue layer of the split flap portion can jeopardize the survival of the buccal papilla left in place.[52] The ideal thickness of the partial-thickness flap has not been studied. Epithelium thickness varies between 111 and 610 µm with a mean of 364 µm.[53] The recommended thickness of free gingival grafts was reported to be 1 to 2 mm.[54,55] Based on the gingival graft studies, a thickness of 1.5 mm was chosen for the split thickness flap in the papilla base incision. The selected thickness resulted in excellent healing results.[52]

Strategies and Procedures

In order to obtain the best possible healing, optimal blood perfusion to all tissues in and around the surgical site is required. As tissues obtain blood supply from various sources, the disruption of one circulation pathway may still allow the tissue to survive if the incision and tissue handling are correct. This means that vertical incisions should be placed parallel to the long axis of the tooth rather than diverging, and they should never converge. In addition, the releasing vertical incision should start paramedial from the papilla and should never be placed either midaxial or through the middle of the papilla. The initial path of the incision must be placed perpendicular to the marginal edge of the gingiva. After reaching the midpapilla area, the scalpel is turned in a vertical direction and continued apically, as the dotted line in Figure 9-11 demonstrates.

The healing capacity of oral tissues is typically excellent. Only rarely are there serious postsurgical complications, such as tissue necrosis, nerve damage, profound bleeding, or serious infections. When general basic rules are followed, adequate healing of the soft tissues can be expected. Healing is influenced by flap shrinkage, which results in tissue tension and difficult reapproximation of wound edges upon closure and requires an increased number of sutures, adding further trauma to the tissues. This is particularly true for submarginal flap types. Keeping the flap moist at all times helps to reduce dehydration and shrinkage. Postoperative gingival recession is a difficult therapeutic dilemma that has increasingly become a clinical concern for the surgeon and patient. With the aid of contemporary techniques such as microscopic magnification, more suitable materials, and the use of microinstruments, soft tissue management has evolved and will result in a more predictable and successful outcome.[38]

Papilla preservation/protection

The interdental papilla, the portion of the gingiva between two adjacent teeth, is critical for functional, phonetic, and esthetic reasons. Complete and predictable restoration of lost interdental papillae is one of the biggest challenges in periodontal reconstructive surgery.[56] Therefore, it is imperative to maintain the integrity of

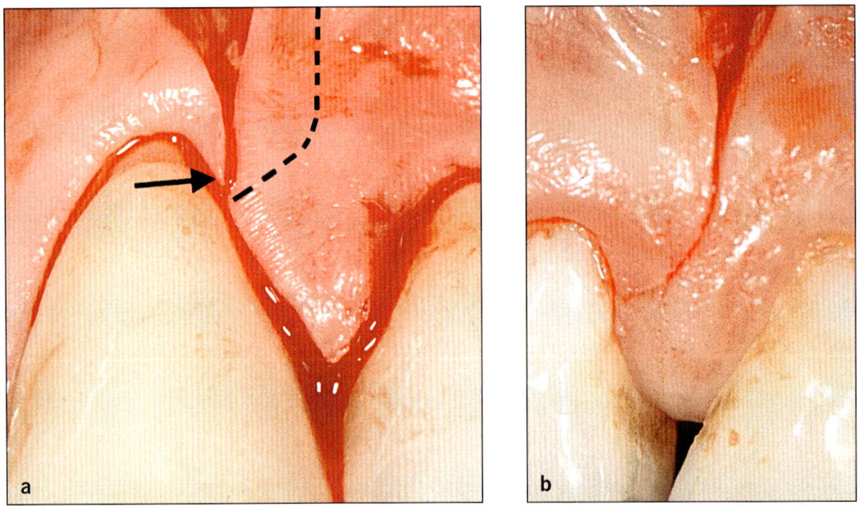

Fig 9-11 *(a)* Vertical releasing incision that creates a compromised tissue area *(arrow)*. The proximal, nonreflected tissue portion will most probably necrotize because of insufficient blood supply. A *dashed line* indicates the desired incision course, beginning perpendicular to the gingival margin. *(b)* Correctly performed vertical incision. (Reprinted from Velvart et al[38] with permission.)

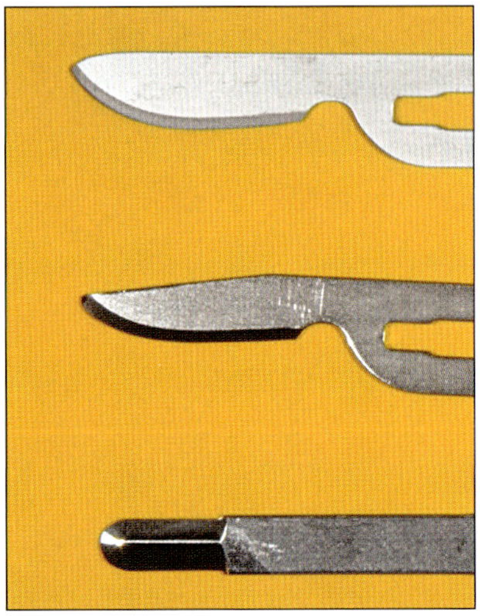

Fig 9-12 Comparison of different sizes of scalpel blades. *(top)* Regular blade size #15. *(middle)* Smaller #15C blade. *(bottom)* Microblade with double-sided cutting edges. (Reprinted from Velvart and Peters[64] with permission.)

the papilla during surgical procedures. Most frequently, a sulcular full-thickness flap is used in periradicular surgery. In this flap technique, the buccal papilla is mobilized and becomes part of the flap.[57] Ideally, a sulcular incision should dissect the buccal from the lingual papilla. In narrow interproximal spaces, complete mobilization of the papilla is often difficult and may cause tissue loss. Shrinkage of the papilla during the healing phase can occur and may initiate the ultimate loss of papilla height. Velvart et al,[58] in a preliminary study, investigated the shrinkage of papillae after sulcular flaps in patients with healthy periodontal tissues. The reduction of papilla height increased gradually during healing. Immediately postoperatively, papilla height loss due to surgical manipulation resulted in a recession ranging from one-fourth (n =14) to one-fourth to one-half (n = 3) of the original height. At suture removal, six sites had a loss of height of up to one-half the original position. None of the 17 sites remained at preoperative levels at any time.

A quantitative study analyzed recession of the interdental papillae in periodontally healthy situations after apical surgery using sulcular flap incisions.[59] All experimental sites exhibited a significant loss of papilla height at 1 month ($P < .003$) and 3 months ($P < .004$). Main loss of papilla height occurred between baseline and the 1-month recall (-1.1 ± 0.8 mm), while a small but significant further loss occurred between the 1- and 3-month recall appointments (-0.2 ± 0.3 mm; $P < .05$). Recall at 3 months showed that retractions increased in 10 sites, while in 3 sites the loss had diminished compared with the value after 1 month. These results suggest that the conventional sulcular flap results in considerable retraction of papilla height after 1 month and 3 months postsurgically.[59]

The issue of papilla preservation has been largely addressed in periodontal therapy. In anterior periodontal surgery, a papillary retention procedure is advocated to maintain papilla height to maximize postoperative esthetics.[60,61] Cortellini et al[62,63] suggested a modification of the papilla preservation technique that allows primary closure of the interdental space over a bioabsorbable membrane. A horizontal incision is performed at the base of the lingual papilla. The papilla is subsequently elevated to the buccal side. After coronal repositioning of the buccal flap over the membrane, the interproximal area is covered with the papilla, which is attached to the buccal flap. Primary closure over the membrane was obtained in all treated sites using the modified preservation technique. Probing attachment level gains and pocket depth reduction were observed after 1 year when using this technique.

The use of the papilla preservation technique in apical surgery is seldom possible, the reason being that the entire papilla, if incised on the lingual aspect as mentioned above, cannot be mobilized under the contact point due to lack of space. This leads to modification of the flap for endodontic surgery. The papilla base incision is performed only on the buccal aspect of the tooth. The procedure requires horizontal and vertical incisions in a specific way. The first incision line should begin perpendicular to the outer contour of the marginal gingiva, as shown and marked with a green line in Fig 9-8.

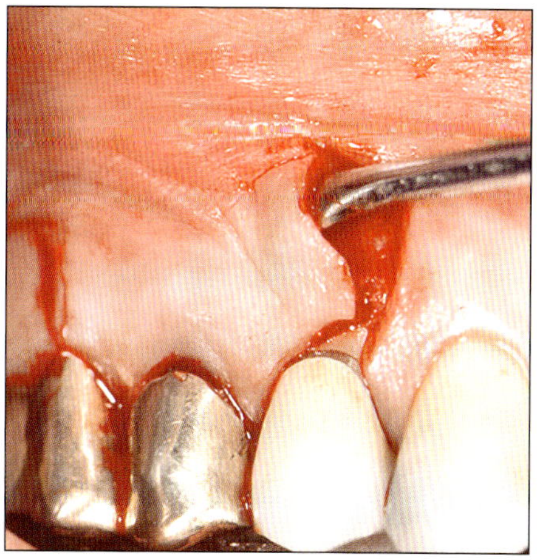

Fig 9-13 Raising a flap from the releasing incision with a distocoronal-directed motion, undermining the periosteum. (Reprinted from Velvart[1] with permission.)

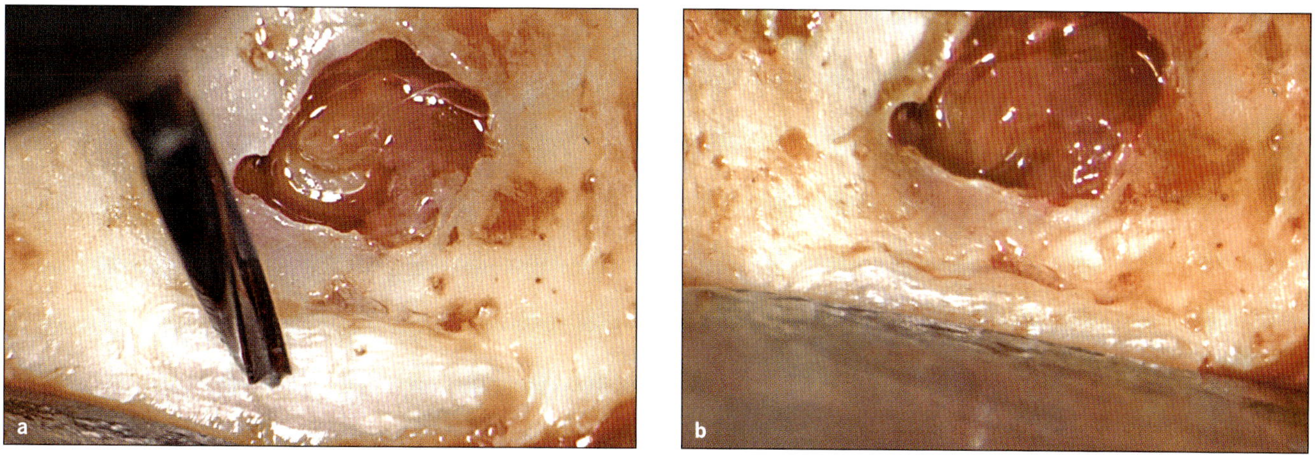

Fig 9-14 *(a and b)* A small groove in the bone at the base of the flap serves as a rest for the periosteal elevator, giving the assistant a safe position for it so that it will not slip and possibly crush the tissues. (Courtesy of Dr Richard Rubinstein, Farmington Hills, Michigan.)

This rule applies to any type of incision to avoid thinning out of tissues and to allow sufficient blood supply to reach the area, promoting better healing. The importance of proper incision and surgical technique in obtaining recession-free and esthetically improved healing was pointed out in a recent clinical study on the papilla base flap.[52] The marginal incision commences by the preparation of the papilla base using a microsurgical blade. The size of the blade should not exceed 2.5 mm in width. Suitable shapes include standard #15C blades or blades with a rounded end (BB 369, Aesculap) (Fig 9-12). The crucial point is a controlled movement of the scalpel blade within the small dimensions of the interproximal space.

The evaluation of healing patterns of the papilla base incisions after 3 months revealed mainly completely undetectable or only partially detectable incision lines and generally demonstrated excellent healing. None of the operated sites displayed any measurable loss of papilla height or other complications.[52]

Flap elevation/mobilization

After the incision, lifting the tissue from the underlying bone should raise the flap. In the process, the periosteum should not be perforated or torn. To optimize healing conditions, maintenance of an intact periosteum is essential because it will protect the surgical cavity from being in direct contact with the mucosal tissue, which otherwise may enter the cavity and prevent complete bone fill. Flap elevation should begin from the releasing incision in an undermining action (Fig 9-13). The elevating instrument then should be directed toward the marginal ridge. If the periosteum cannot be separated completely from the crestal bone, the flap will be freed by carefully dissecting the nonseparated tissue remnants with a scalpel. Once the flap has been retracted, a small groove should be prepared in the bone with a small round bur. This groove serves as a rest for the retractor, to prevent crushing of the flap during the surgery (Fig 9-14).

Conclusion

The introduction of microsurgery to surgical endodontics attempted to minimize trauma and enhance surgical results. Because of the combination of magnification and more delicate instruments, improved and careful tissue handling has become possible. This in turn allows for more predictable healing and less esthetically compromising tissue defects and recessions.

To achieve these goals, several measures are necessary, including accurate preoperative treatment planning in reference to the condition and the quality of the tissue to be manipulated. Although application of basic rules leads to adequate soft tissue healing after endodontic surgery, there is a great potential for improvements in postsurgical esthetic outcome. As in other dental fields, pink esthetics of oral soft tissues become increasingly important, and efforts should be made to minimize scar formation and recessions after surgical procedures. This is even more the case when larger restorations are present and healthy periodontal tissues are reflected as access flaps for periradicular surgeries. Microsurgery alone will not accelerate epithelial healing rates, but through perfect tissue adaptation of wound edges, it can create smaller distances for epithelial migration during the healing process. More rapid soft tissue healing is a result of reduced tissue trauma and enhanced wound closure during microsurgical procedures. Toward this end, minimal trauma should be inflicted during incision and raising of the flap. Both the flap and nonreflected tissue remaining on the tooth surface should be kept moist during the entire procedure, especially in situations where excellent hemostasis can be achieved. The flap design plays an important role in determining how much recession will occur postoperatively. Papilla base flaps have greatly improved the conditions for recession-free healing after endodontic surgery.

References

1. Velvart P. Surgical endodontics. In: Bergenholtz G, Hørsted-Bindslev P, Reit C (eds). Textbook of Endodontology, ed 2. Oxford: Blackwell, 2003:348–365.
2. Jansson L, Sandstedt P, Låftman AC, Skoglund A. A relationship between apical and marginal healing in periradicular surgery. Oral Surg Oral Med Oral Pathol Oral Radiol Endod 1997;83:596–601.
3. Ehnevid H, Jansson L, Lindskog S, Blomlöf L. Periodontal healing in teeth with periapical lesions. A clinical retrospective study. J Clin Periodontol 1993;20:254–258.
4. McLean JW. Long-term esthetic dentistry. Quintessence Int 1989;20:701–708.
5. Allen EP. Use of mucogingival surgical procedures to enhance esthetics. Dent Clin North Am 1988;32:307–330.
6. Gargiulo AW, Wentz FM, Orban B. Dimensions and relations of the dentogingival junction in humans. J Periodontol 1961;32:261–267.
7. Schroeder HE, Listgarten MA. The gingival tissues: The architecture of periodontal protection. Periodontol 2000 1997;13:91–120.
8. Kohl JT, Zander HA. Morphology of interdental gingival tissues. Oral Surg Oral Med Oral Pathol 1961;14:287–295.
9. Pilot T. Macro-morphology of the interdental papilla [in German]. Dtsch Zahnarztl Z 1973;28:1220–1221.
10. Bimstein E, Machtei E, Eidelman E. Dimensional differences in the attached and keratinized gingiva and gingival sulcus in the early permanent dentition: A longitudinal study. J Pedod 1986;10:247–253.
11. Schroeder HE. Oral Structural Biology: Embryology, Structure and Function of Normal Hard and Soft Tissues of the Oral Cavity and Temporomandibular Joints, ed 1. New York: Thieme, 1991.
12. Newcomb GN, Powell RN. Human gingival Langerhans cells in health and disease. J Periodontal Res 1986;21:640–652.
13. Tonetti MS, Straub AM, Lang NP. Expression of the cutaneous lymphocyte antigen and the alpha IEL beta 7 integrin by intraepithelial lymphocytes in healthy and diseased human gingiva. Arch Oral Biol 1995;40:1125–1132.
14. Ayanoglou C, Lécolle S, Septier D, Goldberg M. Cuprolinic blue visualization of cytosolic and membrane-associated glycosaminoglycans in the rat junctional epithelium and gingival epithelia. Histochem J 1994;26:213–225.
15. Bartold PM, Wiebkin OW, Thonard JC. Proteoglycans of human gingival epithelium and connective tissue. Biochem J 1981;211:119–127.
16. Miyasaki KT, Iofel R, Lehrer RI. Sensitivity of periodontal pathogens to the bactericidal activity of synthetic protegrins, antibiotic peptides derived from porcine leukocytes. J Dent Res 1997;76:1453–1459.
17. Schonwetter BS, Stolzenberg ED, Zasloff MA. Epithelial antibiotics induced at sites of inflammation. Science 1995;267(5204):1645–1648.
18. Overall CM. Regulation of tissue inhibitor of matrix metalloproteinase expression. Ann NY Acad Sci 1994;732:51–64.
19. Uitto VJ, Airola K, Vaalamo M, et al. Collagenase-3 (matrix metalloproteinase-13) expression in induced in oral mucosal epithelium during chronic inflammation. Am J Pathol 1998;152:1489–1499.
20. Clark RAF. The Molecular and Cellular Biology of Wound Repair, ed 2. New York: Plenum, 1996.
21. Payne WA, Page RC, Ogilvie AL, Hall WB. Histopathologic features of the initial and early stages of experimental gingivitis in man. J Periodontal Res 1975;10:51–64.
22. Orban B, Wentz F, Everett F, Grant D. Periodontics. St Louis: Mosby, 1958.
23. Holmes CH. Morphology of the interdental papillae. J Periodontol 1965;36:455–460.
24. Tarnow DP, Magner AW, Fletcher P. The effect of the distance from the contact point to the crest of bone on the presence or absence of the interproximal dental papilla. J Periodontol 1992;63:995–996.
25. Nobuto T, Yanagihara K, Teranishi Y, Minamibayashi S, Imai H, Yamaoka A. Periosteal microvasculature in the dog alveolar process. J Periodontol 1989;60:709–715.
26. Velvart P, Hecker H, Tillinger G. Detection of the apical lesion and the mandibular canal in conventional radiography and computed tomography. Oral Surg Oral Med Oral Pathol Oral Radiol Endod 2001;92:682–688.
27. Klinge B, Petersson A, Maly P. Location of the mandibular canal: comparison of macroscopic findings, conventional radiography, and computed tomography. Int J Clin Maxillofac Implants 1989;4:327–332.
28. Patel S, Durack C, Abella F, Shemesh H, Roig M, Lemberg K. Cone beam computed tomography in endodontics—A review. Int Endod J 2015;48:3–15.
29. Cohenca N, Shemesh H. Clinical applications of cone beam computed tomography in endodontics: A comprehensive review. Quintessence Int 2015;46:657–668.
30. Cohenca N, Shemesh H. Clinical applications of cone beam computed tomography in endodontics: A comprehensive review. Quintessence Int 2015;46:465–480.
31. Listgarten MA. Periodontal probing: What does it mean? J Clin Periodontol 1980;7:165–176.
32. Quirinen M, Aventroodt P, Peters W, Pauwels M, Couckel W, van Steenberghe D. Effect of different chlorhexidine formulations in mouthrinses on de novo plaque formation. J Clin Periodontol 2001;28:1127–1136.
33. Schiött CR, Löe H, Jensen SB, Kilian M, Davies RM, Glavind K. The effect of chlorhexidine mouthrinses on the human oral flora. J Periodontal Res 1970;5:84–89.
34. Newman PS, Addy M. A comparison of a periodontal dressing and chlorhexidine gluconate mouthwash after the internal bevelled flap procedure. J Clin Periodontol 1978;49:576–579.
35. Newman PS, Addy M. A comparison of hypertonic saline and chlorhexidine mouthrinses after the inverse bevel flap procedure. J Periodontol 1982;52:315–318.
36. Worrall SF, Knibbs PJ, Glenwright HD. Methods of reducing bacterial contamination of the atmosphere arising from use of an air polisher. Br Dent J 1987;163(4):118–119.

37. Lang NP, Löe H. The relationship between the width of keratinized gingiva and gingival health. J Periodontol 1972;43:623–627.
38. Velvart P, Peters CI, Peters OA. Soft tissue management: Flap design, incision, tissue elevation, and tissue retraction. Endod Topics 2005;11:78–97.
39. von Arx T, Salvi GE, Janner S, Jensen SS. Gingival recession following apical surgery in the esthetic zone: A clinical study with 70 cases. Eur J Esthetic Dent 2009;4:28–45.
40. Caudill RF, Oringer RJ, Langer L, Langer B, Bahat O, Handelsman M. Esthetic periodontics (periodontal plastic surgery). In: Wilson T, Kornmann K (eds). Fundamentals of Periodontics, ed 2. Chicago: Quintessence, 2003:540–561.
41. Pontoriero R, Carnevale G. Surgical crown lengthening: A 12-month clinical wound healing study. J Periodontol 2001;72:841–848.
42. Tibbetts LS, Shanelec D. Current status of periodontal microsurgery. Curr Opin Periodontol 1996;3:118–125.
43. Peters LB, Wesselink PR. Soft tissue management in endodontic surgery. Dent Clin North Am 1997;41:513–528.
44. Gutmann JL, Harrison JW. Flap design and incisions. In: Gutmann JL, Harrison JW (eds). Surgical Endodontics, ed 1. Boston: Blackwell, 1991:162–175.
45. Mörmann W, Ciancio SG. Blood supply of human gingiva following periodontal surgery. A fluorescein angiographic study. J Periodontol 1977;48:681–692.
46. Ohmori S, Kurata K. Experimental studies on the blood supply to various types of skin grafts in rabbits using isotope P32. Plast Reconstr Surg Transplant Bull 1960;25:547–555.
47. Patterson TJ. The survival of skin flaps in the pig. Br J Plast Surg 1968;21:113–117.
48. Luebke RG. Surgical endodontics. Dent Clin North Am 1974;18:379–391.
49. Pihlstrom BL, McHugh RB, Oliphant TH, Ortiz-Campos C. Comparison of surgical and nonsurgical treatment of periodontal disease. A review of current studies and additional results after 6 1/2 years. J Clin Periodontol 1983;10:524–541.
50. von Arx T, Alsaeed M, Salvi GE. Five-year changes in periodontal parameters after apical surgery. J Endod 2011;37:910–918.
51. Velvart P, Peters CI, Peters OA. Soft tissue management: Suturing and wound healing. Endod Topics 2005;11:179–195.
52. Velvart P. Papilla base incision: A new approach to recession-free healing of the interdental papilla after endodontic surgery. Int Endod J 2002;35:453–460.
53. Soehren SE, Allen AL, Cutright DE, Seibert JS. Clinical and histologic studies of donor tissues utilized for free grafts of masticatory mucosa. J Periodontol 1973;44:727–741.
54. Mörmann W, Schaer F, Firestone A. The relationship between success of free gingival grafts and transplant thickness. Revascularization and shrinkage—One-year clinical study. J Periodontol 1981;52:74–80.
55. Wennström J, Pini Prato G. Mucogingival therapy. In: Lindhe J, Karring T, Lang NP (eds). Clinical Periodontology and Implant Dentistry, ed 3. Copenhagen: Blackwell, 1997:550–596.
56. Blatz MB, Hürzeler MB, Strub JR. Reconstruction of the lost interproximal papilla—Presentation of surgical and nonsurgical approaches. Int J Periodontics Restorative Dent 1999;19:395–406.
57. Baumann MA, Beer R. Endodontology. New York: Thieme, 2010.
58. Velvart P, Ebner-Zimmermann U, Ebner JP. Papilla healing following sulcular full thickness flap in endodontic surgery. Oral Surg Oral Med Oral Pathol Oral Radiol 2004;98:365–369.
59. Velvart P, Ebner-Zimmermann U, Pierre Ebner J. Papilla healing following sulcular full thickness flap in endodontic surgery. Oral Surg Oral Med Oral Pathol Oral Radiol Endod 2004;98:365–369.
60. Michaelides PL, Wilson SG. A comparison of papillary retention versus full-thickness flaps with internal mattress sutures in anterior periodontal surgery. Int J Periodontics Restorative Dent 1996;16:388–397.
61. Takei HH, Han TJ, Carranza FA Jr, Kenney EB, Lekovic V. Flap technique for periodontal bone implants. Papilla preservation technique. J Periodontol 1985; 56:204–210.
62. Cortellini P, Pini Prato G, Tonetti MS. The modified papilla preservation technique with bioresorbable barrier membranes in the treatment of intrabony defects. Case reports. Int J Periodontics Restorative Dent 1996;16:546–559.
63. Cortellini P, Prato GP, Tonetti MS. The modified papilla preservation technique. A new surgical approach for interproximal regenerative procedures. J Periodontol 1995;66:261–256.
64. Velvart P, Peters CI. Soft tissue management in endodontic surgery. J Endod 2005;31:4–15.

Chapter Ten

Apical Microsurgery: Application of Armamentaria, Materials, and Methods

Richard Rubinstein, Mohamed I. Fayad

Nonsurgical root canal therapy has proven to be a highly successful procedure when the clinical case is properly diagnosed, treated, and restored. If a conventionally treated case fails and it is determined that the reason for failure is endodontic in origin and not periodontal, traumatic, or restorative in nature, apical microsurgery is often the treatment of choice. Significant advances in the use of magnification and illumination and supportive armamentaria in recent years have benefited treatment protocols in apical surgery such that teeth that might otherwise have been extracted now have a predictable chance for retention.

Case Selection and Treatment Planning

One of the most important caveats in apical microsurgery is in knowing when to perform it. Case selection will impact heavily on treatment outcomes, which then influence future treatment choices and long-term success rates. The most important diagnostic tool to this end has been the introduction of limited field computed tomography (cone beam computed tomography [CBCT]). When utilizing this technology, exploratory or diagnostic surgery

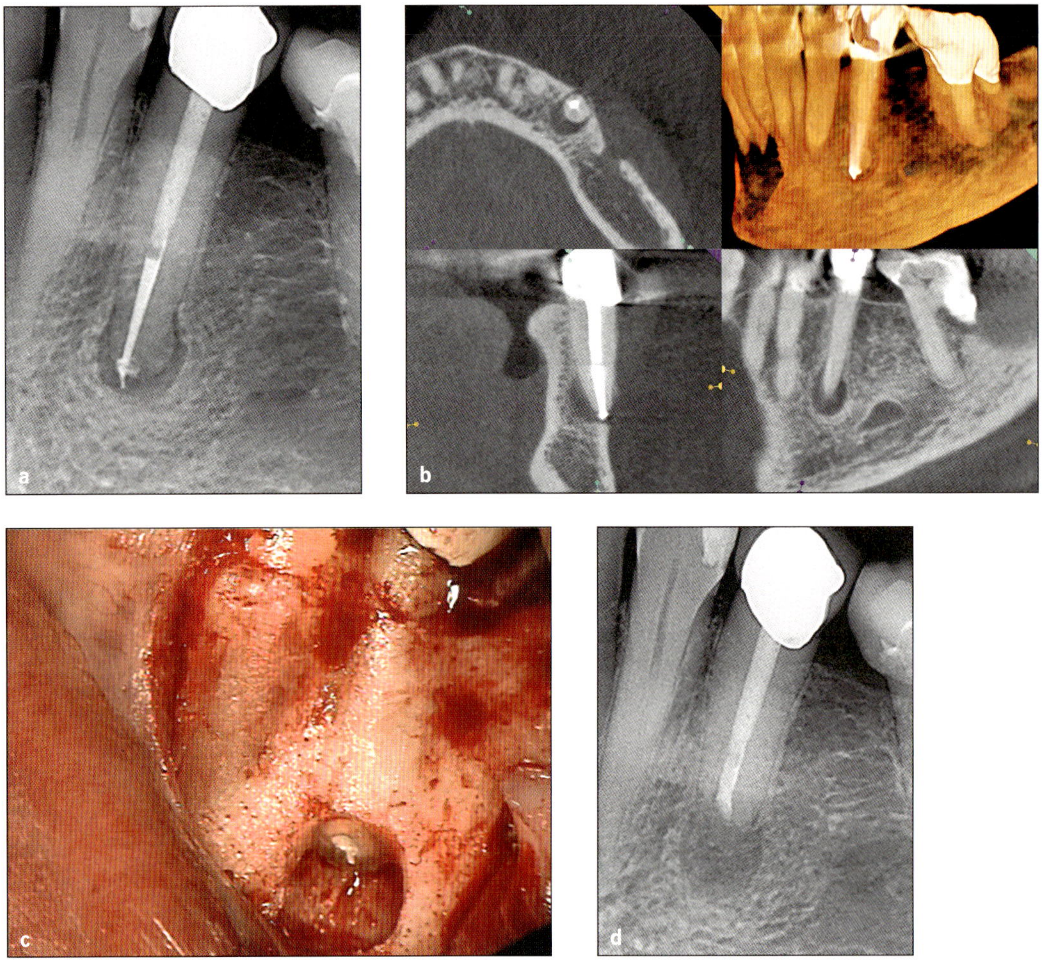

Fig 10-1 *(a)* Preoperative radiograph. *(b)* CBCT scan. *(c)* Apical retrofilling. *(d)* Postoperative radiograph.

becomes a thing of the past as treatment decisions with predictable outcomes can easily be made. In addition, an appropriate armamentarium and strategic approaches can be prepared well in advance of the actual surgery.

CBCT examination can help us treatment plan by revealing the exact position of the apical periodontitis. In Fig 10-1a, a preoperative radiograph shows apical periodontitis. The sagittal view of the CBCT scan also indicates that the periodontitis is apical, but the coronal view shows that the buccal cortical plate is quite thick and that the root is lingually positioned (Fig 10-1b). Knowing this information in advance allows the clinician time to select the appropriate armamentarium to address the position and treatment of the apical periodontitis (Figs 10-1c and 10-1d).

In Fig 10-2a, the coronal view of a CBCT scan shows that the mental nerve is quite close to the location of the apical periodontitis and that root resection should be more coronally positioned to avoid potential paresthesia. Also note the root is inclined to the lingual. This information is not available in the planar two-dimensional (2D) radiograph (Fig 10-2b). Again, knowing this prior to the surgery will allow for proper preparation by the clinician (Figs 10-2c and 10-2d).

In Fig 10-3a, the sagittal view of a CBCT scan shows that there is adequate space between the apical periodontitis and the mandibular canal and that there is little chance of harming the inferior alveolar or mental nerves. Therefore, this case should be fairly routine (Figs 10-3b to 10-3e).

In Fig 10-4a, the axial view of a CBCT scan shows that there is apical periodontitis on all three roots of this maxillary first molar. The coronal view shows that the palatal apical periodontitis is more accessible from the palatal approach and that the buccal apical periodontitis is accessible from the buccal approach. Knowing this in advance of the surgery allows the clinician to treatment plan for both buccal and lingual flaps and plan for a more predictable surgery (Figs 10-4b to 10-4h).

Fig 10-2 *(a)* CBCT scan. *(b)* Preoperative radiograph *(c)* Apical retrofilling. *(d)* Postoperative radiograph.

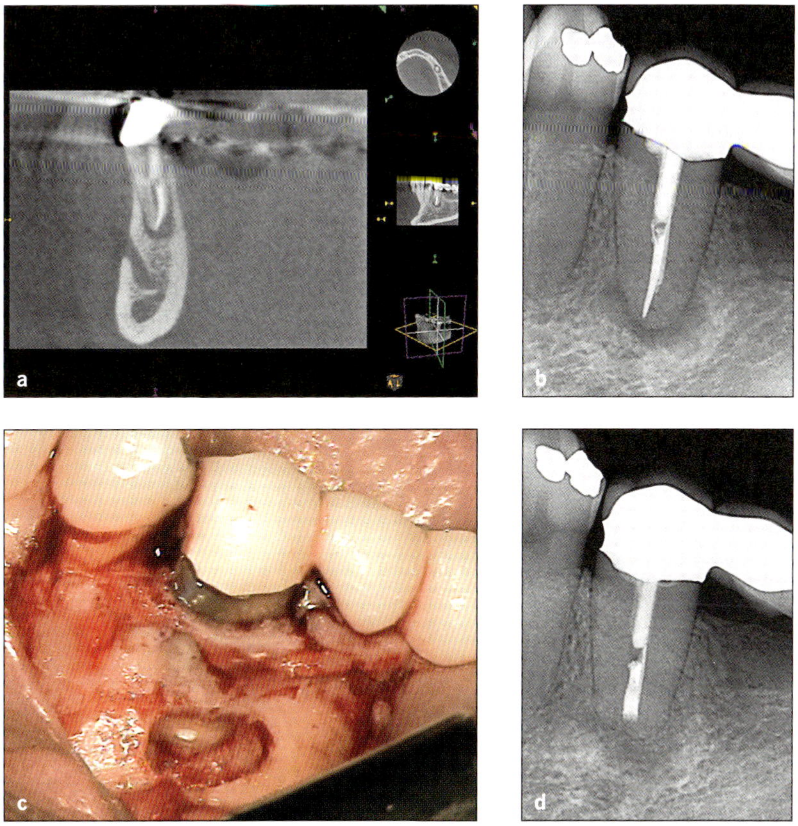

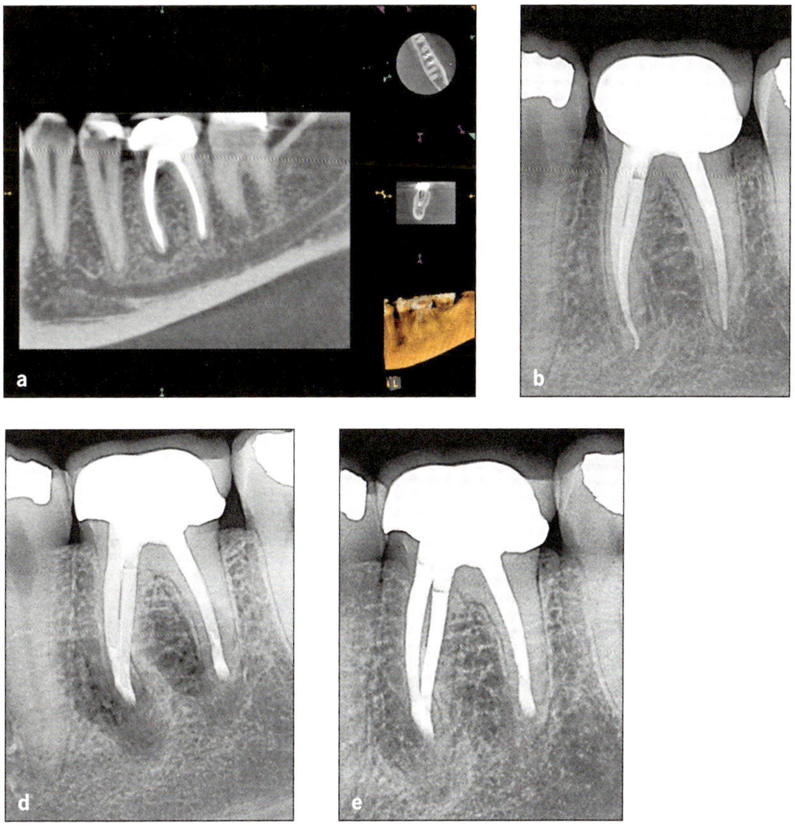

Fig 10-3 *(a)* CBCT scan. *(b)* Preoperative radiograph (note that apical periodontitis is not apparent). *(c)* Apical retrofillings. *(d)* Postoperative radiograph. *(e)* Healing at 6 months.

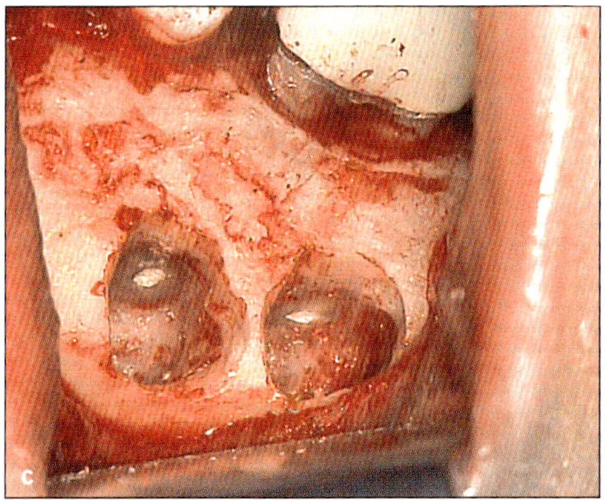

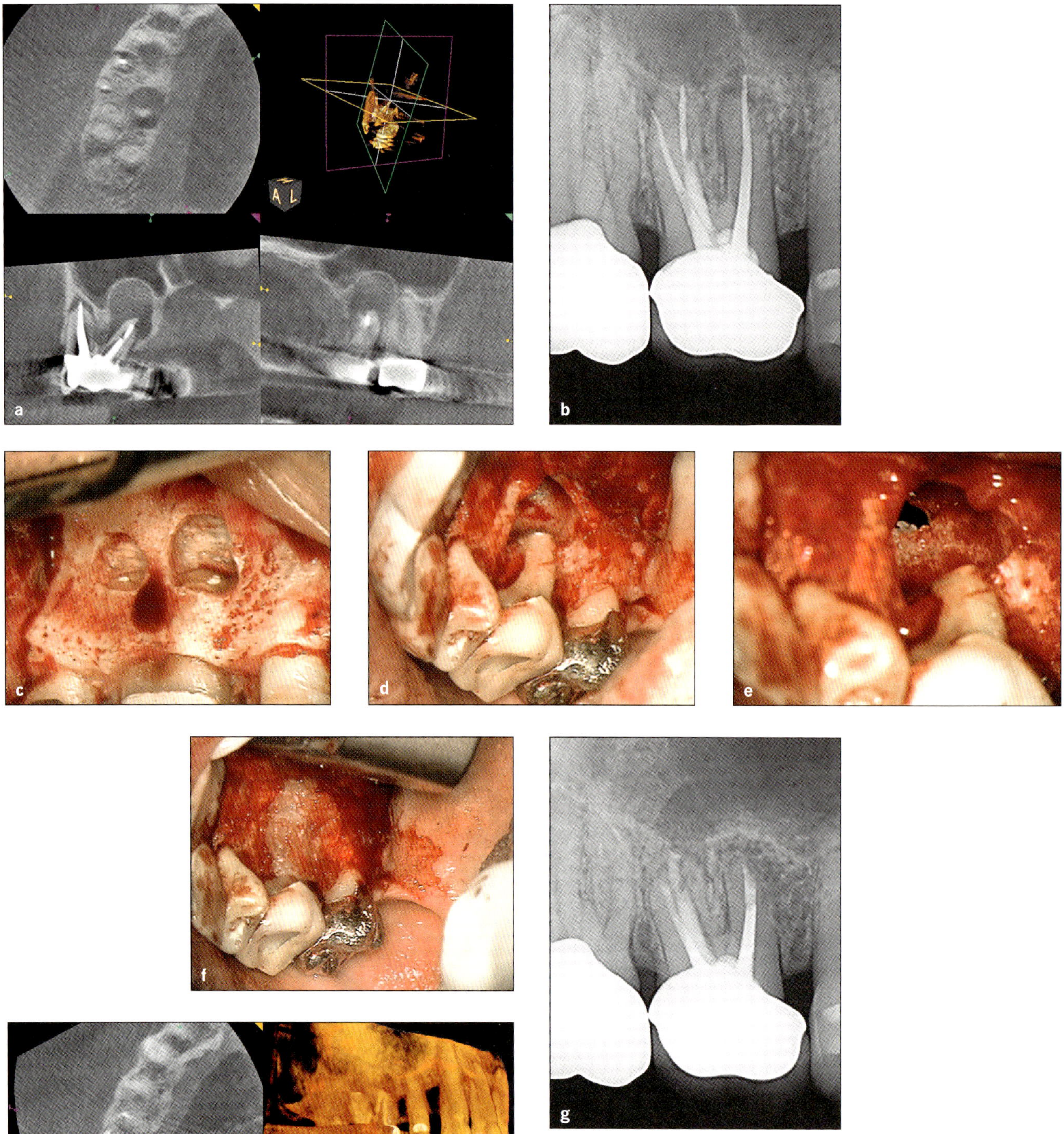

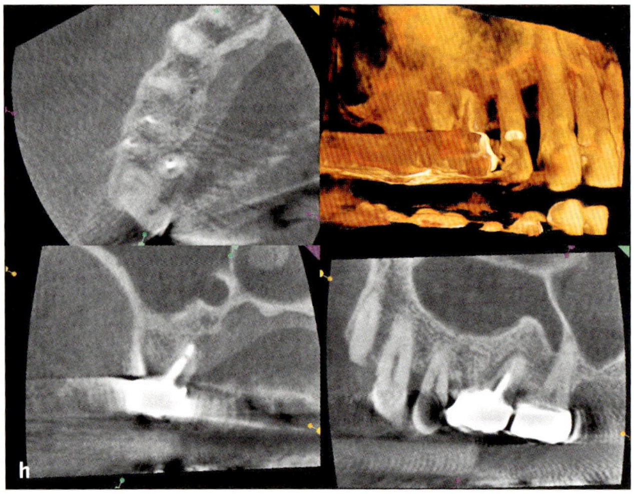

Fig 10-4 *(a)* CBCT scan. *(b)* Preoperative radiograph (note that the 2D planar view does not show the extent of the apical periodontitis). *(c)* Buccal apical retrofillings. *(d)* Palatal retrofill. *(e)* Opening into the maxillary sinus. *(f)* DynaBlast paste graft (Keystone Dental) in situ. *(g)* Postoperative radiograph. *(h)* CBCT scan 1½ years later showing significant healing.

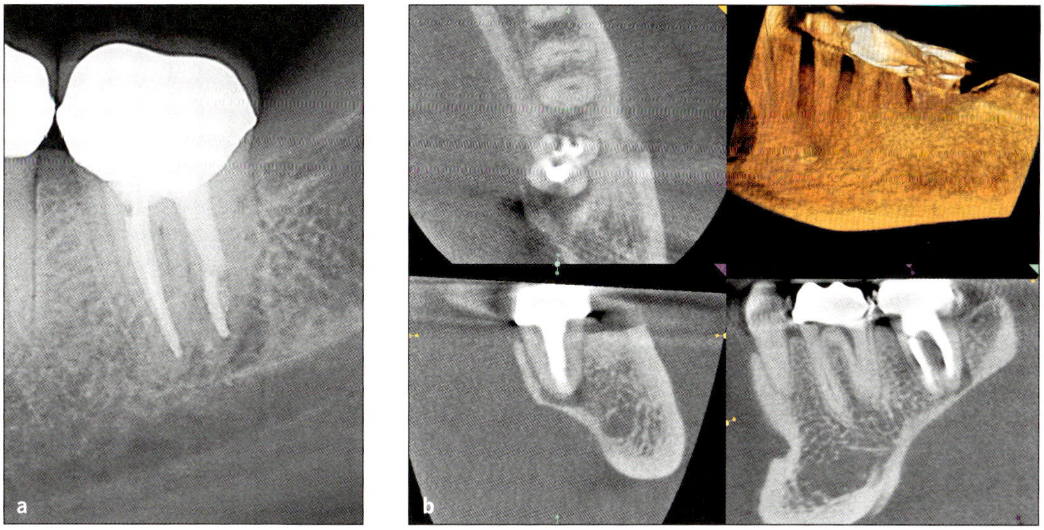

Fig 10-5 *(a)* 2D planar view. *(b)* CBCT scan.

CBCT examination can often help determine when not to take a surgical approach. In Fig 10-5a, the 2D planar view shows a mandibular second molar with apical periodontitis. The clinician might be concerned about the location of the mandibular canal. The coronal view of the CBCT scan (Fig 10-5b) shows that the location of the mandibular canal is apical and buccal to the apical terminus and not of great concern. However, the coronal view also shows that the root is located against the lingual cortical plate of bone and that surgical access is not practical. Orthograde retreatment, intentional replantation, or removal of the tooth with replacement by an implant-retained crown may be a better choice.

Figure 10-6 shows a similar situation. The 2D planar view (Fig 10-6a) shows a mandibular second molar with apical periodontitis. The CBCT scan (Fig 10-6b) shows that there is an untreated mesiobuccal canal. This can be seen in the axial and coronal views. In addition, the roots are positioned against the lingual cortical plate, making the surgical approach impractical. Clearly, orthograde retreatment is the best option as to not entomb the necrotic pulp tissue with a surgical approach (Figs 10-6c and 10-6d).

In Fig 10-7a, a 2D planar film shows a mandibular second premolar with apical periodontitis. The mental foramen can be seen at the periphery of the image. The sagittal view of the CBCT scan (Fig 10-7b) shows an unusual mental foramen and a narrow vertical extension of the nerve canal extending into the proximity of the lesion. Surgical removal of this lesion could very well cause permanent paresthesia. Note that the apical periodontitis on the mandibular first premolar seen in the sagittal section of the CBCT scan does not appear in the 2D planar view. Orthograde retreatment may be the best solution for both the mandibular first and second premolars and in fact was recommended and subsequently performed (Fig 10-7c). The follow-up 2D planar radiograph shows healing at 1 year (Fig 10-7d). The follow-up CBCT scan at 1 year shows significant bone fill in the axial, coronal, and sagittal sections (Fig 10-7e).

These are just a few examples of the benefits of limited field CBCT technology and how it can assist the clinician in treatment planning and making better treatment decisions so that surgical outcomes are more predictable. For further discussion of the use of CBCT in apical microsurgery, see chapter 6.

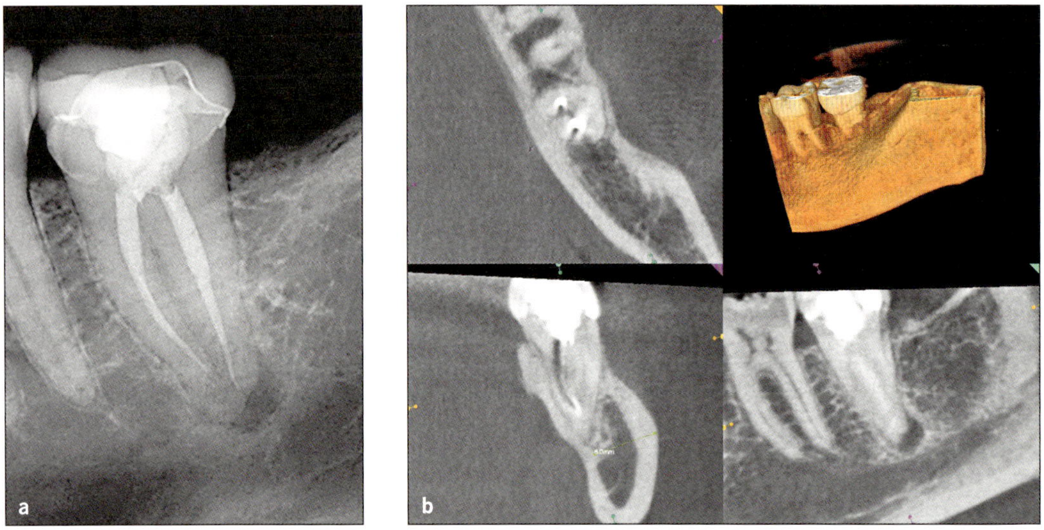

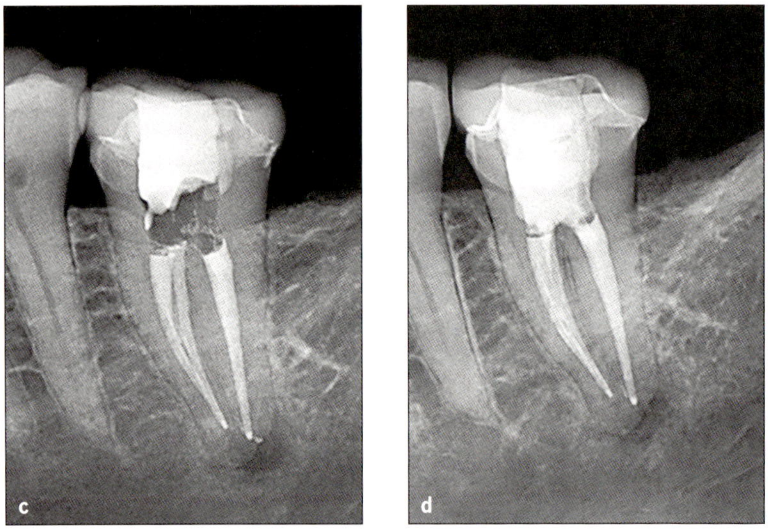

Fig 10-6 *(a)* 2D planar view. *(b)* CBCT scan. *(c)* Postoperative radiograph showing treatment of the untreated mesiobuccal canal. *(d)* Six-month follow-up radiograph showing initial healing.

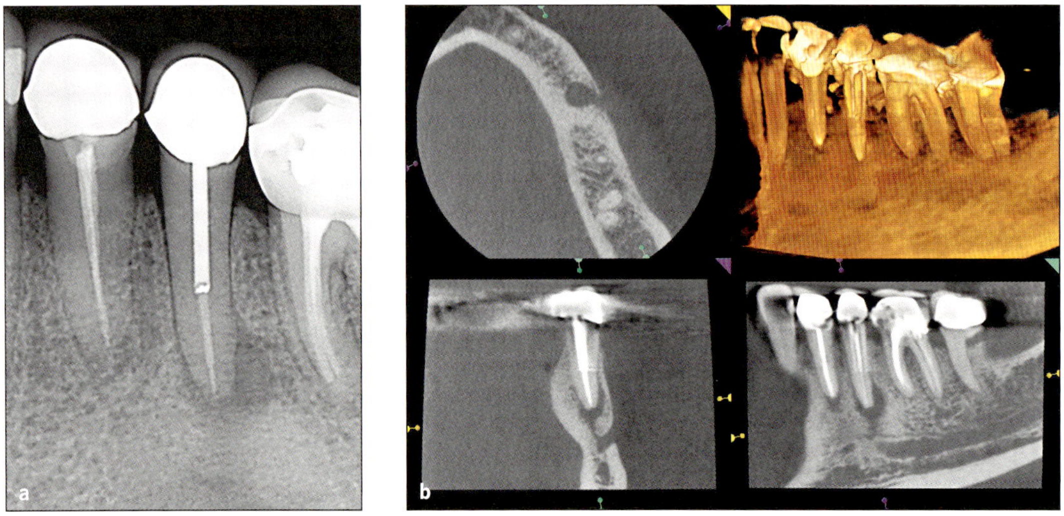

Fig 10-7 *(a)* 2D planar view. *(b)* CBCT scan showing an unusual mental foramen and canal. →

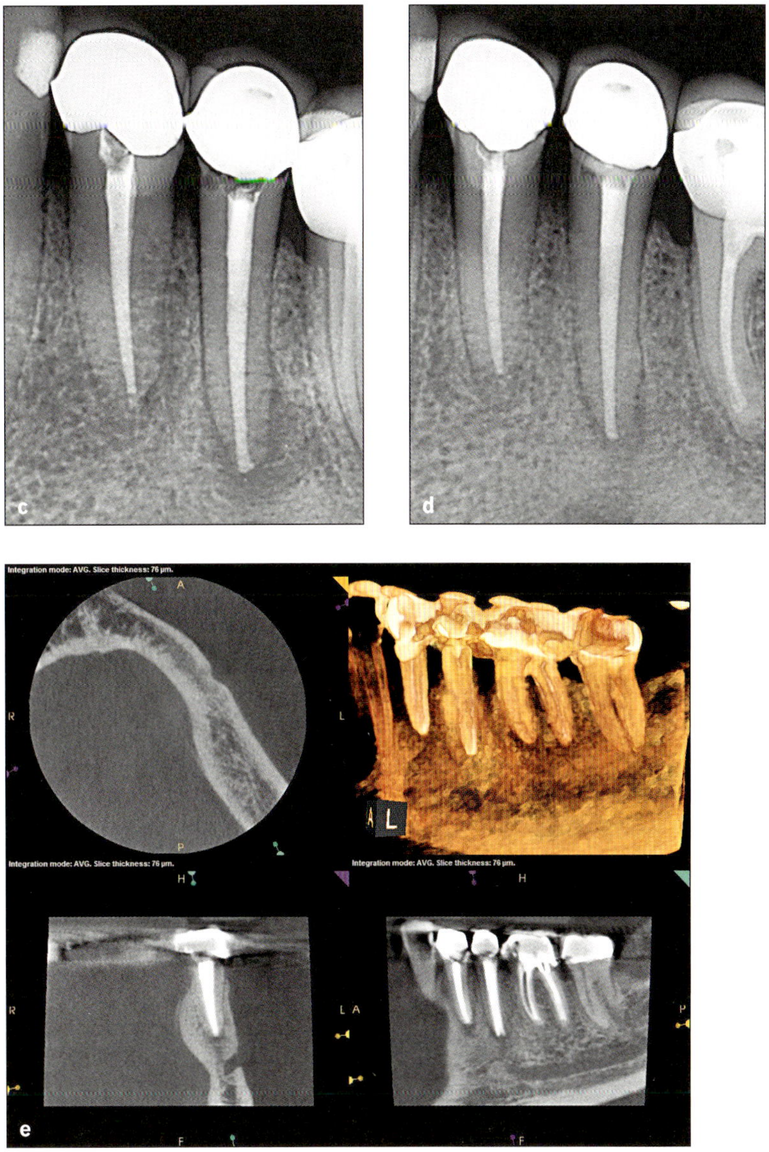

Fig 10-7 *(cont) (c)* Orthograde retreatment of both mandibular premolars. *(d)* One-year follow-up 2D planar view. *(e)* One-year follow-up CBCT scan showing healing in the axial, coronal, and sagittal sections.

Apical Microsurgery

In order to understand the objectives of apical microsurgery and the application of armamentaria, materials, and methods, it is helpful to divide the subject into multiple stages or sections. Among these stages are flap design, flap reflection, flap retraction, osteotomy, periapical curettage, biopsy, hemostasis, apical resection, resected apex evaluation, apical preparation, apical preparation evaluation, drying the apical preparation, selecting retrofilling materials, mixing retrofilling materials, placing retrofilling materials, condensing retrofilling materials, carving retrofilling materials, finishing retrofilling materials, and flap closure.

Flap design, reflection, and retraction

After anesthesia is obtained, and prior to incising the surgical flap, the oral cavity should be rinsed with a disinfectant solution such as chlorhexidine. A 0.12% chlorhexidine rinse has been shown to significantly reduce the bacterial count in the oral cavity in advance of operative procedures.[1] For a complete discussion of anesthesia and hemostasis, see chapter 8.

Microscalpels (Fig 10-8) are used in the design of the free gingival margin flap to delicately and atraumatically incise the interdental papillae when full-thickness flaps are required. Microscalpels cause less trauma than conventional scalpels, thereby resulting in less scarring and

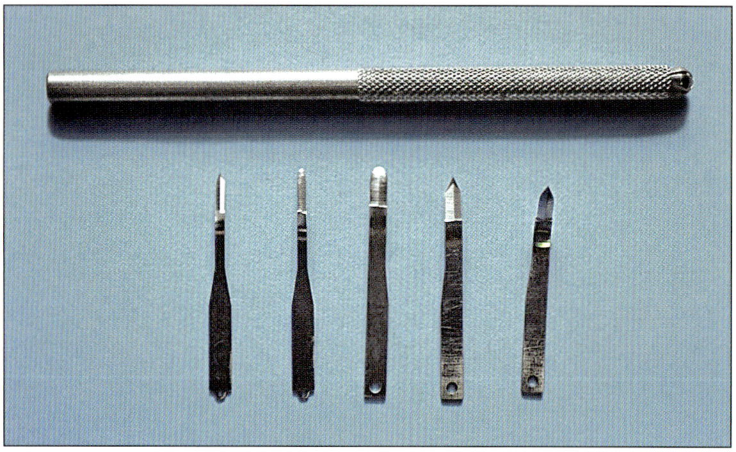

Fig 10-8 A variety of microscalpels sized 1 to 5 used for precise incision (Kerr Endodontics).

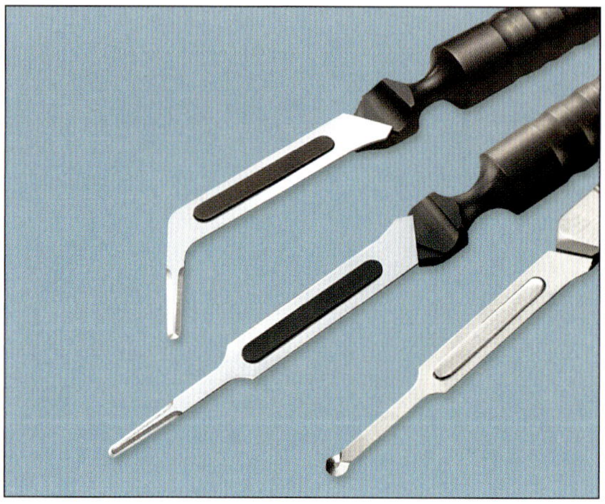

Fig 10-9 Feather Microsurgical Blades. (Courtesy of J. Morita.)

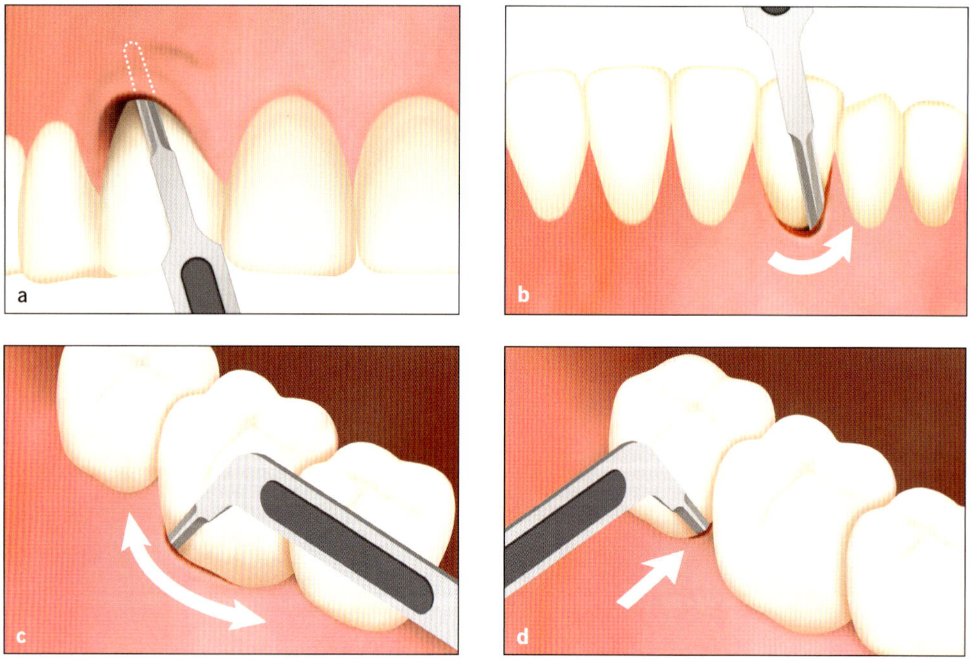

Fig 10-10 *(a to d)* Application of Feather Microsurgical Blades. (Courtesy of J. Morita.)

more favorable cosmetic outcomes. Feather Microsurgical Blades (J. Morita; Fig 10-9) are made of high-quality stainless steel using high-precision grinding technology, which produces ultrasharp cutting edges that work with a variety of handles. These blades allow for a very fine incision and minimize the risk of tissue injury (Fig 10-10). Vertical incisions can be made with a 15c blade in a Bard-Parker handle and are 1.5 to 2 times longer than those in conventional apical surgery to assure that the flap can easily be reflected out of the light path of the microscope.

Historically, flaps have been reflected with a Molt 2/4 curette or variation of the Molt 2/4. This instrument is double ended, and the cross-sectional diameters of the working ends are 3.5 mm and 7 mm. Under low-range magnification, it can readily be seen that even the smallest end of this instrument is too large to place beneath the interdental papilla without causing significant tearing and trauma to the delicate tissues. Rubinstein Mini-Molts (JEDMED; Fig 10-11) are available in two configurations whose working ends are either 2 and 3.5 mm or 2 and 7 mm. The smaller ends of these instruments provide for

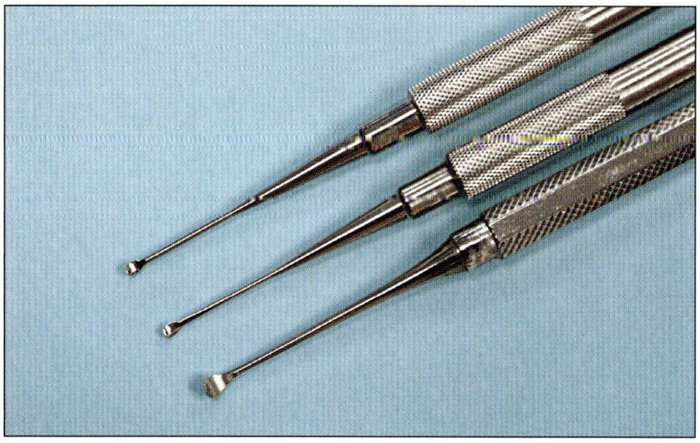

Fig 10-11 A comparison of the small ends of two Mini-Molts *(left)* and a standard Molt 2/4 curette *(right)*.

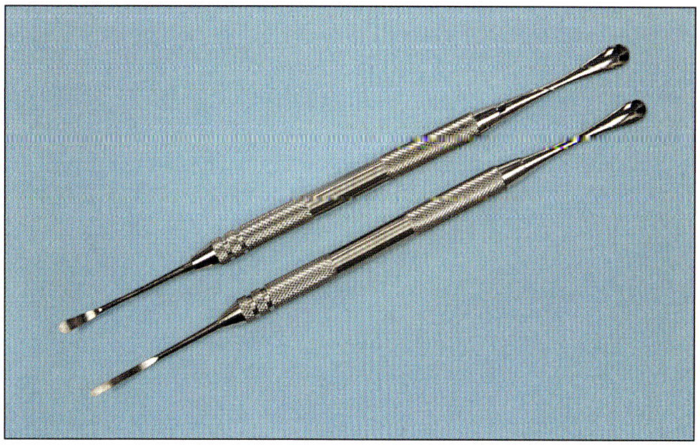

Fig 10-12 PR-1 and PR-2 periosteal elevators.

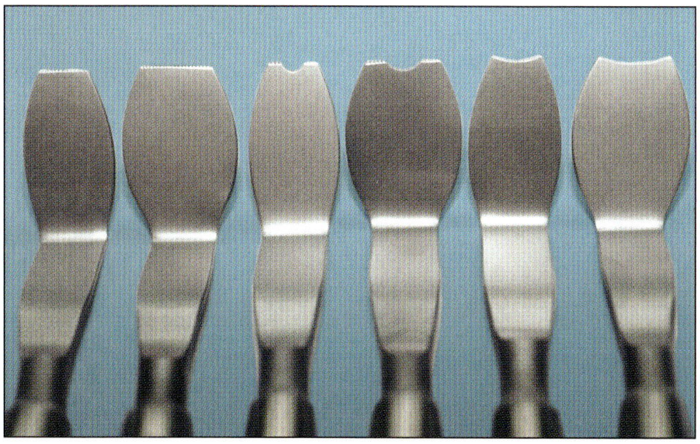

Fig 10-13 Blade and contact surfaces of the Rubinstein Retractors 1 to 6 (JEDMED).

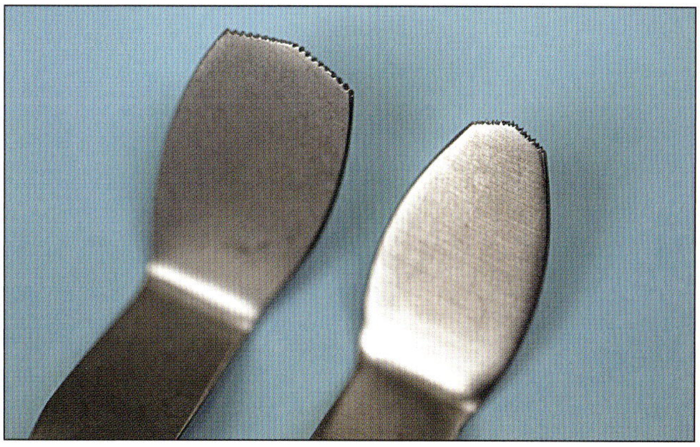

Fig 10-14 Rubinstein Retractors 7 and 8 (universal and universal mini; JEDMED).

atraumatic elevation of the interdental papilla, making flap reflection more predictable and gentle to the tissues. The recently introduced PR-1 and PR-2 (G. Hartzell & Son; Fig 10-12) have similar geometries and also accomplish the goals of atraumatic flap reflection.

Instruments such as the Minnesota retractor have been used to retract the flap away from the surgical field after reflection while assuring visual access. Maintaining pressure on this instrument for even a short period of time often causes restriction of blood flow to the fingers of the operator, and its use can be quite uncomfortable. A series of six retractors from JEDMED (Fig 10-13) and two new universal positioning retractors (Fig 10-14), which offer a variety of serrated contact surfaces that are flat, notched, and recessed, allow the operator several options for secure placement in areas of anatomical concern. Among these are placements over the nasal spine, canine eminence, and mental nerve. These retractors decrease the chance of slippage, which can cause trauma to the flap and delicate gingival mucosa. The blades of the retractors are designed to retract both the flap and the lip and are bent at 110 degrees to keep the retractor and the operator's hand out of the light path of the microscope. The handles are ergonomically designed to decrease cramping and fatigue and can be held in a variety of hand or finger grips. For further discussion of soft tissue management and conventional and contemporary flap designs, see chapter 9.

Osteotomy

Because we can see better with the surgical operating microscope (SOM), bone removal can be more conservative. Handpieces such as the Impact Air 45 (Kerr Endodontics), introduced by oral surgeons to facilitate sectioning of mandibular third molars, are also suggested for apical surgery to gain better access to the apices of maxillary and mandibular molars. When using the handpiece, the water spray is aimed directly into the surgical field, but the airstream is ejected out through the back of the handpiece, thus eliminating much of the splatter that occurs

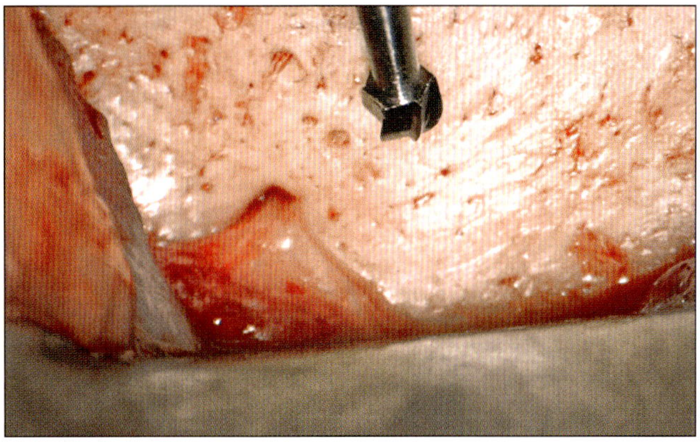

Fig 10-15 Impact Air 45 with high-speed surgical length bur in close proximity to the mental nerve (magnification ×8).

with conventional high-speed handpieces. Because there is no pressurized air or water, the chances of producing pyemia and emphysema are significantly reduced.

Burs such as a Lindemann H161 or H162 bone cutter (Brasseler USA) are extremely efficient and are recommended for hard tissue removal. They are 9 mm in length and have only four flutes, which result in less clogging. With the use of an SOM and an Impact Air 45, high-speed surgical burs can be placed even in areas of anatomical jeopardy with a high degree of confidence and accuracy (Fig 10-15). The size of the osteotomy should be as small as practical so that wound healing will not be impaired, yet large enough to allow for complete debridement of the bony crypt and access for root-end procedures that will follow. If the apical periodontitis has not penetrated the cortical plate of bone, a preoperative CBCT scan of the surgical field will provide the exact location of the root terminus. A premeasured endodontic file can then be positioned over the involved tooth, and the exact location of the terminus can be visualized. Using gentle brushstrokes, the osteotomy should be initiated slightly coronal to the end of the root to avoid encroachment on potentially significant anatomical structures. After several brushstrokes, an endodontic explorer such as a DG16 can "peck and check" for penetration through the bone and into the lesion and can be repeated as necessary until the lesion is located. The osteotomy is then enlarged peripherally to visualize the root, lesion, and bony crypt.

Curettage and biopsy

With the SOM, periapical curettage is facilitated because bony margins can be scrutinized for completeness of tissue removal. A Columbia 13/14 curette is recommended in small bony crypts because it is curved and can reach to the lingual aspect of a root. After the Columbia 13/14 is used, the Jacquette 34/35 scaler is recommended to remove the remainder of granulomatous tissue. Because of its sharp edge, the Jacquette 34/35 is an excellent instrument for removing granulomatous tissue from the junction of the root surface and the bony crypt. The more tissue that can be removed results in less work for the body to do relative to wound healing. Larger lesions can be removed by using curettes such as a Lucas 85. The lesion can be blunt dissected from the bony crypt, scooped out using the concave surface of the instrument, and then delivered to a specimen bottle.

It goes without saying that if tissue warrants removal, it warrants examination and diagnosis by an oral pathologist. At no time should a surgeon remove tissue and accept the responsibility of its diagnosis based on clinical impression, color, or consistency. In addition, any foreign material present in the bony crypt should be removed because it could cause persistent irritation and may prevent complete healing of the tissues.[2] After the bony crypt has been physically debrided, it should be rinsed thoroughly with sterile saline. For further discussion of radiolucent periapical pathosis, see chapter 4.

Apical resection and resected apex evaluation

There is general agreement that the main cause of failure in conventional endodontic treatment is the clinician's inability to adequately shape, disinfect, and obturate the entire root canal system.[3] The majority of this untreated anatomy is located in the apical 3 mm, and for this reason a 3-mm resection is recommended.[4–6] With the introduction of ultrasonics for creating root-end preparations, a second reason for a 3-mm resection has emerged. Several authors have studied the incidence of craze lines, cracks, and fractures in the root and cementum surfaces after ultrasonic root-end preparations.[7–11] While all of these studies showed a statistically significant increase, none

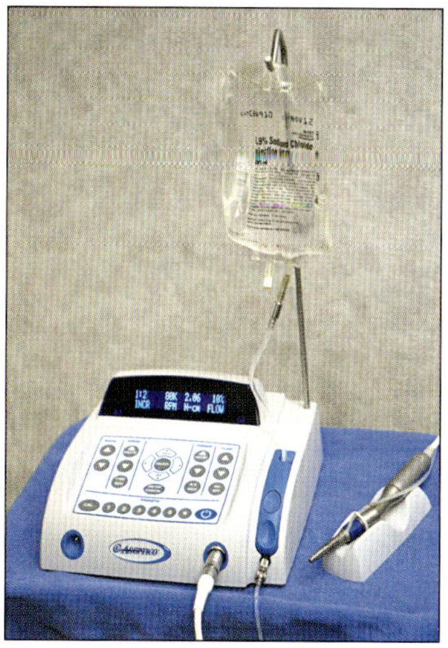

Fig 10-16 Aseptico 7000 motor and NSK 2:1 nose-cone handpiece.

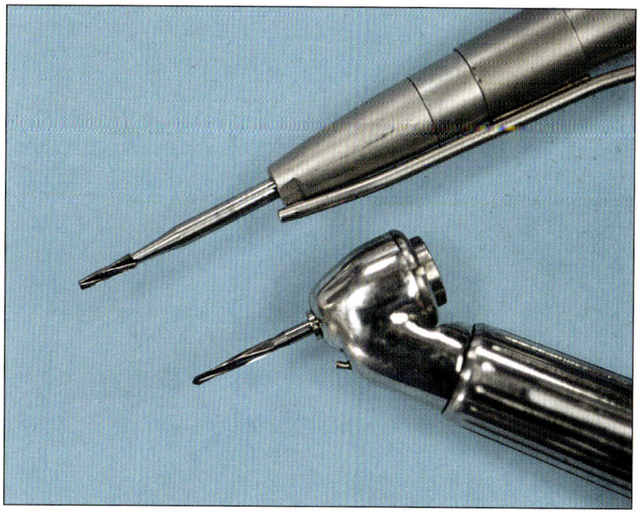

Fig 10-17 A comparison of the Impact Air 45 *(bottom)* and NSK 2:1 nose-cone handpiece *(top)* with surgical length burs.

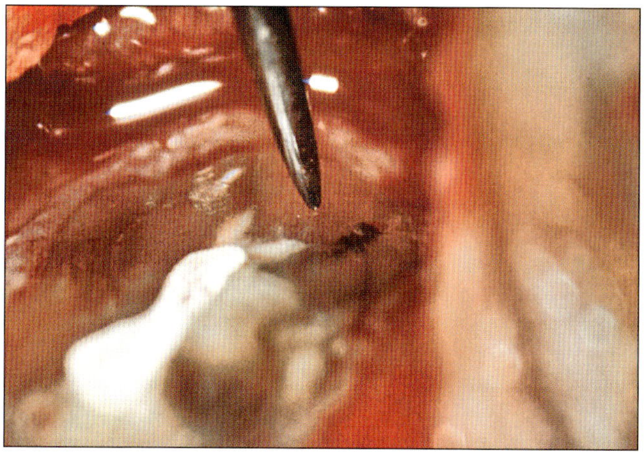

Fig 10-18 CX-1 explorer locating an untreated portal of exit on the beveled surface of a previously retrofilled root (magnification ×20).

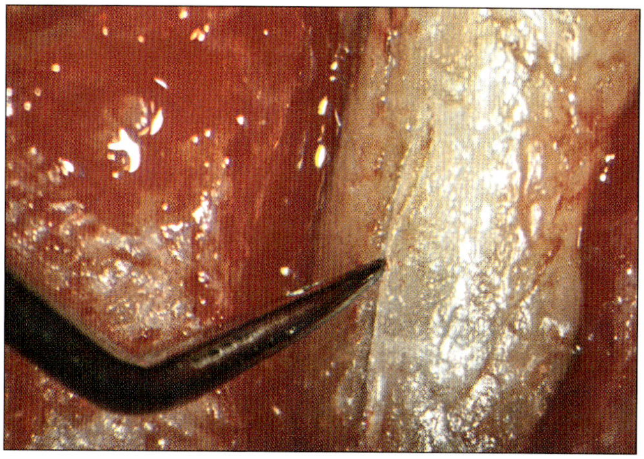

Fig 10-19 CX-1 explorer locating a crack on the facial surface of a root (magnification ×20).

has shown any clinical significance as a result of the findings. In as much as the greatest cross-sectional diameter of a root in the apical 6 mm is typically at the 3-mm level, it is suggested that this be the location of the resection in order to create an adequate buffer or cushion to absorb the potential deleterious effects of ultrasonic energy.

Historically, a long bevel was created in order to provide access for a microhead handpiece. With the introduction of periapical ultrasonics, little to no bevel is needed. This results in fewer cut dentinal tubules and less chance of leakage. The Impact Air 45 handpiece and 170L tapered fissure bur have been the instruments of choice to resect the root. However, because of the size of the head of the handpiece, visual access is often impaired, especially in the posterior regions of the mouth. Recent advancements in electric motor design and straight handpieces afford the clinician opportunities for direct visualization of the root-end while performing root resection and the creation of axial bevels that approximate zero degrees. One such unit is the Aseptico 7000 motor (Aseptico) and NSK 2:1 nose-cone handpiece (NSK) (Figs 10-16 and 10-17). The unit drives the handpiece at 80,000 rpm and is more than sufficient to atraumatically cut cortical bone and root. A variety of burs are available in 44.5-mm and 65-mm lengths, allowing access to difficult-to-reach areas. A saline solution spray is directed over the bur and cools the bone and root surfaces. Saline has the advantage over distilled water and city water in that it is physiologic and sterile. The Aseptico 7000 motor and NSK nose-cone handpiece can also be used to perform the osteotomy.

After the root-end resection has been completed, the beveled surface of the root can be examined under mid-range magnification. Using a small CX-1 micro explorer (Kerr Endodontics), small microfractures, isthmuses, and portals of exit can readily be seen (Figs 10-18 and 10-19).

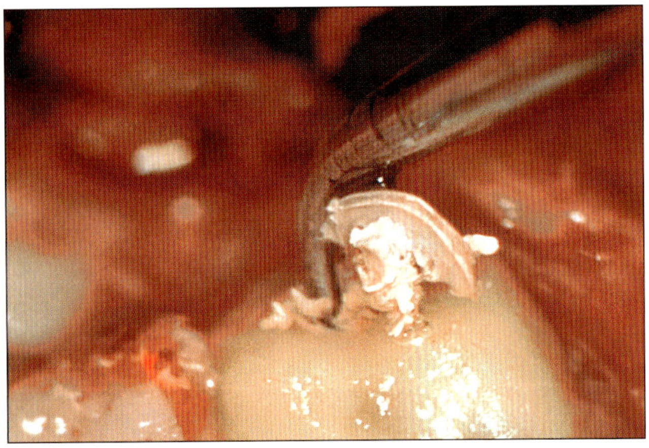

Fig 10-20 Thermoplasticized gutta-percha spinning around a stainless steel tip (magnification ×16).

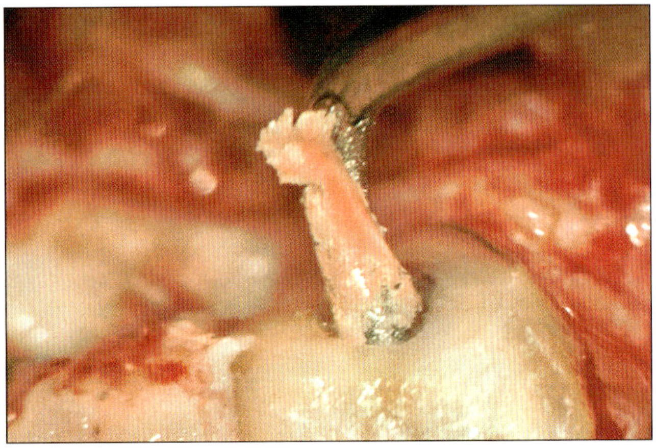

Fig 10-21 Thermoplasticized gutta-percha "walking" out of the preparation (magnification ×16).

Apical preparation

Since the introduction of periapical ultrasonic technology in the early 1990s by Carr, apical preparations have been made with ultrasonic tips.[12] These tips are driven by a variety of commercially available ultrasonic units, which are self-tuning regardless of changes in tip or load for maximum stability during operation. A piezoelectric crystal made of quartz or ceramic located in the handpiece is vibrated at 28,000 to 40,000 cycles per second, and the energy is transferred to the ultrasonic tip in a single plane. Dentin is then abraded microscopically, and gutta-percha is thermoplasticized. Continuous irrigation along the tip cools the cutting surface while maximizing debridement and cleaning.

Since their initial introduction, a variety of tips and tip configurations have been introduced to accommodate virtually any access situation. Most ultrasonic tips are 0.25 mm in diameter and approximately 3 mm in length. When used, they are placed in the long axis of the root so that the walls of the preparation will be parallel and encompass about 3 mm of the apical morphology. As the piezoelectric crystal in the handpiece is activated, the energy is transferred to the ultrasonic tip, which then moves forward and backward in a single plane, and dentin is "brush cut" away in gentle strokes. The combination of the SOM and ultrasonic tips make previously challenging cases routine. By combining magnification and ultrasonic technology, apical preparation can be visualized and executed with a high level of confidence that was previously unattainable.

Brent et al[13] studied the incidence of intradentin and canal cracks in apical preparations made with stainless steel and diamond-coated ultrasonic tips.[13] They found that diamond-coated tips do not result in significant root-end cracking and can remove cracks caused by prior instruments. For this reason, diamond-coated tips are suggested as the last ultrasonic tip to be used in root-end preparation. Furthermore, clinical use of diamond tips has shown that they are more efficient at removing gutta-percha than stainless steel tips. The irregular surface of the diamond coating appears to grab and hold the gutta-percha, facilitating removal. When using smooth-surfaced ultrasonic tips, the gutta-percha just spins on the smooth surface, making removal difficult (Figs 10-20 and 10-21).

Clinicians have observed that not all ultrasonic tips work equally well in every manufacturer's ultrasonic units; this observation has led to the term *tip specificity*. Each individual clinician must determine which tips work best in a given unit. For this reason, it is suggested that the clinician use the lowest possible setting when initiating cutting and increase the setting incrementally until a smooth, chatter-free, efficient stroke is achieved. If the unit is initially set at too high a power setting, the tip may fracture prior to being placed on the beveled surface of the root, so caution is advised.

When using ultrasonic tips, the clinician should use gentle brushstrokes with the smallest tip possible to conserve root dentin. This procedure should be observed while using midrange magnification of the SOM. Pressure on the tip should be gentle. If resistance is met, it is assumed that the tip is lingual verted. The operator should then back off to low-range magnification or look with the unaided eye to check that the tip is aligned in the long axis of the root. If this step is not taken and a lingual-verted path is continued, a perforation of the root might occur (Fig 10-22).

There were no clear guidelines on how to make the apical preparation until Gilheany et al[14] studied the angle of the bevel and the depth of the preparation from the fa-

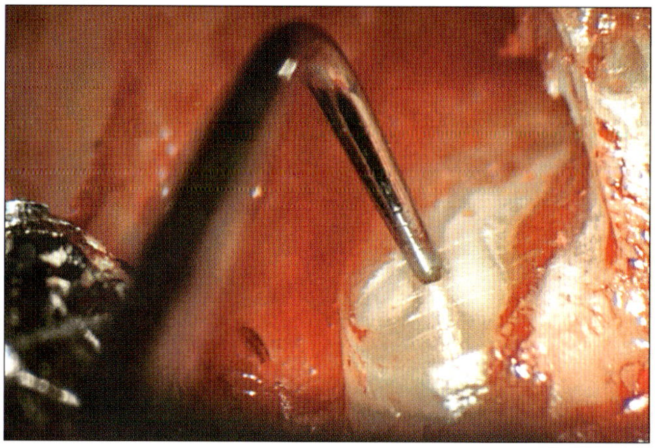

Fig 10-22 Off-axis angulation with ultrasonic tip (magnification ×16).

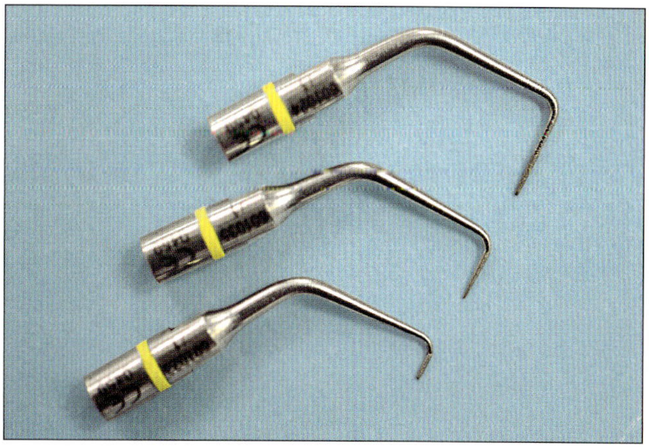

Fig 10-23 Endo Success Apical Surgery Tips.

cial wall necessary to affect an adequate apical seal. They reported that a 1-mm preparation was necessary with a 0-degree bevel, a 2.1-mm preparation was necessary with a 30-degree bevel, and a 2.5-mm preparation was necessary with a 45-degree bevel. They further recommended a 3.5-mm-deep preparation when measured radiographically to account for errors in vertical angulation. This study raised the question as to whether preparation of an isthmus, which is so common, should be treated differently than the preparation of the main canals.[4–6] Clearly, to satisfy the criteria set forth by Gilheany et al,[14] the clinician needs to create a 3-mm circumferential preparation in the long axis of the root, which includes all the anatomical ramifications of the pulp space, including the isthmus.

The inability to adequately clean and disinfect the isthmus with orthograde techniques was shown by Ricucci and Siqueira.[15] This makes the surgical treatment of the isthmus even more critical, and detailed attention must be used to thoroughly treat this space. This presents a conundrum for the clinician performing orthograde treatment or retreatment, as we are seldom able to instrument and irrigate these isthmuses and ramifications. Siqueira[16] proposed that all retreatment cases should be regarded as infected and that the microorganisms reside mainly in the isthmuses, fins, dentin debris, apical deltas, and root-filling voids. These microorganisms are in the form of a biofilm as described by Nair et al.[17] They suggested that biofilms could not be eradicated by the host's defense system or chemotherapy but rather by mechanical dislocation and disruption of the biofilm. The only way to achieve this is to surgically remove the portion of the root containing the isthmus and to ultrasonically clean this space. According to Teixeira et al,[18] most isthmuses are found 3 to 5 mm from the apex. Research by Mannocci et al[19] and Degerness and Bowles[20] support this finding. This is further evidence that a minimum of 3 mm of apical root structure should be removed to eliminate the apical delta. Additional debris and biofilm contained in the isthmus and fins are addressed by retroprepping a minimum of 3 mm coronally to further decrease the number of microorganisms remaining in the root. Currently, we are not able to assess whether the ultrasonic action of retrotips adds to the mechanical removal of biofilm created by the microabrasion of dentinal walls. Assuming that the mechanism of this action is the same as orthograde ultrasonic irrigation, one can assume that most of the bacteria will be removed from the isthmus.[21]

There are clinical situations in which a post has been placed without orthograde treatment. The untreated canal space is usually filled with pulpal remnants, debris, and bacterial contamination. Endo Success Apical Surgery Tips (Acteon; Fig 10-23) address this problem. The tip lengths are 3, 6, and 9 mm. When used in progressive sequence, up to 9 mm of canal space can be cleaned and debrided. Longer pluggers are available to condense retrofilling materials to length.

Piezosurgery

Piezosurgery is a bone-cutting modality with rapidly increasing indications in different surgical fields, including endodontic surgery. The main advantages of Piezosurgery include protection of soft tissues, optimal visualization of the surgical field, decreased blood loss, reduced vibration and noise, increased comfort for the patient, and protection of tooth structures. Some disadvantages of Piezosurgery include the initial financial burden associated with the purchase of the device, the long duration of the sur-

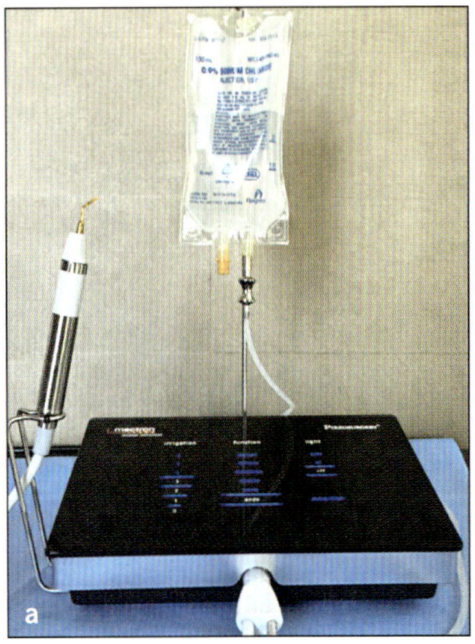

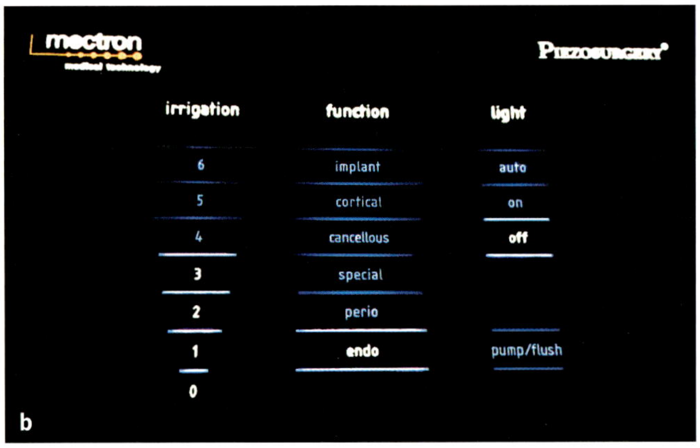

Fig 10-24 *(a)* Piezosurgery Touch (Mectron). *(b)* The control panel allows the clinician to choose the surgical procedure (power) and irrigation types.

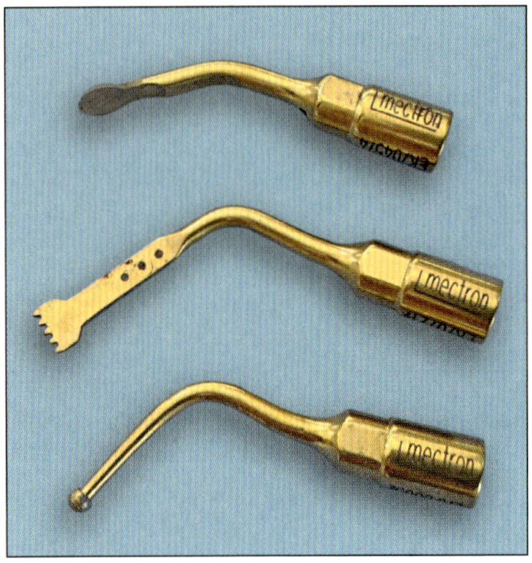

Fig 10-25 Piezosurgical tips. *(top)* OP5 used for lesion enucleation. *(middle)* OT7S-3 used for root resection. *(bottom)* OT5 used for osteotomy.

gical procedure, and the fact that the instruction manuals of many piezoelectric units discourage use of these devices in patients with implanted cardiac pacemakers.[22] The technology was developed in 1998 by the Italian oral surgeon Tomaso Vercellotti to overcome the limitations of conventional bone surgery[23] (Fig 10-24).

This new and innovative method of surgery uses piezoelectric ultrasonic vibrations to perform precise and safe osteotomies and root resections. Piezosurgical tips (Fig 10-25) cut bone and root atraumatically using ultrasonic vibrations and provide an alternative to the mechanical and electrical instruments used in conventional oral surgery. The instrument uses a modulated and ultrasonic frequency that permits the cutting of hard tissues. The vibrations obtained are amplified and transferred to a vibration tip, which when applied with slight pressure to bone (Fig 10-26) or root tissue (Fig 10-27) results in a cavitation phenomenon—a mechanical cutting effect that occurs exclusively in mineralized tissue.[22] Piezosurgical tips designed for Piezosurgery are specifically engineered and are approximately three times as powerful as conventional ultrasonic tips like those used in root-end preparation. Piezosurgery is particularly useful when osteotomies are performed close to important soft tissues, such as nerves, blood vessels, or the sinus membrane, or when mechanical or thermal injury must be avoided. The cutting characteristics of Piezosurgery depend on several factors: *(1)* the degree of bone mineralization or density, *(2)* the design of the cutting tip, *(3)* the pressure applied to the handpiece, and *(4)* the speed of operation.

Piezosurgical devices provide a clear surgical site and maintain a blood-free field during bone cutting through the air-water cavitation effect. In piezoelectric surgery, *cavitation* describes the processes of vaporization, bubble generation, and subsequent bubble implosion into many microscopic gas bubbles. This occurs in a flowing liquid

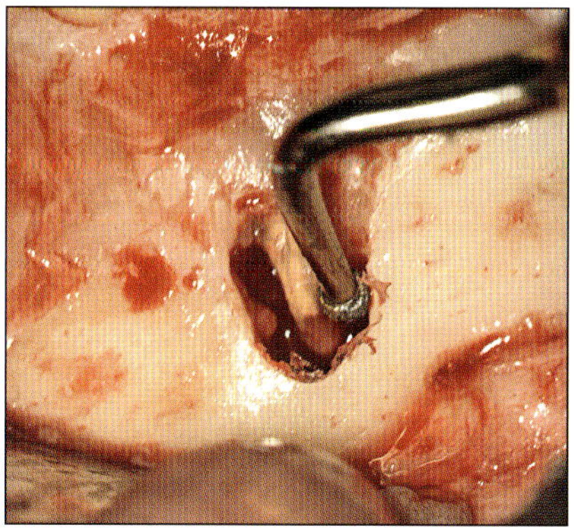

Fig 10-26 Osteotomy performed with the OT5 insert. Note the close proximity to the mental nerve bundle in relation to the periapical lesion and apex of the mandibular right second premolar.

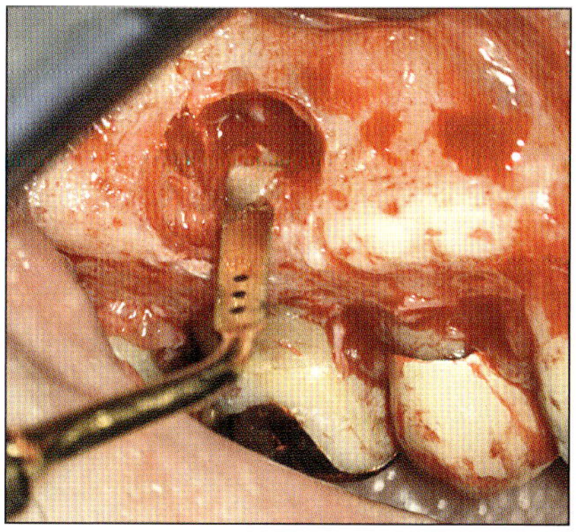

Fig 10-27 Root resection performed with the OT7S-3 insert on the mesiobuccal root of a maxillary right first molar.

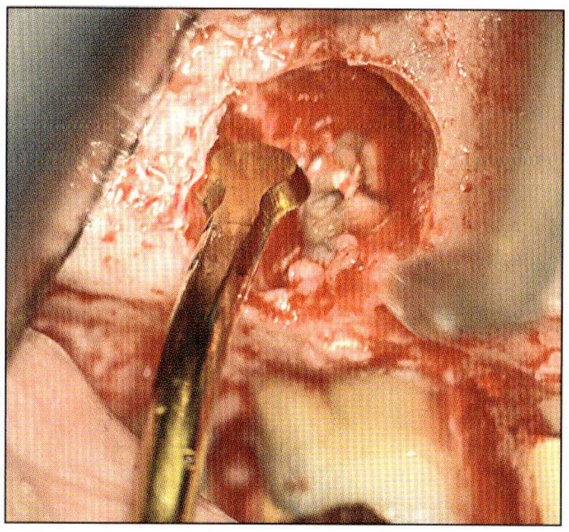

Fig 10-28 Enucleation of the lesion using the OP5 insert in the bony crypt of a maxillary right first molar.

as a result of oscillations in pressure caused by ultrasonic vibrations.[24] Walmsley et al[25] evaluated the cavitation process and concluded that cavitation fragments bacterial cell walls and therefore has an antibacterial function.

One additional advantage and application of Piezosurgery is the ability to completely enucleate radicular cysts, which facilitates the pathologic examination of the entire lesion (Fig 10 28). Most lesions can be removed in their entirety with very little disruption to the adjacent bone and soft tissue.

Apical preparation evaluation and drying the apical preparation

Another development in apical microsurgery has been the introduction of the surgical micromirror. Among the early pioneers of micromirrors was Dr Carlo Zinni, an otorhinolaryngologist from Parma, Italy (Zinni C, personal communication, 1997). Being an early user of the microscope, Zinni recognized the need to indirectly view the pharynx and larynx for proper diagnosis. Zinni crafted the first polished stainless steel mirrors from which the early endodontic micromirrors were developed (Fig 10-29).

Micromirrors come in a variety of shapes and sizes and have diameters ranging from 1 to 5 mm. Many surface materials have been used on micromirrors, including polished stainless steel, polished tungsten carbide, and diamond-like coating. Recently introduced micromirrors utilize a rhodium coating (JEDMED; Fig 10-30). Rhodium is extremely hard and durable and is unsurpassed in reflectivity, clarity, and brightness. They are front-surface scratch resistant and autoclavable. Using the SOM and micromirrors, it is now possible to look up into the apical preparation to check for completeness of tissue removal. Before using micromirrors, it was impossible to assess the thoroughness of apical preparation. Failure to completely remove old root canal filling material and debris from the facial wall of the apical preparation (Fig 10-31) may lead to facial wall leakage and eventual failure if not cleaned before placement of an apical seal. Clearly, it is necessary to circumferentially remove all debris from the apical preparation to satisfy the criteria set forth by Gilheany et al[14] and Ricucci and Siqueira.[15]

Debris can be removed from the facial wall by capturing the maximum cushion of thermoplasticized gutta-percha with a small plugger and condensing it coronally (Fig 10-32). A variety of small pluggers ranging in diameters from 0.25 to 0.75 mm are available for this purpose. Facial wall debris can further be addressed by removal with a back-action ultrasonic tip. Virtually all modern-day ultrasonic tips have some degree of back action in their design. This angle can vary between 70 and 80 degrees. Final inspection should be performed using a micromirror to ensure that the preparation is uniformly clean and free of debris.

Once the apical preparation has been examined, it should be rinsed and dried. Historically, apical preparations were dried with paper points before placing retrofilling materials. This allowed for thorough adaptation of retrofilling materials against the walls of the cavity preparation and decreased the chances of creating material voids. Microcontrol of air and water is now accomplished by using a small blunt microtip irrigating needle (Ultradent) mounted in a Stropko Irrigator (Kerr Endodontics). The irrigator fits over a triflow syringe and allows for the directional microcontrol of air and water (Fig 10-33). Now the beveled root surface and the apical preparation can be completely rinsed and dried before inspection with micromirrors. Anatomical complexities, isthmuses, and tissue remnants are more easily seen when the cut surfaces are thoroughly rinsed and then desiccated (Fig 10-34).

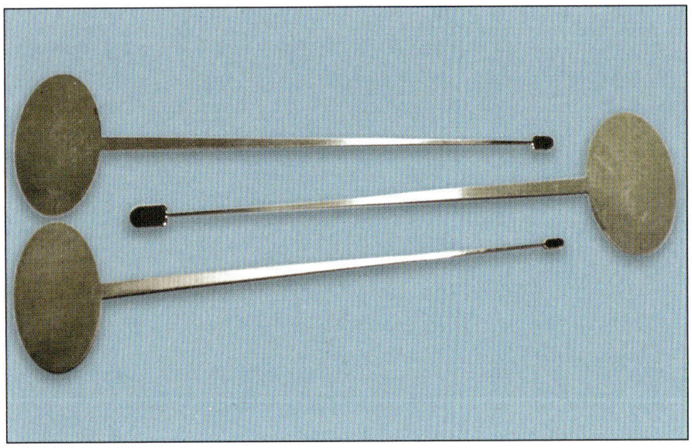

Fig 10-29 Zinni ENT micromirrors.

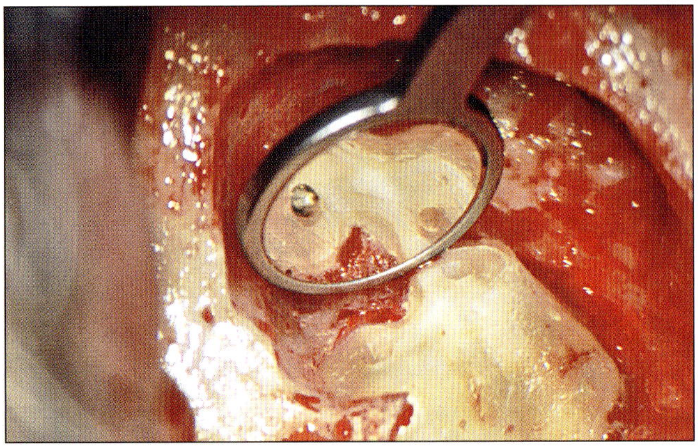

Fig 10-30 Rhodium micromirror view of the beveled surface of the root (magnification ×13).

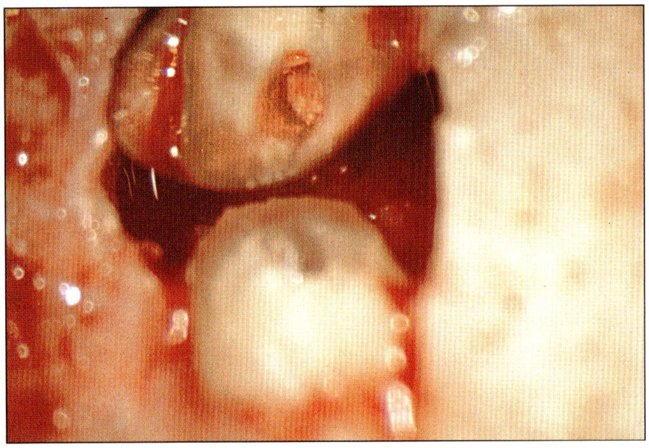

Fig 10-31 Micromirror view of gutta-percha and debris on the facial wall of the apical preparation (magnification ×16).

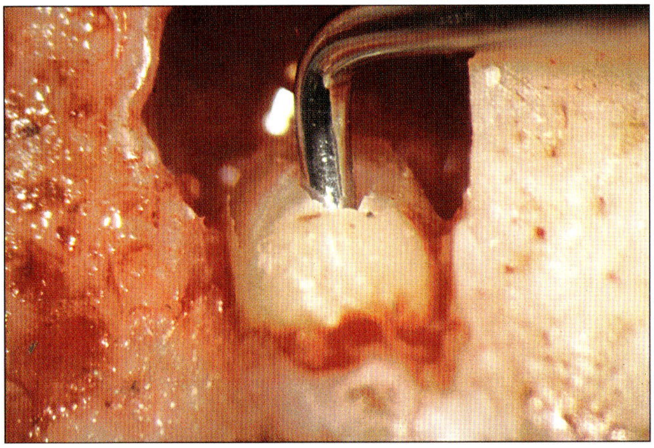

Fig 10-32 Condensing thermoplasticized gutta-percha away from the facial wall and compressing it coronally (magnification ×16).

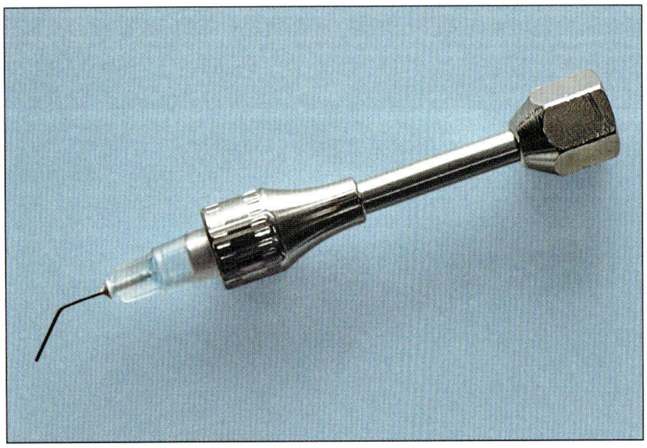

Fig 10-33 Stropko Irrigator with an attached blunt irrigating needle.

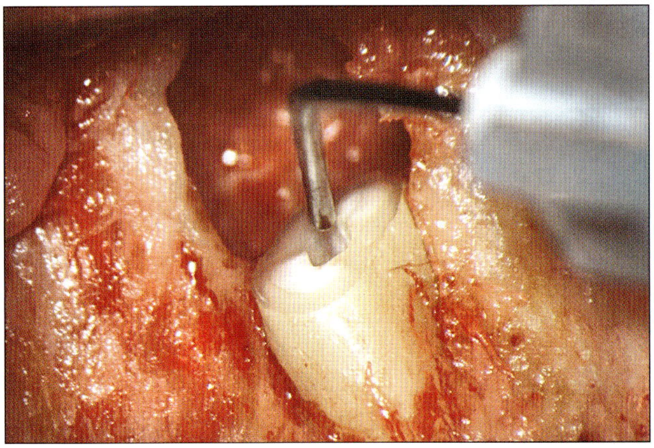

Fig 10-34 Blue Micro Tip (Ultradent) drying the apical preparation (magnification ×13). Note the chalky, dry beveled surface.

Hemostasis

Prior to selecting and placing retrofilling materials, it is essential to have established good hemostasis. Hemostasis begins by obtaining and reviewing the patient's health questionnaire. In addition to the many anticoagulants that patients are prescribed, herbal supplements and a variety of vitamins can complicate hemostasis. Most patients are not aware of the potential surgical complications that are possible from dietary supplements they may be taking. It is critical to evaluate the various pharmaceutical cocktails that patients may be consuming. Patients must be off of daily 81 mg aspirin or fish oil supplements for 7 days in order to reestablish normal platelet function. Consultation with the patient's physician may be necessary. Anesthesia must be profound with adequate vasoconstrictor. In most cases, intraoperative hemostasis is not necessary. Should this not be the case, a variety of materials are available, including ferric sulfate, aluminum chloride, collagen, hemostatic gauze, racemic epinephrine, or electrocautery. When selecting hemostatic agents, one should consider their effect on hard and soft tissue and whether their use could compromise healing. For a complete discussion of local anesthesia and hemostasis, see chapter 8.

Selecting retrofilling materials

After the apical preparation is rinsed and dried and hemostasis is established, retrofilling materials are selected and placed. Historically, amalgam was first suggested for retrofillings by Farrar and reported in *Dental Cosmos* in 1884.[26] This remained the standard until 1959, when Omnell found a cytotoxic precipitate of zinc carbonate, and hence zinc-free amalgam became the retrofilling material of choice.[27] In 1978, Oynick and Oynick observed collagen fibers from the periodontal ligament abutting SuperEBA retrofill cement (Southern Anesthesia & Surgical) and possibly extending into the SuperEBA matrix; they suggested that SuperEBA may promote healing.[28] Based on this single observation, zinc oxide eugenol–based cements such as SuperEBA and desiccated IRM became the materials of choice and were the first modern apical retrofilling materials. Bioceramics such as ProRoot MTA (Dentsply), BioAggregate (Innovative Bioceramix), EndoSequence Root Repair Material (Brasseler USA), Grey MTA Plus (Avalon Biomed), and Biodentine (Septodont USA) were soon to follow. The class of bioceramics includes alumina and zirconia, bioactive glass, glass-ceramics, coatings and composites, calcium silicates, hydroxyapatite, resorbable calcium phosphates, and radiotherapy glasses. The general class is used for joint and tissue replacement and for coating metal implants to improve biocompatibility. They are chemically and physically stable in a biologic environment, and they chemically bond to dentin. ProRoot MTA, BioAggregate, EndoSequence Root Repair Material, and Grey MTA Plus all fit this definition.

The question as to whether SuperEBA has different outcomes than ProRoot MTA was studied by Song et al and reported as a prospective randomized controlled study.[29] They reported that there was no significant difference in the clinical outcomes of endodontic microsurgery when SuperEBA and ProRoot MTA were used as root-end filling materials. The surgical technique may then have a greater bearing on the clinical result than the specific root-end filling material. For a more detailed discussion of root-end filling materials, see chapter 11.

Mixing, placing, condensing, carving, and finishing retrofilling materials

The clinician should select instruments and carriers that allow for direct observation of placement so that he or she can see how the materials perform as they are placed into the apical preparation. Cement-consistency retrofilling materials such as SuperEBA and desiccated IRM are mixed to a putty consistency and carried to the apical preparation in small truncated cones 1 to 2 mm in size on a #12 spoon excavator (Fig 10-35). The cross-sectional diameter of this instrument is 1 mm and therefore does not block the visual access to the apical preparation. The tip of the cone reaches the base of the preparation as the sides of the cone contact the walls. Between each aliquot of material, a small plugger (JEDMED) that will fit inside the apical preparation is used to condense the SuperEBA (Fig 10-36). Additional aliquots of material are added and condensed until there is a slight excess mound of material on the beveled surface of the root. Final compaction is accomplished with a ball burnisher. When the cement has set, a finishing bur or smooth diamond is used to finish the retrofilling. After the SuperEBA has been finished, a CX-1 explorer is used under high magnification to check for marginal integrity and adaptation. Final examination of the retrofilling is performed after the surface has been dried with a Stropko Irrigator, because it is more accurate to check the margins of the preparation when the beveled surface of the root is dry (Fig 10-37). EndoSequence Root Repair Material putty can also be delivered in this fashion. However, finishing EndoSequence Root Repair Material putty is merely done by wiping across the beveled surface of the root with a slightly moistened cotton pellet. The EndoSequence Root Repair Material is also available in syringeable form, which can be injected into the apical preparation, condensed if necessary, and wiped across the beveled surface of the root to finish. The only difference between the putty and syringeable material is the viscosity.

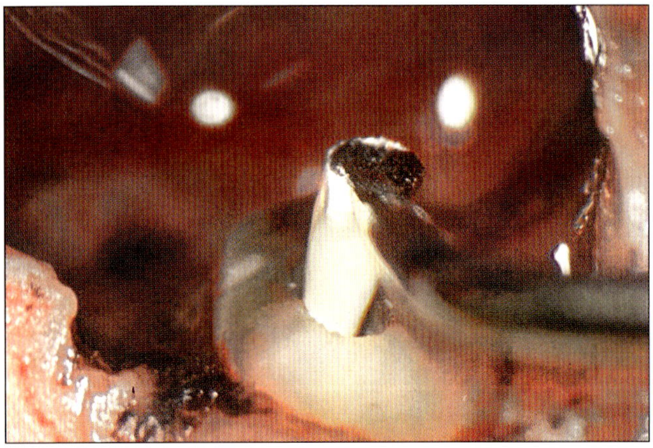

Fig 10-35 Placing SuperEBA into the apical preparation with a #12 spoon excavator (magnification ×16).

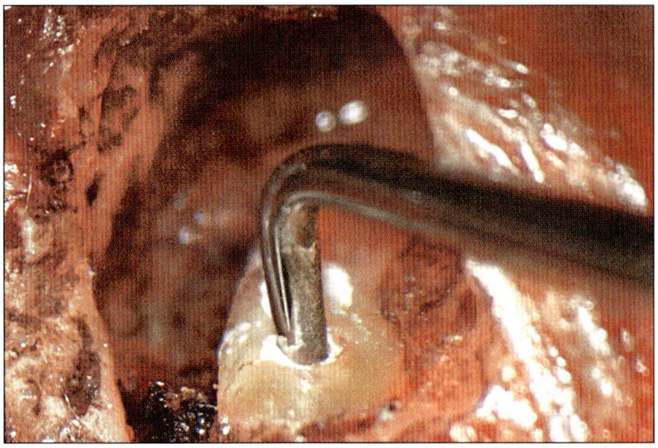

Fig 10-36 Plugging SuperEBA into the apical preparation with a small plugger (magnification ×16).

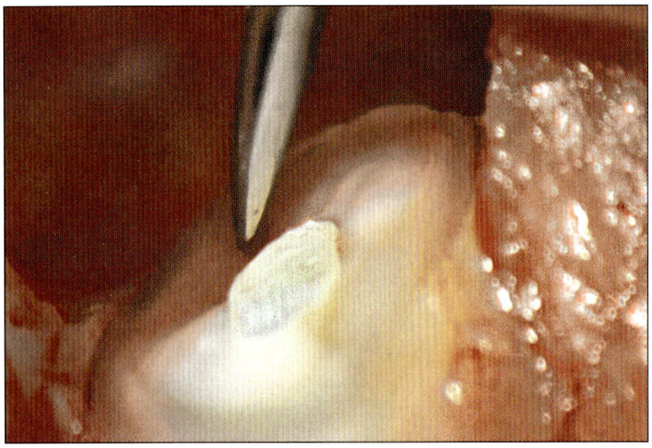

Fig 10-37 Checking for marginal integrity with a CX-1 explorer (magnification ×20).

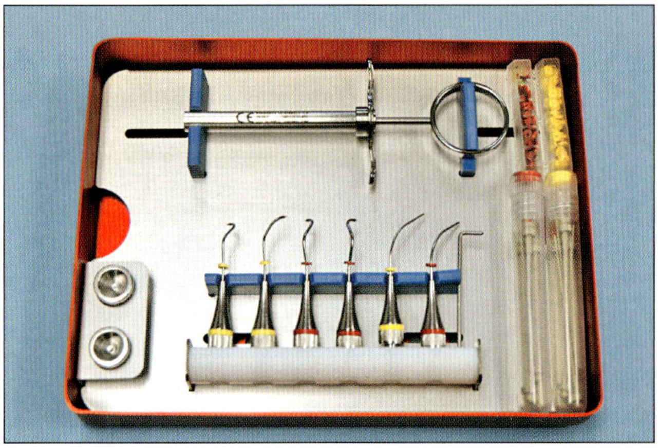

Fig 10-38 Micro Apical Placement System.

Materials such as ProRoot MTA are best delivered to the apical preparation with a carrier-based system. The problems with carriers in the past were that the diameters were too large to fit into the apical preparation, bends were inadequate, and they plugged easily. The Micro Apical Placement (MAP) System (Roydent) addresses these problems (Fig 10-38). This system consists of several delivery tips with cross-sectional diameters ranging from 0.9 mm for small preparations to 1.5 mm for use in large preparations and immature roots. The plungers are made of a poly(ether ether ketone) (PEEK) material, which has a coating similar to Teflon, and therefore retrofilling materials will not stick to the surface. The PEEK plunger can easily navigate a triple-bended carrier. When in use, the carriers should not be packed too tightly, and gentle pressure should be used to express the material. The carriers should be disassembled and cleaned immediately after use; otherwise, mixed materials may set up inside of the tip, and the tip may have to be replaced.

When placing ProRoot MTA, select a carrier that will fit into the apical preparation (Fig 10-39). This will avoid spilling material into the bony crypt. This is mostly a cosmetic issue, because ProRoot MTA is a tricalcium compound. Once it dissolves in tissue fluids, it combines with phosphate ions and produces $CaPO_4$, which is osteoconductive. ProRoot MTA is then condensed with small pluggers that will fit inside the apical preparation to ensure thorough compaction and less chance of leakage. Because ProRoot MTA is cohesive to itself but only slightly adhesive to the walls of the preparation, care must be taken to avoid pulling the material out of the preparation (Fig 10-40). Gentle teasing and drying with a Stropko Irrigator, if necessary, and recapturing and recondensing the material along the walls of the preparation will ensure its complete placement. The recently introduced Grey MTA Plus has a smaller particle size than ProRoot MTA, and as such the mixing and handling properties make it an easy material to use.

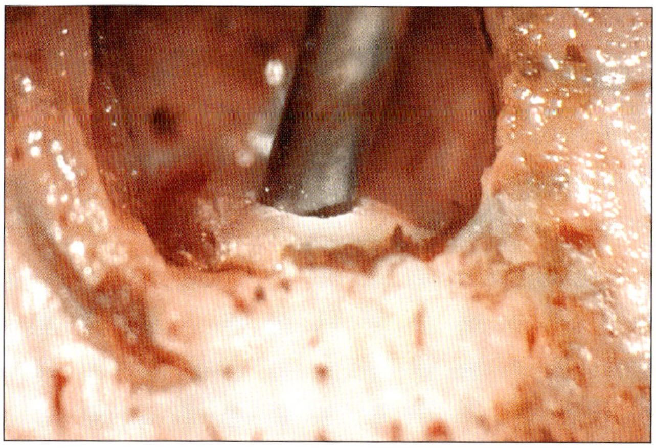

Fig 10-39 MAP carrier placed inside the apical preparation (magnification ×16).

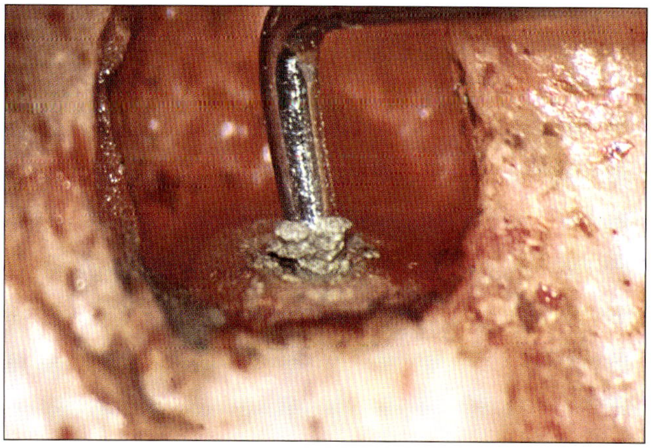

Fig 10-40 ProRoot MTA being pulled out of the apical preparation (magnification ×16).

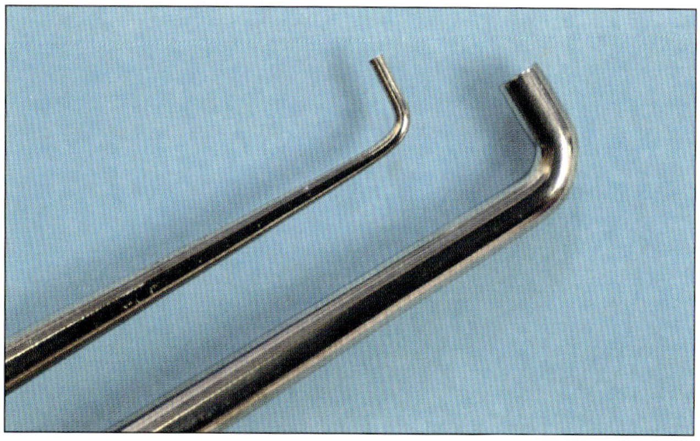

Fig 10-41 Comparison of micro *(left)* and macro *(right)* pluggers.

ProRoot MTA and Grey MTA Plus retrofillings are finished by wiping the beveled surface of the root with a moist cotton pellet. Visual inspection at midrange magnification is used to check for any remaining cotton fibrils and also to check for marginal integrity.

When apical surgery involves immature roots, using small-diameter pluggers to condense retrofilling materials can be inefficient and a waste of time. JEDMED recently introduced three new pluggers. These pluggers incorporate 60- and 90-degree angles, cross-sectional diameters of 1.5 and 2 mm, and a 1-mm ball that address these needs (Fig 10-41). The combination of using a large, 1.5-mm-diameter MAP carrier and a large-diameter plugger provide for efficient retrofilling and condensing of apical preparations made in immature roots or those requiring larger preparations.

Biodentine is a bioactive dentin substitute that has mechanical properties similar to dentin, is highly biocompatible, and has been suggested for use as a retrofilling material. The powder contains tricalcium silicate and, when mixed in an amalgamator for 30 seconds with aqueous calcium chloride, gives the clinician about 12 minutes working time until it sets. The material is carried to the apical preparation in a manner similar to SuperEBA. The main drawback to this material is that it is not very radiopaque and therefore not easily seen on radiograph.

Placing bone grafts and membranes

A frequently asked question is whether a bone graft should be placed in the bony crypt or a membrane placed over the surgical site as a matter of routine. According to a 2011 web-based survey of practicing endodontists by Naylor et al,[30] 40% of the respondents are using guided tissue regeneration (GTR) techniques in conjunction with their root-end surgeries, and a majority of those who did not use GTR indicated that they would consider using these techniques with better evidence and available training. According to the review paper by Lin et al,[31] biologically a clot is a better space filler than all bone grafting materials because it contains the host's own biologic product to provide an excellent scaffold for wound healing. They also concluded that the use of membrane barriers in periapical surgery has not been shown to have a clear benefit in regenerating tissues and that long-term studies designed to provide a high level of evidence are required to provide a better understanding of the use of membrane barriers and bone grafts in periapical surgery. The best application of membrane barriers in periapical surgery appears to be in combined endodontic-periodontal lesions or large periapical lesions communicating with the alveolar crest. They also concluded that there is no conclusive evidence to demonstrate that the application of membrane barriers in large or through-and-through bony lesions has a better long-term outcome than a control group in periapical surgery. While this is true, the cosmetic result from a mature periapical scar can be somewhat disturbing and does present the possibility of a future surgical procedure if the concept of healed by scar is not fully understood.[31]

Molven et al[32] followed 34 cases that were healed by scar at 1 year for 8 to 12 years. Twenty-two remained the same, one healed, and one failed. They concluded that cases that were healed by scar at 1 year could be considered successful in the absence of signs and symptoms.[32] Dahlin et al[33] showed that complete osseous healing of experimentally induced bone defects in rat jaws occurred after 6 weeks when polytetrafluoroethylene (PTFE) membranes were placed on both sides of the defect. Pecora et al[34] repeated the Dahlin study with calcium sulfate as a barrier and found the same results.

If necessary, bone fillers such as DynaBlast paste (Keystone Dental) can be used to graft the bony crypt. This composite graft contains human demineralized bone matrix (DBM) and mineralized cancellous bone from the same donor. The DBM contains bone morphogenetic proteins, which are osteoinductive. The cancellous bone provides the scaffold or matrix. Because this material has a maximum bone chip size of 0.5 mm, it can also be used in periodontal defects. DynaBlast paste is syringeable and can easily be injected into the bony crypt or periodontal defect. DynaBlast putty (Keystone Dental) is a more dense graft material and can be used in larger bony defects, but because the maximum particle size is 1 mm, it cannot be used to treat periodontal defects.

When indicated, membranes such as DynaMatrix membrane (Keystone Dental), harvested from porcine small intestine submucosa, can be used. This material retains its natural composition of collagen plus active tissue proteins, which signal the body to facilitate tissue ingrowth and angiogenesis. When healing is complete, the membrane remodels into the patient's natural tissue and is undetectable. This usually takes 2 to 4 months. DynaMatrix membrane is used for both GTR and guided bone regeneration, is easy to handle, and can be left exposed with no clinical consequences. For further discussion of grafting procedures, see the section on grafting in chapter 15.

Flap closure

The final stage of apical microsurgery is flap closure. Care must be taken to reapproximate the flap in order to promote healing by primary intention. The flap is repositioned by using an Adson tissue forceps. These forceps not only assist in repositioning the flap but also can be used to secure the flap while suturing. Once the flap has been repositioned, a moist sterile 2 × 2 gauze sponge is placed over the flap, and firm finger pressure is applied to restore elasticity to the tissue prior to suturing.

Suturing is a critical part of flap closure. When selecting a suture material, one needs to consider several factors. In addition to securing the flaps closely together, it must be easy to handle, produce little to no inflammation or bacterial contamination, and not dissolve before initial healing is complete. Historically, silk has been the suture of choice for many clinicians due to its excellent handling properties. However, it is a multifilament material, which produces considerable wicking and increased bacterial contamination. Parirokh et al[35] showed significantly more bacterial contamination and physical debris with silk sutures than with polyvinylidene fluoride (PVDF), a monofilament suture, at 3, 5, and 7 days post placement. However, PVDF is difficult to handle and needs to be pulled several times to erase the stiff memory. In addition, patients often complain that the tag ends of the suture are stiff and irritating to the oral mucosa. Tevdek (Teleflex Medical) is a PTFE-coated multifilament suture that acts like a monofilament. This material produces less inflammation and contamination than silk and has the added benefit of having handling properties similar to silk. Because Tevdek is such a soft material, it is suggested that the clinician place an additional throw when tying the surgical knot to maintain its integrity.

While the selection of suture material is important, it is also necessary to consider needle design. Manufacturers have suggested various needle configurations to help the clinician reapproximate the flap and cause as little tissue trauma as possible. Among the choices are reverse cutting needles and tubular side-cutting needles. Reverse cutting needles are more traumatic than tubular side-cutting needles. Because they are sturdier than tubular side-cutting needles, they can withstand occasional contact with interproximal bone if resistance is met while redirecting the needle. On the other hand, the more delicate tubular side-cutting needles may bend if contact is made with bone. Tevdek suture material offers the choice of a double-needled 3/8-inch circle. The KT-1 needle has an arc length of 12.1 mm, making it ideal for reapproximating a vertical incision and for suturing attached gingival flaps. The KT-2 needle has an arc length of 17.8 mm, making it ideal for interproximal suturing. Both of these needles are tubular and site cutting.

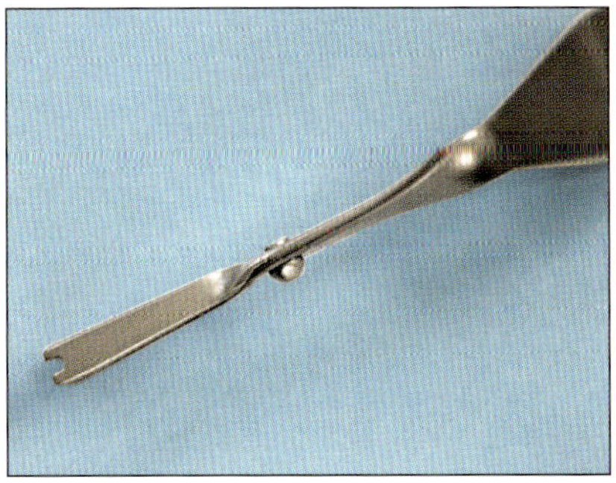

Fig 10-42 Corn Forceps.

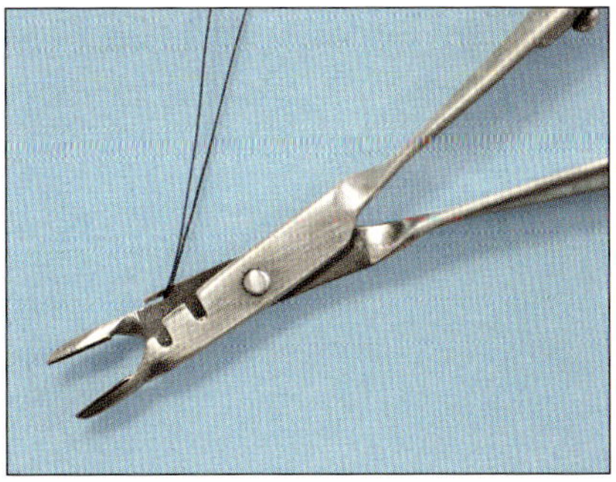

Fig 10-43 Baraquer needle holder/scissors with suture material engaged in the scissors.

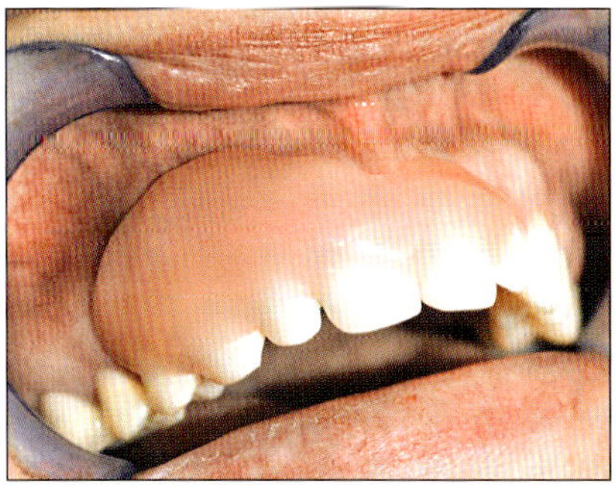

Fig 10-44 Barricaid placed over the surgical wound.

While the Adson tissue forceps can hold the flap firmly while suturing, newer instruments such as the Corn Forceps (Laschal Surgical) are designed for precision needle placement (Fig 10-42). The forceps grasp the tissue, and the needle enters the tissue through an opening in the ends of the forceps.

There are a variety of needle holders available for the clinician. Historically, needle holders were designed to be held like a pair of scissors. Newer designs such as the Mathieu and Castroviejo allow the clinician to place his or her hand closer to the working end of the instrument and allow for more control of the needle. The recently introduced Baraquer needle holder (Laschal Surgical; Fig 10-43) has an additional advantage in that it contains a small scissors that can also cut the suture. Once the knot is tied, the longer portion of the suture material and the tag end of the suture are slid down into the scissors until the needle holder is placed against the knot. Because the needle holder is 2 mm wide, once the scissors is engaged and the suture cut, all tag ends will be the same length. Now the clinician can suture and cut knots with the same instrument.

Once the sutures are placed, the flap should be compressed with a saline-soaked gauze and firm finger pressure for a minimum of 3 minutes. If this is not performed properly, there is a possibility that bleeding may occur under the flap, a hematoma may form, and impaired healing may occur.

If necessary, a periodontal dressing can be placed to protect the surgical site. Historically, zinc oxide eugenol dressings were used for this purpose. However, they were quite messy to mix and difficult to work with. Surgical wound dressings such as Barricaid (Dentsply; Fig 10-44) are much easier to use and are better accepted by the patient. Barricaid is a urethane dimethacrylate resin, which is light cured. The surfaces of the teeth to be covered are dried, and the resin is directly dispensed over the teeth and surgical wound. Using a soapy gloved finger, the material is muscle molded. The dressing is then light cured for 40 to 60 seconds. If necessary, material can be added. The dressing is removed gently with an explorer, with care not to pull the sutures away from the healing site. If the sutures are stuck to the dressing, they should be cut before the dressing is lifted away. For further discussion of suturing and postoperative instructions, see chapter 13.

Suture removal

The key to suture removal is in the healing of the epithelium. Harrison and Jurosky[36] reported that a thin epithelial seal was established in the horizontal incisional wound at 24 hours and that a multilayered epithelial seal was established in the vertical incisional wound between 24 and 48 hours. While some clinicians might infer from this study that sutures could be removed at 48 hours, one must understand that it does not take into account personal habits of patients and their willingness to comply with postoperative directions. Therefore, most clinicians would agree that sutures could be left in place for up to 7 days without causing significant soft tissue irritation. The SOM can be used to facilitate suture removal at low-range magnification. For further discussion on surgical wound healing, see chapter 14.

Microsurgical scissors and tweezers should be used to cut and remove the sutures. The smaller the sutures, the greater the need for microsurgical scissors so as not to damage the flap. Recently introduced for suture removal is the Scissors/Forceps Combination instrument (Laschal Surgical; Fig 10-45). Sutures can now be cut and removed with one hand. The hooked end of the scissors always engages the suture on the right side of the knot, so the forceps side of the instrument faces the knot (Fig 10-46a). If it is engaged on the left side of the knot, you will pull the knot through the flap. On closure, a spring element engages the edge of the scissors and traps the segment of

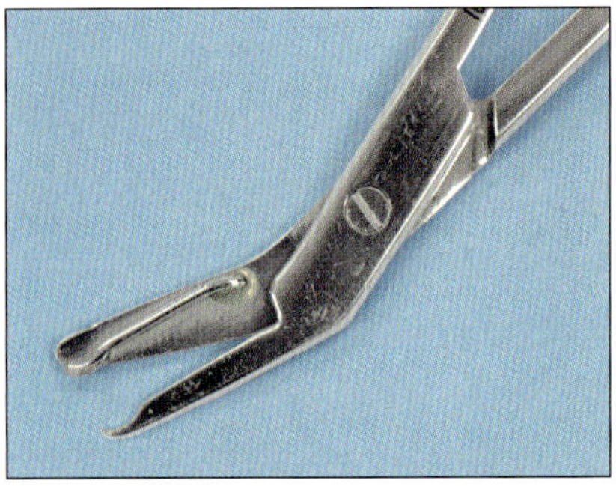

Fig 10-45 Scissors/Forceps Combination suture removal instrument.

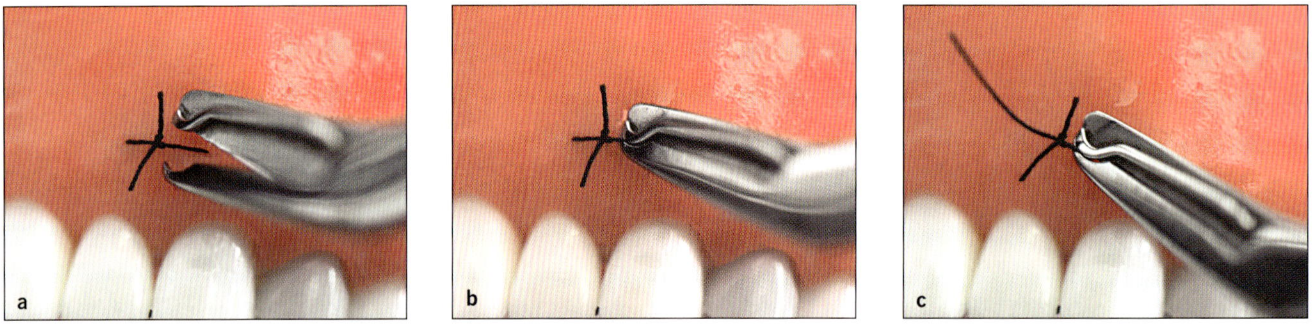

Fig 10-46 *(a)* The hooked end of the Scissors/Forceps Combination suture removal instrument engaging the right side of the knot. *(b)* The spring element engaging the edge of the scissors and trapping the knot. *(c)* Completing the shear, cutting the suture, and lifting it away.

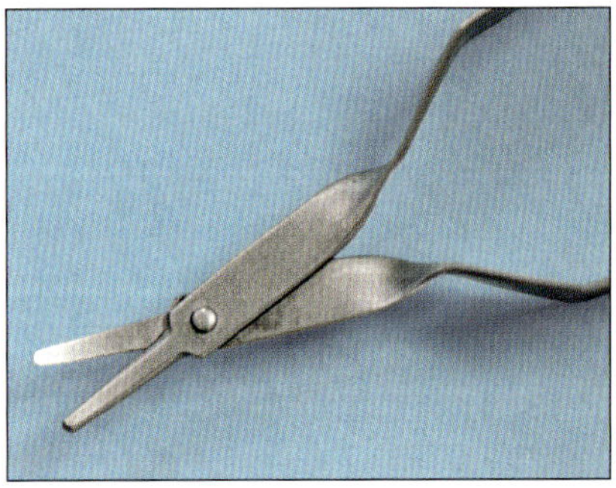

Fig 10-47 Safety-ended suture scissors.

the suture still attached to the knot (Fig 10-46b). Further closure causes the spring element to flex, exposing the sharp blade, completing the shear, and cutting the suture (Fig 10-46c).

If the patient has delayed the time for suture removal and the soft tissue has grown over the knot, suture removal can become problematic. Safety-ended suture scissors (Laschal Surgical; Fig 10-47) have been designed to remove sutures that are buried in edematous or hypertrophic tissue. The blunt rounded blades in the closed position probe to the base of the suture and are then opened to separate the swollen tissue. The scissors are then gently readvanced and the blades closed to cut the suture. The scissors always cut at the very tip of the blades, so the suture is completely severed without shredding.

Does Apical Microsurgery Really Make a Difference?

The SOM was originally introduced as a surgical tool. Almost immediately after its introduction, many clinicians realized its benefit in conventional treatment and nonsurgical retreatment. Consequently, many instruments and devices were developed for use in disassembly, post removal, and removal of separated instruments.

Gorni and Gagliani[37] reported the outcome of 452 nonsurgical retreatment cases 2 years after treatment. The range of magnification used during treatment of the cases was ×3.5 to ×5.5. They reported a success rate of 47% when the root canal morphology had been altered and a success rate of 86.8% when the root canal morphology was respected. The overall success rate reported was 69%.[37] The difficult question to answer when considering a nonsurgical versus a surgical approach is whether the clinician can readdress the original biology of the case. This question may be impossible to answer without actually re-entering the case and possibly rendering the tooth nonrestorable after disassembly. Considering this possible outcome, apical microsurgery may have been a better and more conservative approach. As discussed at the beginning of this chapter, a CBCT study can also assist the clinician in treatment-planning decisions.

Frank et al[38] reported that success rates in apical surgeries sealed with amalgam, which had been considered successful, dropped to 57.7% after 10 years. Friedman et al[39] reported successful treatment results as 44.1% in 136 premolar and molar roots that were observed over a period of 6 months to 8 years. Kvist and Reit[40] in a randomized study compared results of surgically and nonsurgically treated cases. They could find no systematic difference in the outcome of treatment, which ranged in success from 56% to 60%. These studies all used a conventional surgical protocol without the benefit of an SOM and microsurgical armamentarium.

Setzer et al[41,42] in a meta-analysis of the literature compared endodontic microsurgical techniques with and without the use of higher magnification. Weighted pooled success rates calculated from extracted raw data showed an 88% positive outcome for traditional root-end surgery and a 94% positive outcome for apical microsurgery. The difference in probability was statistically significant for molars.

Rubinstein and Kim[43,44] reported the short-term and long-term success rates for apical surgery using the SOM and SuperEBA as the retrofilling material as 96.8% and 91.5%, respectively. The rate of healing independent of lesion size was 7.2 months. Unlike most early conventional surgical studies, which reported the pooled results of multiple clinicians and consisted mostly of anterior teeth, 60% of the cases reported by Rubinstein and Kim consisted of premolar and molar teeth.[45–51]

Several studies have demonstrated a favorable outcome of apical surgery performed with ultrasonic technology similar to that used by Rubinstein and Kim.[43,44,52–55] However, none of these studies used the SOM. Furthermore, the follow-up periods in these studies were considerably shorter, and it must be emphasized that due to variations in treatment and evaluation methods, direct comparisons to the cited studies cannot be made.

More recently, Song et al[56] reported on the long-term outcome of apical microsurgery cases classified as successful when further followed from a previous short-term study. The success rates from the 5-year short-term study were 91.5%. The healed population was then followed for a period of 6 to 10 years. The long-term success for these cases after 6 years was 93.3%.[56] Von Arx et al[57] demonstrated similar results in a 5-year longitudinal assessment of the prognosis of apical microsurgery as 8% poorer than assessed at 1 year.

Assuming that the surgery has been performed properly, it is important to understand the reasons for regression of healing. Some of the reasons for regression have been reported as fracture, periodontal disease, lateral canals, and leaky restorations.[44,56] These are not endodontic in origin and may skew statistics.

Setzer et al[41] showed in a meta-analysis of traditional root-end surgery and endodontic apical microsurgery that the success rate of traditional surgery was 59% and that of apical microsurgery was 94%. The difference was statistically significant, and the relative risk ratio showed that the probability for success for apical microsurgery was 1.58 times the probability of success for traditional surgery.[41] For further discussion on outcomes of endodontic surgery, see chapter 17.

References

1. Veksler AE, Kayrouz GA, Newman MG. Reduction of salivary bacteria by preprocedural rinses with chlorhexidine 0.12%. J Periodontol 1991;62:649–651.
2. Lin LM, Gaengler P, Langeland K. Periradicular curettage. Int Endod J 1996; 29:220–227.
3. Kakehashi S, Stanley HR, Fitzgerald RJ. The effects of surgical exposures of dental pulps in germ-free and conventional laboratory rats. Oral Surg Oral Med Oral Pathol 1965;20:340–349.
4. Weller RN, Niemczyk SP, Kim S. Incidence and position of the canal isthmus. Part 1. Mesiobuccal root of the maxillary first molar. J Endod 1995;21:380–383.
5. West JD. The Relationship Between the Three-Dimensional Endodontic Seal and Endodontic Failures [thesis]. Boston: Boston University, 1975.
6. Kim S, Pecora G, Rubinstein R. Color Atlas of Microsurgery in Endodontics. Philadelphia: Saunders, 2001:21–22.
7. Layton CA, Marshall JG, Morgan LA, Baumgartner JC. Evaluation of cracks associated with ultrasonic root-end preparation. J Endod 1996;22:157–160.
8. Beling KL, Marshall JG, Morgan LA, Baumgartner JC. Evaluation for cracks associated with ultrasonic root-end preparation of gutta-percha filled canals. J Endod 1997;23:323–326.
9. Min MM, Brown CE Jr, Legan JJ, Kafrawy AH. In vitro evaluation of effects of ultrasonic root-end preparation on resected root surfaces. J Endod 1997;23: 624–628.
10. Morgan LA, Marshall JG. A scanning electron microscopic study of in vivo ultrasonic root-end preparations. J Endod 1999;25:567–570.
11. Rainwater A, Jeansonne BG, Sarkar N. Effects of ultrasonic root-end preparation on microcrack formation and leakage. J Endod 2000;26:72–75.
12. Carr GB. Microscopes in endodontics. J Calif Dent Assoc 1992;20(11):55–61.
13. Brent PD, Morgan LA, Marshall JG, Baumgartner JC. Evaluation of diamond-coated ultrasonic instruments for root-end preparation. J Endod 1999;25:672–675.
14. Gilheany PA, Figdor D, Tyas MJ. Apical dentin permeability and microleakage associated with root end resection and retrograde filling. J Endod 1994;20:22–26.
15. Ricucci D, Siqueira JF Jr. Biofilms and apical periodontitis: Study of prevalence and association with clinical and histopathologic findings. J Endod 2010;36:1277–1288.
16. Siqueira JF Jr. Reaction of periradicular tissues to root canal treatment: Benefits and drawbacks. Endod Topics 2005;10:123–147.
17. Nair PN, Henry S, Cano V, Vera J. Microbial status of apical root canal system of human mandibular first molars with primary apical periodontitis after "one-visit" endodontic treatment. Oral Surg Oral Med Oral Pathol Oral Radiol Endod 2005;99:231–252.

18. Teixeira FB, Sano CL, Gomes BP, Zaia AA, Ferraz CC, Souza-Filho FJ. A preliminary in vitro study of the incidence and position of the root canal isthmus in maxillary and mandibular first molars. Int Endod J 2003;36:276–280.
19. Mannocci F, Peru M, Sherriff M, Cook R, Pitt Ford TR. The isthmuses of the mesial root of mandibular molars: A micro-computed tomographic study. Int Endod J 2005;38:558–563.
20. Degerness R, Bowles W. Anatomic determination of the mesiobuccal root resection level in maxillary molars. J Endod 2008;34:1182–1186.
21. Gutarts R, Nusstein J, Reader A, Beck M. In vivo debridement efficacy of ultrasonic irrigation following hand-rotary instrumentation in human mandibular molars. J Endod 2005;31:166–170.
22. Abella F, de Ribot J, Doria G, Duran-Sindreu F, Roig M. Applications of piezoelectric surgery in endodontic surgery: A literature review. J Endod 2014;40:325–332.
23. Vercellotti T. Technological characteristics and clinical indications of piezoelectric bone surgery. Minerva Stomatol 2004;53:207–214.
24. Baldi D, Menini M, Pera F, Ravera G, Pera P. Sinus floor elevation using osteotomes or piezoelectric surgery. Int J Oral Maxillofac Surg 2011;40:497–503.
25. Walmsley AD, Laird WR, Williams AR. Dental plaque removal by cavitational activity during ultrasonic scaling. J Clin Periodontol 1988;15:539–543.
26. Farrar JN. Radical and heroic treatment of alveolar abscess by amputation of roots of teeth, with description and application of the cantalever crown. Dent Cosmos 1884;26:135–139.
27. Omnell KA. Electrolytic precipitation of zinc carbonate in the jaw; An unusual complication after root resection. Oral Surg Oral Med Oral Pathol 1959;12:846–952.
28. Oynick J, Oynick T. A study of a new material for retrograde fillings. J Endod 1978;4:203–206.
29. Song M, Shin SJ, Kim E. Outcomes of endodontic micro-resurgery: A prospective clinical study. J Endod 2011;37:316–320.
30. Naylor J, Mines P, Anderson A, Kwon D. The use of guided tissue regeneration techniques among endodontists: A web-based survey. J Endod 2011;37:1495–1498.
31. Lin L, Chen MY, Ricucci D, Rosenberg PA. Guided tissue regeneration in periapical surgery. J Endod 2010;36:618–625.
32. Molven O, Halse A, Grung B. Incomplete healing (scar tissue) after periapical surgery—Radiographic findings 8 to 12 years after treatment. J Endod 1996; 22:264–268.
33. Dahlin C, Linde A, Gottlow J, Nyman S. Healing of bone defects by guided tissue regeneration. Plast Reconstr Surg 1988;81:672–676.
34. Pecora G, Andreana S, Margarone JE 3rd, Covani U, Sottosanti JS. Bone regeneration with a calcium sulfate barrier. Oral Surg Oral Med Oral Pathol Oral Radiol Endod 1997;84:424–429.
35. Parirokh M, Asgary S, Eghbal MJ, Stowe S, Kakoei S. A scanning electron microscope study of plaque accumulation on silk and PVDF suture materials in oral mucosa. Int Endod J 2004;37:776–781.
36. Harrison JW, Jurosky KA. Wound healing in the tissues of the periodontium following periradicular surgery. I. The incisional wound. J Endod 1991;17:425–435.
37. Gorni FG, Gagliani MM. The outcome of endodontic retreatment: A 2-yr follow-up. J Endod 2004;30:1–4.
38. Frank AL, Glick DH, Patterson SS, Weine FS. Long-term evaluation of surgically placed amalgam fillings. J Endod 1992;18:391–3898.
39. Friedman S, Lustmann J, Shaharabany V. Treatment results of apical surgery in premolar and molar teeth. J Endod 1991;17:30–33.
40. Kvist T, Reit C. Results of endodontic retreatment: A randomized clinical study comparing surgical and nonsurgical procedures. J Endod 1999;25:814–817.
41. Setzer FC, Shah SB, Kohli MR, Karabucak B, Kim S. Outcome of endodontic surgery: A meta-analysis of the literature—Part 1: Comparison of traditional root-end surgery and endodontic microsurgery. J Endod 2010;36:1757–1765.
42. Setzer FC, Kohli MR, Shah SB, Karabucak B, Kim S. Outcome of endodontic surgery: A meta-analysis of the literature—Part 2: Comparison of endodontic microsurgical techniques with and without the use of higher magnification. J Endod 2012;38:1–10.
43. Rubinstein RA, Kim S. Short-term observation of the results of endodontic surgery with the use of a surgical operation microscope and Super-EBA as root-end filling material. J Endod 1999;25:43–48.
44. Rubinstein RA, Kim S. Long-term follow-up of cases considered healed one year after apical microsurgery. J Endod 2002;28:378–383.
45. Dorn SO, Gartner AH. Retrograde filling materials: A retrospective success-failure study of amalgam, EBA, and IRM. J Endod 1990;16:391–393.
46. Finne K, Nord PG, Persson G, Lennartsson B. Retrograde root filling with amalgam and Cavit. Oral Surg Oral Med Oral Pathol 1977;43:621–626.
47. Grung B, Molven O, Halse A. Periapical surgery in a Norwegian county hospital: Follow-up findings of 477 teeth. J Endod 1990;16:411–417.
48. Hirsch JM, Ahlström U, Henrikson PA, Heyden G, Peterson LE. Periapical surgery. Int J Oral Surg 1979;8:173–185.
49. Mattila K, Altonen M. A clinical and roentgenological study of apicoectomized teeth. Odontol Tidskr 1968;76:389–408.
50. Rud J, Andreasen JO, Jensen JE. A follow-up study of 1,000 cases treated by endodontic surgery. Int J Oral Surg 1972;1:215–228.
51. Zuolo ML, Ferreira MO, Gutmann JL. Prognosis in periradicular surgery: A clinical prospective study. Int Endod J 2000;33:91–98.
52. Sumi Y, Hattori H, Hayashi K, Ueda M. Ultrasonic root-end preparation: Clinical and radiographic evaluation of results. J Oral Maxillofac Surg 1996;54:590–593.
53. Sumi Y, Hattori H, Hayashi K, Ueda M. Titanium-inlay—A new root-end filling material. J Endod 1997;23:121–123.
54. Testori T, Capelli M, Milani S, Weinstein RL. Success and failure in periradicular surgery: A longitudinal retrospective analysis. Oral Surg Oral Med Oral Pathol Oral Radiol Endod 1999;87:493–498.
55. von Arx T, Kurt B. Root-end cavity preparation after apicoectomy using a new type of sonic and diamond-surfaced retrotip: A 1-year follow-up study. J Oral Maxillofac Surg 1999;57:656–661.
56. Song M, Chung W, Lee SJ, Kim E. Long-term outcome of the cases classified as successes based on short-term follow-up in endodontic microsurgery. J Endod 2012;38:1192–1196.
57. von Arx T, Jensen SS, Hänni S, Friedman S. Five-year longitudinal assessment of the prognosis of apical microsurgery. J Endod 2012;38:570–579.

Chapter Eleven

Root-End Filling Materials

Masoud Parirokh, Shahrokh Shabahang

Apical surgery is indicated to overcome certain factors that may cause endodontic failure. Short- and long-term evidence-based investigations have shown that placement of a root-end filling improves the outcome of apical surgery.[1,2] A root-end filling material should seal the root-end cavity in order to prevent penetration of microorganisms or their byproducts from the root canal space into the periradicular tissues.[3]

Characteristics of an Ideal Root-End Filling Material

An ideal root-end filling material should be biocompatible, dimensionally stable, nonresorbable, nonmutagenic, easy to handle, insoluble in periradicular tissues, and radiopaque; it should not cause tooth discoloration, it should have reasonable working and setting times, and it should promote cementogenesis.[3,4] Numerous studies have evaluated various dental materials as root-end fillings. These include gutta-percha, polycarboxylate cements, silver cones, amalgam, Cavit (3M ESPE), zinc phosphate cement, gold foil, titanium screws, zinc oxide–eugenol (ZOE) cements (intermediate restorative material [IRM] and SuperEBA [Southern Anesthesia & Surgical]), glass-ionomer cement (GIC), Diaket (3M ESPE), composite resins (Retroplast [Retroplast Trading]), resin–glass ionomer hybrids (Geristore [DenMat]), and mineral trioxide aggregate (ProRoot MTA [Dentsply]). Recently, other bioactive endodontic (BAE) cements have also been evaluated.[3,5] Chemical compositions of currently used materials are listed in Tables 11-1 and 11-2. This chapter highlights results from previous investigations on sealing ability, biocompatibility, and clinical properties of these materials.

Table 11-1 Chemical composition of newly introduced bioactive endodontic cements

Material (manufacturer)	Composition	Regions approved and available for clinical use*
Gray mineral trioxide aggregate (Dentsply)	Tricalcium silicate, dicalcium silicate, bismuth oxide, tricalcium aluminate, calcium sulfate dihydrate (gypsum), and calcium aluminoferrite; liquid: distilled water	FDA, around the world
White mineral trioxide aggregate (Dentsply)	Tricalcium silicate, dicalcium silicate, bismuth oxide, tricalcium aluminate, calcium sulfate dihydrate or gypsum; liquid: distilled water	FDA, around the world
Angelus MTA (Angelus)	Tricalcium silicate, dicalcium silicate, bismuth oxide, tricalcium aluminate, calcium oxide, aluminum oxide, silicon dioxide; liquid: distilled water	FDA 510K clearance; CE Certificate; Health Canada License; JPAL Japanese Certificate; registered in several other countries in Latin America and Asia
BioAggregate (Innovative BioCeramix)	Tricalcium silicate, dicalcium silicate, calcium phosphate monobasic, amorphous silicon oxide and tantalum pentoxides; liquid: deionized water	FDA 510K clearance
Biodentine (Septodont)	Tricalcium silicate, dicalcium silicate, calcium carbonate, zirconium oxide, calcium oxide, iron oxide; liquid: calcium chloride, a hydrosoluble polymer, and water	FDA 510K clearance
Calcium enriched mixture (CEM) cement (BioniqueDent)	Calcium oxide, silicon dioxide, aluminum oxide, magnesium oxide, sulfur trioxide, phosphorus pentoxide, sodium oxide, and chlorine; liquid: water-based solution	Iran Ministry of Health
EndoBinder (Binderware)	Aluminum oxide and calcium oxide	NA
Endocem MTA (Maruchi)	Calcium oxide, aluminum oxide, silicon dioxide, magnesium oxide, iron oxide, sulfur trioxide, titanium dioxide, water/carbon dioxide, and bismuth oxide	CE (Europe), FDA (USA), JET (Japan), TGA (Australia), KFDA (South Korea)
Endocem Zr (Maruchi)	Calcium oxide, silicon dioxide, aluminum oxide, magnesium oxide, ferrous oxide, zirconium oxide	CE (Europe), FDA (USA), TGA (Australia), KFDA (South Korea)
EndoSequence RRM, RRP (Brasseler USA)	Zirconium oxide, calcium silicates, tantalum oxide, calcium phosphate monobasic, and filling and thickening agents	NR
Micro-Mega MTA (Micro-Mega)	Tricalcium silicate, dicalcium silicate, tricalcium aluminate, bismuth oxide, calcium sulfate dehydrate, and magnesium oxide	NR
MTA Bio (Angelus)	Portland cement and bismuth oxide	NR
White MTA Plus (Avalon Biomed)	Tricalcium silicate, dicalcium silicate, bismuth oxide, tricalcium aluminate, and calcium sulfate	Not clear
Gray MTA Plus (Avalon Biomed)	Tricalcium silicate, dicalcium silicate, bismuth oxide, tricalcium aluminate, calcium sulfate, and calcium aluminoferrite	Not clear
Neo MTA Plus (Avalon Biomed)	Tricalcium silicate, dicalcium silicate, tantalite, calcium sulfate, and silica	Not clear
OrthoMTA (BioMTA)	Tricalcium silicate, dicalcium silicate, tricalcium aluminate, tetracalcium aluminoferrite, free calcium oxide, and bismuth oxide	FDA 510K clearance
Quick-Set (Avalon Biomed; patent pending)	Monocalcium aluminate powder that contains bismuth oxide (as a radiopacifier) and hydroxyapatite	NR
RetroMTA (BioMTA)	Calcium carbonate, silicon oxide, aluminum oxide, and hydraulic calcium zirconia complex; liquid: water	FDA 510K clearance
iRoot BP (Innovative BioCeramix)	Zirconium oxide, calcium silicates, tantalum oxide, calcium phosphate monobasic, and filler and thickening agents	FDA 510K clearance
Tech Biosealer RootEnd (Isasan)	Mixture of white CEM, calcium sulfate, calcium chloride, bismuth oxide, and montmorillonite	CE

*An email was sent to all manufacturers regarding regulatory approval for their products as root-end filling materials. NR indicates no response, and NA indicates that no email address was available.

Table 11-2 Chemical composition of other currently used root-end filling materials

Material	Composition
Zinc oxide–eugenol cements	
IRM	Powder: zinc oxide, polymethacrylate; liquid: eugenol and 1% acetic acid
SuperEBA	Powder: zinc oxide, aluminum oxide, natural resins; liquid: eugenol, o-methoxybenzoic acid
Glass-ionomer cement	Powder: calcium aluminosilicate; liquid: polyacrylic acid
Diaket	Powder: zinc oxide, bismuth phosphate; liquid: 2.2-dihydroxy-5.5 dichlorodi-phenylmethane, propionylacetophenone, triethanolamine, caproic acid copolymers of vinyl acetate, and vinyl chloride vinyl isobutylether
Composite resin (Retroplast)	Paste A: Bis-GMA/TEGDMA 1:1, benzoyl peroxide N,N-di-(2-hyydroxyethyl)-p-toluidine, and butylated hydroxytoluene (BHT)
	Paste B: Resin ytterbium trifluoride aerosil ferric oxide; dentin bonding agent: Gluma (Heraeus Kulzer)
Resin-ionomer hybrids	
Geristore (DenMat)	Light cure hydrophilic Bis-GMA (resin-based fluoro alumina silica glass)
Dyract (Dentsply)	Radiopaque fluorosilicate glass in matrix of acidic polymerizable monomers and other light-curing polymers

Sealing Ability

Several methods of testing have been used to evaluate the sealing ability of root-end filling materials. These methods include dye penetration, fluid filtration, protein leakage, glucose concentration test, bacteria and their byproduct penetration tests, and marginal adaptation.[6] All of these methods have certain limitations; nevertheless, they provide some information regarding the ability of the materials to provide an apical seal following root-end resection and preparation.

Dye penetration test

The sealing ability of several root-end filling materials has been evaluated using dye penetration tests.[7,8] Most of these studies have reported that mineral trioxide aggregate (MTA) is more resistant to dye leakage in comparison with SuperEBA, amalgam, or IRM.[6] Composite resin did not show a significant difference in dye leakage compared with GIC.[9] Furthermore, no significant difference in dye leakage was found between white MTA (WMTA) and gray MTA (GMTA) when they were used as root-end filling materials.[10,11] BioAggregate materials (BA) showed significantly lower dye leakage compared with WMTA, IRM, amalgam, and softened gutta-percha.[12]

Dye leakage tests may present significant shortcomings for indicating the sealing ability of a root-end filling material. For instance, methylene blue is one of the commonly used dyes in leakage studies, and its coloring can be impacted by calcium hydroxide (CH). Therefore, methylene blue should not be used to study leakage of materials such as MTA and some BAE cements, which produce CH during hydration.

Another factor that may impact the reliability of dye penetration studies is the effect of tooth storage conditions on future investigations. For example, formalin may influence leakage results. The pH of a dye may also affect leakage results. In contrast to GIC, the porosity and marginal leakage of WMTA may not be affected when immersed in an acidic dye such as rhodamine B.[6]

Despite these shortcomings, a general conclusion from dye penetration studies is that some BAE cements are resistant to dyes when used as root-end filling materials.

Fluid filtration test

Fluid filtration tests have been used to test root-end filling materials and their ability to achieve a good seal. In one study, MTA demonstrated better resistance to fluid penetration than amalgam and SuperEBA.[6] This method has also been used to determine potential improvements in the sealing ability of certain materials depending on the liquid used for hydration. While substitution of 2% chlorhexidine for the normally provided liquid did not significantly improve the sealing ability of Biodentine (BD; Septodont),[13] Calcium Enriched Mixture (CEM) cement (BioniqueDent) showed significantly higher sealing ability when placed in phosphate buffer saline compared with distilled water.[14]

The results obtained with fluid filtration tests have not been consistent with other leakage tests. For instance, when fluid filtration was used to evaluate leakage of WMTA, Fuji IX (GC America), and IRM, Fuji IX showed significantly lower leakage than WMTA and IRM at the 6-month evaluation period; however, when the same researchers employed flow porometry, results showed that IRM and WMTA leak significantly less than Fuji IX.

The type of teeth used (ie, human or bovine) and the size of the cavity preparation may also influence study results when fluid filtration is employed.[6]

Glucose concentration test

The glucose concentration test has also been used as a method to determine the sealing ability of root-end filling materials. Studies using this methodology have shown that WMTA exhibits no significant difference in leakage compared with BA or iRoot BP Plus (Innovative BioCeramix) when used as a root-end filling material.[15,16]

Bacterial and endotoxin penetration tests

A large number of studies have used bacterial penetration as a means to evaluate the sealing ability of root-end filling materials.[6,17] Various species of microorganisms have been used. Earlier studies compared traditional root-end filling materials such as amalgam with newly developed root-end filling materials[6]; however, once MTA was established as a superior material, it soon replaced amalgam as the gold standard for studying and comparing newer root-end filling materials.[17–20]

The available data comparing SuperEBA and MTA with regard to resistance to bacterial penetration is inconsistent. Some investigations have reported significantly higher resistance to bacterial and endotoxin penetration for MTA, while others have found no significant difference between the two materials. On the other hand, compared with IRM, MTA is significantly more resistant to bacterial penetration,[6] while no significant difference has been found between MTA and Resilon, hydroxyapatite, Geristore, composite, or amalgam with ProBond dentin bonding (Dentsply).[6,21]

In one study, results obtained from dye and bacterial penetration did not match when testing BAE cements used as root-end filling materials. While gray MTA showed significantly higher resistance to bacterial penetration compared with CEM cement, no significant difference was found in dye penetration between the same materials.[22]

In another study, both fluid filtration and bacterial leakage tests showed no significant difference between CEM cement and MTA when used as root-end fillings.[23]

Bacterial nutrient leakage test

MTA and EndoSequence Putty (Brasseler USA) showed no significant difference in their sealing ability when a bacterial nutrient leakage test was used to examine their effectiveness.[24]

Factors that may influence sealing ability of root-end filling materials

Environment

BAE cements may interact with their surrounding environment.[4,6] For instance, MTA demonstrated significantly better resistance to bacterial penetration when stored in synthetic tissue fluid compared with samples kept in distilled water.[25] On the other hand, saliva contamination adversely affected the resistance of WMTA to bacterial penetration.[6] In the same study, acidic pH had an adverse effect on the sealing ability of MTA against dye leakage.[6] Interestingly, CEM cement showed significantly lower dye leakage when placed in an environment contaminated with saliva than did MTA.

Dry and blood-contaminated MTA and CEM cement samples showed no significant difference when used as root-end filling materials.[26] CEM cement also showed enhanced sealing ability when placed in phosphate-buffered saline (PBS) compared with distilled water.[14] In another study, blood contamination did not affect the marginal adaptation of MTA, CEM cement, BD, or BA when these materials were placed in root-end cavities.[27]

Thickness of material

Some studies have reported that the thickness of root-end filling materials may have some impact on their sealing ability. Protein leakage studies have shown that root-end filling materials (ie, MTA) placed at less than 4 mm thick with an acidic pH adversely affect sealing ability.[6] In contrast, in other studies, MTA and CEM cement showed no significant difference in dye leakage when 1-, 2-, and 3-mm thicknesses of the materials were tested as root-end fillings.[28,29]

Rinsing root-end cavities with chelating agents

Rinsing root-end cavities prior to placement of root-end filling materials may have an adverse effect on their sealing ability. BA, MTA, and Portland cement (PC) all performed worse in fluid filtration studies when the root-end cavities were rinsed with either MTAD (BioPure, Dentsply) or ethylenediaminetetraacetic acid (EDTA) prior to the material placement; however, rinsing the cavities with either chlorhexidine or distilled water prior to material placement resulted in the lowest amount of apical leakage.[30,31] In contrast, the dye leakage of BD was significantly decreased when the root-end cavities were washed with MTAD prior to placement of the material.[32] More studies are required to determine whether rinsing the root-end cavity preparation prior to placement of the filling material is appropriate.

Placement method

No significant difference in fluid filtration, dye leakage, or bacterial penetration was noted when MTA, WMTA, and CEM cement were placed in an orthograde fashion followed by apical root resection compared with root-end resection and retrograde placement of the materials.[6,33,34] Nevertheless, at least a 3-mm thickness of the material should remain in the root following root resection to provide an optimal seal.[6] Also, sonic vibration during MTA condensation may decrease dye penetration when the material is used as a root-end filling.[35] A recent investigation reported that indirect ultrasonic condensation of MTA can provide a significantly denser root-end filling than placement of the material by manual condensation.[36]

Time

An important issue is the effect of time on the sealing ability of root-end filling materials. BAE cements may interact with the surrounding environment, resulting in formation of crystals on their surface (eg, after immersion in a synthetic tissue fluid).[10,25] Over time, the sealing ability of materials may change. In one study, while Resilon seemed initially more resistant to fluid filtration than WMTA, over time WMTA showed improved sealing ability while Resilon samples showed increased leakage.[37] Therefore, the time elapsed after placement of a particular material should be considered when evaluating data from various studies.

Mixing method

The effect of mixing method on sealing ability of root-end filling materials may depend on the type of material employed. For instance, hand mixing BD induced higher dye leakage when compared with trituration of the material with an amalgamator.[38] In contrast, no significant difference was found among three methods of MTA mixing (ie, trituration with an amalgamator, ultrasonic vibration, and conventional mixing).[18]

Root-end resection, cavity preparation method, and root-end conditioning

In addition to the type of material employed, other factors have been investigated for their potential effects on the sealing properties of root-end filling materials. These include the angle of root-end resection, the device used for root-end preparation, power setting, the type of root-end preparation tip, preconditioning of the root-end cavities, and using finishing burs after placement of the root-end filling.[39–49] No significant difference in dye leakage has been reported between ultrasonic and conventional bur preparation.[39]

GMTA showed significantly less dye leakage than zinc-free silver amalgam when the root end was resected with different bevel angles.[40] When MTA is used as the root-end filling material, the resection angle (45 or 90 degrees) is not a factor as long as the material thickness is 3 mm or more.[41]

The device used for root-end preparation may have an impact on the quality of root-end cavity and sealing ability of the materials. While ultrasonic devices may be a better choice for root-end preparation than certain lasers (ie, Waterlase [Biolase]),[42] the erbium-doped yttrium aluminum garnet (Er:YAG) laser resulted in improved albeit not significantly better resistance to dye leakage around MTA than ultrasonic preparation.[43] When the Er:YAG laser was compared with ultrasonic root-end cavity preparation, cavities filled with MTA resulted in significantly better seal compared with IRM and SuperEBA.[6]

In a more recent investigation, root-end cavities prepared with the Er:YAG laser and filled with BD provided significantly higher resistance to dye leakage than cavities filled with MTA and prepared with the Er:YAG laser or ultrasonics.[44] These results were somewhat refuted by another study that demonstrated significantly higher resistance to dye leakage in root-end cavities prepared with ultrasonic tips and filled with MTA compared with BD.[39]

Lasers can be used either for root-end cavity preparation or for pretreating root-end cavities. One study compared MTA and iRoot BP after pretreatment with EDTA or the erbium, chromium–doped yttrium, scandium, gallium and garnet (Er,Cr:YSGG) laser. Scanning electron microscope (SEM) evaluation showed that while no significant difference in marginal adaptation was found between the two pretreatment protocols for each material, in both conditions MTA provided superior marginal adaptation to iRoot BP.[45]

The presence of cracks originating from the root canal can adversely affect the seal of root-end fillings. Although MTA and GIC show no difference in sealing ability, when cracks are present, MTA provides a better seal.[6]

Type of ultrasonic tip and power setting of the device may also influence leakage following root-end preparation. A glucose leakage investigation showed that when SuperEBA was used for root-end filling, preparation of the root-end cavity with a diamond-coated retro tip with a high power setting provided significantly lower leakage than zirconium nitride–coated and stainless steel ultrasonic retro tips with either low or high power settings.[46]

While acid etching root-end cavity walls prior to MTA placement may improve the marginal adaptation of the material,[47] it did not have a significant influence on the sealing ability of WMTA when used as a root-end filling material.[47]

While some clinicians recommend the use of finishing burs in order to improve marginal adaptation of root-end filling materials, SEM evaluation showed that using finishing burs does not improve the seal of root-end fillings when root-end cavities were filled with MTA; however, SuperEBA and IRM showed significantly better adaptation following the use of finishing burs.[48] In another study, dye penetration was not reduced after using finishing burs on IRM and SuperEBA when used as root-end filling materials.[49]

Marginal Adaptation

One of the main reasons for failure following periapical surgery is inadequate root-end filling or gap formation between the root-end filling materials and the dentin. Both SEM and confocal microscope investigations have been used to evaluate marginal adaptation of root-end filling materials.[50–64]

SEM

Numerous investigations have evaluated the marginal adaptation of root-end filling materials. SEM studies have shown imperfect root-end filling adaptation in the majority of failed cases.[51] Good marginal adaptation has been demonstrated for WMTA by some investigators.[6] Most studies have reported that MTA has a better marginal adaptation than IRM, SuperEBA,[6,48] amalgam,[6,53] and GIC.[6] Nevertheless, one study reported no significant difference in marginal adaptation among MTA, IRM, SuperEBA, and Resilon.[54] Additionally, no significant difference has been found between the marginal adaptation of GMTA and WMTA.[55,56] In other studies, MTA and cold ceramic had similar marginal adaptation[62] while WMTA showed significantly better marginal adaptation than Sealer 26 (Dentsply).[57] It is important to note that MTA is an interactive material, and thus the marginal adaptation of the material may be impacted in certain media (eg, synthetic tissue fluid), which could cause formation of apatite crystals at the material interface.[25,58]

MTA, CEM cement, BD, and BA showed no significant difference in marginal adaptation in the presence of blood.[27] Similarly, no significant difference has been observed in the marginal adaptation of WMTA, OrthoMTA (BioMTA), and RetroMTA (BioMTA) in the presence of PBS.[59] Both MTA and IRM have shown significantly better marginal adaptation than BD.[60]

The type of SEM and the condition of preparing the samples can influence the results of marginal adaptation of root-end filling materials.[6] In addition, evaluating transversal or longitudinal sections may provide different results.[61] In one study, WMTA and two forms of EndoSequence RRM (putty and paste; Brasseler USA) showed similar marginal adaptation in transverse sections; however, WMTA and EndoSequence Putty showed significantly better results than EndoSequence Paste in longitudinal sections.[61]

Confocal laser scanning microscope

The confocal laser scanning microscope is a very useful device to evaluate the marginal adaptation of root-end filling materials.[52] Several investigations have used confocal microscopy to evaluate leakage and marginal adaptation of root-end filling materials. These studies showed excellent marginal adaptation when MTA was used as a root-end filling.[39,43,44,63,64] BD showed significantly better marginal adaptation than white MTA or GIC.[64]

In conclusion, MTA and some BAE cements have shown reasonable marginal adaptation.

Biocompatibility

The biocompatibility of dental materials is evaluated by in vitro and in vivo tests. Cell viability and genotoxicity of dental materials are evaluated by in vitro studies, whereas in vivo tests, including subcutaneous and intraosseous implantation, evaluate the connective tissue response to dental materials.[6,65,66]

Bioactivity of dental materials can be evaluated by in vitro and in vivo tests.[67,68] In recent years, in vitro biocompatibility investigations of biomaterials, particularly BAE cements, have attracted more attention because of their ability to promote cell growth, differentiation, and adhesion.[69–71]

Genotoxicity

Determination of genotoxicity is necessary in order to evaluate possible risks of a dental material on human genetic components.[72] Most investigations have reported

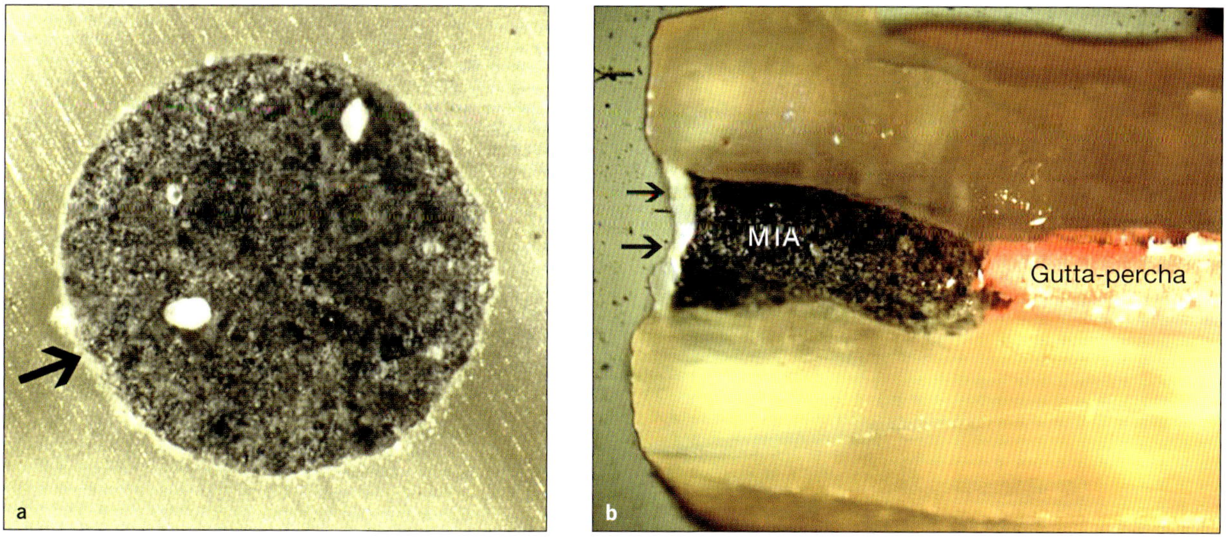

Fig 11-1 *(a)* Precipitation of hydroxyapatite over GMTA when placed as a root-end filling material. The precipitate can also be seen between the material and root canal walls *(arrow)*. *(b)* Precipitation of apatite crystals over MTA when placed as a root-end filling *(arrows)*.

genotoxicity with regard to GIC, amalgam, and composite resins.[73–78] The degree of genotoxicity is not similar in different types of GICs and composite resins.[79–83]

SuperEBA, IRM, MTA, CEM cement, MTA, BD, and EndoSequence BC sealer (Brasseler USA) have demonstrated acceptable biocompatibility in terms of genotoxicity.[84–93] Among BAE cements, currently only MTA Fillapex (Angelus) has shown genotoxicity.[72]

In conclusion, the genotoxicities of various types of BAE cements, composite resins, and GICs are not identical. In addition to the composition of a material, the concentration of any given material may also influence its genotoxicity. Most new BAE cements have not been evaluated for genotoxicity.

Bioactivity

Bioactivity refers to the interaction of materials with the surrounding environment, which is evaluated when the material is immersed in a synthetic tissue fluid.[94] ISO 23317 (in vitro evaluation for apatite-forming ability of implant materials) is used for evaluating bioactivity of a material when immersed in a synthetic tissue fluid (Fig 11-1).

Bioactivity may enhance the sealing ability of root-end filling materials by providing a chemical bond between the material and the surrounding tissues.[4,25,95] Some of the materials used as root-end filling materials, such as amalgam, are not bioactive.[96] In contrast, most BAE cements cause formation of an apatite layer between the material and the surrounding dentinal wall (see Fig 11-1a). MTA, Endocem MTA (Maruchi), Endocem Zr (Maruchi), BA, EndoSequence Putty, CEM cement, and BD have demonstrated bioactivity.[94,97–100]

The level of bioactivity is not similar in all BAE cements. For instance, MTA releases significantly higher levels of calcium and provides a higher calcium-phosphorus ratio in the precipitate compared with Endocem Zr.[98,99] Apatite layer formation between BAE cements and the tooth structure is also considered a sign of bioactivity. One study showed that the thickness of the interface layer in MTA-treated teeth is significantly higher than that found in teeth treated with BD.[98] The amount of calcium and silicate ions incorporated into the dentinal walls may be one of the signs of bioactivity of dental materials. BD and WMTA have demonstrated significantly higher calcium ion release than EndoSequence BC sealer.[101]

The calcium-silicon ratio and the composition of precipitate are not similar when various BAE cements are immersed in PBS.[97,99]

Bioactivity is one of the most important properties of BAE cements, and it is one of reasons that these materials have received more attention in biomedical tissue engineering.[67] The bioactivity of a material also refers to its ability to interact with cells to promote a specific response. These properties can be studied in cell cultures, where biomineralization is assessed through alkaline phosphatase (ALP) activity, and in in vivo studies through the formation of hard tissues.[68,102]

Some BAE cements increase ALP activity, while others have either no effect or diminish the activity (Table 11-3).

For instance, an osteoblast-like cell culture was used to evaluate the effect of MTA and EndoSequence RRM on

Table 11-3 Changes in the gene expression of various signaling molecules and markers following the presence of BAE cements or their extracts

Material	ALP	TGF-β	Col 1	OPN	OCN	OX	OSN	RUNX2	BMP	DSP	BSP	COX2	PGE2	MEP	NO	DMP-1	IL-1β	IL-6	IL-8	VEGF	TNF-α	MMP	ROS
PC	↑	↑	↑	↑	↑	↑	↔	↑	–	↑	↑	–	–	↑	↑	↑	–	–	–	–	–	–	–
AMTA	↑	–	–	–	–	–	–	–	–	–	–	↓	↓	–	↓	–	↑	↓	↓	–	↓	↓	↓
GMTA	↑	↑	↑	↑	↑	↑	↑	↑	↓	↑	–	↓	↓	–	↓	–	↔	↓	↔	↑	↓	–	↓
WMTA	↑	↑	–	↑	–	–	↑	–	–	↑	↑	↑	–	↑	↑	↑	↑	–	–	–	–	–	–
BA	↑	–	↑	↑	–	–	↑	–		–	–	↓	↓	–	↓	–	↓	↓	↓	–	↓	–	–
MM MTA	↑	–	↑	–	–	–	↑	–		–	–	–	↓	–	↓	–	↓	↓	↓	↑	↓	–	–
BD	↔	↑	↔	–	–	–	↑	↔	↑	↔	↑	–	–	–	–	↑	↓	↓	↓	–	↔	↓	↓
Endocem	↑	–	–	↓	–	–	↑	–		↑	–	–	–	–	–	↑	–	–	–	–	–	–	–
CEM cement	↑	–	↑	–	↑	–	–	–	↓	–	–	–	–	–	–	–	–	–	–	–	–	–	–
iRoot BP Plus	↑	–	–	–	–	–	–	–	–	–	–	–	–	–	–	–	–	–	–	–	–	–	–
White MTA Plus	–	–	–	–	–	–	–	–	–	–	–	–	–	–	–	–	–	–	–	–	–	–	↓
Gray MTA Plus	–	–	–	–	–	–	–	–	–	–	–	–	–	–	–	–	–	–	–	–	–	–	↓
Ortho MTA	↑	–	–	↓	↑	–	–	–	–	↑	–	↓	↓	–	↓	–	↓	↓	↓	–	↓	↓	↓
EndoSequence Putty	–	–	–	–	–	–	–	–	–	–	–	–	–	–	–	–	↑	↑	↑	–	↓	–	–
EndoSequence Flow	↑	–	–	–	–	–	–	–	–	–	–	–	–	–	–	–	↑	↑	↑	↑	↓	–	–
TBE	↓	–	–	–	–	–	–	–	–	–	↓	–	–	–	–	–	–	–	–	–	–	–	–
Quick-Set	–	–	–	–	–	–	–	–	–	–	–	–	–	–	–	–	↓	–	–	–	–	–	–

–, no significant change in the marker or it has not been investigated yet; ↑, upregulated; ↓, downregulated; ↔, scarce results (some studies showed upregulation, some downregulation, and some no significant difference to the control); ALP, alkaline phosphatase; TGF-β, transforming growth factor beta; Col 1, collagen 1; OPN, osteopontin; OCN, osteocalcin; OX, Osterix; OSN, osteonectin; RUNX2, Runt-related transcription factor 2; BMP, bone morphogenetic protein; DSP, dentin sialophosphoprotein; BSP, bone sialophosphoprotein; COX2, cyclooxygenase 2; PGE2, prostaglandin E2; MEP, matrix extracellular phosphoglycoprotein; NO, nitrous oxide; DMP-1, dentin matrix protein-1; IL-1β, interleukin 1 beta; IL-6, interleukin 6; IL-8, interleukin 8; VEGF, vascular endothelial growth factor; TNF-α, tumor necrosis factor alpha; MMP, matrix metalloproteinase; ROS, reactive oxygen species; AMTA, Angelus MTA; MM MTA, Micro-Mega MTA; TBE, Tech BioSealer Endo (Isasan).

cellular bioactivity and ALP activity; it showed that EndoSequence RRM significantly lowers bioactivity as well as ALP activity in all time periods, whereas MTA has no effect on these activities.[103]

The long-term benefits of bioactivity may lie in the ability of bioactive materials to induce formation of hard tissues (ie, cementum) over the entire root end. This coverage would provide a double seal layer that would include a biologic seal, further reducing the chance of microleakage of irritants into the periapical tissues. Furthermore, this biologic seal would allow regeneration of the periodontal apparatus surrounding the root structure.

Biologic Mechanism of Action of BAE Cements

MTA can induce cell differentiation, angiogenesis, and mineralization. Several mechanisms have been proposed for these effects. Mitogen-activated protein kinase (MAPK), extracellular signal-regulated kinase (ERK), and c-Jun N-terminal kinase (JNK), as well as nuclear factor kappa B (NFκB), p38, and bone morphogenetic protein (BMP)/Smad signaling pathways are all involved in cell differentiation and the mineralization activity of MTA. Calcium and silica ion release is recognized as one of the main reasons for MTA activity.[104–108]

It should be noted that various biomaterials conduct their activity via various pathways. For instance, inhibiting MAPK and calcium-calmodulin-dependent protein kinase II downregulate the mineralization effect of BD. While p38 MAPK inhibitors have no effect on the mineralization induction of BD, the MAPK inhibitor for ERK 1/2 (U0126) and JNK (SP600125) significantly decrease the mineralization effect of the material in cell culture.[109]

The exact mechanism of action and sequence of gene expression in response to various BAE cements as well as the impact of the chemical composition of these materials on their inherent properties are not completely understood. It is well recognized that the pH and the ability to promote release of ions play important roles in various properties of BAE cements. Calcium and silicate have been shown to have an important influence on cell proliferation, differentiation, and function. Studies on BAE cements including MTA, BD, and BA have shown that these materials can activate osteogenic/odontogenic properties of dental pulp cells via proliferation, angiogenesis, and mineralization. Various systems are responsible for these events, including ERK 1/2, nuclear factor E2-related factor 2, p38, JNK, MAPK, p42/p44 mitogen-activated protein kinase, NFκB, and fibroblast growth factor receptor pathways.[67]

Cell viability

The data regarding cytotoxicity of Geristore is sparse. In a human fibroblast cell culture study, Geristore showed superior cell viability, morphology, adhesion, and attachment compared with MTA and GIC.[110] However, in another study using L929 mouse fibroblast cells to compare Geristore with WMTA, investigators showed no significant difference between the materials up to the 3-week observation period.[111] One may conclude that the cell line may have some impact on the results of cell viability tests.[6]

Several investigations on various cell lines have shown no significant difference between MTA and CEM cement cell viability.[91,112–116] The study length may also influence cell viability results. Two investigations reported higher cell toxicity in CEM cement than in MTA in early time periods, whereas data from later time periods showed no significant difference between the two materials.[117,118] Most cell viability studies have found no significant difference between EndoSequence RRM and WMTA, GMTA, white Angelus MTA (WAMTA), and BD in various cell culture models (dermal fibroblast, L929 fibroblast, gingival human fibroblast, periodontal ligament fibroblast, osteoblast [MG63], and dental cell cultures).[119–124]

IRM has demonstrated significantly higher cytotoxicity than Quick-Set (Avalon Biomed), MM MTA (Micro-Mega), and BA.[125,126] MTA has also shown significantly better cell viability than amalgam.[53] Incorporation of MTA with GIC decreased the cytotoxicity of the GIC.[127] Comparison of EndoBinder (EB; Binderware) with Angelus MTA (AMTA) and WAMTA has shown similar cell viability for all test materials with no significant difference compared with the control group.[128,129] Both WAMTA and MTA-Bio (Angelus) have shown low toxicity with no significant difference from controls. However, MTA-Bio has shown to have an irregular surface with more porosity than WAMTA.[130]

Gene expression of signaling molecules and markers

Numerous investigations have evaluated signaling molecule expression or release when BAE cements or their extracts have been exposed to various cell cultures.[69,114,123,126–128,131–151] BAE cements may either upregulate or downregulate signaling molecules; however, some investigations have reported inconsistent results. Table 11-3 shows a wide range of signaling molecules that may be present or expressed when either the material or its extracts are placed in cell cultures. Some studies have shown that BAE cements increase certain signaling molecules, while others have shown that they have no effect or even downregulate the molecules. The variability in published findings may be a result of the duration of the study and differences in the cell lines that were used.

Reactive oxygen species (ROS) are naturally produced during oxygen metabolism, which may have an important effect in maintaining cell health, multiplication, and signaling. Upregulation of ROS results in cell damage. GMTA may have an influence on ROS because the material significantly downregulates ROS in rat odontoblast-like cells (MPDC-23).[127]

The impact of biomaterials on specific gene expression is an important issue in endodontics. In fact, the materials' properties in cell differentiation, migration, mineralization, and inflammation can be evaluated by their gene expression in cell cultures. Numerous studies have investigated gene expression of various cell lines, including human dental pulp cells, dental pulp stem cells, and murine dental papilla–derived odontoblast-like cell lines (MDPC-23). Some studies evaluated thousands of genes to detect any change on them following exposure to the biomaterials, whereas others have focused on specific genes that have been implicated in various biologic processes (ie, mineralization, differentiation, inflammation, and migration). These studies have shown that MTA, BD, BA, α-tricalcium phosphate (α-TCP), Quick-Set, iRoot BP, iRoot BP Plus, and CEM cement upregulate or downregulate genes involved in differentiation, migration, mineralization, and inflammation.[116,140,150,152–158]

Gene expression in response to MTA and other BAE cements mostly points to specific genes and their changes in cell cultures. These gene products include collagen type 1 (*COL1A1*), *ALP*, Runt-related transcription factor 2 (*RUNX2*), osteocalcin (*OCN*), dexamethasone sodium phosphate (*DSP*), *BMP*, osteonectin (*OSN*), bone sialoprotein (*BSP*), osteopontin (*OPN*), dentin sialophosphoprotein (*DSPP*), heme oxygenase 1 (*HO-1*), vascular endothelial growth factor (*VEGF*), receptor activator of nuclear factor kappa-B (*RANK*), *TRAF6*, *NFκB*, and *NFATC1*.[116,140,152–159]

Investigation of gene expression and signaling molecules in most studies have been focused on the following genes:

- Osteogenic gene products: *OCN*, *BSP*, and *ALP*
- Odontogenic gene expression: *BMP*, *OSN*, *BSP*, *OPN*, *DSPP*, *COL1*, and *HO-1*
- Proinflammatory mediators: nitrous oxide (*NO*), prostaglandin E2 (*PGE2*), cyclooxygenase 2 (*COX-2*), interleukin 1 alpha (*IL-1α*), interleukin 6 (*IL-6*), and interleukin 8 (*IL-8*)

Biomaterials may not induce their effects via similar genes. They may induce their effects by increasing or decreasing expression of different genes.[150,157,159] MTA, BA, and BD upregulate some genes while downregulating others.[154,158,160] For instance, both MTA and BA have shown a significant increase in osteogenic genes in terms of OCN, BSP, and ALP activity compared with controls; however, BD has no significant effect on expression of these genes compared with controls.[161]

In a three-dimensional human stem cell dental pulp cell culture study, BD was compared with MTA to evaluate expression of mineralization-associated genes (*COL1A1*, *ALP*, *DSPP*, and *RUNX2*) for up to 14 days. Both MTA and BD had similar expression patterns of mineralization-associated genes.[150] Significantly higher expression levels of *COL1A1* and *OSN* genes were observed for BD, MTA, and MM MTA compared with the control.[162]

In a 3D Balb/c 3T3 fibroblast cell culture model, WAMTA and BD showed similar cell viability to the control after a 24-hour exposure time. No significant difference was found between the two materials regarding the level of tumor necrosis factor alpha (TNF-α) when compared with the control group; however, IL-1α was significantly upregulated compared with the control for both materials. The limitation of this study was the short evaluation time.[163]

There is some discussion regarding the cell types that should be used for evaluating cytotoxicity and signaling molecules when testing dental materials. Many cell lines have similar responses to dental materials. For instance, MG-63 osteosarcoma cells may produce similar cytokine responses to osteoblasts.[163] Although many studies have used MG-63 cells to evaluate BAE cements,[123,136,155,164–166] because MTA and BAE cements could have an impact on genes, the selection of cell types may be important. For example, the use of human osteosarcoma cells (MG-63 and Saos-2) is not suitable for BAE cements because chromosomal alterations of these cell types may induce abnormal functions in both cellular and molecular levels. Thus, the use of malignant cell lines to assess materials' biologic properties may be unreasonable.[167]

Another important point is the difference in the method of evaluation. In one study, enzyme-linked immunosorbent assay showed higher COL1 and BSP expression on day 6 in response to iRoot SP compared with AH Plus (Dentsply), whereas real-time polymerase chain reaction (PCR) showed no significant difference between the groups in the same period of time.[168]

Certain markers have been identified as early (ALP and OSN), middle (OPN), or late (OCN) differentiation markers.[169] Studies on gene expression of some BAE cements (PC, BD, AMTA, OrthoMTA, Micro-Mega MTA, Endocem) have demonstrated that there is no significant difference in the amount of gene expression among these materials. In contrast, other root-end filling materials (iRoot BP Plus, BA, and CEM cement) have illustrated significantly higher gene expression than MTA; however, MTA provided significantly higher transforming growth factor beta-1 (TGF-β1) than CEM cement.[67]

Differences observed in the amount of secretion of certain cytokines, signaling molecules, and markers in response to biomaterials may vary depending on the statistical analysis method used. In a study on MG-63 osteoblasts, analysis of variance showed no significant difference between MTA and EndoSequence RRM, while a t-test showed a significant difference between the materials.[123]

In conclusion, BAE cements certainly have an impact on the expression of genes and signaling molecules and markers that are involved in cell differentiation, migration, inflammation, and mineralization. Nevertheless, it should be kept in mind that detection of gene expression and signaling molecules following exposure to the cements may depend on various parameters such as the duration of the study period, concentration of the test material(s), time of assessment, number of genes that are to be detected, type of cell culture, and method of statistical analysis used.[123,157]

Subcutaneous implantation

Most investigations on MTA have reported moderate to severe tissue reactions at early time intervals following subcutaneous implantation that eventually subside in later evaluation periods[6,170–172] (Fig 11-2). Most studies have observed a trend in reduction of tissue response

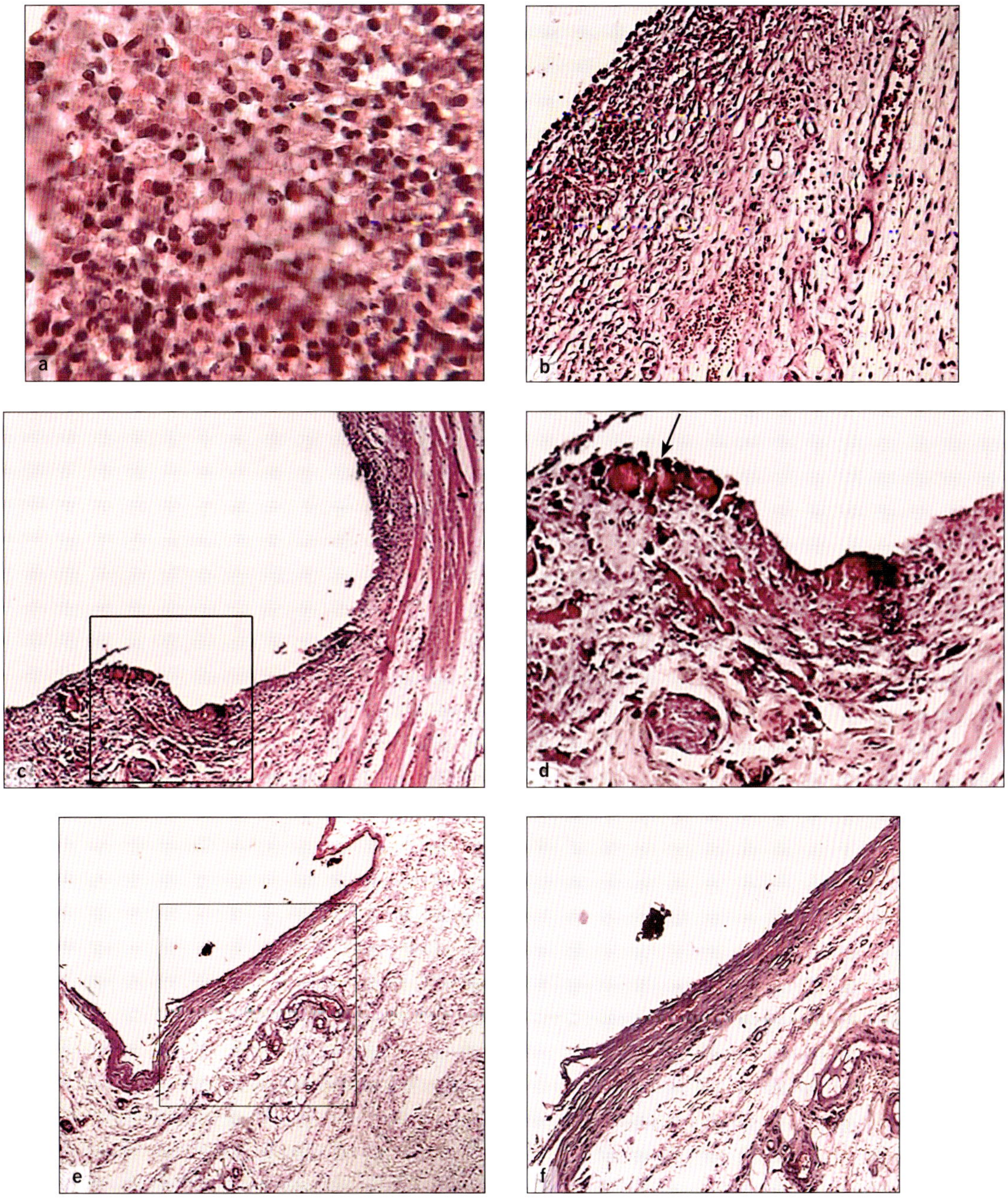

Fig 11-2 *(a)* Polymorphonuclear infiltration and necrosis at an early time period after subcutaneous MTA implantation. *(b)* Moderate infiltration of inflammatory cells and tissue hemorrhage 7 days after subcutaneous MTA implantation. *(c and d)* Formation of calcified structures in the soft tissue *(arrow)* 30 days after subcutaneous MTA implantation (magnification ×10 *[c]*, ×40 *[d, inset of c]*). *(e and f)* No inflammation and capsule formation at 60 days following subcutaneous implantation of MTA (magnification ×10 *[e]*, ×40 *[f, inset of e]*).

to MTA as well as presence of von Kossa positive structures following subcutaneous implantation of the material.[6,65,171,173–176] Resin composites and resin-ionomer hybrids such as Retroplast and Geristore have shown tissue irritation.[177,178] Geristore may induce significantly more inflammation than WAMTA, WMTA, and BA.[178] No significant difference has been found between WAMTA, WMTA, and BA in terms of subcutaneous reaction to the materials.[178,179]

When comparing BA and MTA, the subcutaneous response may be dependent on the type of MTA used in a given study. One study reported higher biocompatibility for BA compared with GMTA,[180] whereas WMTA was significantly more biocompatible than BA in another report.[178] BA and iRoot SP have been shown to be biocompatible following subcutaneous implantation.[180,181] BD has demonstrated significantly higher inflammatory response and tissue reaction than AMTA and controls in the early observation period following implantation (7 days); however, at longer evaluation periods (14 and 30 days), no significant difference was found among the groups. On the other hand, BD and AMTA showed significantly lower tissue reaction than ZOE cement.[182]

CEM cement was compared with WMTA and GMTA in a subcutaneous investigation. Results showed that CEM cement, unlike both GMTA and WMTA, resulted in no tissue necrosis during the study period. The authors stated that all test materials were tolerated well and demonstrated osseoinductive characteristics based on the presence of a calcified precipitate.[65]

EndoBinder has demonstrated a lower inflammatory tissue reaction than gray AMTA (GAMTA).[183] Both GMTA and EndoSequence RRM can induce a significantly greater inflammatory reaction than controls; however, this reaction (degranulation of mast cells and deposition of amyloid protein) is significantly higher with GMTA than with EndoSequence. By the final observation period (30 days), the inflammatory reaction decreased significantly more in the EndoSequence group than in the GMTA group. Specifically, GMTA caused necrosis and abscess formation that were not present adjacent to EndoSequence. The authors attributed this reaction to the exothermic peak of MTA that may increase tissue temperature during setting, causing abscess formation. This conclusion may not be justified because of the likely cooling effect of blood during the implantation process. Furthermore, most of the previous investigations have not reported similar abscess formation.[184]

It is important to note that various types of apatite do not necessarily have the same effect on mineralization in vivo. To compare set and freshly mixed WMTA, apatite formed by WMTA in the laboratory and synthetic hydroxyapatite were evaluated following subcutaneous implantation over a 60-day period. Results showed that both set and fresh MTA as well as synthetic hydroxyapatite induced mineralization. The mineralization activity of the apatite induced by WMTA in laboratory conditions was different than either the synthetic hydroxyapatite or the apatite formed in vivo. Similar to the previous studies referenced, the observed inflammatory reaction subsided over time. No significant difference was found among the groups in terms of the intensity of the inflammatory response observed. Furthermore, while no significant difference in induction of calcification was reported between set and freshly mixed WMTA, set WMTA showed significantly higher frequency of dystrophic calcification than the freshly mixed material.[185] Apaydin et al[186] compared freshly placed MTA as a root-end filling with set MTA placed in an orthograde fashion followed by root resection. While they did not find significant differences between the two in terms of the quantity of cementum formation or osseous healing, they did report a significantly higher frequency of cementum coverage over the freshly placed MTA.[186] This finding may suggest a potential inductive effect in the early stages of setting of MTA when placed in vivo after mixing.

Subcutaneous implantation of dentin tubes filled with AMTA, MTA-Bio, and PC showed significantly higher biomineralization adjacent to MTA-Bio and AMTA compared with PC.[68] In addition, formation of the dentin-cement interface and intratubular mineralization was significantly quicker for MTA-Bio and AMTA than for PC. Surprisingly, the addition of $CaCl_2$ to PC to reduce its setting time[187,188] also reduced its bioactivity.[68]

The use of PC as a root-end filling material has been a matter of controversy among researchers. Several investigators have reported no significant difference between PC and MTA in terms of biocompatibility.[171,172] Some investigators believe that because PC is a main component of MTA, it can be used for the same clinical indications; however, others have refuted its utility for clinical use because of the presence of noxious elements in its composition.[6,189] The presence of arsenic in MTA-based materials is a matter of concern among some researchers. Based on ISO standards (ISO 9917-1), the total content of arsenic in a dental material should not exceed 2 mg/kg. Nevertheless, atomic absorption spectrophotometry has shown arsenic levels in GAMTA as high as 5.01 mg/kg and in two types of gray PC (GPC) as high as 10.73 and 18.46 mg/kg. Subcutaneous implantation of GPC, a white PC (WPC) with low arsenic content, and GAMTA showed that one of the PCs that had higher arsenic content induced a significantly higher inflammatory reaction at 60 days. Despite lower amounts of arsenic in WPC, the inflammatory reaction to the material is not as good as with GAMTA.[190]

Systemic Effect of Some BAE Cements

To evaluate systemic effects, WAMTA and BA were implanted in subcutaneous tissues of rats. Blood samples were obtained, and histologic evaluation of the kidneys and livers were conducted. In this study, animals with implanted MTA demonstrated inflammatory changes as well as higher function (ie, urea and creatinine levels in the kidneys and serum alanine aminotransferase and aspartate aminotransferase levels in the livers) in the liver and kidney compared with controls throughout the study.[191] On the other hand, despite early negative findings in the BA group, longer evaluation periods demonstrated a decrease in the inflammatory response and high function of these organs. However, the investigators reported no permanent damage to these organs.

In conclusion, results of biocompatibility tests such as cytotoxic evaluation in cell cultures and subcutaneous implantation may be similar or different.[6,192] A potential explanation for variations reported in subcutaneous implantation studies may be differences in the methods used for evaluating the specimens by various pathologists. There are two popular methods for evaluating subcutaneous implantation of dental materials. These include the Federation Dentaire International (FDI) recommendation[193] and recommendations made by Cox et al.[194] The FDI recommendation determines the inflammatory reaction by counting inflammatory cells in various areas of microscopic sections. The method introduced by Cox et al determines the inflammatory reactions by identifying several variables such as density of inflammatory cells, tissue reactions (eg, fibrosis), vascular responses (eg, congestion), and fibrin extravasation. In a study conducted to evaluate the same specimens with these two methodologies, Vosoughhosseini et al[192] concluded that the FDI method is significantly more reliable than the Cox method for evaluating inflammation following subcutaneous implantation of materials.

Time of evaluation may also be an important factor. For example, during early time intervals MTA induces intense tissue response that decreases with time.[173]

Biomineralization of Root-End Filling Materials

Biomineralization induced by BAE cements has been confirmed by von Kossa positive structures observed after subcutaneous implantation of MTA sealer, PC, WAMTA, GMTA, AMTA, Endo CPM (EGEO SRL), and BA.[171,174,175,179] OPN is a known glycoprotein that is present in mineralized as well as pathologic calcifications of tissues. There is some evidence that OPN mediates bone cell adhesion, migration, and differentiation as well as initial bone matrix formation and mineralization. Expression of OPN was observed in the cytoplasm of fibroblasts in the capsule adjacent to implanted materials 14 days following implantation. Presence of von Kossa positive structures was confirmed starting 7 days following implantation of MTA sealer, PC, and WAMTA.[171]

One of the reasons that MTA is known as a bioactive material is the presence of calcium ions, which are released from the material after mixture with distilled water and when the material comes in direct contact with interstitial fluids. Another reason is its high pH.[4]

It is important to note that the early tissue response to implanted materials can be a result of the surgical procedure, including dissection of living tissues. True irritation of the implanted material would manifest itself in later observation times. Therefore, a material would be considered biocompatible if it provides a moderate to severe reaction in early periods after implantation followed by a significant reduction in tissue response over time. Control samples obtained from tissues that have undergone identical surgical procedures are necessary to compare with implanted test materials.[65] In subcutaneous implantation procedures, similar to experiments involving placement of MTA in synthetic tissue fluid, calcium ions are produced. The resultant CH serves as an irritant to the surrounding tissues that may persist long after MTA implantation.[183] In response to long-standing irritation, a fibrous capsule may form around the implanted material. Capsule thickness is one of the criteria that is evaluated in subcutaneous implantation studies. Some researchers postulate that thickness of the fibrous capsule may be an indication of inflammation and thus may have an inverse relation to the biocompatibility of a material.[184] In contrast, others believe that presence of a capsule, particularly at early time periods following implantation, illustrates tissue tolerance to a dental material.[195]

Another important point to note is that few studies have evaluated biomaterials for adequate time periods.[68,170,196,197] In fact, ISO 7405 standards require evaluation periods of no less than 84 days to allow proper comparison of the early tissue reaction to a given material's long-term response.[183]

Subcutaneous Implantation and Signaling Molecules

WMTA upregulates proinflammatory cytokines in a time-dependent manner. On the first day following implantation, the expression of myeloperoxidase, NFκB, activating protein-1, COX-2, inducible nitric oxide synthase (iNOS), and VEGF is upregulated as detected by immunohistochemical analysis. SEM observation has shown the formation of apatite-like crystals with the passage of time and the resultant formation of a dense layer of apatite over dentin tubes containing WMTA. Therefore, it seems that after WMTA implantation, both proinflammatory and healing markers are present simultaneously during the first week following the procedure.[198]

Another subcutaneous implantation study using WMTA and CH showed that during the first 3 days following implantation, several cytokines (TNF-α, IL-1β, and IL-10) expressed significantly increased levels compared with controls. One difference between the WMTA and CH groups was higher levels of TNF-α in the WMTA group. In addition, WMTA led to significantly higher expression levels of NFκB (a factor that modulates COX-2 expression), COX-2, VEGF, and iNOS compared with the control group. The detected genes may be classified as proinflammatory (IL-1β, VEGF, and TNF-α), anti-inflammatory (IL-10), pro–wound healing (IL-1β and VEGF), and anti–wound healing (TNF-α and IL-10). Different peak levels of each cytokine at various time intervals indicate various functions for each in temporal fashion. For instance, peak levels of TNF-α observed at 12 hours following implantation showed a proinflammatory effect during this time period, whereas reduced expression of TNF-α and significant elevation in the expression of IL-1β exhibited proinflammatory and pro–wound healing effects of the latter cytokine. IL-10 expression decreases over time because IL-10 exerts an anti-inflammatory/anti–wound healing effect. TNF-α may initiate an inflammatory cascade followed by increased expression of IL-1β, which stimulates inflammatory cells as well as fibroblasts. At the same time, production of IL-10 further suppresses the activity of inflammatory cells, causing a shift from acute phase to chronic phase. It is important to note that due to the extensive coagulation necrosis that is caused by CH, the repair process is delayed in comparison to that observed with MTA.[199]

In one study, WMTA and Life (a hard-setting CH-based material; Kerr) were subcutaneously implanted for 14 days. The harvested specimens were immunostained for macrophages (CD68), M2 macrophages (CD163), and CD34 (a marker for vascularization and wound healing). Real-time PCR was used for mannose receptor C type 1 (an M2 macrophage marker), CD34, and CD163 messenger RNA (mRNA). Results showed that WMTA significantly increases CD34, CD163, and CD68 markers at the site of implantation compared with Life and control specimens. The authors concluded that WMTA promotes healing by upregulating M2 macrophages and neovascularization by CD34-expressing cells. Several reasons have been described for the upregulation of M2 macrophages at the site of implantation. These include calcium ion release, a higher pH level than that of Life (12 vs 8), and the presence of silica.[200]

In another study, subcutaneously implanted EB+20% wt ZnO as a radiopacifier was compared with WAMTA and a hard-setting CH for up to 90 days. Throughout the study, all tested materials showed a similar inflammatory reaction. Gene expression of the following mediators were evaluated: IL-1β, TNF-α, IL-4, IL-10, and prostaglandin E synthase 2 (PTGES2). Only PTGES2 and IL-10 gene expression were detected in the specimens. At 7 days post implantation, EB led to significantly higher mRNA expression for *PTGES2* (the gene encoding COX-2) and IL-10 (a cytokine expressed during chronic inflammatory reactions) compared with WAMTA. At 30 days, both materials resulted in downregulation of both mediators, particularly EB, which was statistically significant.[197]

Another investigation compared subcutaneously implanted MTA with WPC for up to 30 days. Results showed that control samples had a significantly lower inflammatory response than either material. The test materials showed no significant difference to each other in terms of inflammatory response. The lack of a difference between control samples and the test materials at 7 days illustrates the potential impact of trauma induced by the surgery itself. The authors attributed the presence of a thick capsule around the implanted tubes to the factors released from leukocytes. These factors may be cytokines involved in collagen synthesis, including IL-1 and IL-4, as well as growth factors such as platelet-derived growth factor and TGF-β.[172]

Intraosseous Implantation

Several studies have illustrated the biocompatibility of AMTA following intraosseous implantation.[197,201,202] Two investigations with different time intervals evaluated AMTA after tooth extraction and after placement of the material in fresh extraction sockets. Mineralization and new bone formation were seen starting at the 7th day following implantation until the final day of the experiment. Dystrophic calcification was also observed in AMTA samples.[201,202] Another study showed that irrigation of rat mandibular bone defects with a solution containing CH prior to AMTA placement would improve osseous healing.[203]

Light-cured MTA elicited similar bone reaction to that observed with AMTA when it was placed in fresh extraction sockets in rats; however, dystrophic calcification was not observed in light-cured MTA specimens.[201,202]

In another study, CEM cement and MTA were placed in cavities prepared in the femoral bone of rats. All control and test materials caused downregulation of inflammatory cells and upregulation of bone formation throughout the study, with no significant differences among the various groups.[204]

EB, AMTA, and CH were placed in cavities prepared in rat tibias. Tissues were evaluated histologically for up to 90 days following surgery. All groups showed new bone formation throughout the study. Bone formation was significantly higher at the 60- and 90-day intervals in the AMTA and EB groups compared with the control.[205] MTA showed significantly better bone response than light-cured composite and ZOE.[206]

To evaluate bone formation, WMTA and an experimental nano-WMTA were implanted in the mandibles of rabbits for up to 40 days.[207] Both materials were used with and without tricalcium aluminate. The authors used dual-energy x-ray absorptiometry to analyze bone mass with respect to bone mineral content (BMC) and bone mineral density (BMD). Both BMC and BMD were significantly higher in the experimental groups than in the control group. Nano-WMTA resulted in significantly higher BMD and BMC compared with the commercial form of WMTA. Moreover, the addition of tricalcium aluminate significantly enhanced BMD and BMC levels. While in this study histologic responses were not evaluated, a recent investigation showed that nano-WMTA and WMTA result in similar tissue response when bone repair is evaluated up to 60 days following implantation in rabbit mandibles.[208]

To investigate the impact of certain materials on bone in response to irritation, BA and MTA were implanted in mice calvaria for up to 7 days prior to being challenged with lipopolysaccharide (LPS).[209] BA and MTA significantly downregulated osteoclast proliferation and bone resorption. Both materials decreased expression of cathepsin K, nuclear factor of activated T cell cytoplasmic 1, and c-Fos in LPS-induced mouse calvaria.

Another animal study evaluated the combination of laser phototherapy with BMPs, AMTA, and guided bone regeneration in rat tibia bone defects.[210] Results showed that the combination of AMTA as a graft material in bone defects with laser phototherapy provided significantly better results in terms of new bone formation and maturation compared with the other therapeutic combinations.

Skin test

Both observational and histologic examinations following subcutaneous implantation of CEM cement and WMTA showed significantly lower erythematous reaction and inflammatory cell infiltration to the former material during the 72-hour observation period.[211,212]

Analgesic effect

In an entirely different model evaluating another aspect of these materials, a group of investigators injected WMTA, eugenol, and ketoprofen in the lips of rats. In some of the samples, 2.5% formalin was subsequently injected in the lips 20 minutes later.[213] The authors evaluated the nociceptive response of the animals based on behavioral observation. Results showed that injection of WMTA did not elicit a nociceptive response; however, similar to ketoprofen, the material did have some analgesic effects on pain produced by formalin.

Effect on nerve activity

In order to evaluate the effect of root canal sealers on nerve activity, an in vitro study exposed rat trigeminal nerves to freshly mixed or set forms of Roth Root sealer (Pearson Dental), AH Plus, EndoSequence BC sealer, or RealSeal SE (SybronEndo).[214] Results showed that all concentrations of freshly mixed Roth Root sealer and higher concentrations of the set material caused significant upregulation of calcitonin gene-related peptide (CGRP). AH Plus upregulated CGRP levels only in the freshly mixed samples and in a lower concentration. In contrast, set and freshly mixed EndoSequence BC sealer and RealSeal significantly downregulated CGRP levels. It is important to note that the exposure times to the sealers in this study were short.

Evaluation of neural cell excitability and electrical properties on F1 nerve cells demonstrated that neural cell exposure to WMTA induces changes in resting potential to hyperpolarization conditions.[215] Moreover, CEM cement and WMTA alter the duration and potency of action potentials. Both materials cause significant upregulation in the hyperpolarization amplitude and area; however, the impact of WMTA is higher than that of CEM cement. The authors attributed these effects to the induced outward flow of K^+ across the cell membrane.

Vascular effect

MTA does not have adverse effects on microcirculation and blood vessel contraction based on dose-dependent studies.[216,217]

In vivo studies

Variables that may influence the outcome of periapical surgeries may include the quality of coronal restoration, tooth type, location of the tooth, type of root-end filling material, size of the periapical lesion, and presence or absence of root canal retreatment prior to the surgical treatment. For many years, amalgam was the material of choice for root-end filling. Several reasons have led to the need to introduce new materials to replace amalgam. These include leakage of the material, high corrosion of amalgam that can result in the displacement of the material into the periradicular tissues, unsatisfactory long-term outcomes[218] (Fig 11-3), as well as some concerns regarding the material's systemic safety.[219]

In clinical practice, IRM, SuperEBA, and MTA are among the materials that have received more attention among practitioners in recent years. Because of the superiority of MTA in laboratory and clinical research studies, in recently published papers, MTA has been used as the gold standard to be compared with newly developed root-end filling materials.[220]

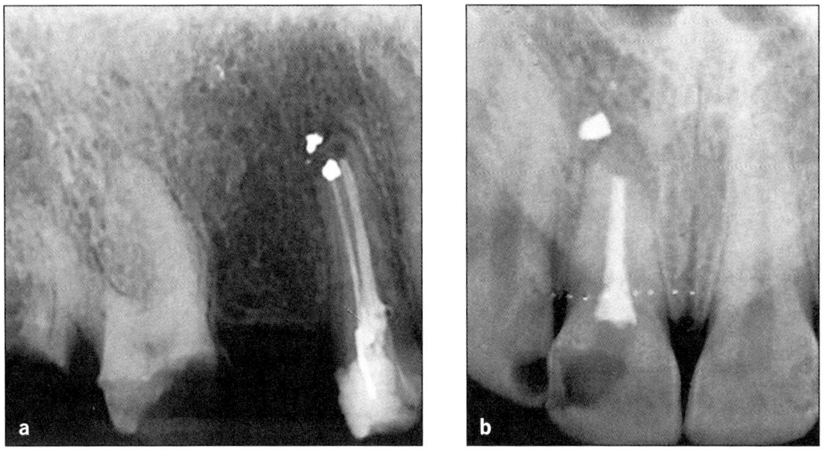

Fig 11-3 *(a and b)* Displacement of amalgam when placed as a root-end filling, potentially causing periapical leakage and failure of periapical surgery.

Animal studies

In animal studies, MTA has demonstrated similar or better outcomes than SuperEBA, amalgam, IRM, ZOE, and thermoplasticized gutta-percha in terms of bone healing and regeneration of periodontal ligaments.[221–229] Unlike the other materials listed, MTA promotes deposition of cementum over the material.[4,226,227] Some other materials that may promote cementum formation include Diaket, CEM cement, EndoSequence RRM, and Quick-Set.[230–233]

In addition to cementum formation, tissue response is an important factor to consider when using a material for root-end filling. MTA and CEM cement have shown similar tissue responses following their use as root-end filling materials.[231] In contrast, Quick-Set has been shown to result in significantly higher inflammation compared with MTA.[232]

Other materials such as EndoSequence RRM have shown promising results as root-end fillers in terms of histopathology as well as cone beam computed tomography (CBCT) and microCT image analyses.[233]

In general, more recent animal studies have focused primarily on BAE cements. Unfortunately, many of these animal studies have had several shortcomings such as short evaluation time, lack of controls, performing the procedure in intact teeth with no previous history of infection, and placing the materials as root-end fillings in teeth without prior root canal therapy. The number of animal studies on BAE cements is very limited.

Human investigations

Most of the published papers regarding recently introduced root-end filling materials are case reports and case series. These studies have illustrated favorable outcomes following the use of MTA and some other BAE cements, including PC, AMTA, BD, Tech Biosealer (Isasan), and CEM cement, as root-end filling materials during periapical surgery or intentional replantation and transplantation[234–256] (Figs 11-4 to 11-6).

Some studies have indicated that the type of root-end filling material may be an important prognostic factor for periapical surgeries.[256–263] Nevertheless, there are few studies that have specifically evaluated the impact of the type of root-end filling material on the final outcome of periapical surgery. For instance, reports comparing IRM and MTA as root-end fillings is sparse. Some have reported no significant difference between the two.[264,265] One study with a 5-year follow-up period reported significantly better outcomes with MTA than SuperEBA,[266] whereas another study reported no significant difference in success rates between the materials in a 4-year follow-up period.[267]

Anatomical variations may also affect the healing outcome when comparing certain types of root-end filling materials used following apical microsurgery. For instance, teeth treated with MTA do not show different outcomes depending on specific anatomical location; however, Retroplast results in higher failure in mandibular premolar and molar teeth. In addition, the percentage of cases with doubtful prognosis may be dependent on the type of root-end filling material.[268] In the Retroplast group, the number of cases with doubtful healing condition during the follow-up period after periapical surgery was much higher than that in the MTA group.[268] The use of MTA as a root-end filling material also provides significantly better short-term and long-term outcomes compared with burnished gutta-percha with a heated instrument.[1,2] No significant difference was reported between MTA and EndoSequence when used as root-end filling materials.[269]

Fig 11-4 *(a)* Post placement and compromised root canal obturation resulting in a periapical lesion. *(b)* Follow-up 6 months after placement of MTA as a root-end filling. (c) Follow-up at 2 years. *(d)* Follow-up at 4 years. (Courtesy of Dr Hamed Manochehrifar, Kerman, Iran.)

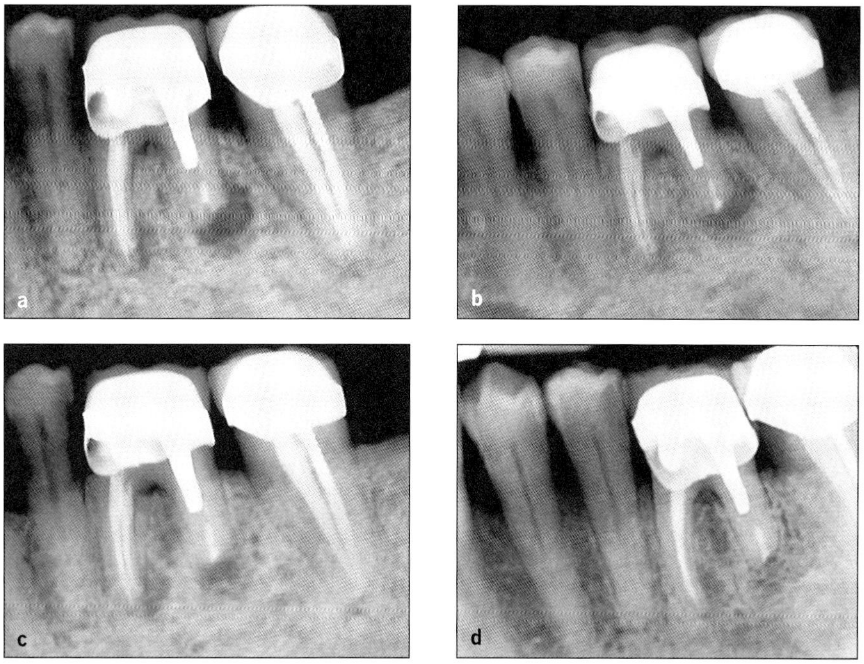

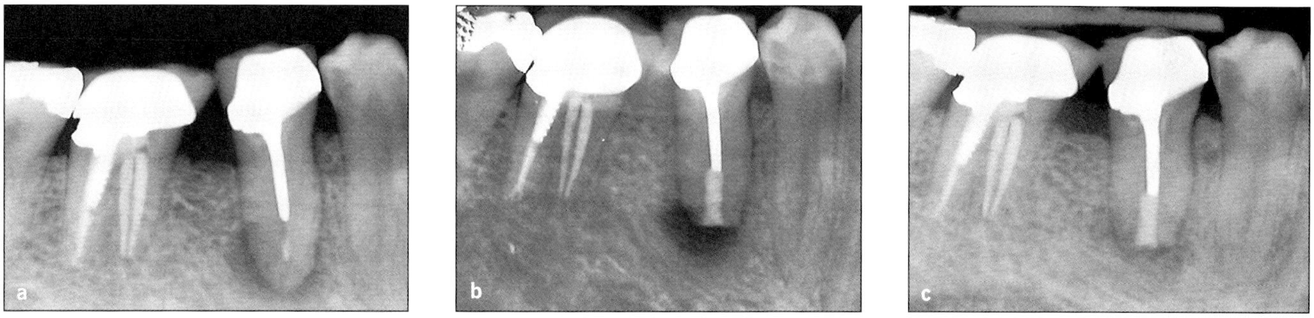

Fig 11-5 *(a)* Post placement and incomplete root canal obturation resulting in formation of a symptomatic periapical lesion. *(b)* Immediately after placing MTA as a root-end filling during intentional implantation. *(c)* Follow-up at 18 months. (Courtesy of Dr Hamed Manochehrifar, Kerman, Iran.)

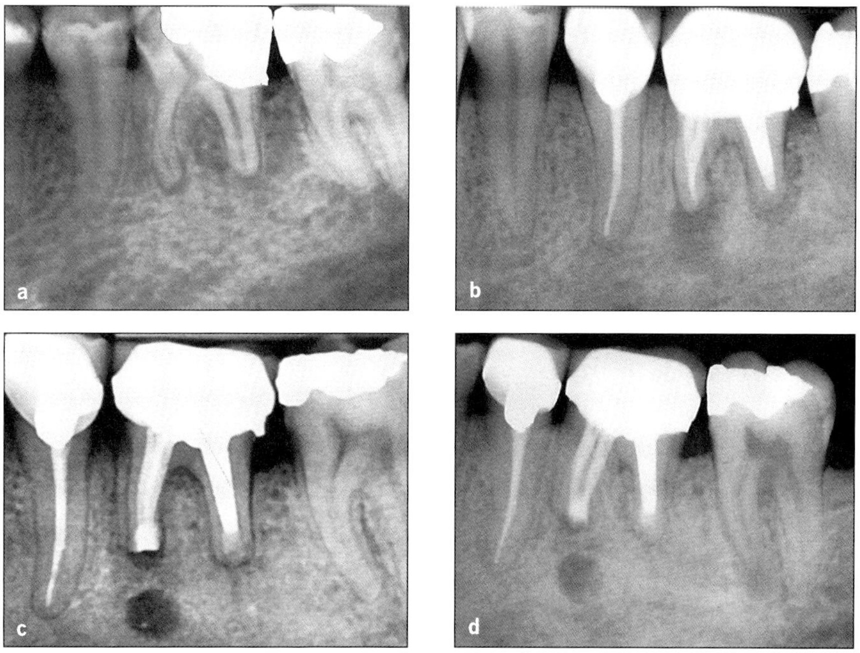

Fig 11-6 *(a)* Mandibular left first molar prior to root canal treatment. *(b)* Failure of root canal treatment 11 years posttreatment. *(c)* Placement of CEM cement as a root-end filling during intentional replantation. *(d)* Periapical healing 4 years after treatment.

One retrospective study focused on the impact of modern technologic tools (eg, use of the surgical microscope, GMTA as a root-end filling material, and piezoelectric devices for osteotomy and root-end resection) on the final outcome of periapical surgery. This relatively large study (938 teeth) showed that use of modern endodontic tools results in a fivefold increase in success compared with the traditional technique for periapical surgery.[270]

Some investigators have employed certain adjuncts in armamentaria in efforts to improve the outcomes of periapical surgery and the impact on overall quality of life. One example is the use of diode laser irradiation prior to placement of MTA root-end fillings. While no controls were included, this study reported reduction of the lesion size following the treatment.[271]

With regard to clinical symptoms, one study reported no significant difference in pain following periapical surgery when MTA or IRM was used as a root-end filling material.[272] Another study found that placement of plasma-rich growth factors over root ends filled with MTA, within the surgical bone defect, and over the sutures during periapical surgery resulted in a reduction in pain, swelling, and analgesic consumption. Furthermore, patients reported an improvement in daily life activities such as mouth opening, chewing, speaking, sleeping, working, and other daily routines.[273] A lower frequency of swelling has also been reported in patients following placement of MTA as a root-end filling material when compared with cold-burnished gutta-percha following apical surgery.[1]

Several systematic reviews and meta-analyses have evaluated the effect of root-end filling materials on the final outcome of periapical surgery.[274–277] The results of these studies are inconsistent. One systematic review and meta-analysis reported that the type of root-end filling material (MTA, IRM, SuperEBA) has no significant influence on the outcome of periapical surgeries[274]; however, other systematic reviews and meta-analyses have reported that the type of root-end filling material may have some impact on the final outcome of periapical surgeries.[275–277] Two systematic reviews and meta-analyses reported a significantly better outcome when IRM or MTA was used as a root-end filling material compared with amalgam, GIC, or gutta-percha,[275,276] whereas another systematic review and meta-analysis found that only MTA has a significant positive influence on the final outcome of periapical surgery.[277]

Based on studies published between 1980 and 2007, a higher percentage of teeth that received MTA as a root-end filling healed compared with teeth filled with other root-end filling materials.[275] The difference in results among old and recently published systematic reviews and meta-analyses may be due to more recent studies including higher sample sizes.[220]

In conclusion, studies evaluating the type of root-end filling material as a prognostic factor in apical surgery are limited. Most of these studies have had several important shortcomings, including being retrospective, having small sample sizes, presenting no interexaminer and intraexaminer reliability and validity data, lacking kappa score presentation, as well as having short-term follow-up periods and low recall rates. Therefore, the risk of case selection bias, incomplete recording, and postoperative examiner bias could be high in their results.[278]

Based on current literature and data, MTA has been supported by investigations with higher levels of evidence as the material of choice for root-end filling. A survey among active diplomates of the American Board of Endodontics in the United States showed that MTA is the most popular root-end filling material (61.4%), followed by SuperEBA (34.3%), amalgam (3.4%), and GIC (0.8%).[279] Despite certain drawbacks of the material (long setting time, high cost, discoloration potential, and handling difficulties), MTA is currently the material of choice for root-end filling. Future studies should focus on comparing newly introduced materials with MTA by designing rigorous randomized clinical trials and cohorts.

References

1. Christiansen R, Kirkevang LL, Hørsted-Bindslev P, Wenzel A. Randomized clinical trial of root-end resection followed by root-end filling with mineral trioxide aggregate or smoothing of the orthograde gutta-percha root filling—1-year follow-up. Int Endod J 2009;42:105–114.
2. Kruse C, Spin-Neto R, Christiansen R, Wenzel A, Kirkevang LL. Periapical bone healing after apicoectomy with and without retrograde root filling with mineral trioxide aggregate: A 6-year follow-up of a randomized controlled trial. J Endod 2016;42:533–537.
3. Torabinejad M, Pitt Ford TR. Root end filling materials: A review. Endod Dent Traumatol 1996;12:161–178.
4. Parirokh M, Torabinejad M. Mineral trioxide aggregate: A comprehensive literature review--Part III: Clinical applications, drawbacks, and mechanism of action. J Endod 2010;36:400–413.
5. Prati C, Gandolfi MG. Calcium silicate bioactive cements: Biological perspectives and clinical applications. Dent Mater 2015;31:351–370.
6. Torabinejad M, Parirokh M. Mineral trioxide aggregate: A comprehensive literature review--Part II: Leakage and biocompatibility investigations. J Endod 2010;36:190–202.
7. de Martins GR, Carvalho CA, Valera MC, de Oliveira LD, Buso L, Carvalho AS. Sealing ability of castor oil polymer as a root-end filling material. J Appl Oral Sci 2009;17:220–223.
8. Shi S, Zhang DD, Chen X, Bao ZF, Guo YJ. Apical sealing ability of bioceramic paste and mineral trioxide aggregate retrofillings: A dye leakage study. Iran Endod J 2015;10:99–103.
9. Chohan H, Dewan H, Annapoorna BM, Manjunath MK. Comparative evaluation of sealing ability of glass ionomer-resin continuum as root-end filling materials: An in vitro study. Int Soc Prev Community Dent 2015;5:488–493.
10. Lotfi M, Vosoughhosseini S, Saghiri MA, et al. Effect of synthetic tissue fluid on microleakage of grey and white mineral trioxide aggregate as root-end filling materials: An in vitro study. Sultan Qaboos Univ Med J 2012;12:323–329.
11. Shahi S, Yavari HR, Rahimi S, Eskandarinezhad M, Shakouei S, Unchi M. Comparison of the sealing ability of mineral trioxide aggregate and Portland cement used as root-end filling materials. J Oral Sci 2011;53:517–522.
12. El Sayed M, Saeed M. In vitro comparative study of sealing ability of Diadent BioAggregate and other root-end filling materials. J Conserv Dent 2012;15:249–252.

13. Suri NK, Nikhil V, Jha P, Jaiswal S. Evaluation of effect of addition of 2% chlorhexidine on the sealing ability of Biodentine: An in vitro study. J Conserv Dent 2015;18:479–482.
14. Ghorbani Z, Kheirieh S, Shadman B, Eghbal MJ, Asgary S. Microleakage of CEM cement in two different media. Iran Endod J 2009;4:87–90.
15. Leal F, De-Deus G, Brandão C, Luna AS, Fidel SR, Souza EM. Comparison of the root-end seal provided by bioceramic repair cements and White MTA. Int Endod J 2011;44:662–668.
16. Leal F, De-Deus G, Brandão C, Luna A, Souza E, Fidel S. Similar sealability between bioceramic putty ready-to-use repair cement and white MTA. Braz Dent J 2013;24:362–366.
17. Nair U, Ghattas S, Saber M, Natera M, Walker C, Pileggi R. A comparative evaluation of the sealing ability of 2 root-end filling materials: An in vitro leakage study using *Enterococcus faecalis*. Oral Surg Oral Med Oral Pathol Oral Radiol Endod 2011;112:e74–e77.
18. Shahi S, Jeddi Khajeh S, Rahimi S, et al. Effect of different mixing methods on the bacterial microleakage of calcium-enriched mixture cement. Minerva Stomatol 2016;65:269–275.
19. Medeiros PL, Bernardineli N, Cavenago BC, et al. Sealing ability of MTA, CPM, and MBPc as root-end filling materials: A bacterial leakage study. J Appl Oral Sci 2016;24:148–152.
20. Espir CG, Guerreiro-Tanomaru JM, Spin-Neto R, Chávez-Andrade GM, Berbert FL, Tanomaru-Filho M. Solubility and bacterial sealing ability of MTA and root-end filling materials. J Appl Oral Sci 2016;24:121–125.
21. Ashraf H, Faramarzi F, Paymanpour P. Sealing ability of Resilon and MTA as root-end filling materials: A bacterial and dye leakage study. Iran Endod J 2013;8:177–181.
22. Kazem M, Mahjour F, Dianat O, Fallahi S, Jahankhah M. Root-end filling with cement-based materials: An in vitro analysis of bacterial and dye microleakage. Dent Res J (Isfahan) 2013;10:46–51.
23. Moradi S, Lomee M, Gharechahi M. Comparison of fluid filtration and bacterial leakage techniques for evaluation of microleakage in endodontics. Dent Res J (Isfahan) 2015;12:109–114.
24. Antunes HS, Gominho LF, Andrade-Junior CV, et al. Sealing ability of two root-end filling materials in a bacterial nutrient leakage model. Int Endod J 2016;49:960–965.
25. Parirokh M, Askarifard S, Mansouri S, Haghdoost AA, Raoof M, Torabinejad M. Effect of phosphate buffer saline on coronal leakage of mineral trioxide aggregate. J Oral Sci 2009;51:187–191.
26. Hasheminia M, Loriaei Nejad S, Asgary S. Sealing ability of MTA and CEM cement as root-end fillings of human teeth in dry, saliva or blood-contaminated conditions. Iran Endod J 2010;5:151–156.
27. Bolhari B, Ashofteh Yazdi K, Sharifi F, Pirmoazen S. Comparative scanning electron microscopic study of the marginal adaptation of four root-end filling materials in presence and absence of blood. J Dent (Tehran) 2015;12:226–234.
28. Rahimi S, Shahi S, Lotfi M, Yavari HR, Charehjoo ME. Comparison of microleakage with three different thicknesses of mineral trioxide aggregate as root-end filling material. J Oral Sci 2008;50:273–277.
29. Rahimi S, Asgary S, Samiei M, Bahari M, Vahid Pakdel SM, Mahmoudi R. The effect of thickness on the sealing ability of CEM cement as a root-end filling material. J Dent Res Dent Clin Dent Prospects 2015;9:6–10.
30. Bayram HM, Saklar F, Bayram E, Orucoglu H, Bozkurt A. Determination of the apical sealing abilities of mineral trioxide aggregate, Portland cement, and bioaggregate after irrigation with different solutions. J Int Oral Health 2015;7:13–17,
31. Kubo CH, Gomes AP, Mancini MN. In vitro evaluation of apical sealing in root apex treated with demineralization agents and retrofiled with mineral trioxide aggregate through marginal dye leakage. Braz Dent J 2005;16:187–191.
32. Naik MM, de Ataide Ide N, Fernandes M, Lambor R. Assessment of apical seal obtained after irrigation of root end cavity with MTAD followed by subsequent retrofilling with MTA and Biodentine: An in vitro study. J Conserv Dent 2015; 18:132–135.
33. Moradi S, Disfani R, Ghazvini K, Lomee M. Sealing ability of orthograde MTA and CEM cement in apically resected roots using bacterial leakage method. Iran Endod J 2013;8:109–113.
34. Moradi S, Disfani R, Lomee M, Naghavi N. Effect of root resection on sealing ability of orthograde apical plugs of mineral trioxide aggregate and calcium enriched mixture. J Dent (Tehran) 2014;11:447–454.
35. Bernabé PF, Gomes-Filho JE, Bernabé DG, et al. Sealing ability of MTA used as a root end filling material: Effect of the sonic and ultrasonic condensation. Braz Dent J 2013;24:107–110.
36. Friedl CC, Williamson AE, Dawson DV, Gomez MR, Liu W. Comparison of mechanical and indirect ultrasonic placement technique on mineral trioxide aggregate retrofill density in simulated root-end surgery. J Endod 2016;42:650–653.
37. De Bruyne MA, De Moor RJ. Long-term sealing ability of Resilon apical root-end fillings. Int Endod J 2009;42:884–892.
38. Gupta PK, Garg G, Kalita C, Saikia A, Srinivasa TS, Satish G. Evaluation of sealing ability of Biodentine as retrograde filling material by using two different manipulation methods: An in vitro study. J Int Oral Health 2015;7:111–114.
39. Mandava P, Bolla N, Thumu J, Vemuri S, Chukka S. Microleakage evaluation around retrograde filling materials prepared using conventional and ultrasonic techniques. J Clin Diagn Res 2015;9:ZC43–ZC46.
40. Post LK, Lima FG, Xavier CB, Demarco FF, Gerhardt-Oliveira M. Sealing ability of MTA and amalgam in different root-end preparations and resection bevel angles: An in vitro evaluation using marginal dye leakage. Braz Dent J 2010;21:416–419.
41. Garip H, Garip Y, Oruçoğlu H, Hatipoğlu S. Effect of the angle of apical resection on apical leakage, measured with a computerized fluid filtration device. Oral Surg Oral Med Oral Pathol Oral Radiol Endod 2011;111:e50–e55.
42. Batista de Faria-Junior N, Tanomaru-Filho M, Guerreiro-Tanomaru JM, de Toledo Leonardo R, Camargo Villela Berbert FL. Evaluation of ultrasonic and ErCr:YSGG laser retrograde cavity preparation. J Endod 2009;35:741–744.
43. Girish CS, Ponnappa K, Girish T, Ponappa M. Sealing ability of mineral trioxide aggregate, calcium phosphate and polymethylmethacrylate bone cements on root ends prepared using an Erbium: Yttrium aluminium garnet laser and ultrasonics evaluated by confocal laser scanning microscopy. J Conserv Dent 2013; 16:304–308.
44. Nanjappa AS, Ponnappa KC, Nanjamma KK, Ponappa MC, Girish S, Nitin A. Sealing ability of three root-end filling materials prepared using an erbium: Yttrium aluminum garnet laser and endosonic tip evaluated by confocal laser scanning microscopy. J Conserv Dent 2015;18:327–330.
45. Onay EO, Gogos C, Ungor M, et al. Effect of Er,Cr:YSGG laser irradiation on apical sealing ability of calcium silicate-containing endodontic materials in root-end cavities. Dent Mater J 2014;33:570–575.
46. Gunes B, Aydinbelge HA. Effects of ultrasonic root-end cavity preparation with different surgical-tips and at different power-settings on glucose-leakage of root-end filling material. J Conserv Dent 2014;17:476–480.
47. Al-Fouzan K, Al-Garawi Z, Al-Hezaimi K, Javed F, Al-Shalan T, Rotstein I. Effect of acid etching on marginal adaptation of mineral trioxide aggregate to apical dentin: Microcomputed tomography and scanning electron microscopy analysis. Int J Oral Sci 2012;4:202–207.
48. Gondim E, Zaia AA, Gomes BP, Ferraz CC, Teixeira FB, Souza-Filho FJ. Investigation of the marginal adaptation of root-end filling materials in root-end cavities prepared with ultrasonic tips. Int Endod J 2003;36:491–499.
49. Gondim E Jr, Kim S, de Souza-Filho FJ. An investigation of microleakage from root-end fillings in ultrasonic retrograde cavities with or without finishing: A quantitative analysis. Oral Surg Oral Med Oral Pathol Oral Radiol Endod 2005;99:755–760.
50. Parirokh M, Behdani F, Eghbal MJ, Asgari S. A comparative investigation of marginal adaptation and surface defects of MTA and Root MTA as two root-end filling materials. J Kerman Uni Med Sci 2006;12:22–28.
51. Taschieri S, Bettach R, Lolato A, Moneghini L, Fabbro MD. Endodontic surgery failure: SEM analysis of root-end filling. J Oral Sci 2011;53:393–396.
52. Torres-Lagares D, Rodríguez-Martos R, Castellanos-Cosano L, Yáñez-Vico R, Segura-Egea JJ, Gutiérrez-Pérez JL. Confocal microscopy: A valid approach to evaluate the three-dimensional characteristics of root-end cavities. Med Oral Pathol Oral Cir Bucal 2013;18(3):e542–e546.
53. Badr AE. Marginal adaptation and cytotoxicity of bone cement compared with amalgam and mineral trioxide aggregate as root-end filling materials. J Endod 2010;36:1056–1060.
54. Oliveira HF, Gonçalves Alencar AH, Poli Figueiredo JA, Guedes OA, de Almeida Decurcio D, Estrela C. Evaluation of marginal adaptation of root-end filling materials using scanning electron microscopy. Iran Endod J 2013;8:182–186.
55. Bidar M, Moradi S, Jafarzadeh H, Bidad S. Comparative SEM study of the marginal adaptation of white and grey MTA and Portland cement. Aust Endod J 2007; 33:2–6.
56. Baranwal AK, Paul ML, Mazumdar D, Adhikari HD, Vyavahare NK, Jhajharia K. An ex-vivo comparative study of root-end marginal adaptation using grey mineral trioxide aggregate, white mineral trioxide aggregate, and Portland cement under scanning electron microscopy. J Conserv Dent 2015;18:399–404.
57. Munhoz MF, Marchesan MA, Cardoso DR, Silva SR, Silva-Sousa YT, Sousa-Neto MD. Quantitative 3D profilometry and SEM analysis of the adaptation of root-end filling materials placed under an optical microscope. Int Endod J 2011;44:560–566.
58. Bird DC, Komabayashi T, Guo L, Opperman LA, Spears R. In vitro evaluation of dentinal tubule penetration and biomineralization ability of a new root-end filling material. J Endod 2012;38:1093–1096.

59. Ghorbanzadeh A, Shokouhinejad N, Fathi B, Raoof M, Khoshkhounejad M. An in vitro comparison of marginal adaptation of MTA and MTA-like materials in the presence of PBS at one-week and two-month intervals. J Dent (Tehran) 2014; 11:560–568.
60. Soundappan S, Sundaramurthy JL, Raghu S, Natanasabapathy V. Biodentine versus mineral trioxide aggregate versus intermediate restorative material for retrograde root end filling: An in vitro study. J Dent (Tehran) 2014;11:143–149.
61. Shokouhinejad N, Nekoofar MH, Ashoftehyazdi K, Zahraee S, Khoshkhounejad M. Marginal adaptation of new bioceramic materials and mineral trioxide aggregate: A scanning electron microscopy study. Iran Endod J 2014;9:144–148.
62. Mokhtari F, Modaresi J, Javadi G, Davoudi A, Badrian H. Comparing the marginal adaptation of cold ceramic and mineral trioxide aggregate by means of scanning electron microscope: An in vitro study. J Int Oral Health 2015;7(9):7–10.
63. Torabinejad M, Watson TF, Pitt Ford TR. Sealing ability of a mineral trioxide aggregate when used as a root end filling material. J Endod 1993;19:591–595.
64. Ravichandra PV, Vemisetty H, Deepthi K, et al. Comparative evaluation of marginal adaptation of Biodentine and other commonly used root end filling materials—An in vitro study. J Clin Diagn Res 2014;8:243–245.
65. Parirokh M, Mirsoltani B, Raoof M, Tabrizchi H, Haghdoost AA. Comparative study of subcutaneous tissue responses to a novel root-end filling material and white and grey mineral trioxide aggregate. Int Endod J 2011;44:283–289.
66. Parirokh M, Forghani FR, Paseban H, Asgary S, Askarifard S, Esmaeeli Mahani S. Cytotoxicity of two resin-based sealers and a fluoride varnish on human gingival fibroblasts. Iran Endod J 2015;10:89–92.
67. Rathinam E, Rajasekharan S, Chitturi RT, Martens L, De Coster P. Gene expression profiling and molecular signaling of dental pulp cells in response to tricalcium silicate cements: A systematic review. J Endod 2015;41:1805–1817.
68. Dreger LA, Felippe WT, Reyes-Carmona JF, Felippe GS, Bortoluzzi EA, Felippe MC. Mineral trioxide aggregate and Portland cement promote biomineralization in vivo. J Endod 2012;38:324–329.
69. Hsu TT, Yeh CH, Kao CT, et al. Antibacterial and odontogenesis efficacy of mineral trioxide aggregate combined with CO2 laser treatment. J Endod 2015;41:1073–1080.
70. Liu CH, Hung CJ, Huang TH, Lin CC, Kao CT, Shie MY. Odontogenic differentiation of human dental pulp cells by calcium silicate materials stimulating via FGFR/ERK signaling pathway. Mater Sci Eng C Mater Biol Appl 2014;43:359–366.
71. Shie MY, Ding SJ. Integrin binding and MAPK signal pathways in primary cell responses to surface chemistry of calcium silicate cements. Biomaterials 2013;34:6589–6606.
72. Bin CV, Valera MC, Camargo SE, et al. Cytotoxicity and genotoxicity of root canal sealers based on mineral trioxide aggregate. J Endod 2012;38:495–500.
73. Müller BP, Eisenträger A, Jahnen-Dechent W, Dott W, Hollender J. Effect of sample preparation on the in vitro genotoxicity of a light curable glass ionomer cement. Biomaterials 2003;24:611–617.
74. Bakopoulou AA, Triviai IN, Tsiftsoglou AS, Garefis PD. In vitro assessment of cytotoxicity of resin-based dental restorative materials on WEHI 13 var fibroblasts. Int J Prosthodont 2006;19:13–16.
75. Ribeiro DA, Marques ME, Salvadori DM. Genotoxicity and cytotoxicity of glass ionomer cements on Chinese hamster ovary (CHO) cells. J Mater Sci Mater Med 2006;17:495–500.
76. Ribeiro DA, Marques ME, Salvadori DM. Biocompatibility of glass-ionomer cements using mouse lymphoma cells in vitro. J Oral Rehabil 2006;33:912–917.
77. Visalli G, Baluce B, La Maestra S, et al. Genotoxic damage in the oral mucosa cells of subjects carrying restorative dental fillings. Arch Toxicol 2013;87:179–187.
78. Tadin A, Galic N, Mladinic M, Marovic D, Kovacic I, Zeljezic D. Genotoxicity in gingival cells of patients undergoing tooth restoration with two different dental composite materials. Clin Oral Investig 2014;18:87–96.
79. Bakopoulou A, Mourelatos D, Tsiftsoglou AS, Giassin NP, Mioglou E, Garefis P. Genotoxic and cytotoxic effects of different types of dental cement on normal cultured human lymphocytes. Mutat Res 2009;672:103–112.
80. Angelieri F, Joias RP, Bresciani E, Noguti J, Ribeiro DA. Orthodontic cements induce genotoxicity and cytotoxicity in mammalian cells in vitro. Dent Res J (Isfahan) 2012;9:393–398.
81. Marovic D, Tadin A, Mladinic M, Juric-Kacunic D, Galic N. In vitro detection of DNA damage in human leukocytes induced by combined effect of resin composites and adhesive systems. Am J Dent 2014;27:35–41.
82. Gallorini M, Cataldi A, di Giacomo V. HEMA-induced cytotoxicity: Oxidative stress, genotoxicity and apoptosis. Int Endod J 2014;47:813–818.
83. Pettini F, Savino M, Corsalini M, Cantore S, Ballini A. Cytogenetic genotoxic investigation in peripheral blood lymphocytes of subjects with dental composite restorative filling materials. J Biol Regul Homeost Agents 2015;29:229–233.
84. Ribeiro DA, Matsumoto MA, Duarte MA, Marques ME, Salvadori DM. In vitro biocompatibility tests of two commercial types of mineral trioxide aggregate. Braz Oral Res 2005;19:183–187.
85. Ribeiro DA, Matsumoto MA, Duarte MA, Marques ME, Salvadori DM. Ex vivo biocompatibility tests of regular and white forms of mineral trioxide aggregate. Int Endod J 2006;39:26–30.
86. da Silva GN, Braz MG, de Camargo EA, Salvadori DM, Ribeiro DA. Genotoxicity in primary human peripheral lymphocytes after exposure to regular and white mineral trioxide aggregate. Oral Surg Oral Med Oral Pathol Oral Radiol Endod 2006;102:e50–e54.
87. Laurent P, Camps J, De Méo M, Déjou J, About I. Induction of specific cell responses to a Ca(3)SiO(5)-based posterior restorative material. Dent Mater 2008;24:1486–1494.
88. Brzovic V, Miletic I, Zeljezic D, et al. In vitro genotoxicity of root canal sealers. Int Endod J 2009;42:253–263.
89. Ding SJ, Kao CT, Chen CL, Shie MY, Huang TH. Evaluation of human osteosarcoma cell line genotoxicity effects of mineral trioxide aggregate and calcium silicate cements. J Endod 2010;36:1158–1162.
90. Zeferino EG, Bueno CE, Oyama LM, Ribeiro DA. Ex vivo assessment of genotoxicity and cytotoxicity in murine fibroblasts exposed to white MTA or white Portland cement with 15% bismuth oxide. Int Endod J 2010;43:843–848.
91. Naghavi N, Ghoddusi J, Sadeghnia HR, Asadpour E, Asgary S. Genotoxicity and cytotoxicity of mineral trioxide aggregate and calcium enriched mixture cements on L929 mouse fibroblast cells. Dent Mater J 2014;33:64–69.
92. Samiei M, Asgary S, Farajzadeh M, et al. Investigating the mutagenic effects of three commonly used pulpotomy agents using the Ames test. Adv Pharm Bull 2015;5:121–125.
93. Candeiro GT, Moura-Netto C, D'Almeida-Couto RS, et al. Cytotoxicity, genotoxicity and antibacterial effectiveness of a bioceramic endodontic sealer [epub ahead of print 17 August 2015]. Int Endod J doi:10.1111/iej.12523.
94. Gandolfi MG, Siboni F, Primus CM, Prati C. Ion release, porosity, solubility, and bioactivity of MTA Plus tricalcium silicate. J Endod 2014;40:1632–1637.
95. Sarkar NK, Caicedo R, Ritwik P, Moiseyeva R, Kawashima I. Physicochemical basis of the biologic properties of mineral trioxide aggregate. J Endod 2005;31:97–100.
96. Chen S, Cai Y, Engqvist H, Xia W. Enhanced bioactivity of glass ionomer cement by incorporating calcium silicates. Biomatter 2016;6:e1123842.
97. Shokouhinejad N, Nekoofar MH, Razmi H, et al. Bioactivity of EndoSequence root repair material and bioaggregate. Int Endod J 2012;45:1127–1134.
98. Kim JR, Nosrat A, Fouad AF. Interfacial characteristics of Biodentine and MTA with dentine in simulated body fluid. J Dent 2015;43:241–247.
99. Han L, Kodama S, Okiji T. Evaluation of calcium-releasing and apatite-forming abilities of fast-setting calcium silicate-based endodontic materials. Int Endod J 2015;48:124–130.
100. Asgary S, Eghbal MJ, Parirokh M, Ghoddusi J. Effect of two storage solutions on surface topography of two root-end fillings. Aust Endod J 2009;35:147–152.
101. Han L, Okiji T. Bioactivity evaluation of three calcium silicate-based endodontic materials. Int Endod J 2013;46:808–814.
102. Mestieri LB, Gomes-Cornélio AL, Rodrigues EM, et al. Biocompatibility and bioactivity of calcium silicate-based endodontic sealers in human dental pulp cells. J Appl Oral Sci 2015;23:467–471.
103. Modareszadeh MR, Di Fiore PM, Tipton DA, Salamat N. Cytotoxicity and alkaline phosphatase activity evaluation of EndoSequence root repair material. J Endod 2012;38:1101–1105.
104. Zhao X, He W, Song Z, Tong Z, Li S, Ni L. Mineral trioxide aggregate promotes odontoblastic differentiation via mitogen-activated protein kinase pathway in human dental pulp stem cells. Mol Biol Rep 2012;39:215–220.
105. Woo SM, Hwang YC, Lim HS, et al. Effect of Nifedipine on the differentiation of human dental pulp cells cultured with mineral trioxide aggregate. J Endod 2013;39:801–805.
106. Yan M, Wu J, Yu Y, et al. Mineral trioxide aggregate promotes the odonto/osteogenic differentiation and dentinogenesis of stem cells from apical papilla via nuclear factor kappa B signaling pathway. J Endod 2014;40:640–647.
107. Huang SC, Wu BC, Kao CT, Huang TH, Hung CJ, Shie MY. Role of the p38 pathway in mineral trioxide aggregate-induced cell viability and angiogenesis-related proteins of dental pulp cell in vitro. Int Endod J 2015;48:236–245.
108. Woo SM, Kim WJ, Lim HS, et al. combination of mineral trioxide aggregate and platelet-rich fibrin promotes the odontoblastic differentiation and mineralization of human dental pulp cells via BMP/Smad signaling pathway. J Endod 2016;42:82–88.
109. Luo Z, Kohli MR, Yu Q, Kim S, Qu T, He WX. Biodentine induces human dental pulp stem cell differentiation through mitogen-activated protein kinase and calcium-/calmodulin-dependent protein kinase II pathways. J Endod 2014;40:937–942.

110. Gupta SK, Saxena P, Pant VA, Pant AB. Adhesion and biologic behavior of human periodontal fibroblast cells to resin ionomer Geristore: A comparative analysis. Dent Traumatol 2013;29:389–393.
111. Modareszadeh MR, Chogle SA, Mickel AK, et al. Cytotoxicity of set polymer nano composite resin root-end filling materials. Int Endod J 2011;44:154–161.
112. Ghoddusi J, Tavakkol Afshari J, Donyavi Z, Brook A, Disfani R, Esmaeelzadeh M. Cytotoxic effect of a new endodontic cement and mineral trioxide aggregate on L929 line culture. Iran Endod J 2008;3:17–23.
113. Ghasemi N, Rahimi S, Lotfi M, et al. Effect of mineral trioxide aggregate, calcium enriched mixture cement and mineral trioxide aggregate with disodium hydrogen phosphate on BMP-2 production. Iran Endod J 2014;9:220–224.
114. Hengameh A, Reyhaneh D, Nima MM, Hamed H. Effects of two bioactive materials on survival and osteoblastic differentiation of human mesenchymal stem cells. J Conserv Dent 2014;17:349–353.
115. Jaberiansari Z, Naderi S, Tabatabaei FS. Cytotoxic effects of various mineral trioxide aggregate formulations, calcium-enriched mixture and a new cement on human pulp stem cells. Iran Endod J 2014;9:271–276.
116. Asgary S, Nazarian H, Khojasteh A, Shokouhinejad N. Gene expression and cytokine release during odontogenic differentiation of human dental pulp stem cells induced by 2 endodontic biomaterials. J Endod 2014;40:387–392.
117. Mozayeni MA, Milani AS, Marvasti LA, Asgary S. Cytotoxicity of calcium enriched mixture cement compared with mineral trioxide aggregate and intermediate restorative material. Aust Endod J 2012;38:70–75.
118. Khedmat S, Dehghan S, Hadjati J, Masoumi F, Nekoofar MH, Dummer PM. In vitro cytotoxicity of four calcium silicate-based endodontic cements on human monocytes, a colorimetric MTT assay. Restor Dent Endod 2014;39:149–154.
119. Alanezi AZ, Jiang J, Safavi KE, Spångberg LS, Zhu Q. Cytotoxicity evaluation of EndoSequence root repair material. Oral Surg Oral Med Oral Pathol Oral Radiol Endod 2010;109(3):e122–e125.
120. Damas BA, Wheater MA, Bringas JS, Hoen MM. Cytotoxicity comparison of mineral trioxide aggregates and EndoSequence bioceramic root repair materials. J Endod 2011;37:372–375.
121. Hirschman WR, Wheater MA, Bringas JS, Hoen MM. Cytotoxicity comparison of three current direct pulp-capping agents with a new bioceramic root repair putty. J Endod 2012;38:385–388.
122. Ma J, Shen Y, Stojicic S, Haapasalo M. Biocompatibility of two novel root repair materials. J Endod 2011;37:793–798.
123. Ciasca M, Aminoshariae A, Jin G, Montagnese T, Mickel A. A comparison of the cytotoxicity and proinflammatory cytokine production of EndoSequence root repair material and ProRoot mineral trioxide aggregate in human osteoblast cell culture using reverse-transcriptase polymerase chain reaction. J Endod 2012;38:486–489.
124. Machado J, Johnson JD, Paranjpe A. The effects of EndoSequence root repair material on differentiation of dental pulp cells. J Endod 2016;42:101–105.
125. Wei W, Qi YP, Nikonov SY, et al. Effects of an experimental calcium aluminosilicate cement on the viability of murine odontoblast-like cells. J Endod 2012;38:936–942.
126. Chang SW, Lee SY, Kum KY, Kim EC. Effects of ProRoot MTA, Bioaggregate, and Micromega MTA on odontoblastic differentiation in human dental pulp cells. J Endod 2014;40:113–118.
127. Chen S, Mestres G, Lan W, Xia W, Engqvist H. Cytotoxicity of modified glass ionomer cement on odontoblast cells. J Mater Sci Mater Med 2016;27:116.
128. Silva EJ, Herrera DR, Almeida JF, Ferraz CC, Gomes BP, Zaia AA. Evaluation of cytotoxicity and up-regulation of gelatinases in fibroblast cells by three root repair materials. Int Endod J 2012;45:815–820.
129. Silva EJ, Herrera DR, Rosa TP, et al. Evaluation of cytotoxicity, antimicrobial activity and physicochemical properties of a calcium aluminate-based endodontic material. J Appl Oral Sci 2014;22:61–67.
130. Lessa FC, Aranha AM, Hebling J, Costa CA. Cytotoxic effects of White-MTA and MTA-Bio cements on odontoblast-like cells (MDPC-23). Braz Dent J 2010;21:24–31.
131. Min KS, Kim HI, Park HJ, Pi SH, Hong CU, Kim EC. Human pulp cells response to Portland cement in vitro. J Endod 2007;33:163–166.
132. Min KS, Lee SI, Lee Y, Kim EC. Effect of radiopaque Portland cement on mineralization in human dental pulp cells. Oral Surg Oral Med Oral Pathol Oral Radiol Endod 2009;108(4):e82–e86.
133. Gomes-Filho JE, Watanabe S, Gomes AC, Faria MD, Lodi CS, Penha Oliveira SH. Evaluation of the effects of endodontic materials on fibroblast viability and cytokine production. J Endod 2009;35:1577–1559.
134. Lee SK, Lee SK, Lee SI, et al. Effect of calcium phosphate cements on growth and odontoblastic differentiation in human dental pulp cells. J Endod 2010;36:1537–1542.
135. Gomes-Filho JE, Gomes AC, Watanabe S, Oliveira SH, Bernabé PF, Percinoto C. Evaluation of tissue reaction, cell viability and cytokine production induced by Sealapex Plus. J Appl Oral Sci 2011;19:329–336.
136. Bidar M, Zarrabi MH, Tavakol Afshari J, et al. Osteoblastic cytokine response to gray and white mineral trioxide aggregate. Iran Endod J 2011;6:111–115.
137. Eid AA, Gosier JL, Primus CM, et al. In vitro biocompatibility and oxidative stress profiles of different hydraulic calcium silicate cements. J Endod 2014;40:255–260.
138. Salles LP, Gomes-Cornélio AL, Guimarães FC, et al. Mineral trioxide aggregate-based endodontic sealer stimulates hydroxyapatite nucleation in human osteoblast-like cell culture. J Endod 2012;38:971–976.
139. Lee SY, Min KS, Choi GW, et al. Effects of simvastatin and enamel matrix derivative on Portland cement with bismuth oxide-induced growth and odontoblastic differentiation in human dental pulp cells. J Endod 2012;38:405–410.
140. Seo MS, Hwang KG, Lee J, Kim H, Baek SH. The effect of mineral trioxide aggregate on odontogenic differentiation in dental pulp stem cells. J Endod 2013;39:242–248.
141. Hakki SS, Bozkurt BS, Ozcopur B, Gandolfi MG, Prati C, Belli S. The response of cementoblasts to calcium phosphate resin-based and calcium silicate-based commercial sealers. Int Endod J 2013;46:242–252.
142. Güven EP, Taşlı PN, Yalvac ME, Sofiev N, Kayahan MB, Sahin F. In vitro comparison of induction capacity and biomineralization ability of mineral trioxide aggregate and a bioceramic root canal sealer. Int Endod J 2013;46:1173–1182.
143. Chang SW, Lee SY, Ann HJ, Kum KY, Kim EC. Effects of calcium silicate endodontic cements on biocompatibility and mineralization-inducing potentials in human dental pulp cells. J Endod 2014;40:1194–1200.
144. Chang SW, Lee SY, Kang SK, Kum KY, Kim EC. In vitro biocompatibility, inflammatory response, and osteogenic potential of 4 root canal sealers: Sealapex, Sankin apatite root sealer, MTA Fillapex, and iRoot SP root canal sealer. J Endod 2014;40:1642–1648.
145. Braga JM, Oliveira RR, Martins RC, Ribeiro Sobrinho AP. The effects of a mineral trioxide aggregate-based sealer on the production of reactive oxygen species, nitrogen species and cytokines by two macrophage subtypes. Int Endod J 2014;47:909–919.
146. Park SJ, Heo SM, Hong SO, Hwang YC, Lee KW, Min KS. Odontogenic effect of a fast-setting pozzolan-based pulp capping material. J Endod 2014;40:1124–1131.
147. Corral Nuñez CM, Bosomworth HJ, Field C, Whitworth JM, Valentine RA. Biodentine and mineral trioxide aggregate induce similar cellular responses in a fibroblast cell line. J Endod 2014;40:406–411.
148. Kim M, Yang W, Kim H, Ko H. Comparison of the biological properties of ProRoot MTA, OrthoMTA, and Endocem MTA cements. J Endod 2014;40:1649–1653.
149. Ozdemir Y, Kutukculer N, Topaloglu-Ak A, Kose T, Eronat C. Comparative evaluation of pro-inflammatory cytokine levels in pulpotomized primary molars. J Oral Sci 2015;57:145–150.
150. Widbiller M, Lindner SR, Buchalla W, et al. Three-dimensional culture of dental pulp stem cells in direct contact to tricalcium silicate cements. Clin Oral Investig 2016;20:237–246.
151. Chang SW, Bae WJ, Yi JK, et al. Odontoblastic differentiation, inflammatory response, and angiogenic potential of 4 calcium silicate-based cements: Micromega MTA, ProRoot MTA, RetroMTA, and experimental calcium silicate cement. J Endod 2015;41:1524–1529.
152. Paranjpe A, Zhang H, Johnson JD. Effects of mineral trioxide aggregate on human dental pulp cells after pulp-capping procedures. J Endod 2010;36:1042–1047.
153. Hakki SS, Bozkurt SB, Ozcopur B, Purali N, Belli S. Periodontal ligament fibroblast response to root perforations restored with different materials: A laboratory study. Int Endod J 2012;45:240–248.
154. Zanini M, Sautier JM, Berdal A, Simon S. Biodentine induces immortalized murine pulp cell differentiation into odontoblast-like cells and stimulates biomineralization. J Endod 2012;38:1220–1226.
155. Varalakshmi PR, Kavitha M, Govindan R, Narasimhan S. Effect of statins with α-tricalcium phosphate on proliferation, differentiation, and mineralization of human dental pulp cells. J Endod 2013;39:806–812.
156. Eid AA, Niu LN, Primus CM, et al. In vitro osteogenic/dentinogenic potential of an experimental calcium aluminosilicate cement. J Endod 2013;39:1161–1166.
157. Öncel Torun Z, Torun D, Demirkaya K, et al. Effects of iRoot BP and white mineral trioxide aggregate on cell viability and the expression of genes associated with mineralization. Int Endod J 2015;48:986–993.
158. Tian J, Qi W, Zhang Y, et al. Bioaggregate inhibits osteoclast differentiation, fusion, and bone resorption in vitro. J Endod 2015;41:1500–1506.
159. Zhang S, Yang X, Fan M. BioAggregate and iRoot BP Plus optimize the proliferation and mineralization ability of human dental pulp cells. Int Endod J 2013;46:923–929.

160. Kim YS, Min KS, Jeong DH, Jang JH, Kim HW, Kim EC. Effects of fibroblast growth factor-2 on the expression and regulation of chemokines in human dental pulp cells. J Endod 2010;36:1824–1830.
161. Lee BN, Lee KN, Koh JT, et al. Effects of 3 endodontic bioactive cements on osteogenic differentiation in mesenchymal stem cells. J Endod 2014;40:1217–1222.
162. Margunato S, Taşlı PN, Aydın S, Karapınar Kazandağ M, Şahin F. in vitro evaluation of proroot MTA, Biodentine, and MM-MTA on human alveolar bone marrow stem cells in terms of biocompatibility and mineralization. J Endod 2015;41:1646–1652.
163. Silva EJ, Senna PM, De-Deus G, Zaia AA. Cytocompatibility of Biodentine using a three-dimensional cell culture model. Int Endod J 2016;49:574–580.
164. Lee BN, Son HJ, Noh HJ, et al. Cytotoxicity of newly developed ortho MTA root-end filling materials. J Endod 2012;38:1627–1630.
165. Ko H, Yang W, Park K, Kim M. Cytotoxicity of mineral trioxide aggregate (MTA) and bone morphogenetic protein 2 (BMP-2) and response of rat pulp to MTA and BMP-2. Oral Surg Oral Med Oral Pathol Oral Radiol Endod 2010;109:e103–e108.
166. Attik GN, Villat C, Hallay F, et al. In vitro biocompatibility of a dentine substitute cement on human MG63 osteoblasts cells: Biodentine versus MTA. Int Endod J 2014;47:1133–1141.
167. Ahmed HM, Luddin N, Kannan TP, Mokhtar KI, Ahmad A. Cell attachment properties of Portland cement-based endodontic materials: Biological and methodological considerations. J Endod 2014;40:1517–1523.
168. Zhang W, Li Z, Peng B. Effects of iRoot SP on mineralization-related genes expression in MG63 cells. J Endod 2010;36:1978–1982.
169. Bae WJ, Chang SW, Lee SI, Kum KY, Bae KS, Kim EC. Human periodontal ligament cell response to a newly developed calcium phosphate-based root canal sealer. J Endod 2010;36:1658–1663.
170. Shahi S, Rahimi S, Yavari HR, et al. Effect of mineral trioxide aggregates and Portland cements on inflammatory cells. J Endod 2010;36:899–903.
171. Viola NV, Guerreiro-Tanomaru JM, da Silva GF, Sasso-Cerri E, Tanomaru-Filho M, Cerri PS. Biocompatibility of an experimental MTA sealer implanted in the rat subcutaneous: quantitative and immunohistochemical evaluation. J Biomed Mater Res B Appl Biomater 2012;100:1773–1781.
172. Karanth P, Manjunath MK, Roshni, Kuriakose ES. Reaction of rat subcutaneous tissue to mineral trioxide aggregate and Portland cement: A secondary level biocompatibility test. J Indian Soc Pedod Prev Dent 2013;31(2):74–81.
173. Yang WK, Ko HJ, Kim MR. Evaluation of the rat tissue reaction to experimental new resin cement and mineral trioxide aggregate cement. Restor Dent Endod 2012;37:194–200.
174. Gomes-Filho JE, Watanabe S, Bernabé PF, de Moraes Costa MT. A mineral trioxide aggregate sealer stimulated mineralization. J Endod 2009;35:256–260.
175. Scarparo RK, Haddad D, Acasigua GA, Fossati AC, Fachin EV, Grecca FS. Mineral trioxide aggregate-based sealer: Analysis of tissue reactions to a new endodontic material. J Endod 2010;36:1174–1178.
176. Bramante CM, Kato MM, Assis GF, et al. Biocompatibility and setting time of CPM-MTA and white Portland cement clinker with or without calcium sulfate. J Appl Oral Sci 2013;21:32–36.
177. Hammad HM, Hamadah MA, Al-Omari WM. Histological evaluation of rat tissue response to GMTA, Retroplast, and Geristore retrograde filling materials. Aust Endod J 2011;37:18–25.
178. Saghiri MA, Tanideh N, Garcia-Godoy F, Lotfi M, Karamifar K, Amanat D. Subcutaneous connective tissue reactions to various endodontic biomaterials: An animal study. J Dent Res Dent Clin Dent Prospects 2013;7:15–21.
179. Bósio CC, Felippe GS, Bortoluzzi EA, Felippe MC, Felippe WT, Rivero ER. Subcutaneous connective tissue reactions to iRoot SP, mineral trioxide aggregate (MTA) Fillapex, DiaRoot BioAggregate and MTA. Int Endod J 2014;47:667–674.
180. Batur YB, Acar G, Yalcin Y, Dindar S, Sancakli H, Erdemir U. The cytotoxic evaluation of mineral trioxide aggregate and bioaggregate in the subcutaneous connective tissue of rats. Med Oral Pathol Oral Cir Bucal 2013;18(4):e745–e751.
181. Zhang W, Peng B. Tissue reactions after subcutaneous and intraosseous implantation of iRoot SP, MTA and AH Plus. Dent Mater J 2015;34:774–780.
182. Mori GG, Teixeira LM, de Oliveira DL, Jacomini LM, da Silva SR. Biocompatibility evaluation of Biodentine in subcutaneous tissue of rats. J Endod 2014;40:1485–1488.
183. Aguilar FG, Roberti Garcia LF, Panzeri Pires-de-Souza FC. Biocompatibility of new calcium aluminate cement (EndoBinder). J Endod 2012;38:367–371.
184. Khalil WA, Abunasef SK. Can mineral trioxide aggregate and nanoparticulate EndoSequence root repair material produce injurious effects to rat subcutaneous tissues? J Endod 2015;41:1151–1156.
185. Danesh F, Tootian Z, Jahanbani J, et al. Biocompatibility and mineralization activity of fresh or set white mineral trioxide aggregate, biomimetic carbonated apatite, and synthetic hydroxyapatite. J Endod 2010;36:1036–1041.
186. Apaydin ES, Shabahang S, Torabinejad M. Hard-tissue healing after application of fresh or set MTA as root-end-filling material. J Endod 2004;30:21–24.
187. Parirokh M, Torabinejad M. Mineral trioxide aggregate: A comprehensive literature review—Part I: Chemical, physical, and antibacterial properties. J Endod 2010; 36:16–27.
188. Parirokh M, Asgary S, Eghbal MJ, Kakoei S, Samiee M. A comparative study of using a combination of calcium chloride and mineral trioxide aggregate as the pulp-capping agent on dogs' teeth. J Endod 2011;37:786–788.
189. Parirokh M, Torabinejad M. Calcium Silicate–Based Cements. In: Torabinejad M (ed). Mineral Trioxide Aggregate: Properties and Clinical Applications. Oxford: Wiley, 2014:284–320.
190. Minotti PG, Ordinola-Zapata R, Midena RZ, et al. Rat subcutaneous tissue response to calcium silicate containing different arsenic concentrations. J Appl Oral Sci 2015; 23:42–48.
191. Khalil WA, Eid NF. Biocompatibility of BioAggregate and mineral trioxide aggregate on the liver and kidney. Int Endod J 2013;46:730–737.
192. Vosoughhosseini S, Lotfi M, Moradzadeh M, et al. Comparison of two histopathologic methods for evaluating subcutaneous reaction to mineral trioxide aggregate. Med Oral Patol Oral Cir Bucal 2012;17(1):e41–e44.
193. Fédération Dentaire International, Commission of Dental Materials, Instruments, Equipment and Therapeutics. Recommended standard practices for biological evaluation of dental materials. Int Dent J 1980;30:140–188.
194. Cox CF, Sübay RK, Suzuki S, Suzuki SH, Ostro E. Biocompatibility of various dental materials: Pulp healing with a surface seal. Int J Periodontics Restorative Dent 1996;16:240–251.
195. Derakhshan S, Adl A, Parirokh M, Mashadiabbas F, Haghdoost AA. Comparing subcutaneous tissue responses to freshly mixed and set root canal sealers. Iran Endod J 2009;4:152–157.
196. Yavari HR, Shahi S, Rahimi S, et al. Connective tissue reaction to white and gray MTA mixed with distilled water or chlorhexidine in rats. Iran Endod J 2009;4: 25–30.
197. Garcia Lda F, Huck C, Menezes de Oliveira L, de Souza PP, de Souza Costa CA. Biocompatibility of new calcium aluminate cement: Tissue reaction and expression of inflammatory mediators and cytokines. J Endod 2014;40:2024–2029.
198. Reyes-Carmona JF, Santos AS, Figueiredo CP, et al. Host-mineral trioxide aggregate inflammatory molecular signaling and biomineralization ability. J Endod 2010;36:1347–1353.
199. Reyes-Carmona JF, Santos AR, Figueiredo CP, Felippe MS, Felippe WT, Cordeiro MM. In vivo host interactions with mineral trioxide aggregate and calcium hydroxide: Inflammatory molecular signaling assessment. J Endod 2011;37:1225–1235.
200. Ito T, Kaneko T, Yamanaka Y, Shigetani Y, Yoshiba K, Okiji T. M2 macrophages participate in the biological tissue healing reaction to mineral trioxide aggregate. J Endod 2014;40:379–383.
201. Gomes-Filho JE, de Moraes Costa MT, Cintra LT, et al. Evaluation of alveolar socket response to Angelus MTA and experimental light-cure MTA. Oral Surg Oral Med Oral Pathol Oral Radiol Endod 2010;110(5):e93–e97.
202. Gomes-Filho JE, de Moraes Costa MM, Cintra LT, et al. Evaluation of rat alveolar bone response to Angelus MTA or experimental light-cured mineral trioxide aggregate using fluorochromes. J Endod 2011;37:250–254.
203. do Nascimento C, Issa JP, Iyomasa MM, et al. Bone repair using mineral trioxide aggregate combined to a material carrier, associated or not with calcium hydroxide in bone defects. Micron 2008;39:868–874.
204. Rahimi S, Mokhtari H, Shahi S, et al. Osseous reaction to implantation of two endodontic cements: Mineral trioxide aggregate (MTA) and calcium enriched mixture (CEM). Med Oral Patol Oral Cir Bucal 2012;17(5):e907–e911.
205. Garcia Lda F, Huck C, Scardueli CR, de Souza Costa CA. Repair of bone defects filled with new calcium aluminate cement (EndoBinder). J Endod 2015;41:864–870.
206. Sousa CJ, Loyola AM, Versiani MA, Biffi JC, Oliveira RP, Pascon EA. A comparative histological evaluation of the biocompatibility of materials used in apical surgery. Int Endod J 2004;37:738–748.
207. Saghiri MA, Orangi J, Tanideh N, Janghorban K, Sheibani N. Effect of endodontic cement on bone mineral density using serial dual-energy x-ray absorptiometry. J Endod 2014;40:648–651.
208. Saghiri MA, Orangi J, Tanideh N, et al. Repair of bone defect by nano-modified white mineral trioxide aggregates in rabbit: A histopathological study. Med Oral Pathol Oral Cir Bucal 2015;20(5):e525–e531.
209. Zhang J, Zhu L, Peng B. Effect of BioAggregate on osteoclast differentiation and inflammatory bone resorption in vivo. Int Endod J 2015;48:1077–1085.

210. Pinheiro AL, Aciole GT, Cangussú MC, Pacheco MT, Silveira L Jr. Effects of laser photherapy on bone defects grafted with mineral trioxide aggregate, bone morphogenetic proteins, and guided bone regeneration: A Raman spectroscopic study. J Biomed Mater Res A 2010;95:1041–1047.
211. Tabarsi B, Pourghasem M, Moghaddamnia A, et al. Comparison of skin test reactivity of two endodontic biomaterials in rabbits. Pak J Biol Sci 2012;15:250–254.
212. Shokravi M, Tabarsi B, Moghaddamnia A, Sohanfaraji A, Pourghasem M. Comparison of skin reaction between MTA (Produced in Iran) and CEM in rabbit. Int J Mol Cell Med 2012;1:94–98.
213. Abbasipour F, Bakhtiar H, Vatanpour M, Khalilkhani H, Torabzadeh H, Janahmadi M. A comparative study on anti-hyperalgesia effect of MTA and Ketoprofen in inflammatory pain. Iran Endod J 2009;4:81–86.
214. Ruparel NB, Ruparel SB, Chen PB, Ishikawa B, Diogenes A. Direct effect of endodontic sealers on trigeminal neuronal activity. J Endod 2014;40:683–687.
215. Abbasipour F, Akheshteh V, Rastqar A, Khalilkhani H, Asgary S, Janahmadi M. Comparing the effects of mineral trioxide aggregate and calcium enriched mixture on neuronal cells using an electrophysiological approach. Iran Endod J 2012;7:79–87.
216. Masuda YM, Wang X, Hossain M, et al. Evaluation of biocompatibility of mineral trioxide aggregate with an improved rabbit ear chamber. J Oral Rehabil 2005; 32:145–150.
217. Tunca YM, Aydin C, Ozen T, Seyrek M, Ulusoy HB, Yildiz O. The effect of mineral trioxide aggregate on the contractility of the rat thoracic aorta. J Endod 2007; 33:823–826.
218. Frank AL, Glick DH, Patterson SS, Weine FS. Long-term evaluation of surgically placed amalgam fillings. J Endod 1992;18:391–398.
219. Saatchi M, Shadmehr E, Talebi SM, Nazeri M. A prospective clinical study on blood mercury levels following endodontic root-end surgery with amalgam. Iran Endod J 2013;8:85–88.
220. von Arx T. Apical surgery: A review of current techniques and outcome. Saudi Dent J 2011;23:9–15.
221. Torabinejad M, Hong CU, Lee SJ, Monsef M, Pitt Ford TR. Investigation of mineral trioxide aggregate for root-end filling in dogs. J Endod 1995;21:603–608.
222. Torabinejad M, Pitt Ford TR, McKendry DJ, Abedi HR, Miller DA, Kariyawasam SP. Histologic assessment of mineral trioxide aggregate as a root-end filling in monkeys. J Endod 1997;23:225–228.
223. Bernabe PF, Gomes-Filho JE, Rocha WC, Nery MJ, Otoboni-Filho JA, Dezan Junior E. Histological evaluation of MTA as a root-end filling material. Int Endod J 2007;40:758–65.
224. Bernabé PF, Holland R, Morandi R, et al. Comparative study of MTA and other materials in retrofilling of pulpless dogs' teeth. Braz Dent J 2005;16:149–155.
225. Tawil PZ, Trope M, Curran AE, et al. Periapical microsurgery: An in vivo evaluation of endodontic root-end filling materials. J Endod 2009;35:357–362.
226. Baek SH, Lee WC, Setzer FC, Kim S. Periapical bone regeneration after endodontic microsurgery with three different root-end filling materials: Amalgam, SuperEBA, and mineral trioxide aggregate. J Endod 2010;36:1323–1325.
227. Otani K, Sugaya T, Tomita M, et al. Healing of experimental apical periodontitis after apicoectomy using different sealing materials on the resected root end. Dent Mater J 2011;30:485–492.
228. Wälivaara DÅ, Abrahamsson P, Isaksson S, Salata LA, Sennerby L, Dahlin C. Periapical tissue response after use of intermediate restorative material, gutta-percha, reinforced zinc oxide cement, and mineral trioxide aggregate as retrograde root-end filling materials: A histologic study in dogs. J Oral Maxillofac Surg 2012; 70:2041–2047.
229. Bernabé PF, Gomes-Filho JE, Cintra LT, et al. Histologic evaluation of the use of membrane, bone graft, and MTA in apical surgery. Oral Surg Oral Med Oral Pathol Oral Radiol Endod 2010;109:309–314.
230. Regan JD, Gutmann JL, Witherspoon DE. Comparison of Diaket and MTA when used as root-end filling materials to support regeneration of the periradicular tissues. Int Endod J 2002;35:840–847.
231. Asgary S, Eghbal MJ, Ehsani S. Periradicular regeneration after endodontic surgery with calcium-enriched mixture cement in dogs. J Endod 2010;36:837–841.
232. Kohout GD, He J, Primus CM, Opperman LA, Woodmansey KF. Comparison of Quick-Set and mineral trioxide aggregate root-end fillings for the regeneration of apical tissues in dogs. J Endod 2015;41:248–252.
233. Chen I, Karabucak B, Wang C, et al. Healing after root-end microsurgery by using mineral trioxide aggregate and a new calcium silicate-based bioceramic material as root-end filling materials in dogs. J Endod 2015;41:389–399.
234. Asgary S. Autogenous transplantation of mandibular third molar to replace tooth with vertical root fracture. Iran Endod J 2009;4:117–121.
235. Ozbas H, Subay RK, Ordulu M. Surgical retreatment of an invaginated maxillary central incisor following overfilled endodontic treatment: A case report. Eur J Dent 2010;4:324–328.
236. García B, Peñarrocha M, Peñarrocha MA, Von Arx T. Apical surgery of a maxillary molar creating a maxillary sinus window using ultrasonics: A clinical case. Int Endod J 2010;43:1054–1061.
237. Kahler B. Microsurgical endodontic retreatment of post restored posterior teeth: A case series. Aust Endod J 2010;36:114–121.
238. Kahler B. Microsurgical endodontic retreatment of a maxillary molar with a separated file: A case report. Aust Dent J 2011;56:76–81.
239. Komabayashi T, Jiang J, Zhu Q. Apical infection spreading to adjacent teeth: A case report. Oral Surg Oral Med Oral Pathol Oral Radiol Endod 2011;111:e15–e20.
240. de Carvalho FB, Gonçalves PS, Lima RK, Guerreiro-Tanomaru JM, Rasquin LC, Tanomaru-Filho M. Use of cone-beam tomography and digital subtraction radiography for diagnosis and evaluation of traumatized teeth treated with endodontic surgery and MTA. A case report. Dent Traumatol 2013;29:404–409.
241. Vier-Pelisser FV, Pelisser A, Recuero LC, Só MV, Borba MG, Figueiredo JA. Use of cone beam computed tomography in the diagnosis, planning and follow up of a type III dens invaginatus case. Int Endod J 2012;45:198–208.
242. Pawar AM, Kokate SR, Shah RA. Management of a large periapical lesion using Biodentine as retrograde restoration with eighteen months evident follow up. J Conserv Dent 2013;16:573–575.
243. Pasqualini D, Scotti N, Ambrogio P, Alovisi M, Berutti E. Atypical facial pain related to apical fenestration and overfilling. Int Endod J 2012;45:670–677.
244. Floratos SG, Kratchman SI. Surgical management of vertical root fractures for posterior teeth: Report of four cases. J Endod 2012;38:550–555.
245. Kheirieh S, Fazlyab M, Torabzadeh H, Eghbal MJ. Extraoral retrograde root canal filling of an orthodontic-induced external root resorption using CEM Cement. Iran Endod J 2014;9:149–152.
246. Sharada HL, Deo B, Briget B. Gemination of a permanent lateral incisor—A case report with special emphasis on management. J Int Oral Health 2013;5:49–53.
247. Asgary S, Ehsani S. Periradicular surgery of human permanent teeth with calcium-enriched mixture cement. Iran Endod J 2013;8:140–144.
248. Bernabé PF, Azuma MM, Ferreira LL, Dezan-Júnior E, Gomes-Filho JE, Cintra LT. Root reconstructed with mineral trioxide aggregate and guided tissue regeneration in apical surgery: A 5-year follow-up. Braz Dent J 2013;24:428–432.
249. Moradi Majd N, Arvin A, Darvish A, Aflaki S, Homayouni H. Treatment of necrotic calcified tooth using intentional replantation procedure. Case Rep Dent 2014; 2014:793892.
250. Asgary S, Alim Marvasti L, Kolahdouzan A. Indications and case series of intentional replantation of teeth. Iran Endod J 2014;9:71–78.
251. Kourkouta S, Bailey GC. Periradicular regenerative surgery in a maxillary central incisor: 7-year results including cone-beam computed tomography. J Endod 2014;40:1013–1039.
252. Sübay RK, Sübay MO, Balkaya CM. Intentional replantation of a mandibular canine with multiple iatrogenic endodontic complications. Oral Health Dent Manag 2014;13:811–814.
253. Caron G, Azérad J, Faure MO, Machtou P, Boucher Y. Use of a new retrograde filling material (Biodentine) for endodontic surgery: Two case reports. Int J Oral Sci 2014;6:250–253.
254. Parirokh M, Farzaneh S, Hallajmofrad AR. Conservative management of unset mineral trioxide aggregate root-end filling: A case report. Iranian Endod J 2016;11:241–245.
255. da Silva SR, da Silva Neto JD, Veiga DF, Schnaider TB, Ferreira LM. Portland cement versus MTA as a root-end filling material. A pilot study. Acta Cir Bras 2015;30:160–164.
256. Lieblich SE. Current concepts of periapical surgery. Oral Maxillofac Surg Clin North Am 2015;27:383–392.
257. Song M, Shin SJ, Kim E. Outcomes of endodontic micro-resurgery: A prospective clinical study. J Endod 2011;37:316–320.
258. Song M, Jung IY, Lee SJ, Lee CY, Kim E. Prognostic factors for clinical outcomes in endodontic microsurgery: A retrospective study. J Endod 2011;37:927–933.
259. Song M, Kim E. A prospective randomized controlled study of mineral trioxide aggregate and super ethoxy-benzoic acid as root-end filling materials in endodontic microsurgery. J Endod 2012;38:875–879.
260. Song M, Kim SG, Shin SJ, Kim HC, Kim E. The influence of bone tissue deficiency on the outcome of endodontic microsurgery: A prospective study. J Endod 2013;39:1341–1345.
261. Song M, Kim SG, Lee SJ, Kim B, Kim E. Prognostic factors of clinical outcomes in endodontic microsurgery: A prospective study. J Endod 2013;39:1491–1497.
262. Song M, Nam T, Shin SJ, Kim E. Comparison of clinical outcomes of endodontic microsurgery: 1 year versus long-term follow-up. J Endod 2014;40:490–494.
263. Lui JN, Khin MM, Krishnaswamy G, Chen NN. Prognostic factors relating to the outcome of endodontic microsurgery. J Endod 2014;40:1071–1076.

264. Chong BS, Pitt Ford TR, Hudson MB. A prospective clinical study of mineral trioxide aggregate and IRM when used as root-end filling materials in endodontic surgery. Int Endod J 2003;36:520–526.
265. Lindeboom JA, Frenken JW, Kroon FH, van den Akker HP. A comparative prospective randomized clinical study of MTA and IRM as root-end filling materials in single-rooted teeth in endodontic surgery. Oral Surg Oral Med Oral Pathol Oral Radiol Endod 2005;100:495–500.
266. von Arx T, Jensen SS, Hänni S, Friedman S. Five-year longitudinal assessment of the prognosis of apical microsurgery. J Endod 2012;38:570–579.
267. Kim S, Song M, Shin SJ, Kim E. A randomized controlled study of mineral trioxide aggregate and super ethoxybenzoic acid as root-end filling materials in endodontic microsurgery: Long-term outcomes. J Endod 2016;42:997–1002.
268. von Arx T, Hänni S, Jensen SS. Clinical results with two different methods of root-end preparation and filling in apical surgery: Mineral trioxide aggregate and adhesive resin composite. J Endod 2010;36:1122–1129.
269. Tortorici S, Difalco P, Caradonna L, Tetè S. Traditional endodontic surgery versus modern technique: A 5-year controlled clinical trial. J Craniofac Surg 2014; 25:804–807.
270. Shinbori N, Grama AM, Patel Y, Woodmansey K, He J. Clinical outcome of endodontic microsurgery that uses EndoSequence BC root repair material as the root-end filling material. J Endod 2015;41:607–612.
271. Garcez AS, Arantes-Neto JG, Sellera DP, Fregnani E. Effects of antimicrobial photodynamic therapy and surgical endodontic treatment on the bacterial load reduction and periapical lesion healing. Three years follow up. Photodiagnosis Photodyn Ther 2015;12:575–580.
272. Chong BS, Pitt Ford TR. Postoperative pain after root-end resection and filling. Oral Surg Oral Med Oral Pathol Oral Radiol Endod 2005;100:762–766.
273. Del Fabbro M, Ceresoli V, Lolato A, Taschieri S. Effect of platelet concentrate on quality of life after periradicular surgery: A randomized clinical study. J Endod 2012;38:733–739.
274. Tsesis I, Faivishevsky V, Kfir A, Rosen E. Outcome of surgical endodontic treatment performed by a modern technique: A meta-analysis of literature. J Endod 2009;35:1505–1511.
275. von Arx T, Peñarrocha M, Jensen S. Prognostic factors in apical surgery with root-end filling: A meta-analysis. J Endod 2010;36:957–973.
276. Tang Y, Li X, Yin S. Outcomes of MTA as root-end filling in endodontic surgery: A systematic review. Quintessence Int 2010;41:557–566.
277. Serrano-Giménez M, Sánchez-Torres A, Gay-Escoda C. Prognostic factors on periapical surgery: A systematic review. Med Oral Pathol Oral Cir Bucal 2015; 20(6):e715–e722.
278. Fleming PS, Lynch CD, Pandis N. Randomized controlled trials in dentistry: Common pitfalls and how to avoid them. J Dent 2014;42:908–914.
279. Lee M, Winkler J, Hartwell G, Stewart J, Caine R. Current trends in endodontic practice: Emergency treatments and technological armamentarium. J Endod 2009;35:35–39.

Chapter Twelve

Surgical Endodontics and the Maxillary Sinus

Roderick W. Tataryn

The close proximity of the maxillary posterior root apices to the maxillary sinus predisposes many surgical endodontic procedures to maxillary sinus communication and thus requires careful consideration when performing periapical surgery in this region. A thorough knowledge of the anatomy and physiology of the sinuses, both in healthy and diseased states, as well as an understanding of the effects of periradicular inflammation on the sinus tissues are requisite for the endodontic surgeon. Expertise in modern surgical techniques, an appreciation for complex maxillary posterior canal morphology, and an understanding of appropriate management and the sequelae of sinus involvement are critical. Proficiency in radiographic interpretation of both two-dimensional (2D) and three-dimensional (3D) imaging is also essential for diagnosis, presurgical planning, and postsurgical healing evaluation.

The Maxillary Sinus: Anatomy and Physiology

The paranasal sinuses are hollow air spaces in the skull surrounding the nasal cavity. There are four pairs of paranasal sinuses: the maxillary, frontal, ethmoid, and sphenoid (Fig 12-1). The primary purpose of the sinuses is immune defense via the production of mucus to filter inspired air. The sinuses also warm and humidify inhaled air, reduce the weight of the skull and protect it from trauma, and act as resonance chambers to amplify the voice and give it unique tonal quality.[1]

The maxillary sinus, also called the *antrum*, is located within the body of the maxilla and is the largest of the paranasal sinuses. The size of the adult maxillary sinus is widely variable; the capacity ranges from 9.5 to 20 mL, and the average capacity is 14.75 mL.[2] In children, the sinus floor lies at or above the level of the floor of the nasal cavity, whereas in the adult the sinus floor may be 5 to 10 mm below that of the nasal fossa. Growth and development of the maxillary sinus includes a period of rapid expansion between ages 7 and 18 years, with much of the growth related to invasion of the alveolar process following eruption of the related permanent dentition.[1] A computed tomographic (CT) study found that growth of the maxillary sinus continues until the third decade in males and the second decade in females.[3] The shape of the maxillary sinus in an adult is generally described as a four-sided pyramid, with the base of the pyramid forming the lateral nasal wall and its rounded apex extending into

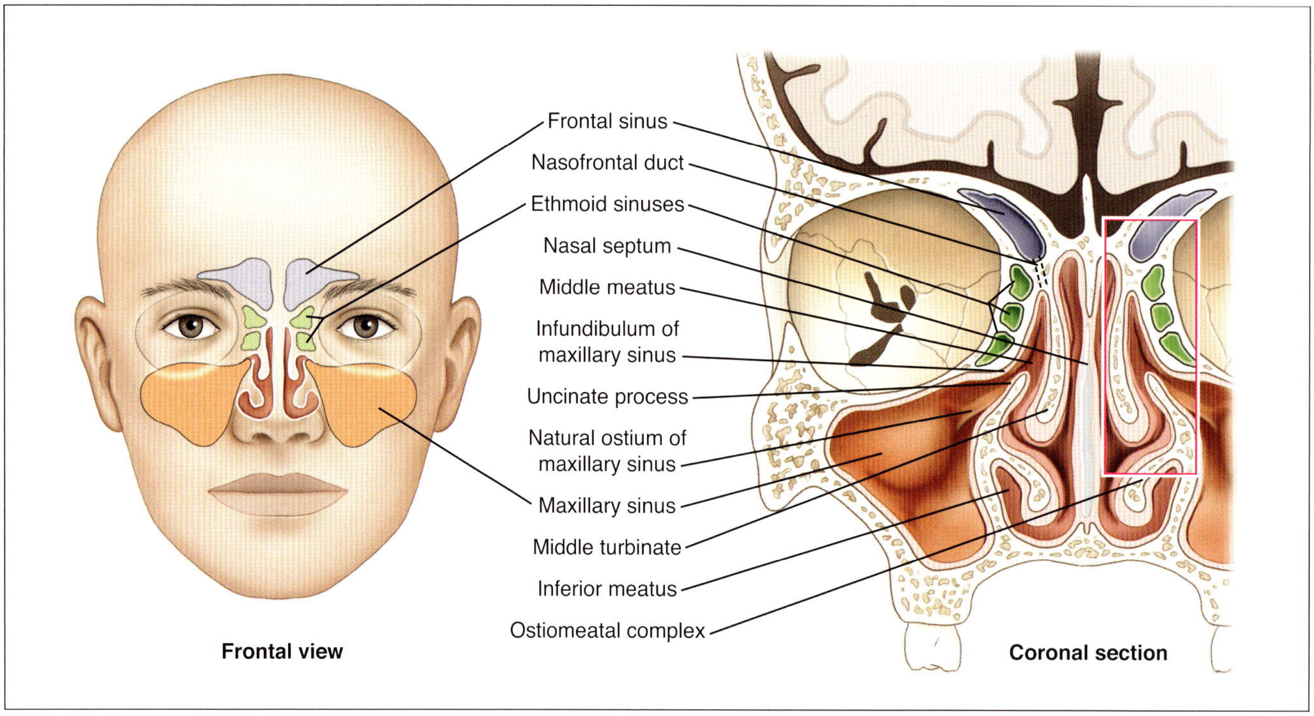

Fig 12-1 The paranasal sinuses and surrounding anatomical structures.

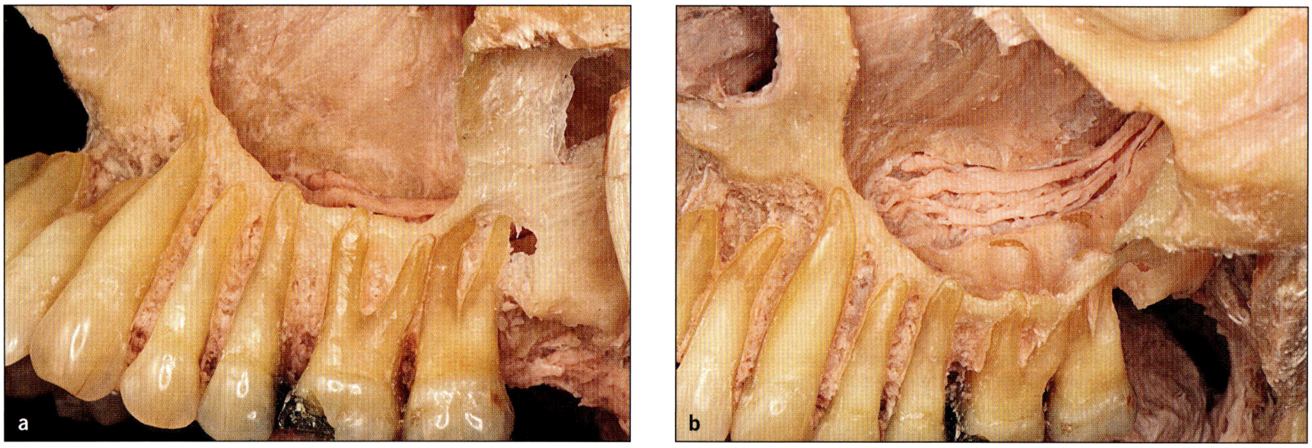

Fig 12-2 *(a)* Cadaver dissection of a highly pneumatized maxillary sinus revealing the intimate proximity of the posterior maxillary root apices to the lateral antral wall and floor. *(b)* The sinus extends inferiorly between the molar roots, and there is a lack of bony partition between the molar palatal root apices and the antrum.

the zygoma. The roof of the sinus forms the floor of the orbit, the concave anterior sinus wall forms the canine fossa, and the posterior wall is adjacent to the infratemporal and pterygopalatine fossae. The floor of the maxillary sinus is composed of the maxillary alveolar process and the palatine process.[2] In larger, more highly pneumatized sinuses, the sinus floor may expand inferiorly deep into the maxillary alveolar process, extending between the individual roots of the maxillary posterior teeth and occasionally extending as far anterior as the maxillary canine (Fig 12-2). The maxillary sinus communicates with the nasal cavity through a main opening in the upper and anterior third of the medial sinus wall called the *ostium*. The ostium enters the middle meatus of the nasal cavity and typically ranges from 1 to 4 mm in diameter. In 10% to 30% of sinuses, an additional opening or accessory ostium is present.[1]

The inner surface of the sinus is lined by the mucoperiosteum, consisting of mucosa, also known as the *sinus membrane*, and the underlying periosteum. The mucosa

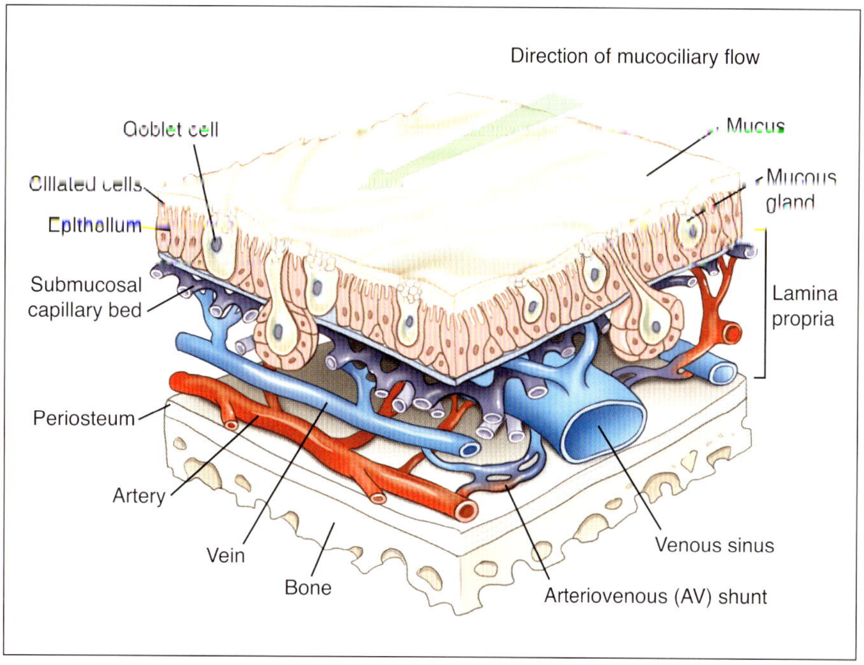

Fig 12-3 Illustration of the cellular layers and structures that compose the mucoperiosteum of the sinus wall.

of the paranasal sinuses is continuous with but is thinner and less vascular than the nasal mucosa. A healthy sinus mucosa generally ranges between 0.13 and 0.5 mm in thickness[4] but will become significantly thicker when inflamed from sinus disease, allergic phenomena, or dental pathosis.[5] The mucosa is made up of a surface layer of pseudostratified, ciliated, and nonciliated columnar epithelial cells, basal cells, an underlying basal membrane, and the lamina propria (Fig 12-3). The lamina propria attaches directly to the periosteum of the underlying cortical bone. The lamina propria provides support and nutrition to the epithelium. It consists of loose connective tissue, a significant vascular network, and a varied population of immune cells including fibroblasts, lymphocytes, plasma cells, macrophages, eosinophilic leukocytes, and mast cells, making it capable of significant expansion and a key location for immune responses to occur.[6] The sinus epithelium is interspersed with mucus-producing goblet cells as well as serous and mucinous glands located below the basement membrane and within the lamina propria that continuously produce and excrete mucinous fluid to the surface of the membrane. The mucinous fluid is composed of 96% water but also contains immune cells, antibodies, and antibacterial proteins, making it an important part of the immune defense by trapping and filtering particles such as inspired dust, spores, viruses, and bacteria. The viscosity of the mucus varies in response to the signals from the autonomic nervous system and in response to inflammation.[7]

Functional cilia are essential to sinus health. The cilia of the epithelial cells beat rapidly, at an average of 16 beats per second, in a coordinated, rhythmic, wavelike pattern that moves the mucus in a spiraling direction upward toward the sinus ostium and into the nasal cavity. From there the mucus is moved to the back of the throat by the ciliated cells lining the nasal cavity, where it is ultimately swallowed and dissolved by digestive acids.[7] A new mucinous blanket is formed approximately every 20 to 30 minutes, and the average adult will produce between 1 and 2 liters of mucus per day. The healthy maxillary sinus is aseptic, containing neither bacteria nor any foreign material.[8] The cilia and associated mucinous flow are typically only able to transport and remove small foreign bodies and other small particulate matter found in inspired air. Larger particles such as surgical debris, tooth roots, and root filling materials are usually too large to be removed via the cilia and ostial pathway.[9]

The maxillary sinus has an extensive vascular network from both endosseous and periosteal supplies. Endosseous vessels run along the buccal antral wall supplied by an anastomosis of the posterior superior and infraorbital arteries. Periosteal vessels are supplied by the posterior superior, infraorbital, and palatine arteries. Maxillary sinus venous drainage occurs via the facial vein, the sphenopalatine vein, and the pterygoid plexus.[9] The vascular drainage joins typical pathways in the maxilla to the jugular veins, but it can also drain upward into the ethmoid and frontal sinuses and eventually reach the cavernous sinus in the floor of the brain, posing a serious complication to the potential spread of maxillary sinus infections.[10]

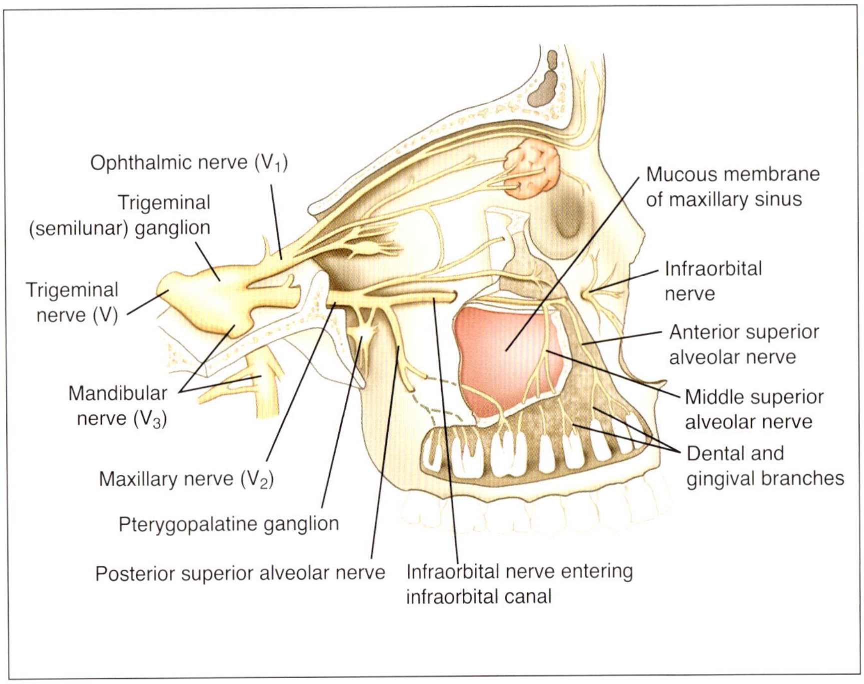

Fig 12-4 Nerve supply to the maxillary sinus.

Sensory innervation of the maxillary sinus mucosal tissues originates directly from the maxillary division of the trigeminal nerve (Fig 12-4). The posterior and middle superior alveolar branches travel along the inner wall of the sinus below the mucous membrane and innervate the posterior antral wall together with the molar and premolar teeth. The anterior superior alveolar nerve travels along the anterior sinus wall innervating the anterior sinus along with the maxillary anterior teeth. Innervation to the orbital wall of the maxillary sinus is via the infraorbital nerve, which travels along a groove in the central portion of the roof of the sinus. Branches of the pterygopalatine ganglion and sphenopalatine ganglion also innervate the sinus mucosa.[1,9]

Rhinosinusitis

Epidemiology

Rhinosinusitis is defined as inflammation of the mucous membrane lining the paranasal sinuses and nasal cavity.[11] Rhinosinusitis is one of the most prevalent chronic illnesses in the United States, affecting 14% of the population and accounting for an estimated 30 million physician visits per year with a direct treatment cost of up to $11 billion annually.[12] More than 20% of all antibiotics prescribed to adults are for the treatment of rhinosinusitis.[13] The terms *rhinosinusitis* and *sinusitis* are used interchangeably in the medical literature; however, the term *rhinosinusitis* is often considered more appropriate because sinus inflammation rarely occurs without concomitant inflammation of the contiguous nasal mucosa.[11,14]

Pathophysiology

The pathophysiology of rhinosinusitis is multifactorial.[15] The primary etiologies are due to obstruction of the sinus ostium and pathophysiologic changes in the mucociliary transport mechanism.[16] It is also well established that odontogenic infections, including periradicular abscesses and periodontal infections, are etiologic factors in a significant percentage of rhinosinusitis cases.[17,18] Trauma and other iatrogenic factors such as sinus wall fractures, endodontic procedures, and extractions may also induce maxillary sinusitis by damaging the integrity of the sinus wall and membrane.[19] The primary cause of ostial obstruction is inflammatory edema of the sinus mucosa, typically in response to a viral infection, an allergen, or bacteria. The sinus ostia are generally small, and even a minimal amount of mucosal swelling can lead to obstruction and prevention of normal sinus drainage. Edema of the sinus mucosa occurs as a result of vasodilation of vessels within the lamina propria; the infiltration of polymorphic neutrophils (PMNs), mast cells, and lymphocytes; and the subsequent release of chemical mediators such as histamines and prostaglandins into the mucosal tissue.[20] The ostia can also be obstructed by

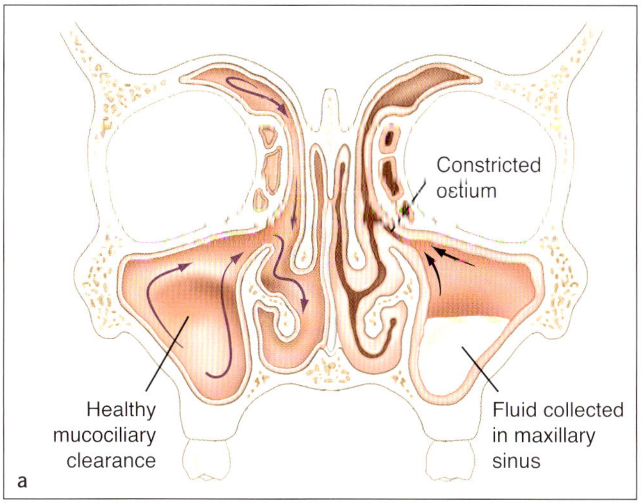

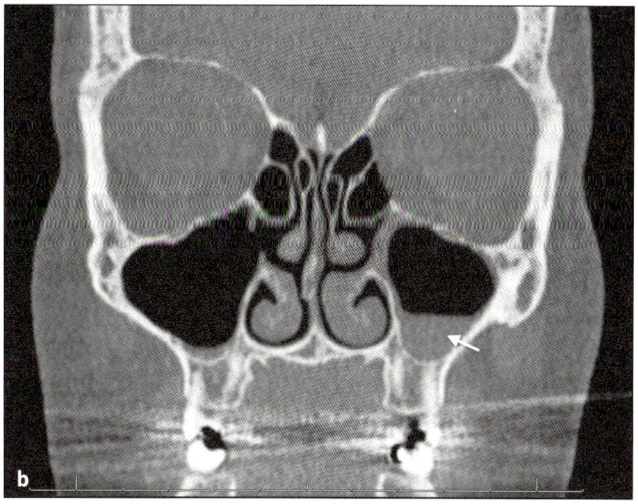

Fig 12-5 Rhinosinusitis. *(a)* Mucosal edema constricts the sinus ostium and prevents normal mucociliary clearance, causing an accumulation of secretions within the sinus. *(b)* Coronal CT image showing mucosal edema and mucous accumulation in the left maxillary sinus *(arrow)*.

other factors including polyps, septal deviation, foreign bodies, or tumors of the nasal cavity. Once obstructed, mucous secretions begin to accumulate within the sinus (Fig 12-5). The lack of sinus ventilation results in a lower oxygen tension and a lower pH, creating a favorable environment for bacterial pathogens to colonize within the sinus. As the condition progresses, the mucus thickens and stagnates, causing ciliary function to be reduced and eventually halted. With time, the epithelial tissue becomes damaged, making a long-standing chronic condition far more difficult to resolve, and an even more opportune environment develops for further bacterial colonization.[15]

Acute and chronic rhinosinusitis

Rhinosinusitis is typically classified based on the duration of patient symptoms: A condition lasting less than 4 weeks is considered *acute* rhinosinusitis (ARS), while a condition lasting more than 12 weeks is considered *chronic* rhinosinusitis (CRS).[11] Symptoms of sinusitis lasting between 4 and 12 weeks fall under the category *subacute* rhinosinusitis, but this condition is rarely distinguished in clinical practice guidelines other than to represent a transition from ARS to CRS.[13] The primary symptoms associated with ARS are nasal congestion, obstruction, and facial pain or pressure, and as such, ARS can generally be diagnosed adequately on the basis of clinical findings alone. Rhinosinusitis may be further classified by etiology into *bacterial* or *viral* rhinosinusitis. The predominant florae isolated in acute bacterial rhinosinusitis are *Streptococcus pneumoniae*, *Moraxella catarrhalis*, and *Haemophilus influenzae*. ARS is most commonly viral in origin and usually disappears in the majority of cases within 10 to 14 days with no medical or surgical intervention. Clinical studies have confirmed that roughly 60% of presumed acute bacterial rhinosinusitis cases resolve spontaneously, yet recent data indicate that antibiotics are prescribed in 81% to 92% of ARS cases.[14]

The bacterial flora of chronic rhinosinusitis is typically a mixed infection, with *Staphylococcus aureus* and anaerobes including *Prevotella* sp, *Porphyromonas* sp, *Fusobacterium nucleatum*, and *Peptostreptococcus* sp being the more frequent isolates.[21] Symptoms of CRS can be more difficult to recognize as they are often milder and more variable in presentation. They include potential major symptoms of mucopurulent drainage, nasal obstruction, facial pain and pressure (though rarely severe), and a decreased sense of smell. Minor symptoms can include halitosis, dental pain, cough, fever, and fatigue.[11]

The role of fungal involvement in CRS continues to be a focus of research and debate. Fungal balls or mycetomas are isolated fungal infections typically occurring in a single sinus cavity and are mostly found in the maxillary sinus. *Aspergillus* is the most commonly found fungus in fungal sinusitis. Certain fungal infections can be either allergic in nature or invasive and more serious, particularly in patients who are immunocompromised or in patients with poorly controlled diabetes.[22,23]

Diagnosis

A definitive diagnosis of rhinosinusitis or other conditions involving diseases of the maxillary sinus falls within the scope of an otorhinolaryngologist, or ear, nose, and throat (ENT) physician. Most sinus infections are initially diagnosed based on patient history and clinical examination. In chronic cases, further tests such as nasal endoscopy, needle aspiration, culture and sensitivity tests, and CT imaging may also be performed.[11] CT sinus imaging can reveal ostial blockage, mucosal edema, and the level of retained fluid within the sinus that may indicate sinus disease and its possible cause (see Fig 12-5b). Although CT imaging has a high sensitivity, it has a low specificity for demonstrating rhinosinusitis. Havas et al[24] have found that sinus abnormalities were found on sinus CT in 42.5% of patients with no symptoms or clinical suspicion of sinus disease. It is also important to note that sinus inflammation and symptoms can occur in the absence of significant CT findings. Fungal sinus infections are usually diagnosed by fungal culture and microscopic identification and can also show characteristic radiopaque findings on CT imaging due to the presence of calcium and traces of metallic elements within the fungal ball.[25]

Treatment

Because obstruction of the ostium is the focal point of maxillary sinus disease, the re-establishment of ostial patency and sinus aeration via a reduction in mucosal edema is the primary goal in the treatment of rhinosinusitis.[13,20] Successful management of most cases of ARS requires only conservative therapy and oral antibiotics for specific bacterial cases. In cases of CRS, with the longer progression of sinus disease and the bacterial flora becoming more anaerobic, treatment includes the administration of broad-spectrum antibiotics such as amoxicillin-clavulanate, clindamycin, or a combination of penicillin and metronidazole.[21] Adjunctive treatments include the use of steroid nasal sprays, decongestants, and saline rinses. If antibiotic therapy and adjunctive treatments are ineffective, then endoscopic sinus surgery is often indicated to surgically enlarge the natural ostium and re-establish drainage by removing any ostial blockage.[15,20] Fungal rhinosinusitis is an absolute indication for sinus surgery.[20,22,26]

Maxillary sinusitis of dental origin

The pathologic extension of dental disease into the maxillary sinus is well established and widely reported in both the dental and medical literatures.[10,17–19,27–45] The literature reports that between 60% and 87.8% of periradicular infections of the maxillary posterior teeth will induce some level of maxillary sinus pathology.[40–44] There are also numerous case reports in the literature showing the full resolution of varying degrees of sinus disease following endodontic treatment or extraction of the source tooth.[10,17,30,32,37,39,45] A commonly quoted incidence for odontogenic sinusitis is 10% to 12% of cases of maxillary sinusitis; however, the source document provides no epidemiologic support for this figure.[28] The actual incidence of odontogenic sinusitis is unknown, likely because diagnostic methods, definitions of disease, and terms used vary widely among investigators; however, several researchers estimate the incidence to be higher than the often-repeated figure of 10% to 12%.[17,18,31,34,35,39] In a study by Melen et al[34] including 198 patients with 244 cases of chronic bacterial maxillary sinusitis, a dental etiology was found in 40.6% of the cases. Lindahl et al[31] found a 47% incidence of dental infections after careful ENT and oral examination of 62 patients with chronic maxillary sinusitis. Maillet et al[35] reviewed 82 cone beam CT (CBCT) scans with 135 instances of maxillary sinusitis and found that 98 occurrences (73%) were tooth associated, with the maxillary first and second molars 11 times more likely to be involved than premolars. Failure to recognize or adequately treat the odontogenic source allows sinusitis to persist and in many cases leads to the failure of medical and surgical sinusitis therapy.[17,18,37,46]

Odontogenic sinus infections may be asymptomatic or produce only mild symptoms for months or even years, inducing only a minimal local reaction in the antral mucosa.[37] A pathologically altered mucosa is presumably less resistant than an intact one to infection and is a pathogenic factor in rhinosinusitis.[31] Depending on the degree of dental infection, the extent of mucosal edema, and ostial patency, sinus obstruction may occur, leading to more serious infections such as severe rhinosinusitis or pansinusitis and, in rare cases, orbital cellulitis, blindness, meningitis, subdural empyema, brain abscess, or cavernous sinus thrombosis.[47–57] These infections can occur along several possible pathways. Infection may spread from the maxillary sinus through bone erosion of the orbit, via infraorbital canals, or through the ethmoid sinus. Infection may also spread into the infratemporal and pterygopalatine fossa and then into the orbit through the inferior orbital fissure. Thirdly, infection can spread along the facial vein and the ophthalmic vein by hematogenous regurgitation because the veins of the face, eyes, nasal cavity, and sinus are all connected without valves.[53]

Despite the abundant literature, high incidence, and serious potential complications of odontogenic sinusitis, this condition frequently goes unrecognized by radiologists, otolaryngologists, and dentists alike. In two separate case series evaluating odontogenic sinusitis, approximately two-thirds of the identifiable dental pathology went unreported by radiologists on sinus CT scans.[17,39] It was also found that routine general dental examination using periapical radiographs failed to diagnose odontogenic maxillary sinusitis in 86% of the cases.[17] CBCT imaging has been shown to significantly improve the ability to detect odontogenic sources for sinusitis.[58,59] The radiographic appearances of the effects of periradicular inflammation on the sinus periosteum and respiratory mucosal tissues are distinctly different than that of endodontic disease found in strictly osseous tissues and can

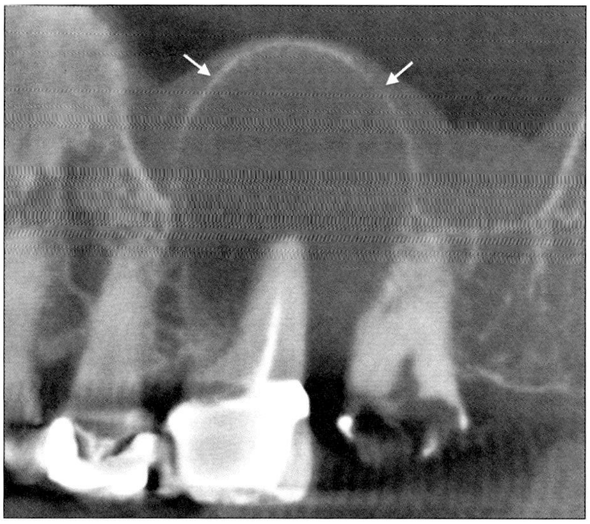

Fig 12-6 Periapical osteoperiostitis ("halo" lesion). Sagittal CBCT image of a failing root canal treatment and distal periodontal defect of the maxillary left first molar. Periradicular periodontitis has displaced the periosteum into the floor of the maxillary sinus, and new cortical bone has formed on the periphery of the disease process as a result of the periosteal reaction to the inflammatory stimulus *(arrows)*.

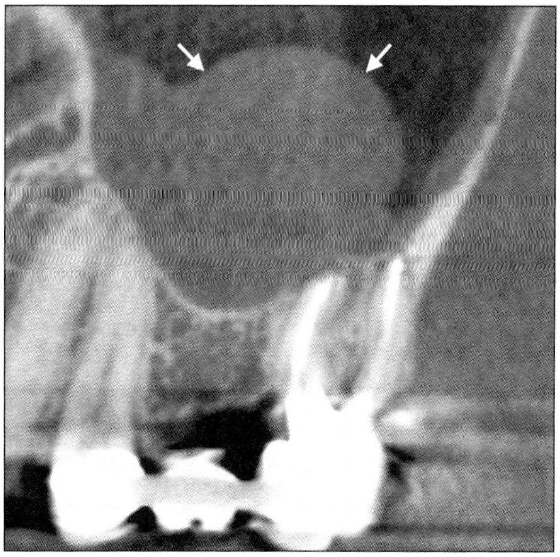

Fig 12-7 Periapical mucositis. Sagittal CBCT image of a failing root canal treatment of the maxillary left second molar. Apical periodontitis has perforated the antral cortex and associated periosteum, causing a localized inflammatory edema of the adjacent sinus mucosa *(arrows)*. Note the lack of any evident osseous changes in the alveolar bone or sinus floor.

mimic sinogenic lesions that do not have a dental etiology. It is imperative that the endodontic surgeon has a comprehensive understanding of the various radiographic and clinical manifestations of odontogenic sinusitis in order to accurately diagnose and treat this condition.

Periapical osteoperiostitis

The presence of apical periodontitis adjacent to the maxillary sinus cortical floor will often expand the sinus periosteum, displace it upward into the sinus, and subsequently induce a periosteal reaction that continues to deposit a thin layer of new bone on the inner periphery of the disease process as it expands. The periosteum is a dense connective tissue membrane consisting of an outer fibrous layer and an inner cellular layer called the *cambium*. The cambium contains progenitor cells that develop into osteoblasts and begin to produce new bone when irritated by inflammatory stimuli. This thin, hard tissue dome on the sinus floor has been termed *periapical osteoperiostitis* and presents on radiographs and CT images as a radiopaque "halo" appearance[60] (Fig 12-6). If the inflammatory process continues, the bone deposits can become thicker and expand deeper into the maxillary sinus. Periapical osteoperiostitis lesions may be accompanied by varying degrees of adjacent mucosal edema and sinus fluid levels, particularly if a break or perforation occurs in the periosteum and osseous halo or dome.

Periapical mucositis

Infected roots that are in direct contact with antral mucosa, or periapical inflammation that has perforated the periosteum, can produce a localized tissue edema in the mucosa without causing osseous damage. This localized odontogenic edema of the sinus mucosal tissue has been termed *periapical mucositis* and is often seen on periapical radiographs and CT imaging as a mucosal thickening or soft tissue expansion in the floor of the sinus directly adjacent to the infected root apex[60] (Fig 12-7). Periradicular inflammation from dental roots not directly adjacent to the sinus mucosa can also cause periapical mucositis without any evident inflammatory bone resorption via extension of inflammatory mediators through bone marrow, blood vessels, and lymphatics.[27] Without evident osseous damage, odontogenic infections involving only the sinus mucosa are more difficult to recognize radiographically than those causing obvious alveolar bone changes or osteoperiostitis lesions. Mucosal edema on the sinus floor and particularly dome-shaped mucosal swellings directly over dental root apices should raise the suspicion of a dental etiology, even in the absence of osseous changes.

Differential diagnosis

It is important to note that sinogenic mucosal thickening, mucous retention cysts, and antral polyps are common findings that can mimic periapical mucositis; therefore, careful clinical endodontic examination is indicated to distinguish a routine mucosal abnormality from periapical mucositis. Mucous retention cysts are benign, dome-shaped lesions caused by either a blocked seromucinous gland duct or invagination of sinus epithelium.[61] They are routinely seen on sinus imaging and are considered incidental findings, normally not requiring intervention.[62] Sinogenic mucosal thickening is also routinely seen on CT imaging and is common in the general population.[24,63,64] Several studies, however, show a strong positive correlation between apical periodontitis and sinus mucosal thickening.[43,63,65–68] Lu et al,[43] in a CBCT study of 508 sinuses, found that the prevalence of maxillary sinus mucosal thickening was 41.5% in patients without apical periodontitis, more than 70% in patients with mild and moderate apical periodontitis, and 100% for those with severe apical periodontitis. Shanbhag et al,[67] reviewing 485 sinuses with CBCT, found that posterior maxillary teeth with periapical lesions were 9.75 times more likely to be associated with mucosal thickening than those without. Bomeli et al,[65] in a CT review of 202 maxillary sinuses, found that increases in mucosal thickening and sinus fluid levels were more likely to have an identifiable dental source. If sinus mucosal hyperplasia is seen radiographically, particularly on the sinus floor or adjacent to a specific dental root, it should raise the suspicion for a potential dental etiology; however, it is not conclusive in the absence of appropriate clinical endodontic examination.

Relationship of the Maxillary Teeth to the Maxillary Sinus

In order to understand the pathologic connection between endodontic disease and sinusitis, as well as for precise planning and execution of periapical surgery, it is crucial to understand the anatomical relationships of the roots, sinus, and neighboring anatomical structures. As mentioned previously, the dimensions of the maxillary sinus vary widely in the population, with highly pneumatized sinuses expanding inferiorly deep into the maxillary alveolar process extending to, around, and in between the individual roots of the maxillary posterior teeth, often leaving only the respiratory mucosa separating the sinus cavity from the dental roots. This unique anatomical relationship has been carefully studied by many investigators for nearly a century. According to a paper by Killey and Kay,[69] a Danish study in 1925 by Von Bonsdorff examined 84 human skulls and measured the distance of various root apices from the sinus floor and the frequency of their root apices being within 0.5 mm of the sinus floor. He found that the second molar averaged 1.3 mm and 45.5%, the first molar 2.6 mm and 30.4%, the second premolar 2.9 mm and 19.7%, and the first premolar 7.6 mm and 0%. Many more current studies using CT report similar findings and confirm that the root apices of the maxillary second molar are generally the closest to the sinus floor and have the highest percentage of protrusion into the sinus, followed by the maxillary first molar, second premolar, and lastly the first premolar.[70–75] In agreement with these findings, other studies have investigated the maxillary sinus volume and concluded that the lowest point of the sinus floor, or area of maximum pneumatization, was related to the second molar in 93% of the cases.[38,76] Minor dimensional differences reported between measurement studies are likely due to factors such as group selection, race, and age.[73] Tian et al[77] assessed root proximity according to age and found that patients over the age of 40 years showed a decreased likelihood of root protrusion into the sinus floor, which is in agreement with other studies reporting that the maxillary sinus reaches maximum volume at approximately age 20 years and then begins decreasing with age.[3,78–80]

Another important anatomical consideration in periapical surgery is the thickness of the buccal and palatal bone to the root apices. This is important in terms of reaching instruments to the surgical site as well as securing the surgical field. A study by Kang et al[81] found that although the apices of the mesiobuccal roots of the second molars had the shortest mean vertical distance to the maxillary sinus floor, they also had the thickest mean horizontal distance to the buccal cortical plate. Jin et al[78] reported that the average distance from the mesiobuccal root of the second molar to the buccal plate was 4.63 mm, the average distances from the palatal apex of the maxillary first and second molars to the buccal bone plate were 10.69 and 10.17 mm, respectively, while, from the palatal bone plate, average distances of 3.15 and 3.08 mm were measured. Other studies confirm these findings with similar reported measurements.[70,71,82,83]

Spatial relationships between the roots of the posterior maxillary teeth and the maxillary sinus may be as crucial to presurgical planning as specific dimensional measurements. Several investigators have devised classification systems for these various relationships.[71,81,82,84,85] Jung and Cho[71] examined 332 maxillary molars with CBCT imaging and proposed four types of vertical relationships between the roots of maxillary molars and the sinus floor with the incidence of each: In Type 0, the root is separate from the sinus floor (25%); in Type 1, the root is in contact with the sinus floor (19%); in Type 2, the root is projecting laterally along the sinus cavity (21.4%); and in Type 3, the root is projecting into the sinus cavity (34.6%) (Fig 12-8). Understanding the case-specific anatomical relationship of the tooth and sinus prior to surgical intervention is imperative in the prevention, minimization, and management of sinus involvement during endodontic surgical treatment.

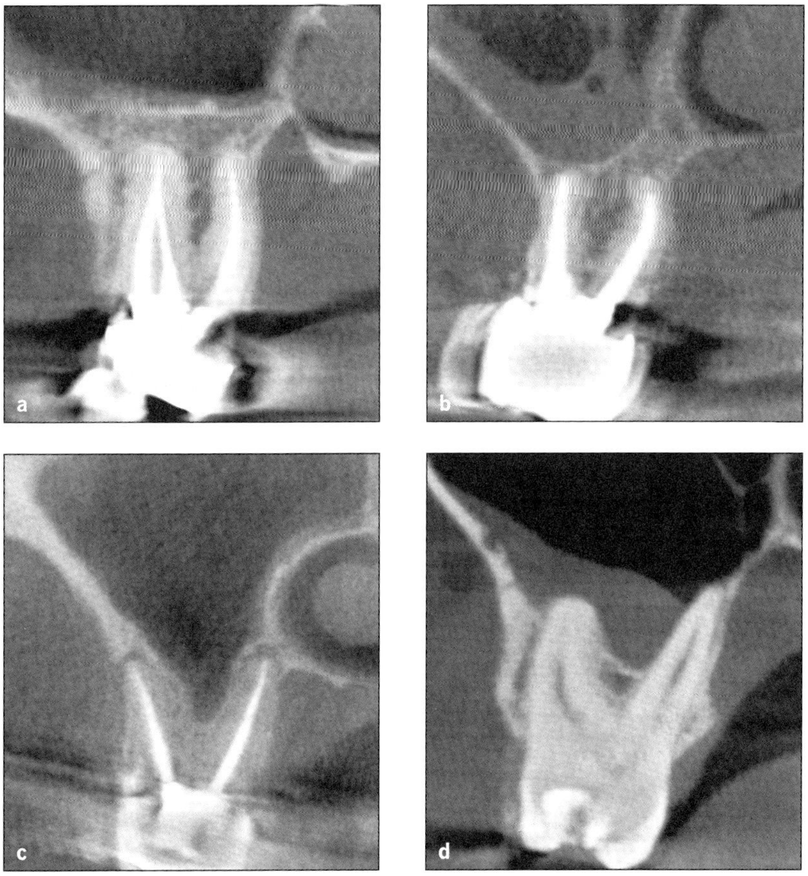

Fig 12-8 Coronal CBCT images showing the four types of vertical relationships described by Jung and Cho.[71] *(a)* Type 0: The root is separate from the sinus floor. *(b)* Type 1: The root is in contact with the sinus floor. *(c)* Type 2: The root is projecting laterally along the sinus cavity wall but is outside the sinus borders. *(d)* Type 3: The root is projecting into the sinus cavity.

Anatomical complexity of the maxillary molars

Effective surgical as well as nonsurgical endodontic therapy depends on a comprehensive understanding of root morphology and the complex anatomy found in root canal systems. In the endodontic literature, the mesiobuccal root of the maxillary first molar has generated more research and clinical investigation than any other root.[85] Considering the close proximity of this highly complex root canal system to the maxillary sinus, and the potential need for surgical intervention to adequately treat it, a thorough understanding of its morphology is crucial for the endodontic surgeon. A literature review of the canal morphology of the maxillary first molar, including 8,399 teeth from 34 studies, indicated that the incidence of two canals in the mesiobuccal root was 56.8%.[85] Hsu and Kim[86] noted that at the 3-mm level from the apex, 90% of the mesiobuccal roots of maxillary first molars have an isthmus. Studies of serial sections as well as microCT analysis indicate that when two canals are present, anastomoses and an isthmus are present in virtually all mesiobuccal root systems, along with accessory canals, apical deltas, and loops, with many variations falling outside of established classification systems[87-91] (Fig 12-9).

It is also known that a significant percentage of maxillary posterior teeth have fused roots. In reviews of eight studies including 1,714 first molars and seven studies including 1,960 second molars, the incidence of root fusion in maxillary first molars was 6.2%, and the incidence of root fusion in maxillary second molars was 25.8%.[92] Root fusion can exist in any or all of the molar roots, and in various configurations, and the incidence of fused roots may differ between ethnic populations.[93,94] It can be expected that teeth with fused roots have an isthmus or weblike connection that must be cleaned, shaped, and filled as any other canal system.[95-97] The inability of instruments, irrigating solutions, and root filling materials to penetrate into the isthmus region can lead to endodontic failure. In these cases, accurate surgical management of this isthmus anatomy may be indicated and necessary for periapical healing[86] (Fig 12-10). Failure to properly manage isthmus anatomy, either in the multicanal mesiobuccal root or in fused maxillary roots, could allow for persistent periapical inflammation and associated odon-

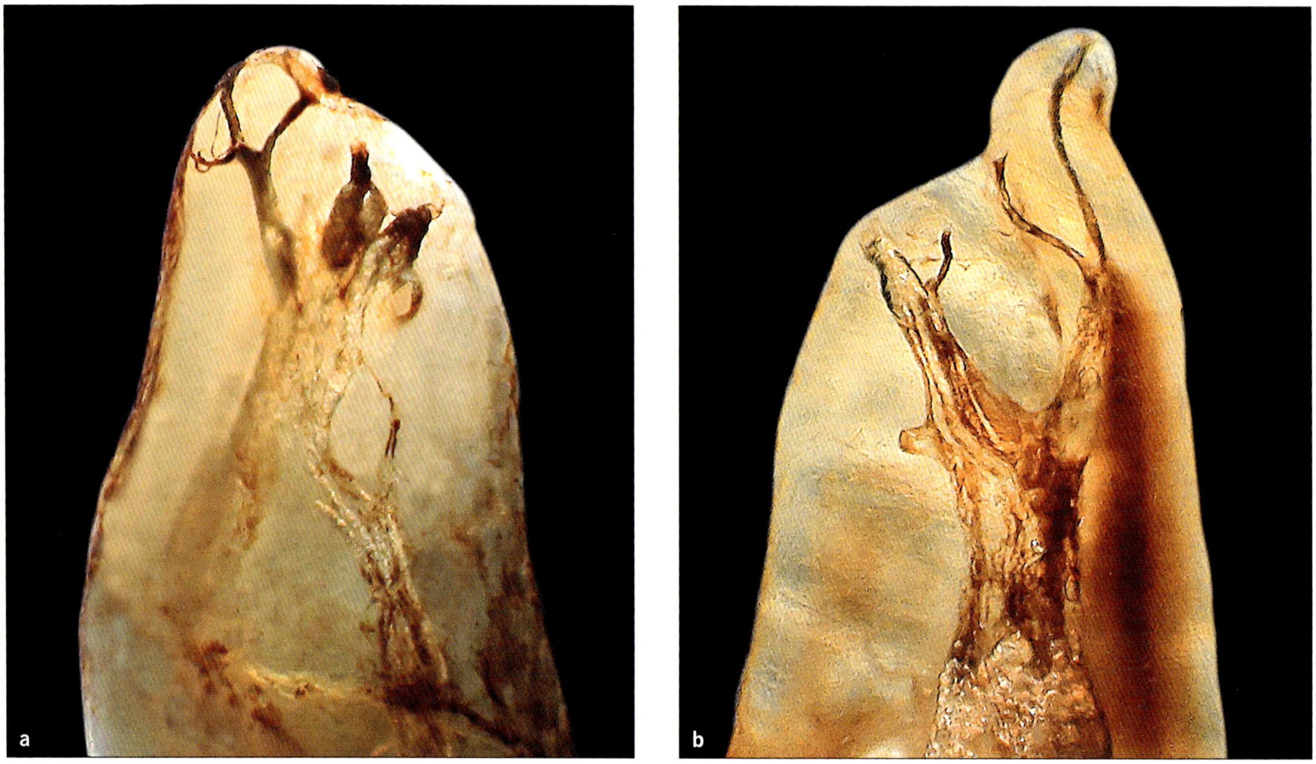

Fig 12-9 Cleared specimens of maxillary first molar mesiobuccal roots showing the complex canal anatomy and endodontic treatment task. The apices of these complex systems are often in close proximity or direct contact with the sinus mucosa, facilitating potential sinus infection in the event of endodontic failure and increasing the difficulty of endodontic surgical procedures. *(a)* Maxillary right first molar mesiobuccal root system. *(b)* Maxillary left first molar mesiobuccal root system. (Courtesy of Dr Craig Barrington, Waxahachie, Texas.)

togenic sinusitis. Considering the intimate relationship between these complex maxillary posterior molar roots and the floor of the maxillary sinus, it is incumbent on the endodontic surgeon to have a clear understanding of the various complex root morphologies in the maxillary posterior dentition and be skilled in their proper surgical management in order to prevent or bring about healing of persistent secondary sinus disease.

Diagnostic imaging in the posterior maxilla

Periapical radiographs are the most widely used imaging modality in endodontics, yet their many limitations can lead clinicians to radiographic misinterpretation, misdiagnosis, and potential mistreatment.[98] The posterior maxilla presents significant and unique interpretation challenges when using conventional 2D imaging. The zygomatic and palatal processes, maxillary sinus cortical floor, and buccal cortical plate are often superimposed onto the dental roots, obscuring or concealing periradicular lesions and root morphology. Also, periapical radiographs are subject to geometric distortion, causing elongation and foreshortening errors, and in the posterior maxilla the irradiation geometry often cannot be made optimal due to a low palatal vault.[99] Conventional periapical radiographs do not consistently reveal mucosal soft tissue changes, periapical osteoperiostitis, or air-fluid levels in the sinus, which can be of great diagnostic value in cases of odontogenic sinusitis. Finally, periapical radiographs cannot be used as predictors for potential perforations of the maxillary sinus,[8] as the positional relationships of the dental roots to the maxillary sinus cannot be reliably assessed.[100]

Current literature has demonstrated the many benefits of CBCT for presurgical planning of periapical surgery in the posterior maxilla.[98–108] In a study by Low et al[101] comparing periapical radiography and CBCT for preoperative diagnosis in 74 posterior maxillary teeth consecutively referred for apical surgery, CBCT revealed 34% more lesions than periapical radiography as well as significantly more expansion of lesions into the maxillary sinus, sinus membrane thickening, and missed canals. The authors

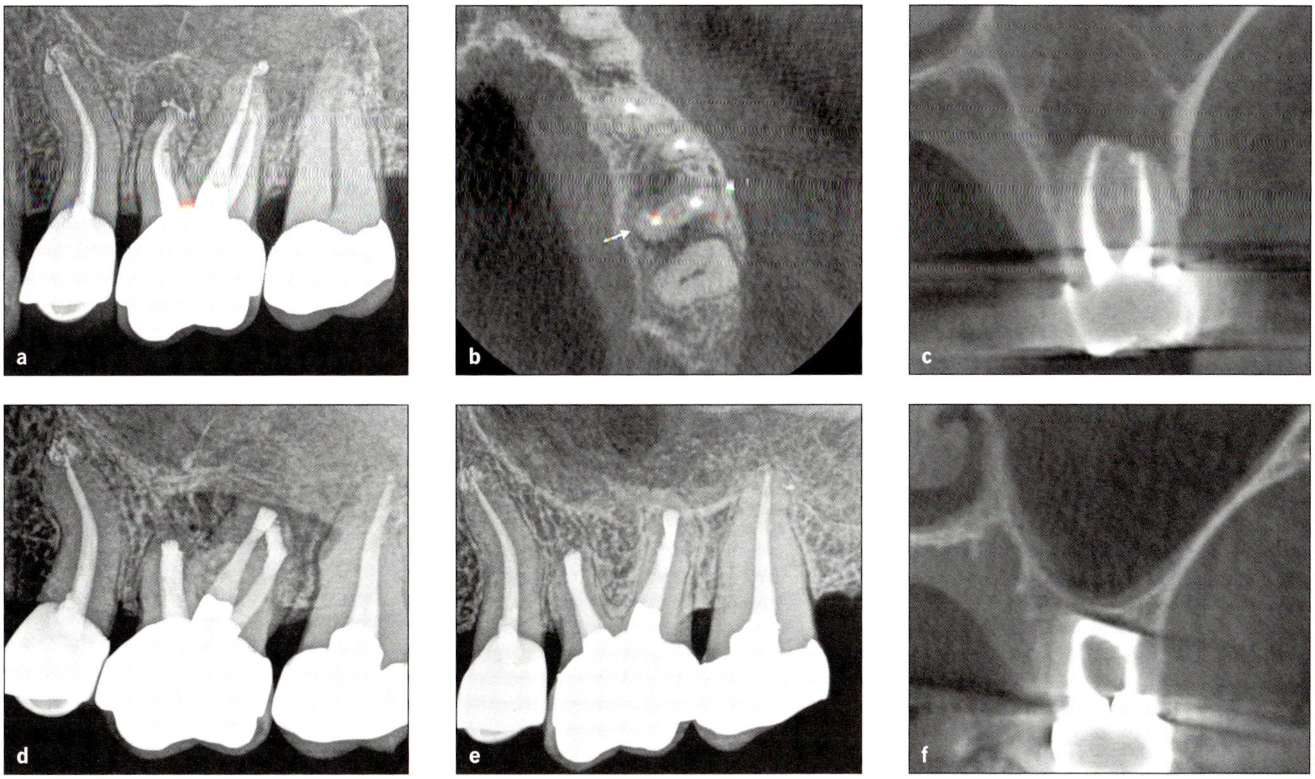

Fig 12-10 Endodontic surgical management of maxillary molar isthmus anatomy. *(a)* Periapical radiograph of a persistent periapical infection of the maxillary left first molar despite two orthograde endodontic treatments. *(b)* Axial CBCT image of the fused distobuccal-palatal (DB-P) root and associated isthmus canal system *(arrows)*. *(c)* Coronal CBCT image of the fused DB-P root system and evident periapical osteoperiostitis lesion. *(d)* Periapical radiograph following surgical retrofilling of the isthmus in the fused DB-P root system, as well as the mesiobuccal 1–mesiobuccal 2 system. Histopathologic evaluation revealed the presence of *Actinomyces* in the periapical lesion. *(e)* Periapical radiograph at the 1-year postsurgical follow-up. *(f)* Coronal CBCT image at the 2-year postsurgical follow-up showing full resolution of the buccal osteotomy, cortical sinus floor, osteoperiostitis lesion, and sinus mucosal edema.

concluded that CBCT offers great advantage compared with conventional radiographs for presurgical treatment planning in the posterior maxilla. Lofthag-Hansen et al[99] compared CBCT and intraoral radiography for the diagnosis of periapical pathology, and all observers agreed that in 70% of the cases CBCT provided clinically relevant information not found in the periapical radiographs. They concluded that when endodontic surgery is planned for multirooted teeth, additional radiographic examination using a 3D technique should be considered. Shahbazian et al,[102] examining 145 dental records, found that periapical radiography could only spot approximately 40% of apical periodontitis on posterior maxillary teeth and 3% of all apical infections extending into the sinus that were seen on CBCT. They also concluded that periapical radiographs are not adequate in observing the anatomical relationship between maxillary molars and the sinus floor. Comparison studies conclude that clinicians cannot accurately determine whether dental roots are protruding into the sinus, or are merely superimposed over them, when using 2D imaging techniques, while CT imaging allows an accurate interpretation of the true relationships of the teeth roots to the sinus.[8,71,75,82,85] A study by Sharan and Madjar,[107] comparing panoramic radiography with CT imaging, found that only 39% of the teeth roots that projected on the sinus cavity in panoramic radiographs showed protrusion into the sinus with CT. CBCT also allows precise measurement of cortical bone thickness[78,81] and accurate presurgical assessment of root morphology, including mesiobuccal root complexities, root fusions, and detection of potential ithmi.[93,94] Considering the importance of precise preoperative planning and execution of endodontic surgery, CT imaging is an indispensable tool for anatomical assessment and case selection, particularly in the posterior maxilla. It offers the ability to accurately view root morphology and sinus relationships and precisely measure distances in multiple planes, without superimposition of adjacent roots or anatomical structures such as the zygoma or palatal process.[108]

Periapical Surgery Involving the Maxillary Sinus

Periradicular surgery of maxillary molars can present unique surgical challenges to the clinician. In addition to management of potential maxillary sinus exposure, a low zygomatic process, a shallow palatal vault, complex root morphology, or wide root divergences can create difficulties in accessing root ends. Despite these challenges, precise and safe endodontic surgical intervention can be performed in posterior maxillary teeth provided the surgeon has an accurate diagnosis, has a clear understanding of case-specific anatomical relationships and root morphology, and uses appropriate surgical techniques.

Care should always be taken to avoid perforation of an intact sinus membrane whenever possible, because any oroantral communication facilitates microbial contamination of the maxillary sinus, increasing the chance of postoperative sinusitis.[109] However, risk of sinus infringement should not be a deterrent for periapical surgery, as there are well-tested techniques to manage it.[95,110] Periapical surgery performed on roots anatomically projecting into the maxillary sinus or with an existing pathologic exposure of the sinus will inevitably result in maxillary sinus communication. In these cases, sinus perforation is not an iatrogenic event or accident but an unavoidable occurrence,[8,111] and as such, the clinician should be able to recognize and treat maxillary sinus exposures as a routine event in surgical endodontic practice. In a retrospective study of 276 patients after periradicular surgery, Ericson et al[112] reported the incidence of oroantral communication as follows: canines 7.7%, first premolars 8.8%, second premolars 26.1%, and molars 40%. Ioannades and Borstlap[113] reported the incidence of oroantral communication as 14.8% in 47 maxillary molar apicoectomies. Freedman and Horowitz[110] reported an incidence of 10.4% in periapical surgeries of 472 maxillary molars and premolars. Watzek et al[9] reported that perforation of the sinus occurred in 28% of 146 maxillary posterior apicoectomies. Oberli et al[8] recorded a perforation rate of 9.6% of 113 periapical surgeries of maxillary premolars and molars.

Prior to periapical surgery involving the maxillary sinus, the physiologic status of the sinus should be determined. Considering the high incidence of odontogenic sinusitis, it is very likely that some amount of sinus inflammation or mucosal edema will exist prior to most periapical surgical procedures. The literature provides no supported contraindications to performing periapical surgery on patients experiencing sinusitis or even presenting with total sinus obstruction with ostial blockage. Rud and Rud[114] have reported that if secretions in the antrum are removed at the same time as the operation of the tooth, it speeds up the healing of the sinusitis. In their findings from 200 periapical surgeries of maxillary first molars, with sinus perforations in half of the cases, 42% had acute or subacute sinus infections when they were operated on. In one of the cases, 15 mL of purulent exudate was drained from the sinus. All but two cases responded with no postoperative signs of sinusitis, one of these cases being an undiagnosed root fracture. Antibiotics were not routinely prescribed before or after treatment.

Surgical communication into the maxillary sinus does not appear to result in permanent alteration of either the sinus membrane or its physiologic function, nor a reduced prognosis for periapical healing.[9,112,115–117] However, the impact of a perforation on sinus physiology and the exact time needed for recovery of proper function has never been assessed.[118] Benninger et al[16] observed that the mucous membrane, complete with cilia, will regenerate in about 5 months after its total surgical removal. Watzek et al[9] reported that antral perforation caused during endodontic surgery constitutes no risk to the sinus, even when a transantral approach is used to treat the palatal root. In a total of 112 sinuses with oroantral communications, they found no increases in pathologic sinus changes compared with the total population. They also found no significant difference in the periapical healing rate between patients with and without intraoperative sinus exposures, reporting complete healing in 89.2% of cases with sinus exposure compared with 85.3% of cases without sinus exposure. These findings were consistent with those reported by Ericson et al,[119] who found no difference in prognosis in 159 surgical cases with and without oroantral communication, and Persson,[120] who also observed no relationship between membrane perforation and surgical outcome in 18 cases reviewed. A review article of the literature on periapical surgery by Garcia et al[121] confirms that none of the included studies found a significant difference in the healing outcome or the postoperative sequelae when oroantral communication had occurred.

If the sinus cavity is exposed during periapical surgery, it is extremely important that a meticulous technique is used to prevent surgical debris, root tips, infected tissue, and surgical materials such as hemostatic agents, cotton pellets, or root-end filling materials from entering the sinus.[8,111,122,123] The introduction of bacteria associated with surgical debris or endodontic materials into the maxillary sinus is well known in the literature to produce an inflammatory response in the sinus mucosa, causing varying symptoms and possibly leading to the need for sinus surgery.[122,124–131] Certain root canal filling materials, particularly those containing zinc oxide, have been implicated as causative agents of maxillary sinus aspergillosis, a fungal infection.[22,132–141] It is believed that these materials act as a foreign body that paralyzes the cilia and affects mucociliary clearance, creating a status of secretions and accumulation of fungal waste that favor the growth

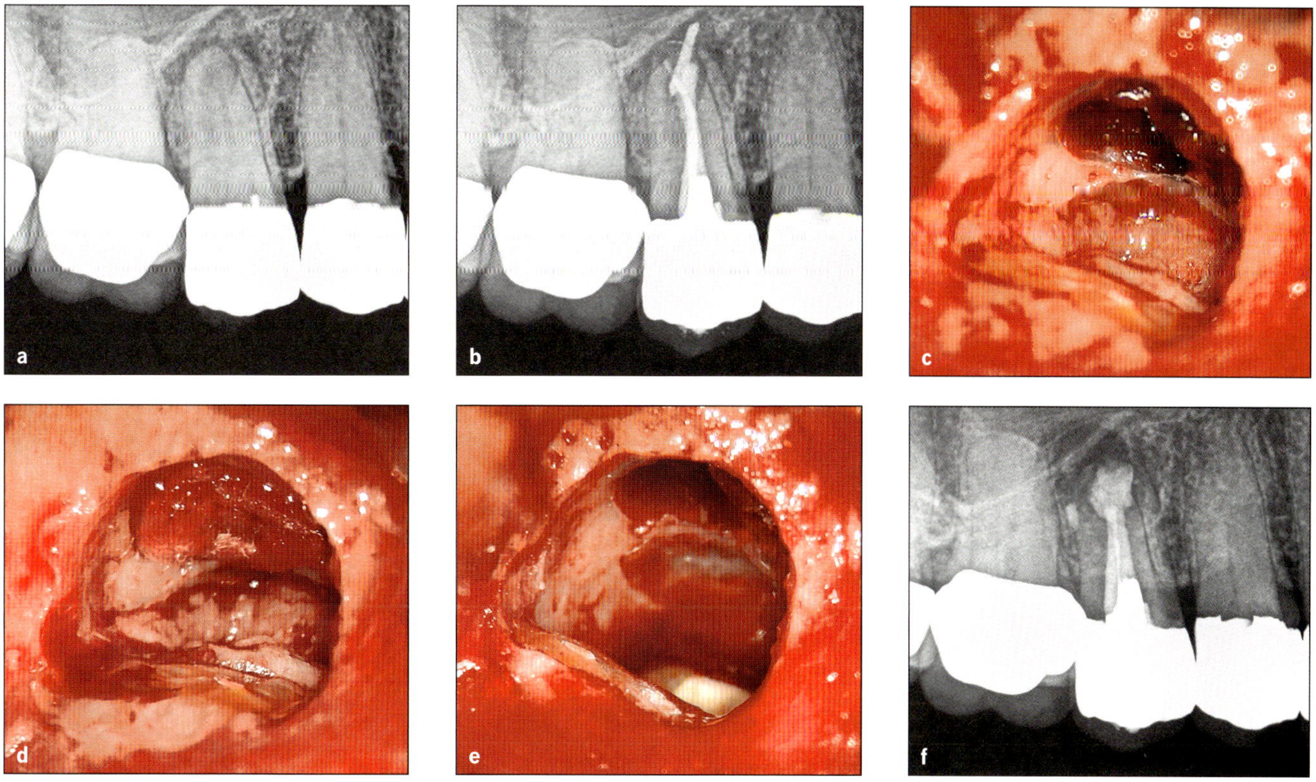

Fig 12-11 Sinus perforation during periapical surgery. *(a)* Preoperative periapical radiograph of a three-canal maxillary right second premolar with a calcified DB canal and inflammatory resorption of the palatal root apex. *(b)* Periapical radiograph of the orthograde root canal treatment with overextension of root canal filling material. *(c)* Surgical osteotomy and buccal root resection exposes a perforation into the maxillary sinus. *(d)* Iodine gauze placed over the defect to prevent surgical debris from entering the maxillary sinus. *(e)* Removal of the gauze following placement of bioceramic retrofillings. *(f)* Postoperative periapical radiograph of the completed orthograde and surgical endodontic treatment.

of *Aspergillus*. Of significance are sealer fragments and the zinc contained in them, which is indispensable for *Aspergillus* growth.[138–140] These studies are associated with orthograde extrusion of obturation materials in the sinus; however, care should be exercised during surgical treatment to prevent endodontic sealer debris from entering the sinus, particularly when surgically treating teeth with extruded or overfilled orthograde root canal fillings.

Displacement of surgical debris, particularly if the artifacts are large and unable to be cleared by the mucociliary mechanism, have the potential to cause maxillary sinus obstruction and severe rhinosinusitis.[142,143] In a healthy sinus, small particles and fluids will be safely expelled by normal sinus clearance; however, larger objects usually remain in the sinus and can cause chronic sinus inflammation, ostial obstruction, and possible interruption of sinus drainage.[9,142,144] There are, however, some case reports of larger displaced foreign objects, such as gutta-percha points, tooth roots, and even titanium implants migrating out of the maxillary sinus and being displaced into deeper structures such as the ethmoid and sphenoid sinuses, requiring more involved endoscopic retrieval.[144–146] Attempting to retrieve displaced objects from the sinus is difficult due to the limited access and potential for additional trauma and inflammation.[111] If a foreign object is introduced into the sinus during periapical surgery and is irretrievable, the patient should be informed, the object's location documented radiographically, and an antibiotic prescribed, and the patient should be referred to an oral and maxillofacial surgeon or an otorhinolaryngologist for further evaluation and treatment.[19] The patient will most likely require surgical removal of the foreign object through a Caldwell-Luc procedure, endoscopic sinusotomy, or mucoperiosteal pedicle window.[143,147–154] Displacement of surgical debris and foreign objects into the sinus can be prevented by minimizing the size of the exposure and placing a barrier such as a cotton pellet tied securely with a suture or an iodine gauze strip or pad for larger defects[95,111] (Fig 12-11). Taschieri et al[118] have advocated the use of an absorbable hemostatic gelatin sponge to isolate the sinus from debris for the added hemostatic benefit. Saline rinsing of the maxillary sinus following surgery is acceptable, if necessary, to flush and remove any surgical debris that may have entered the sinus during treatment.

Postoperative oroantral fistula development is seldom a problem following periapical surgery with sinus ex-

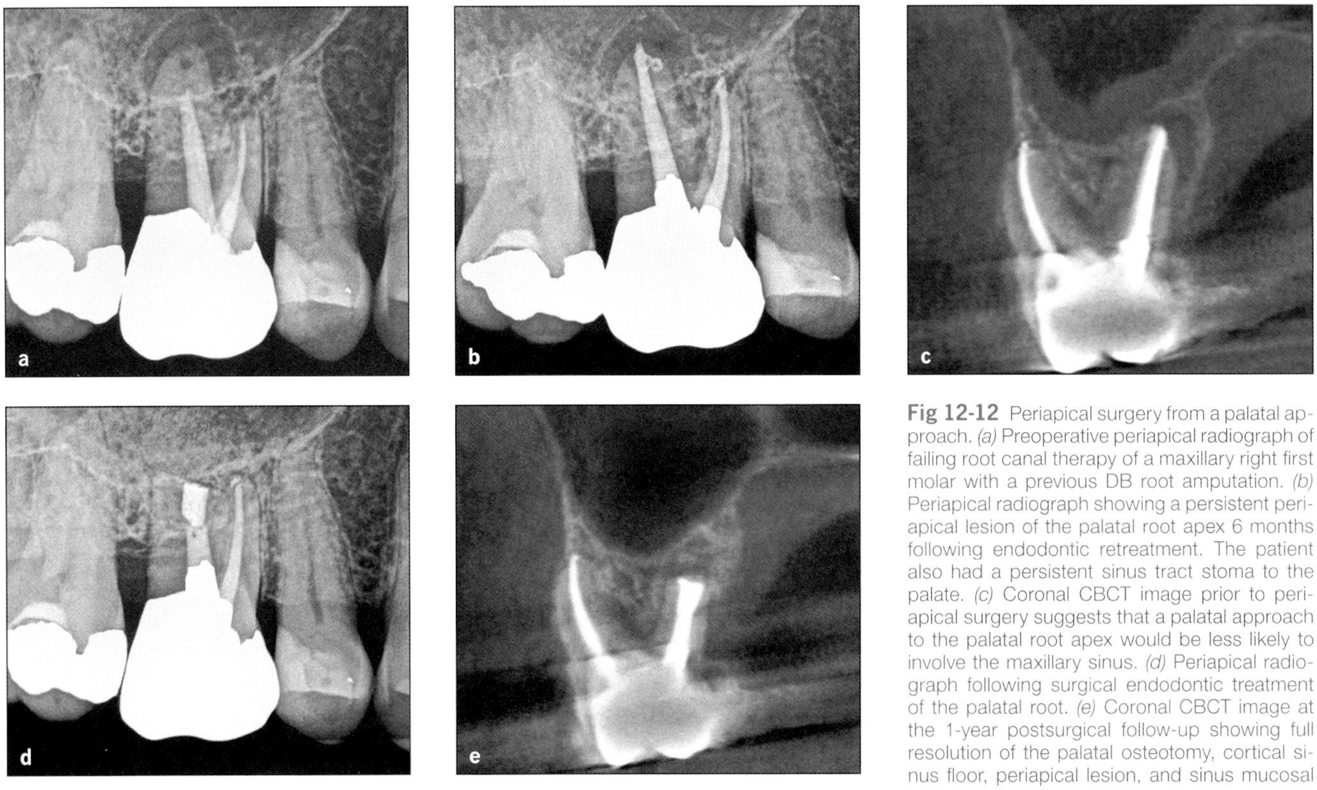

Fig 12-12 Periapical surgery from a palatal approach. *(a)* Preoperative periapical radiograph of failing root canal therapy of a maxillary right first molar with a previous DB root amputation. *(b)* Periapical radiograph showing a persistent periapical lesion of the palatal root apex 6 months following endodontic retreatment. The patient also had a persistent sinus tract stoma to the palate. *(c)* Coronal CBCT image prior to periapical surgery suggests that a palatal approach to the palatal root apex would be less likely to involve the maxillary sinus. *(d)* Periapical radiograph following surgical endodontic treatment of the palatal root. *(e)* Coronal CBCT image at the 1-year postsurgical follow-up showing full resolution of the palatal osteotomy, cortical sinus floor, periapical lesion, and sinus mucosal edema.

posure. Proper reapproximation of a full-thickness mucoperiosteal flap over the sinus perforation is all that is required to prevent an oroantral fistula from developing. There is no indication for membrane placement over the defect to reduce the chance of oroantral fistula, nor is there evidence supporting the use of prophylactic antibiotics or antihistamines prior to, or postoperatively following, exposure of the maxillary sinus. Postoperative instructions are the same as for any other periapical surgery, with the added instruction to avoid nose blowing for the first several days during flap reattachment and to expect possible nosebleeds or nasal drainage of surgical irrigants.

Buccal transantral versus palatal approach for palatal root surgery

Palatal roots of maxillary molars present increased surgical challenges due to their anatomical location. Treatment decisions for the most effective and least invasive surgical approaches to the palatal roots of maxillary molars must be based on individual patient and anatomical factors as well as a careful review of preoperative CBCT imaging. The literature presents differing opinions regarding the optimal approach for access to the palatal root, presenting advantages and disadvantages for each method.

Lin et al[123] have suggested that antral perforations be avoided whenever possible and have advocated a palatal approach to molar palatal roots (Fig 12-12). The palatal approach, however, can provide technical difficulties that are not found with the buccal transantral approach. The palatal tissue is much thicker and less elastic than the buccal mucosa and has a more tenacious fibrous attachment to the palatal alveolar bone, which increases the difficulty of flap management. Also, care must be taken to avoid damaging the greater palatine vessels and nerve when raising a palatal flap. In cases of a shallow palatal vault or a limited jaw opening, the level of difficulty of the palatal approach is increased, often requiring removal of a significant amount of bone and resection of more of the palatal root due to the limited access and visibility. Although the average distance from the palatal cortical plate to the palatal root apex is only about 3 mm compared with an average of 10 mm from the buccal cortical plate,[78,83,155,156] the palatal root often curves toward the buccal and is usually in closer approximation to the maxillary sinus than the palate, making sinus perforation a significant risk, especially in cases with limited access and visibility.[9,116]

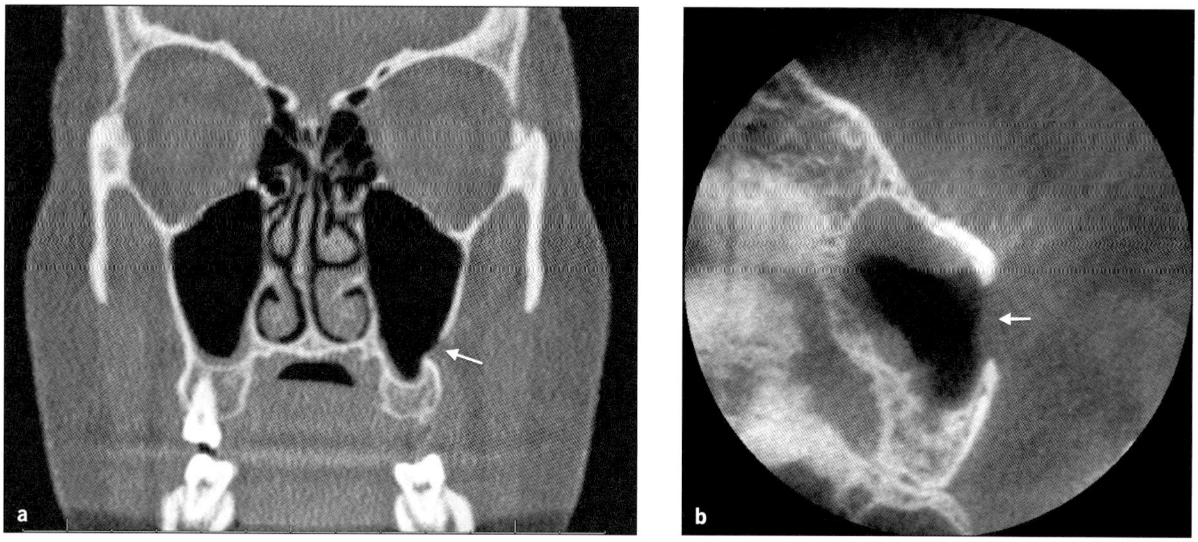

Fig 12-13 Fibrous scar tissue defect in the lateral antral wall. *(a)* Coronal sinus CT image showing lack of osseous healing in the lateral sinus wall following a failed periapical surgery of the maxillary left second molar 5 years prior. The tooth has been extracted, but the lateral wall scar tissue defect remains *(arrow)*. *(b)* Axial CBCT image showing the same osseous defect 8 years postsurgery *(arrow)*.

Approaching the palatal root from the buccal or vestibular aspect will frequently involve exposure of the maxillary sinus due to the sinus floor extending between the individual roots of the molar teeth in approximately 50% of adults.[115] The transantral approach has the advantage of using a single flap and cortical access window to treat all of the roots. This approach also poses no danger to major neural or vascular structures, although it does involve smaller branches of the superior alveolar nerves that travel in the sinus wall innervating the related teeth.[116] Although a subperiosteal method has been presented in the literature,[157,158] the primary concerns with a buccal transantral approach to the palatal root are the necessarily large size of the antral osteotomy, the increased potential for sinus membrane perforation, and the potential introduction of foreign bodies and bacteria into the sinus. Careful management of surgical debris, resected root tips, and dental materials must be exercised to minimize postoperative sinus inflammation.

The degree of osseous regeneration of the sinus wall following surgical endodontic antral perforations has been questioned. Ericson et al[119] demonstrated that while periapical radiographs interpreted complete bone regeneration following oroantral communication during apical surgery, 15% of the cases showed no bony partition between the apical area and the maxillary sinus when viewed with CT. Ericson et al[112] further showed that oroantral communications often lead to permanent bone defects in the alveolar process and in the cortical margin of the maxillary sinus, adding that the defects probably consist of fibrous scar tissue possibly caused by loss of continuity of the periosteum during closure. Tataryn et al,[159] in a study on dogs, found that experimentally induced sinus wall exposures appeared to show osseous healing radiographically, but histologic specimens displayed only partial osseous regeneration interspersed with multiple areas of fibrous connective tissue that were approximately one-tenth the thickness of the presurgical sinus wall. Resorbable collagen membranes did not improve osseous repair. These findings are consistent with investigations of post Caldwell-Luc defects, indicating that fibrous scar tissue grows across the antral wall osteotomies in 100% of cases.[160,161] Sinus wall fibrous scar defects following transantral palatal root approaches may be of significant concern if the tooth requires future extraction and a subsequent sinus elevation surgery becomes necessary (Fig 12-13).

In many cases, maxillary posterior teeth requiring periapical surgery have significant osteoperiostitis lesions that expand the sinus periosteum superiorly and essentially lift the sinus floor and associated mucosa away from the root end.[162] In these cases that exhibit evident periapical osteoperiostitis, periapical surgery performed below the level of the expanded periosteum will not necessarily involve the maxillary sinus, even when treating the palatal root from a vestibular access. Surgical procedures in these patients present little to no risk of displacing surgical debris into the sinus and have the expectation of full regeneration of the buccal cortical plate, alveolar bone, and sinus cortical floor without fibrous scarring, provided that the surgical osteotomy is made below the level of the periosteum (Fig 12-14). Careful CBCT assessment of

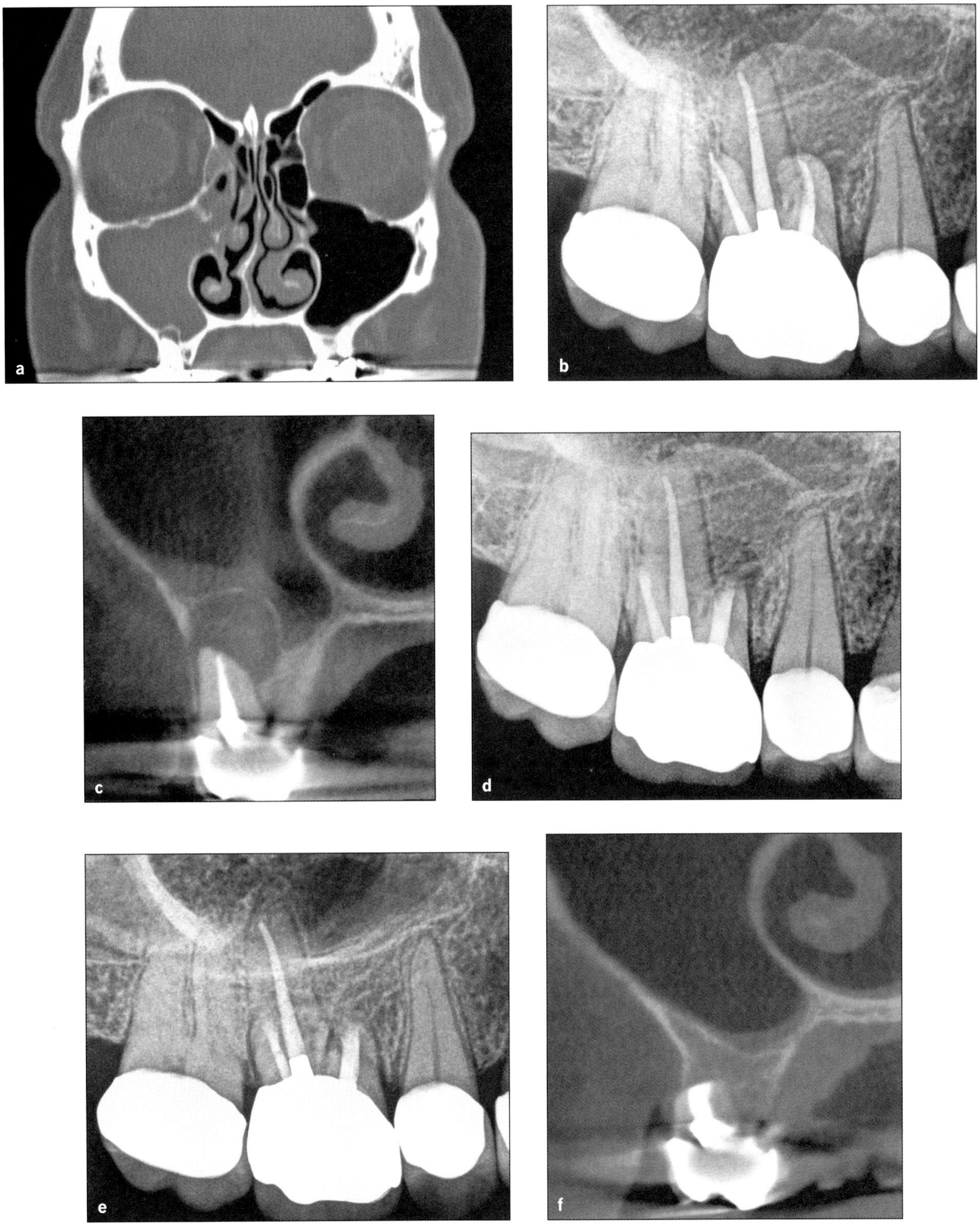

Fig 12-14 Periapical surgery of an odontogenic rhinosinusitis with a periapical osteoperiostitis lesion. *(a)* Sinus CT image of a fully obstructed right maxillary sinus and involvement of the right ethmoid sinuses. Medical therapies had failed, and endoscopic sinus surgery was planned. Note the osteoperiostitis lesion in the floor of the right maxillary sinus suggestive of an odontogenic source. *(b)* Periapical radiograph of a failing endodontic treatment despite the apparently well-filled canal system. *(c)* Coronal CBCT image of the osteoperiostitis lesion in the floor of the right maxillary sinus. *(d)* Postoperative periapical radiograph of the endodontic surgery. *(e)* One-year recall radiograph following periapical surgery shows evident healing. *(f)* Coronal CBCT image at the 1-year postsurgical follow-up showing full resolution of the buccal osteotomy, cortical sinus floor, periapical osteoperiostitis lesion, and odontogenic rhinosinusitis. The patient's rhinosinusitis symptoms resolved completely, and the planned sinus surgery was not performed.

osteoperiostitis lesions should be made prior to periapical surgical procedures in the posterior maxilla, with a careful effort made to perform the osteotomy and surgical procedure below the periosteum whenever possible.

Despite the inherent challenges in performing periapical surgery in the posterior maxilla, modern surgical techniques and imaging combined with requisite surgical skills have been shown to provide a decisive option for addressing endodontic disease and saving the natural tooth.[163]

References

1. Amedee RG. Anatomy, physiology, and evaluation of the paranasal sinuses. In: Ballenger JJ (ed). Diseases of the Nose, Throat, Ear, Head and Neck, ed 14. Philadelphia: Lea and Febiger, 1991:168–183.
2. Alberti PW. Applied surgical anatomy of the maxillary sinus. Otolaryngol Clin North Am 1976;9:3–20.
3. Jun BC, Song SW, Park CS, Lee DH, Cho KJ, Cho JH. The analysis of maxillary sinus aeration according to aging process; Volume assessment by 3-dimensional reconstruction by high-resolutional CT scanning. Otolaryngol Head Neck Surg 2005;132:429–434.
4. Drettner B. Pathophysiology of paranasal sinuses with clinical implications. Clin Otolaryngol Allied Sci 1980;5:277–284.
5. Bornstein MM, Wasmer J, Sendi P, Janner SF, Buser D, von Arx T. Characteristics and dimensions of the Schneiderian membrane and apical bone in maxillary molars referred for apical surgery: A comparative radiographic analysis using limited cone beam computed tomography. J Endod 2012;38:51–57.
6. Kato A. Immunopathology of chronic rhinosinusitis. Allerg Int 2015;64:121–130.
7. Beule AG. Physiology and pathophysiology of respiratory mucosa of the nose and paranasal sinuses. GMS Curr Top Otorhinolaryngol Head Neck Surg 2010;9:Doc07.
8. Oberli K, Bornstein MM, von Arx T. Periapical surgery and the maxillary sinus: Radiographic parameters for clinical outcome. Oral Surg Oral Med Oral Pathol Oral Radiol Endod 2007;103:848–853.
9. Watzek G, Bernhart T, Ulm C. Complications of sinus perforations and their management in endodontics. Dent Clin North Am 1997;41:563–583.
10. Selden HS. The interrelationship between the maxillary sinus and endodontics. Oral Surg Oral Med Oral Pathol 1974;38:623–629.
11. Lanza DC, Kennedy DW. Adult rhinosinusitis defined. Otolaryngol Head Neck Surg 1997;117(3 pt 2):S1–S7.
12. Pleis JR, Lucas JW, Ward BW. Summary health statistics for U.S. adults: National Health Interview Survey, 2008. Vital Health Stat 10 2009;242:1–157.
13. Rosenfeld RM, Piccirillo JF, Chandrasekhar SS, et al. Clinical practice guideline (update): Adult sinusitis executive summary. Otolaryngol Head Neck Surg 2015;152:598–609.
14. Meltzer EO, Hamilos DL. Rhinosinusitis diagnosis and management for the clinician: A synopsis of recent consensus guidelines. Mayo Clin Proc 2011;86:427–443.
15. Benninger MS, Anon J, Mabry RL. The medical management of rhinosinusitis. Otolaryngol Head Neck Surg 1997;117(3 pt 2):S41–S49.
16. Benninger MS, Sebek BA, Levine HL. Mucosal regeneration of the maxillary sinus after surgery. Otolaryngol Head Neck Surg 1989;101:33–37.
17. Longhini AB, Ferguson BJ. Clinical aspects of odontogenic maxillary sinusitis: A case series. Int Forum Allergy Rhinol 2011;1:409–415.
18. Patel NA, Ferguson BJ. Odontogenic sinusitis: An ancient but under-appreciated cause of maxillary sinusitis. Curr Opin Otolaryngol Head Neck Surg 2012;20:24–28.
19. Kretzschmar DP, Kretzschmar JL. Rhinosinusitis: Review from a dental perspective. Oral Surg Oral Med Oral Pathol Oral Radiol Endod 2003;96:128–135.
20. White JA. Paranasal sinus infections. In: Ballenger JJ (ed). Diseases of the Nose, Throat, Ear, Head and Neck, ed 14. Philadelphia: Lea and Febiger, 1991:184–202.
21. Brook I. Microbiology of acute and chronic maxillary sinusitis associated with an odontogenic origin. Laryngoscope 2005;115:823–825.
22. De Foer C, Fossion E, Vaillant JM. Sinus aspergillosis. J Craniomaxillofac Surg 1990;18:33–40.
23. Mensi M, Salgarello S, Pinsi G, Piccioni M. Mycetoma of the maxillary sinus: Endodontic and microbiological correlations. Oral Surg Oral Med Oral Pathol Oral Radiol Endod 2004;98:119–123.
24. Havas TE, Motbey JA, Gullane PJ. Prevalence of incidental abnormalities on computed tomographic scans of the paranasal sinuses. Arch Otolaryngol Head Neck Surg 1988;114:856–859.
25. Stammberger H, Jakse R, Beaufort F. Aspergillosis of the paranasal sinuses. X-ray diagnosis, histopathology, and clinical aspects. Ann Otol Rhinol Laryngol 1984;93:251–256.
26. Costa F, Polini F, Zerman N, Robiony M, Toro C, Politi M. Surgical treatment of *Aspergillus mycetomas* of the maxillary sinus: A review of the literature. Oral Surg Oral Med Oral Pathol Oral Radiol Endod 2007;103(6):e23–e29.
27. Bauer WH. Maxillary sinusitis of dental origin. Am J Orthod Oral Surg 1943;29:133–151.
28. Maloney PL, Doku HC. Maxillary sinusitis of odontogenic origin. J Can Dent Assoc 1968;34:591–603.
29. Waite DE. Maxillary sinus. Dent Clin North Am 1971;15:349–368.
30. Selden HS. Endo-antral syndrome and various endodontic complications. J Endod 1999;25:389–393.
31. Lindahl L, Melen I, Ekedahl C, Holm SE. Chronic maxillary sinusitis. Differential diagnosis and genesis. Acta Otolaryngol 1982;93:147–150.
32. Dodd RB, Dodds RN, Hocomb JB. An endodontically induced maxillary sinusitis. J Endod 1984;10:504–506.
33. Mehra P, Murad H. Maxillary sinus disease of odontogenic origin. Otolaryngol Clin North Am 2004;37:347–364.
34. Melen I, Lindahl L, Andréasson L, Rundcrantz H. Chronic maxillary sinusitis. Definition, diagnosis and relation to dental infections and nasal polyposis. Acta Otolaryngol 1986;101:320–327.
35. Maillet M, Bowles WR, McClanahan SL, John MT, Ahmad M. Cone-beam computed tomography evaluation of maxillary sinusitis. J Endod 2011;37:753–757.
36. Brook I. Sinusitis of odontogenic origin. Otolaryngol Head Neck Surg 2006;135:349–355.
37. Legert KG, Zimmerman M, Stierna P. Sinusitis of odontogenic origin: Pathophysiological implications of early treatment. Acta Otolaryngol 2004;124:655–663.
38. Nimigean VR, Nimigean V, Maru N, Andressakis D, Balatsouras DG, Danielidis V. The maxillary sinus and its endodontic implications: Clinical study and review. B-ENT 2006;2:167–175.
39. Pokorny A, Tataryn R. Clinical and radiologic findings in a case series of maxillary sinusitis of dental origin. Int Forum Allergy Rhinol 2013:3:973–979.
40. Abrahams JJ, Glassberg RM. Dental disease: A frequently unrecognized cause of maxillary sinus abnormalities? Am J Roentenol 1996;166:1219–1223.
41. Matilla K. Roentgenological investigations of the relation between periapical lesions and conditions of the mucous membrane of the maxillary sinuses. Acta Odontolog Scand 1965;23:42–46.
42. Obayashi N, Ariji Y, Goto M, et al. Spread of odontogenic infection originating in the maxillary teeth: Computerized tomographic assessment. Oral Surg Oral Med Oral Pathol Oral Radiol Endod 2004;98:223–331.
43. Lu Y, Liu Z, Zhang L, et al. Associations between maxillary sinus mucosal thickening and apical periodontitis using cone-beam computed tomography scanning: A retrospective study. J Endod 2012;38:1069–1074.
44. Ariji Y, Obayashi N, Goto M, et al. Roots of the maxillary first and second molars in horizontal relation to alveolar cortical plates and maxillary sinus: Computed tomography assessment for infection spread. Clin Oral Investig 2006;10:35–41.
45. Cymerman JJ, Cymerman DH, O'Dwyer RS. Evaluation of odontogenic maxillary sinusitis using cone-beam computed tomography: Three case reports. J Endod 2011;37:1465–1469.
46. Kulacz R, Fishman G, Levine H. An unsuccessful sinus surgery caused by dental involvement within the floor of the maxillary sinus. Oper Techniques Otolaryngol Head Neck Surg 2004;15:2–3.
47. Kim IK, Kim JR, Jang KS, Moon YS, Park SW. Orbital abscess from an odontogenic infection. Oral Surg Oral Med Oral Pathol Oral Radiol Endod 2007;103(1):e1–e6.
48. DeCroos FC, Liao JC, Ramey NA, Li I. Management of odontogenic orbital cellulitis. J Med Life 2011;4:314–317.
49. Gallagher RM, Gross CW, Phillips CD. Suppurative intracranial complications of sinusitis. Laryngoscope 1998;108:1635–1642.
50. Younis RT, Lazar RH, Anand VK. Intracranial complications of sinusitis: A 15-year review of 39 cases. Ear Nose Throat J 2002;81:636–644.
51. Youssef OH, Stefanyszyn MA, Bilyk JR. Odontogenic orbital cellulitis. Ophthal Plast Reconstr Surg 2008;24:29–35.

52. Gold RS, Sager E. Pansinusitis, orbital cellulitis, and blindness as a sequelae of delayed treatment of dental abscess. J Oral Surg 1974;32:40–43.
53. Park CH, Jee DH, La TY. A case of odontogenic orbital cellulitis causing blindness by severe tension orbit. J Korean Med Sci 2013;28:340–343.
54. de Medeiros EH, Pepato AO, Sverzut CE, Trivellato AE. Orbital abscess during endodontic treatment: A case report. J Endod 2012;38:1541–1543.
55. Koch F, Breil P, Marroquin BB, Gawehn J, Kunkel M. Abscess of the orbit arising 48 h after root canal treatment of a maxillary first molar. Int Endod J 2006;39:657–664.
56. Mehra P, Caiazzo A, Bestgen S. Odontogenic sinusitis causing orbital cellulitis. J Am Dent Assoc 1999;130:1086–1092.
57. Ogundiya DA, Keith DA, Mirowski J. Cavernous sinus thrombosis and blindness as complications of an odontogenic infection: Report of a case and review of literature. J Oral Maxillofac Surg 1989;47:1317–1321.
58. Nair UP, Nair MK. Maxillary sinusitis of odontogenic origin: cone-beam volumetric computerized tomography-aided diagnosis. Oral Surg Oral Med Oral Pathol Oral Radiol Endod 2010;110:e53–e57.
59. Guerra-Pereira I, Vaz P, Faria-Almeida R, Braga AC, Felino A. CT maxillary sinus evaluation—A retrospective cohort study. Med Oral Patol Oral Cir Bucal 2015; 20(4):e419–e426.
60. Worth HM, Stoneman DW. Radiographic interpretation of antral mucosal changes due to localized dental infection. J Can Dent Assoc 1973;38:111–115.
61. Gardner DG. Pseudocysts and retention cysts of the maxillary sinus. Oral Surg Oral Med Oral Pathol 1984;58:561–567.
62. Wang JH, Jang YJ, Lee BJ. Natural course of retention cysts of the maxillary sinus: Long-term follow-up results. Laryngoscope 2007;117:341–344.
63. Vallo J, Suominen-Taipale L, Huumonen S, Soikkonen K, Norblad A. Prevalence of mucosal abnormalities of the maxillary sinus and their relationship to dental disease in panoramic radiography: Results from the Health 2000 Health Examination Survey. Oral Surg Oral Med Oral Pathol Oral Radiol Endod 2010;10(3):e80–e87.
64. Ritter L, Lutz J, Neugebauer J, et al. Prevalence of pathologic findings in the maxillary sinus in cone-beam computerized tomography. Oral Surg Oral Med Oral Pathol Oral Radiol Endod 2011;111:634–640.
65. Bomeli SR, Branstetter BF 4th, Ferguson BJ. Frequency of a dental source for acute maxillary sinusitis. Laryngoscope 2009;119:580–584.
66. Nunes CA, Guedes OA, Alencar AH, Peters OA, Estrela CR, Estrela C. Evaluation of periapical lesions and their association with maxillary sinus abnormalities on cone-beam computed tomographic images. J Endod 2016;42:42–46.
67. Shanbhag S, Karnik P, Shirke P, Shanbhag V. Association between periapical lesions and maxillary sinus mucosal thickening: A retrospective cone-beam computed tomographic study. J Endod 2013;39:853–857.
68. Brüllmann DD, Schmidtmann I, Hornstein S, Schulze RK. Correlation of cone beam computed tomography (CBCT) findings in the maxillary sinus with dental diagnoses: A retrospective cross-sectional study. Clin Oral Investig 2012;16: 1023–1029.
69. Killey HC, Kay LW. An analysis of 250 cases of oro-antral fistula treated by the buccal flap operation. Oral Surg Oral Med Oral Pathol 1967;24:726–739.
70. Eberhardt JA, Torabinejad M, Christiansen EL. A computed tomographic study of the distances between the maxillary sinus floor and the apices of the maxillary posterior teeth. Oral Surg Oral Med Oral Pathol 1992;73:345–346.
71. Jung YH, Cho BH. Assessment of the relationship between the maxillary molars and adjacent structures using cone beam computed tomography. Imaging Sci Dent 2012;42:219–224.
72. von Arx T, Fodich I, Bornstein MM. Proximity of premolar roots to maxillary sinus: A radiographic survey using cone-beam computed tomography. J Endod 2014;40:1541–1548.
73. Pagin O, Centurion BS, Rubira-Bullen IR, Alvares Capelozza AL. Maxillary sinus and posterior teeth: Accessing close relationship by cone-beam computed tomographic scanning in a Brazilian population. J Endod 2013;39:748–751.
74. Georgescu CE, Rusu MC, Sandulescu M, Enache AM, Didilescu AC. Quantitative and qualitative bone analysis in the maxillary lateral region. Surg Radiol Anat 2012;34:551–558.
75. Kilic C, Kamburoglu K, Yuksel SP, Ozen T. An assessment of the relationship between the maxillary sinus floor and the maxillary posterior teeth root tips using dental cone-beam computerized tomography. Eur J Dent 2010;4:462–467.
76. Hamdy RM, Abdel-Wahed N. Three-dimensional linear and volumetric analysis of maxillary sinus pneumatization. J Adv Res 2014;5:387–395.
77. Tian XM, Qian L, Xin XZ, Wei B, Gong Y. An analysis of the proximity of maxillary posterior teeth to the maxillary sinus using cone-beam computed tomography. J Endod 2016;42:371–377.
78. Jin GC, Kim KD, Roh BD, Lee CY, Lee SJ. Buccal bone plate thickness of the Asian people. J Endod 2005;31:430–434.
79. Ariji Y, Kuroki T, Moriguchi S, Ariji E, Kanda S. Age changes in the volume of the human maxillary sinus: A study using computed tomography. Dentomaxillofacial Radiol 1994;23:163–168.
80. Ariji Y, Ariji E, Yoshiura K, Kanda S. Computed tomographic indices for maxillary sinus size in comparison with the sinus volume. Dentomaxillofac Radiol 1996; 25:19–24.
81. Kang SH, Kim BS, Kim Y. Proximity of posterior teeth to the maxillary sinus and buccal bone thickness: A biometric assessment using cone-beam computed tomography. J Endod 2015;41:1839–1846.
82. Kwak HH, Park HD, Yoon HR, Kang MK, Koh KS, Kim HJ. Topographic anatomy of the inferior wall of the maxillary sinus in Koreans. Int J Oral Maxillofac Surg 2004;33:382–388.
83. Kalender A, Aksoy U, Basmaci F, Orhan K, Orhan AI. Cone-beam computed tomography analysis of the vestibular surgical pathway to the palatine root of the maxillary first molar. Eur J Dent 2013;7:35–40.
84. Ok E, Güngör E, Colak M, Itunsoy M, Nur BG, Ağlarci OS. Evaluation of the relationship between the maxillary posterior teeth and the sinus floor using cone-beam computed tomography. Surg Radiol Anat 2014;36:907–914.
85. Cleghorn BM, Christie WH, Dong CC. Root and root canal morphology of the human permanent maxillary first molar: A literature review. J Endod 2006;32: 813–821.
86. Hsu YY, Kim S. The resected root surface. The issue of canal isthmuses. Dent Clin North Am 1997;41:529–540.
87. Weller RN, Niemczyk SP, Kim S. Incidence and position of the canal isthmus. Part 1. Mesiobuccal root of the maxillary first molar. J Endod 1995;21:380–383.
88. Verma P, Love RM. A micro CT study of the mesiobuccal root canal morphology of the maxillary first molar tooth. Int Endod J 2011;44:210–217.
89. Somma F, Leoni D, Plotino G, Grande NM, Plasschaert A. Root canal morphology of the mesiobuccal root of maxillary first molars: A micro-computed tomographic analysis. Int Endod J 2009;42:165–174 [erratum 2009;42:954].
90. Park J, Lee J, Ha B, Choi JH, Perinpanayagam H. Three-dimensional analysis of maxillary first molar mesiobuccal root canal configuration and curvature using microcomputed tomography. Oral Surg Oral Med Oral Pathol Oral Radiol Endod 2009;108:437–442.
91. Degerness RA, Bowles WR. Dimension, anatomy and morphology of the mesiobuccal root canal system in maxillary molars. J Endod 2010;36:985–989.
92. Cleghorn BM, Goodacre CG, Christie WH. Morphology of teeth and their root canal systems. In: Ingle JI, Bakland LK, Baumgartner JC (eds). Ingle's Endodontics, ed 6. Hamilton, ON: BC Decker, 2007:151–220.
93. Kim Y, Lee SJ, Woo J. Morphology of maxillary first and second molars analyzed by cone-beam computed tomography in a Korean population: Variations in the number of roots and canals and the incidence of fusion. J Endod 2012;38:1063–1068.
94. Silva EJ, Nejaim Y, Silva AI, Haiter-Neto F, Zaia AA, Cohenca N. Evaluation of root canal configuration of maxillary molars in a Brazilian population using cone-beam computed tomographic imaging: An in vivo study. J Endod 2014;40:173–176.
95. Kim S, Kratchman S. Modern endodontic surgery concepts and practice: A review. J Endod 2006;32:601–623.
96. Teixeira FB, Sano CL, Gomes BP, Zaia AA, Ferraz CC, Souza-Filho FJ. A preliminary in vitro study of the incidence and position of the root canal isthmus in maxillary and mandibular first molars. Int Endod J 2003;36:276–280.
97. von Arx T. Frequency and type of canal isthmuses in first molars detected by endoscopic inspection during periradicular surgery. Int Endod J 2005;38:160–168.
98. Ball RL, Barbizam JV, Cohenca N. Intraoperative endodontic applications of cone-beam computed tomography. J Endod 2013;39:548–557.
99. Lofthag-Hansen S, Huumonen S, Gröndahl K, Gröndahl HG. Limited cone-beam CT and intraoral radiography for the diagnosis of periapical pathology. Oral Surg Oral Med Oral Pathol Oral Radiol Endod 2007;103:114–119.
100. Hassan BA. Reliability of periapical radiographs and orthopantomograms in detection of tooth root protrusion in the maxillary sinus: Correlation results with cone beam computed tomography. J Oral Maxillofac Res 2010;1:e6.
101. Low K, Dula K, Bürgin W, von Arx T. Comparison of periapical radiography and limited cone-beam tomography in posterior maxillary teeth referred for apical surgery. J Endod 2008;34:557–562.
102. Shahbazian M, Vandewoude C, Wyatt J, Jacobs R. Comparative assessment of periapical radiography and CBCT imaging for radiodiagnostics in posterior maxilla. Odontology 2015;103:97–104.
103. Cotton TP, Geisler TM, Holden DT, Schwartz SA, Schindler WG. Endodontic applications of cone-beam volumetric tomography. J Endod 2007;33:1121–1132.
104. Patel S, Dawood A, Ford TP, Whaites E. The potential applications of cone beam computed tomography in the management of endodontic problems. Int Endod J 2007;40:818–830.

105. Scarfe WC, Levin MD, Gane D, Farman AG. Use of cone beam computed tomography in endodontics. Int J Dent 2009;2009:6345–6367.
106. Tyndall DA, Kohltfarber H. Application of cone beam volumetric tomography in endodontics. Aust Dent J 2012;57(suppl 1):72–81.
107. Sharan A, Madjar D. Correlation between maxillary sinus floor topography and related root position of posterior teeth using panoramic and cross-sectional computed tomography imaging. Oral Surg Oral Med Oral Pathol Oral Radiol Endod 2006;102:375–381.
108. Nakata K, Naitoh M, Izumi M, Inamoto K, Ariji E, Nakamura H. Effectiveness of dental computed tomography in diagnostic imaging of periradicular lesion of each root of a multirooted tooth. A case report. J Endod 2006;32:583–587.
109. Pommer B, Unger E, Sütö D, Hack N, Watzek G. Mechanical properties of the Schneiderian membrane in vitro. Clin Oral Implants Res 2009;20:633–637.
110. Freedman A, Horowitz I. Complications after apicoectomy in maxillary premolar and molar teeth. Int J Oral Maxillofac Surg 1999;28:192–194.
111. Jerome CE, Hill AV. Preventing root tip loss in the maxillary sinus during endodontic surgery. J Endod 1995;21:422–424.
112. Ericson S, Finne K, Persson G. A clinical-radiographic review of treated oro-antral communications. Int J Oral Surg 1973;2:185–195.
113. Ioannides C, Borstlap WA. Apicoectomy on molars: A clinical and radiographical study. Int J Oral Surg 1983;12:73–79.
114. Rud J, Rud V. Apicoectomy on molars: A clinical and radiographical study. J Endod 1998;24:260–261.
115. Hauman CH, Chandler NP, Tong DC. Endodontic implications of the maxillary sinus: A review. Int Endod J 2002;35:127–141.
116. Wallace JA. Transantral endodontic surgery. Oral Surg Oral Med Oral Pathol Oral Radiol Endod 1996;82:80–83.
117. Garcia B, Penarrocha M, Martí E, Martínez JM, Gay-Escoda C. Periapical surgery in maxillary premolars and molars: Analysis in terms of the distance between the lesion and the maxillary sinus. J Oral Maxillofac Surg 2008;66:1212–1217.
118. Taschieri S, Fabbro MD, Corbella S, Weinstein T, Rosano G, Tsesis I. Endoscopic minimally invasive management of a periradicular lesion invading the maxillary sinus. J Oral Sci 2011;53:533–538.
119. Ericson S, Finne K, Persson G. Results of apicoectomy of maxillary canines, premolars and molars with special reference to oroantral communication as a prognostic factor. Int J Oral Surg 1974;3:386–393.
120. Persson G. Periapical surgery of molars. Int J Oral Surg 1982;11:96–100.
121. Garcia B, Martorell L, Martí E, Peñarrocha M. Periapical surgery of maxillary posterior teeth. A review of the literature. Med Oral 2006;11(2):e146–e150.
122. Kim JW, Cho KM, Park SH, Park SR, Lee SS, Lee SK. Chronic maxillary sinusitis caused by root canal overfilling of Calcipex II. Restor Dent Endod 2014;39:63–67.
123. Lin L, Chance K, Shovlin F, Skribner J, Langeland K. Oroantral communication in periapical surgery of maxillary posterior teeth. J Endod 1985;11:40–44.
124. Bjornland T, Haanaes HR, Margrethe E, Beyer-Olsen S. Sinusitis caused by endodontic materials displaced into the maxillary sinus. Endod Dent Traumatol 1987;3:37–40.
125. Ektefaie MR, David HT, Poh CF. Surgical resolution of chronic tissue irritation caused by extruded endodontic filling material. J Can Dent Assoc 2005;71:487–490.
126. Brooks JK, Kleinman JW. Retrieval of extensive gutta-percha extruded into the maxillary sinus: Use of 3-dimensional cone-beam computed tomography. J Endod 2013;39:1189–1193.
127. Yaltirik M, Koçak Berberoglu H, Koray M, Dulger O, Yildirim S, Aydil BA. Orbital pain and headache secondary to overfilling of a root canal. J Endod 2003;29:771–772.
128. Yamaguchi K, Matsunaga T, Hayashi Y. Gross extrusion of endodontic obturation materials into the maxillary sinus: A case report. Oral Surg Oral Med Oral Pathol Oral Radiol Endod 2007;104:131–134.
129. Haidar Z. Facial pain of uncommon origin. Oral Surg Oral Med Oral Pathol 1987;63:748–749.
130. Donlon WC. Reamer in the maxillary antrum: A complication of periapical surgery. Oral Surg Oral Med Oral Pathol 1989;68:122–123.
131. Liston PN, Walters RF. Foreign bodies in the maxillary antrum: A case report. Aust Dent J 2002;47:344-6.
132. Beck-Mannagetta J. Zinc and aspergillus. Oral Surg Oral Med Oral Pathol Oral Radiol Endod 1996;81:138–140.
133. Beck-Mannagetta J, Necek D. Radiologic findings in aspergillosis of the maxillary sinus. Oral Surg Oral Med Oral Pathol 1986;62:345–349.
134. Khongkhunthian P, Reichart PA. Aspergillosis of the maxillary sinus as a complication of overfilling root canal material into the sinus: Report of two cases. J Endod 2001;27:476–478.
135. Guivarc'h M, Ordioni U, Catherine JH, Campana F, Camps J, Bukiet F. Implications of endodontic-related sinus aspergillosis in a patient treated by infliximab: A case report. J Endod 2015;41:125–129.
136. Giardino L, Pontieri F, Savoldi E, Tallarigo F. *Aspergillus mycetoma* of the maxillary sinus secondary to overfilling of a root canal. J Endod 2006;32:692–694.
137. Falworth MS, Herold J. Aspergillosis of the paranasal sinuses. A case report and radiographic review. Oral Surg Oral Med Oral Pathol Oral Radiol Endod 1996;81:255–260.
138. Mensi M, Piccioni M, Marsili F, Nicolai P, Sapelli PL, Latronico N. Risk of maxillary fungus ball in patients with endodontic treatment on maxillary teeth: A case-control study. Oral Surg Oral Med Oral Pathol Oral Radiol Endod 2007;103:433–436.
139. Kobayashi A. Asymptomatic aspergillosis of the maxillary sinus associated with foreign body of endodontic origin. Report of a case. Int J Oral Maxillofac Surg 1995;24:243–244.
140. Legent F, Billet J, Beauvillain C, Bonnet J, Miegeville M. The role of dental canal fillings in the development of *Aspergillus* sinusitis: A report of 85 cases. Arch Otorhinolaryngol 1989;246:318–320.
141. Park GY, Kim HY, Min JY, Dhong HJ, Chung SK. Endodontic treatment: A significant risk factor for development of maxillary fungal ball. Clin Exp Otorhinolaryngol 2010;3:136–140.
142. Costa F, Robiony M, Toro C, Sembronio S, Politi M. Endoscopically assisted procedure for removal of a foreign body from the maxillary sinus and contemporary endodontic surgical treatment of the tooth. Head Face Med 2006;2:37.
143. Tsodoulos S, Karabouta I, Voulgaropoulou M, Georgiou C. Atraumatic removal of an asymptomatic migrated dental implant into the maxillary sinus: A case report. J Oral Implantol 2012;38:189–193.
144. González-García A, González-García J, Diniz-Freitas M, García-García A, Bullón P. Accidental displacement and migration of endosseous implants into adjacent craniofacial structures: A review and update. Med Oral Patol Oral Cir Bucal 2012;17(5):e769–e774.
145. Ishikawa M, Mizuno T, Yamazaki Y, Satoh T, Notani K, Fukuda H. Migration of gutta-percha point from a root canal into the ethmoid sinus. Br J Oral Maxillofac Surg 2004;42:58–60.
146. Felisati G, Lozza P, Chiapasco M, Borloni R. Endoscopic removal of an unusual foreign body in the sphenoid sinus: An oral implant. Clin Oral Implants Res 2007;18:776–780.
147. Biglioli F, Chiapasco M. An easy access to retrieve dental implants displaced into the maxillary sinus: The bony window technique. Clin Oral Implants Res 2014;25:1344–1351.
148. Biglioli F, Goisis M. Access to the maxillary sinus using a bone flap on a mucosal pedicle: Preliminary report. J Craniomaxillofac Surg 2002;30:255–259.
149. Costa F, Emanuelli E, Robiony M, Zerman N, Polini F, Politi M. Endoscopic surgical treatment of chronic maxillary sinusitis of dental origin. J Oral Maxillofac Surg 2007;65:223–228.
150. Choi BH, Yoo JH, Sung KJ. Radiographic comparison of osseous healing after maxillary sinusotomy performed with and without a periosteal pedicle. Oral Surg Oral Med Oral Pathol Oral Radiol Endod 1996;82:375–378.
151. Choung PH, Choung YH. Vasculized bone flap for access to the maxillary sinus. J Oral Maxillofac Surg 1997;55:832–825.
152. Lazaridis N, Tilaveridis I, Venetis G, Lazaridou M. Maxillary sinus osteoplasty with vascularized pedicled bone flap. Oral Surg Oral Med Oral Pathol Oral Radiol Endod 2008;106:828–832.
153. Uckan S, Buchbinder D. Sinus lift approach for the retrieval of root fragments from the maxillary sinus. Int J Oral Maxillofac Surg 2003;32:87–90.
154. Yura S, Kato T, Ooi K, Izumiyama Y. Access to the maxillary sinus using a bone flap with sinus mucosal and mucoperiosteal pedicles. Oral Surg Oral Med Oral Pathol Oral Radiol Endod 2010;109(2):e8–e12.
155. Huumonen S, Kvist T, Gröndahl K, Molander A. Diagnostic value of computed tomography in re-treatment of root fillings in maxillary molars. Int Endod J 2006;39:827–833.
156. Rigolone M, Pasqualini D, Bianchi L, Berutti E, Bianchi SD. Vestibular surgical access to the palatine root of the superior first molar: "Low-dose cone-beam" CT analysis of the pathway and its anatomic variations. J Endod 2003;29:773–775.
157. Altonen M. Transantral subperiosteal resection of the palatal root of maxillary molars. Int J Oral Surg 1975;4:277–283.
158. Kurt SN, Üstün Y, Erdogan Ö, Evlice B, Yoldas O, Öztunc H. Outcomes of periradicular surgery of maxillary first molars using a vestibular approach: A prospective, clinical study with one year of follow-up. J Oral Maxillofac Surg 2014;72:1049–1061.
159. Tataryn RW, Torabinejad M, Boyne PJ. Healing potential of osteotomies of the nasal sinus in the dog. Oral Surg Oral Med Oral Pathol Oral Radiol Endod 1997;84:196–202.

160. Akuamoa-Boateng E, Niederdellmann H, Fabinger A. Reconstruction of the facial fenestration in the Caldwell-Luc maxillary sinus operation. Rhinology 1979;17: 237–243.
161. Nemec SF, Peloschek P, Koelblinger C. Sinonasal imaging after Caldwell-Luc surgery: MDCT findings of an abandoned procedure in times of functional endoscopic sinus surgery. Eur J Radiol 2009;70:31–34.
162. Tataryn RW. Rhinosinusitis and endodontic disease. In: Ingle JI, Bakland LK, Baumgartner JC (eds). Ingle's Endodontics, ed 6. Hamilton, ON: BC Decker, 2007:626–637.
163. Tsesis I, Rosen E, Taschieri S, Telishevsky Strauss Y, Ceresoli V, Del Fabbro M. Outcomes of surgical endodontic treatment performed by a modern technique: An updated meta-analysis of the literature. J Endod 2013;39:332–339.

Chapter Thirteen

Suturing and Postoperative Instructions

Erik Sahl, Bonnie Retamozo

The final steps of a surgical treatment are closure of the surgical site or wound and management of the patient during the early postsurgical period when critical wound healing events are occurring. Following surgery, postsurgical examinations are necessary to ensure a successful outcome. Wound closure is critical to that outcome and, if not properly managed, can result in delayed healing of the wound. Postsurgical patient management is imperative because it not only informs the patient of expected outcomes but can also provide essential elements that promote rapid healing of the wound and minimize the risk for undesirable postsurgical sequelae.

Wound Closure

After the completion of apical microsurgery, the final step is to position and secure the surgical flap. The tissue should be replaced as close as possible to the original position and secured. The type of flap design may impact the ease with which reapproximation is accomplished. A full mucoperiosteal flap generally provides less resistance to reapproximation than limited mucoperiosteal flaps. In addition, the ease of reapproximation influences the number of sutures required for stabilization.

Prior to and immediately following the placement of sutures, compression of the tissue with a moistened gauze is advised. This enhances clotting in the severed blood vessels and prevents clot formation between the flap and alveolar bone. Ideal suturing techniques will enable hemostasis, aiding healing of the wound by primary intention and reducing the patient's postoperative discomfort and morbidity. A radiograph should also be taken before the flap is secured to allow for detection of foreign objects adhering to the internal surface of the flap or the crypt.

Selection of Suture Materials

There are numerous suture materials and sizes available on the market. Each material and size of suture has inherent characteristics that not only alter the handling properties but also affect the healing process as well as the tissue response associated with the suture. The ideal suture should be biocompatible, have the appropriate tensile strength for its purpose, be easy to handle surgically, and prevent premature untying or loosening of the surgical knot. A suture size of 5-0 is commonly used for apical surgery, but some clinicians may prefer a slightly larger size (4-0) or smaller size (6-0). It should be noted that suture sizes smaller then 6-0 have the tendency to "cut" through the fragile oral tissue when tension is applied to tie the suture.

The tensile strength of the suture selected is dependent on the surgical procedure and amount of time the suture needs to remain in place. For larger or more complex surgical procedures where tissue healing time is increased, a slower-absorbing suture is recommended. The conventional polyglycolic acid sutures are more durable, having the ability to be retained for roughly 14 days and thereafter resorbing in 3 to 4 weeks, and are therefore recommended for long-term use. Surgical gut sutures, on the other hand, are digested by intraoral enzymes, are rapidly resorbed, and lose their strength in 1 to 2 days, which is the same rate at which the tissue increases its strength. Gut sutures can also be coated with a chromic salt compound that decreases the absorption rate to 7 to 10 days. In patients with acidic intraoral conditions due to systemic medical conditions, the resorption rate of these sutures is also increased.

Another method for wound closure is the use of tissue adhesives, such as cyanoacrylate and fibrin glues. However, currently available research is too limited to provide a recommendation for routine replacement of traditional suture materials with these adhesives.[1,2]

Silk

Silk sutures are comprised of a braided fiber affixed to a sericin fiber. Because of its braided nature, as with all braided types of suture material, it will attract and accumulate plaque and bacteria within the braids. Topical mouthrinses along with excellent oral hygiene practices can minimize this effect on the overall healing of the surgical wound. Additionally, extra care should be given when removing silk sutures. Cleansing and disinfecting the site prior to removal can reduce the introduction of plaque under the wound margin, which could potentially lead to a prolonged healing response.

Polypropylene

Polypropylene is a monofilament, extruded nylon material. Polypropylene is nonabsorbable and elicits a minimal inflammatory effect on living tissues. As a monofilament (nonbraided material), this type of suture is resistant to plaque adherence and bacterial infiltration. Also, this material is resistant to tissue adherence, so removal can be facilitated with a simple pull-out technique. Alternatively, this material has a higher likelihood of knot loosening, resulting in a recommendation for numerous knots when tying.

ePTFE

Commercially known as GORE-TEX (Gore Medical), ePTFE is expanded polytetrafluoroethylene. This polymer cannot be dissolved, and its unique chemical properties make it an extremely biologically inert substance. Being a monofilament material, ePTFE is resistant to plaque accumulation. An additional benefit of this material is that it allows the clinician to tie knots on top of the original knot and further cinch the knot to enhance flap immobilization as well as knot stability.

Catgut

This material is composed of collagen and will be readily absorbed within a matter of days in vascular tissue. Because of its absorbability properties, a major indication for the use of gut sutures is to eliminate the need for suture removal. However, this property can be unpredictable, and resorption rates can vary significantly between manufacturers. Gut suture is significantly more difficult to work with intraorally than other suture materials, resulting in curling and difficulty in maneuverability. This property can be improved by simply soaking the material in sterile water for 5 minutes prior to use to displace the alcohol remnants from packaging. If a longer absorption rate is desired, gut suture is available with a coating of a chromic salt compound, resulting in an extension of tensile strength for up to 7 days.

The surgeon needs to understand the benefits and limitations of each material as well as the goal of the procedure prior to determining which material to select.

Knots

There are two main types of surgical knots used in suturing after surgical procedures: the slip surgical knot and the surgeon's knot. The type of surgical knot to be used by the surgeon is dependent on the type of suture material used. The slip surgical knot (Fig 13-1a) should be performed when using suturing materials such as silk, ePTFE, chromic gut, and plain gut. The surgeon's knot (Fig 13-1b) is appropriate when suturing with synthetic materials so as to prevent untying.

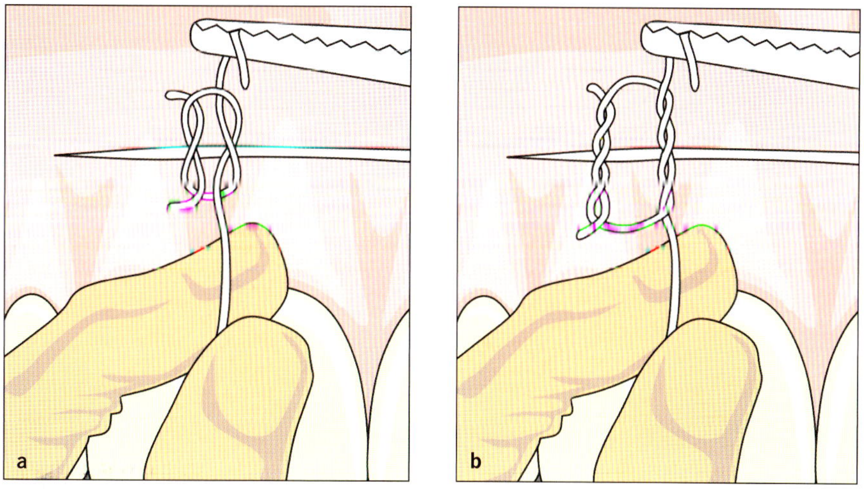

Fig 13-1 *(a)* Slip surgical knot. *(b)* Triple-loop surgeon's knot.

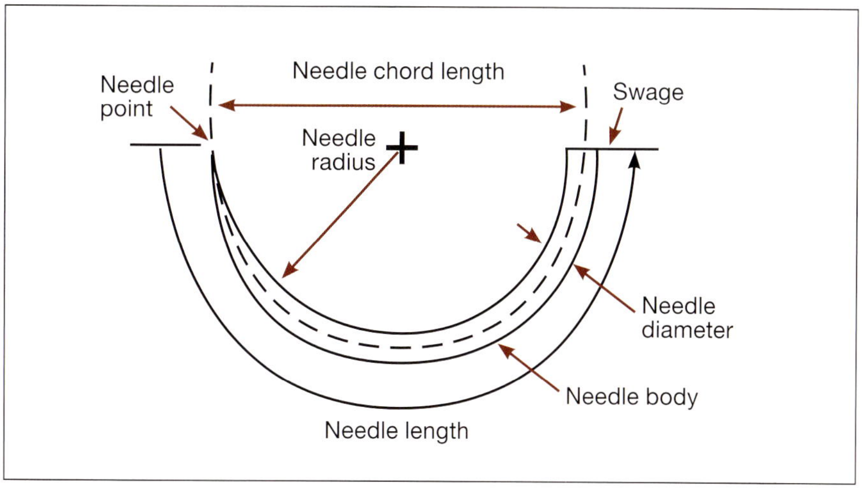

Fig 13-2 Suture needle anatomy.

Needles

In addition to careful selection of a suture material, needle selection is crucial. Selection is based on a combination of factors including the suture technique employed, the tensile strength of the tissue, the width of attached gingiva, the size and shape of the interdental embrasure, and the flap design. The arc of the needle should be based on the curvature needed to penetrate the tissues on both sides of the incision. The radius of the needle arc should allow the clinician to pass from the buccal surface to the lingual surface in one motion by simply rotating the needle on a central axis. This is beneficial when placing sutures in the posterior areas where the interproximal contacts are broader. The most commonly used suture needles to accomplish this are the ⅜ and ½ circle needles.[3]

Needles normally consist of three main parts: the needle point, body, and swaged end (Fig 13-2). Designs for the body include reverse cutting edge, tapered point, tapered cut, or conventional cut. The most commonly used type is the reverse cutting edge, because it usually results in less tissue tearing as the needle point passes through the tissue. The swaged end is press fitted around the suture line to allow smooth passage through the tissue. To avoid needle damage and allow maximum control over the needle, needle holders should grasp the

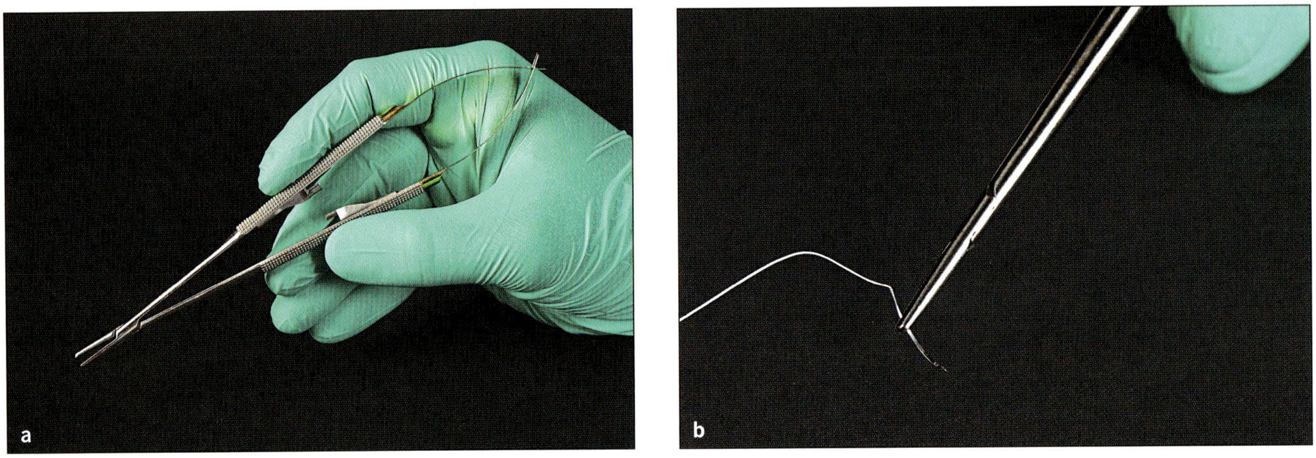

Fig 13-3 *(a and b)* Needle handling.

needle approximately two-thirds the length of the needle from the needle point, approximately 3 mm from the tip of the needle holder (Fig 13-3).

Suturing Techniques

A few concepts should be considered when suturing oral mucosa:

- *Avoid excessive tension on sutures/tissues:* This concept is clinically demonstrated in the form of tissue blanching on the wound margins, which occurs when the vascular flow to the margins is decreased, subsequently resulting in tissue necrosis (Fig 13-4). Developing small tissue cuts known as *tracks* is another complication when clinicians attempt primary closure without sufficient flap release.
- *Position knots away from the wound edges:* Knots are considered the weakest part of sutures. Therefore, placing them at the wound margin might compromise the closure as subsequent swelling may cause pressure on this link and jeopardize the closure achieved by opening the knots. Furthermore, knots are common areas that have a high tendency for plaque accumulation. Such problems will cause the bacterial plaque to be positioned at the flap margins and compromise the granulation process required for maintaining primary closure and optimal tissue healing.
- *Use the least amount of sutures possible to achieve proper wound stabilization:* Excessive and unnecessary suturing will cause multiple needle entries to the flap margins and may compromise the flap integrity and blood supply.
- *Select appropriate starting and ending points:* Whenever possible, suturing should be done from movable to nonmovable tissues. This will enable proper flap approximation and accommodate more predictable tissue management.

The following sections describe common suturing techniques.[5]

Simple interrupted (simple loop)

The simple interrupted suture is the most commonly used suturing technique to close vertical and horizontal incisions for tissue stabilization.

Step-by-step technique

1. Pierce the outer surface of the buccal flap with the suture needle (Fig 13-5a).
2. Thread the needle under the interproximal contact, and pierce the inner aspect of the lingual tissue with the suture needle (Fig 13-5b).
3. Pass the suture needle under the interproximal contact toward the buccal aspect (Fig 13-5c).
4. Tie off the free ends of the suture. Cut off the suture, leaving 2 to 3 mm of suture material (tail) (Fig 13-5d and Video 13-1).

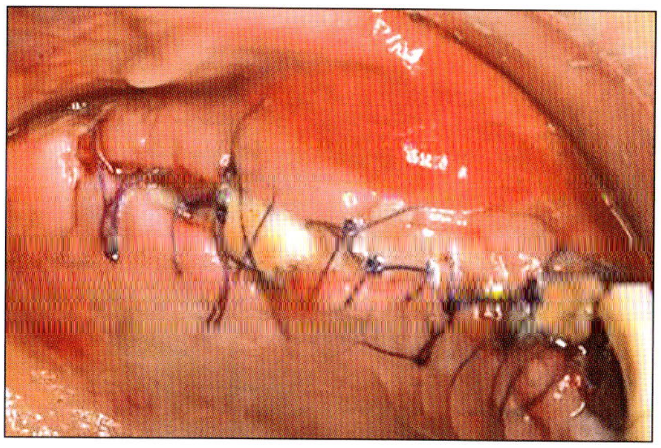

Fig 13-4 Flap necrosis due to excessive tension. (Reprinted from Griffin et al[4] with permission.)

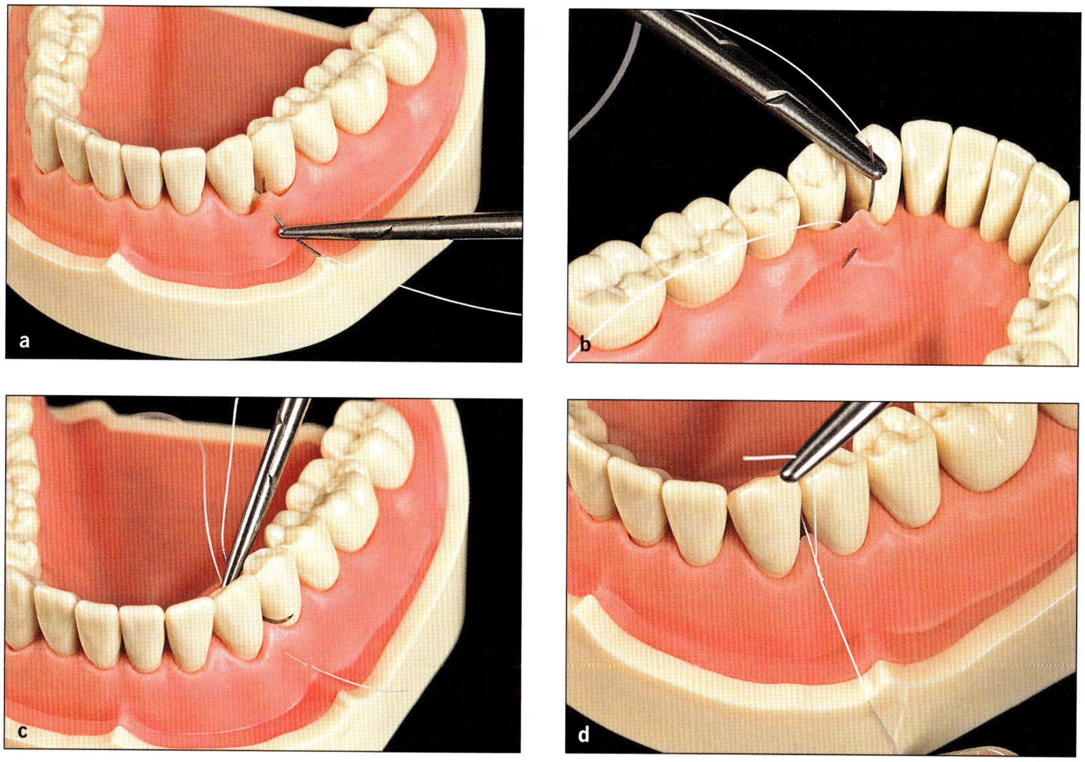

Fig 13-5 *(a to d)* Simple interrupted suture.

Interrupted figure-eight

The interrupted figure-eight suture is the second most commonly used suturing technique. The main advantage gained from using this technique is the ease of access between teeth. On the other hand, the main disadvantage is the interposition of suture material between the flaps, resulting in less-than-ideal tissue approximation.

Step-by-step technique

1. Pierce the outer surface of the buccal flap with the suture needle (Fig 13-6a).
2. Thread the needle under the interproximal contact, and pierce the outer aspect of the lingual tissue with the suture needle (Figs 13-6b and 13-6c).
3. Pass the suture needle through the interproximal contact, and tie and cut off the remaining suture, leaving 2 to 3 mm as a tail (Figs 13-6d and 13-6e and Video 13-2).

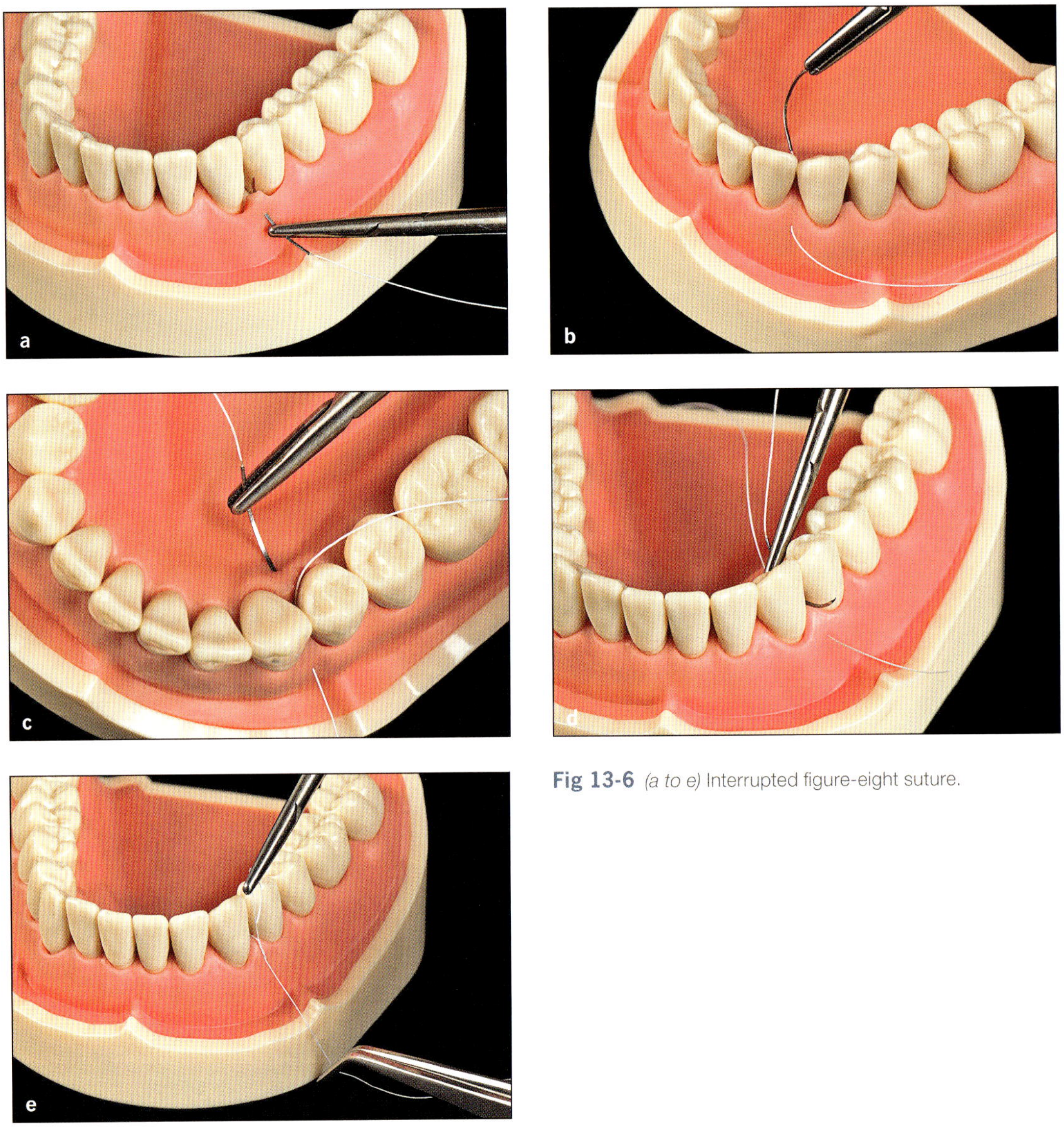

Fig 13-6 *(a to e)* Interrupted figure-eight suture.

Interrupted single sling suture

The interrupted single sling suture is advised when planning for coronal flap repositioning. This is usually achieved by gaining anchorage from lingual contours of the teeth.

Step-by-step technique

1. Pierce the outer aspect of the flap at its mesial end, and pass the needle under the interproximal contact (Figs 13-7a and 13-7b).
2. Wrap the suture around the lingual aspect of the tooth, and pass the needle through the distal interproximal contact (Fig 13-7c).
3. Pierce the inner aspect of the buccal flap, with the needle emerging on the buccal (Fig 13-7d).
4. Thread the suture needle back through the distal interproximal contact, and wrap the suture around the tooth, going mesially (Figs 13-7e and 13-7f).
5. Pass the suture needle back through the mesial interproximal contact, and tie and cut the suture, leaving 2 to 3 mm of suture material as a tail (Fig 13-7g and Video 13-3).

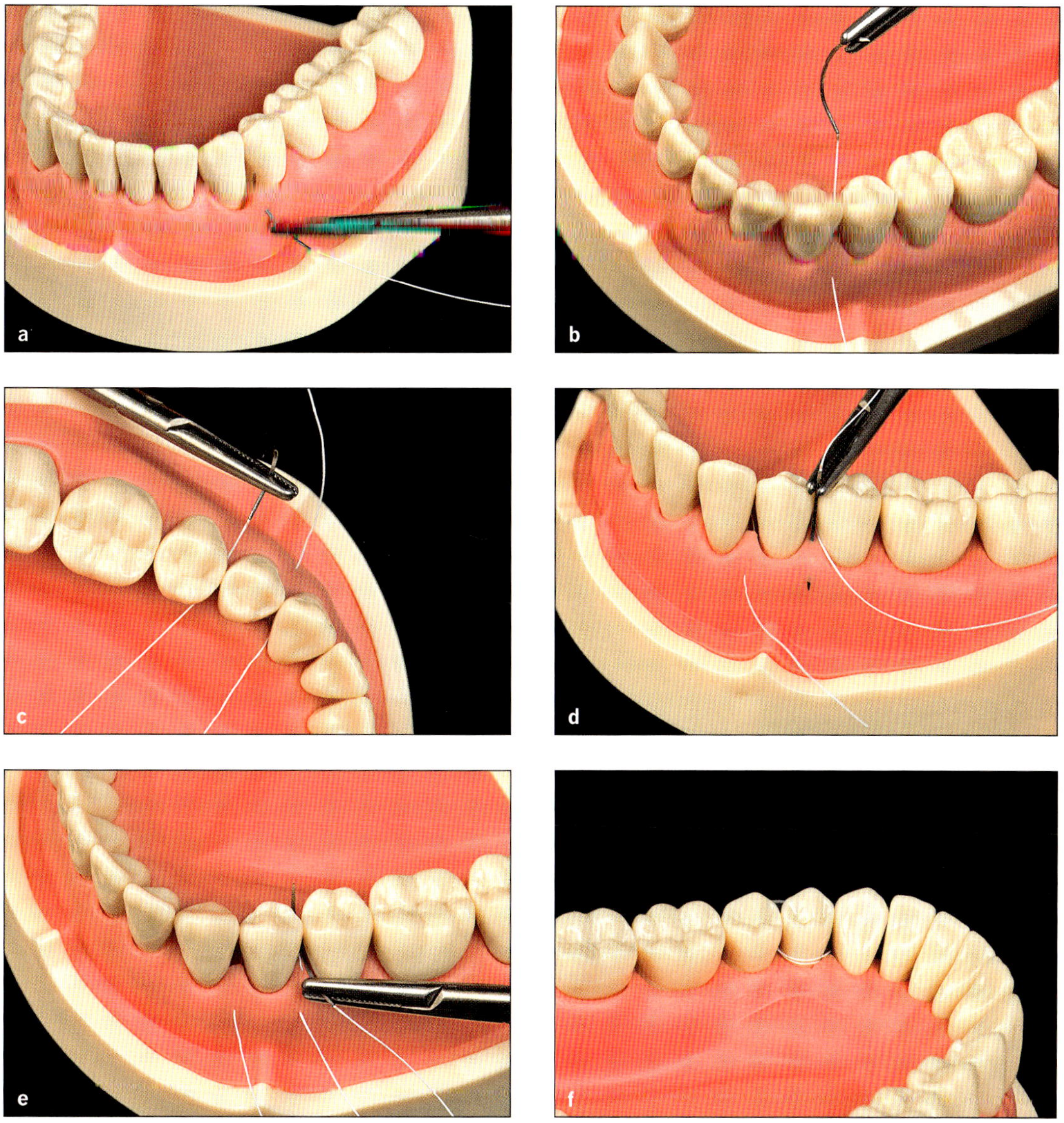

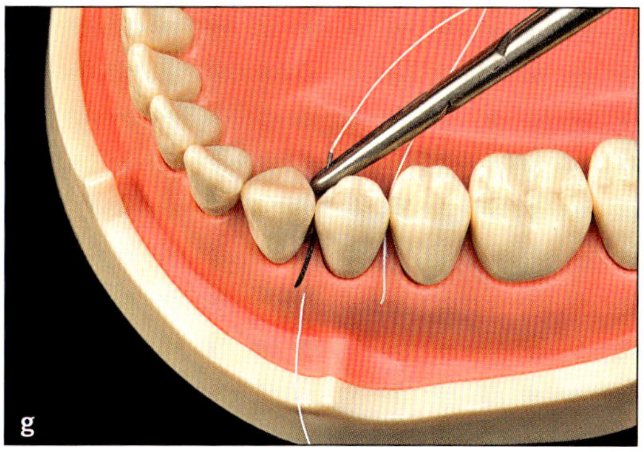

Fig 13-7 *(a to g)* Interrupted single sling suture.

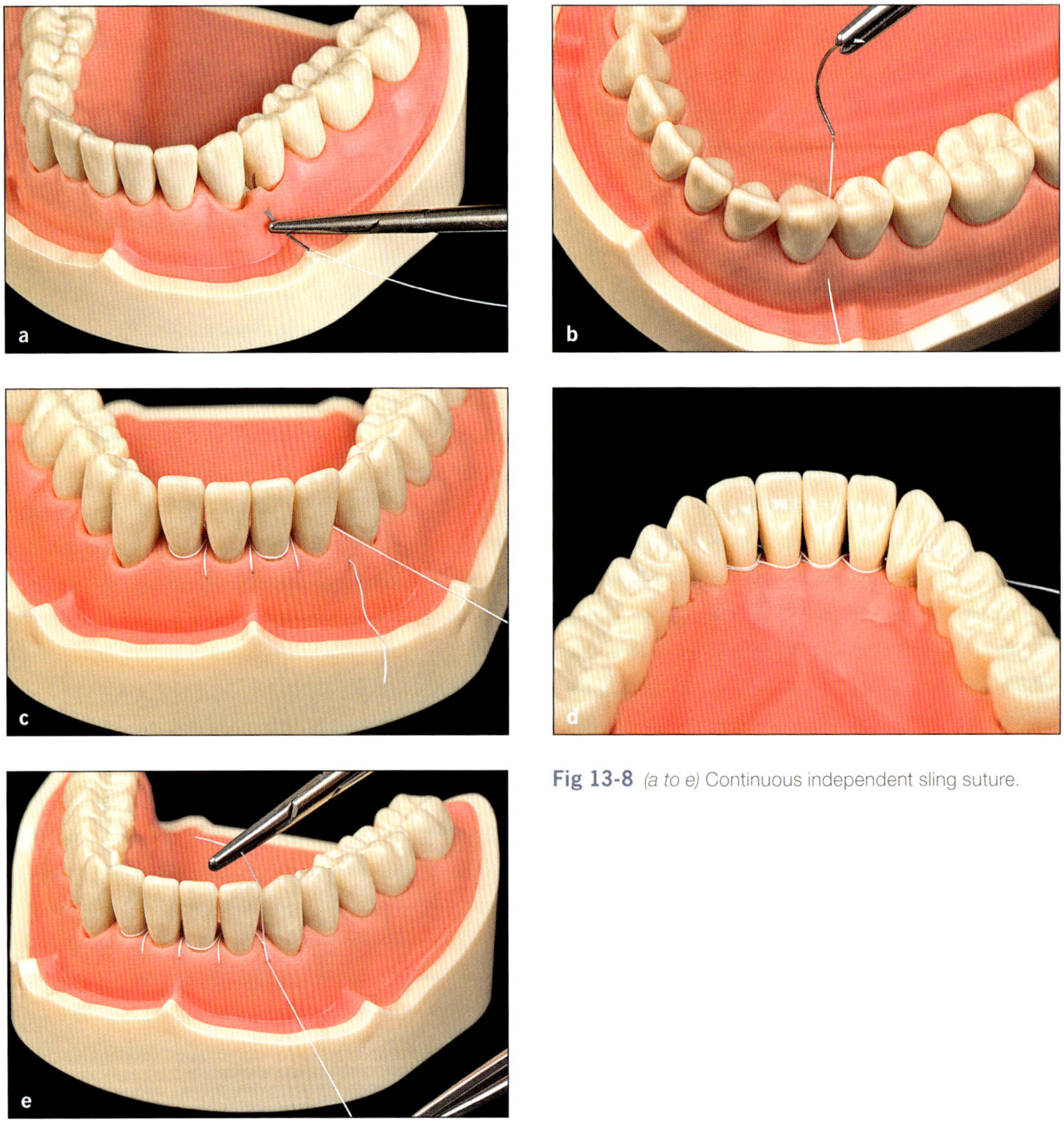

Fig 13-8 *(a to e)* Continuous independent sling suture.

Continuous independent sling suture

The continuous independent sling suture uses continuous sutures to attach two surgical flap edges or to secure multiple interproximal papillae of one flap independently of the other flap. This technique offers the advantage of fewer individual suture ties; however, there are significant disadvantages associated with this technique. If one knot or loop breaks, the integrity of the entire surgical site will be compromised. For this reason, more control can be gained using individually placed interrupted, sling, criss-cross, or mattress sutures in lieu of placing one large continuous suture.[4] The advantage of using this technique is that it minimizes the number of knots needed, thereby shortening the time required for achieving the closure needed. At the same time, however, this brings the disadvantage of relying on one knot for flap closure.

Step-by-step technique

1. Enter the outer aspect of the buccal flap from the mesial aspect, and leave a free end (Fig 13-8a).
2. Pass the needle through the contact area, first piercing the opposite-side tissue from the inner aspect and then returning the needle to the buccal aspect, and then tie off the remaining free end. The papillae should be anchored by piercing 2 to 3 mm from the flap margins (Fig 13-8b).
3. Continue the sling around the lingual aspect, and pierce the buccal flap from the outer aspect (Fig 13-8c).
4. Return the needle to the buccal aspect, and then wrap around the tooth to enter the contact area of the next distal tooth (Fig 13-8d).
5. Return through the contact area, where a sling is formed distally and then the inner aspect of the buc-

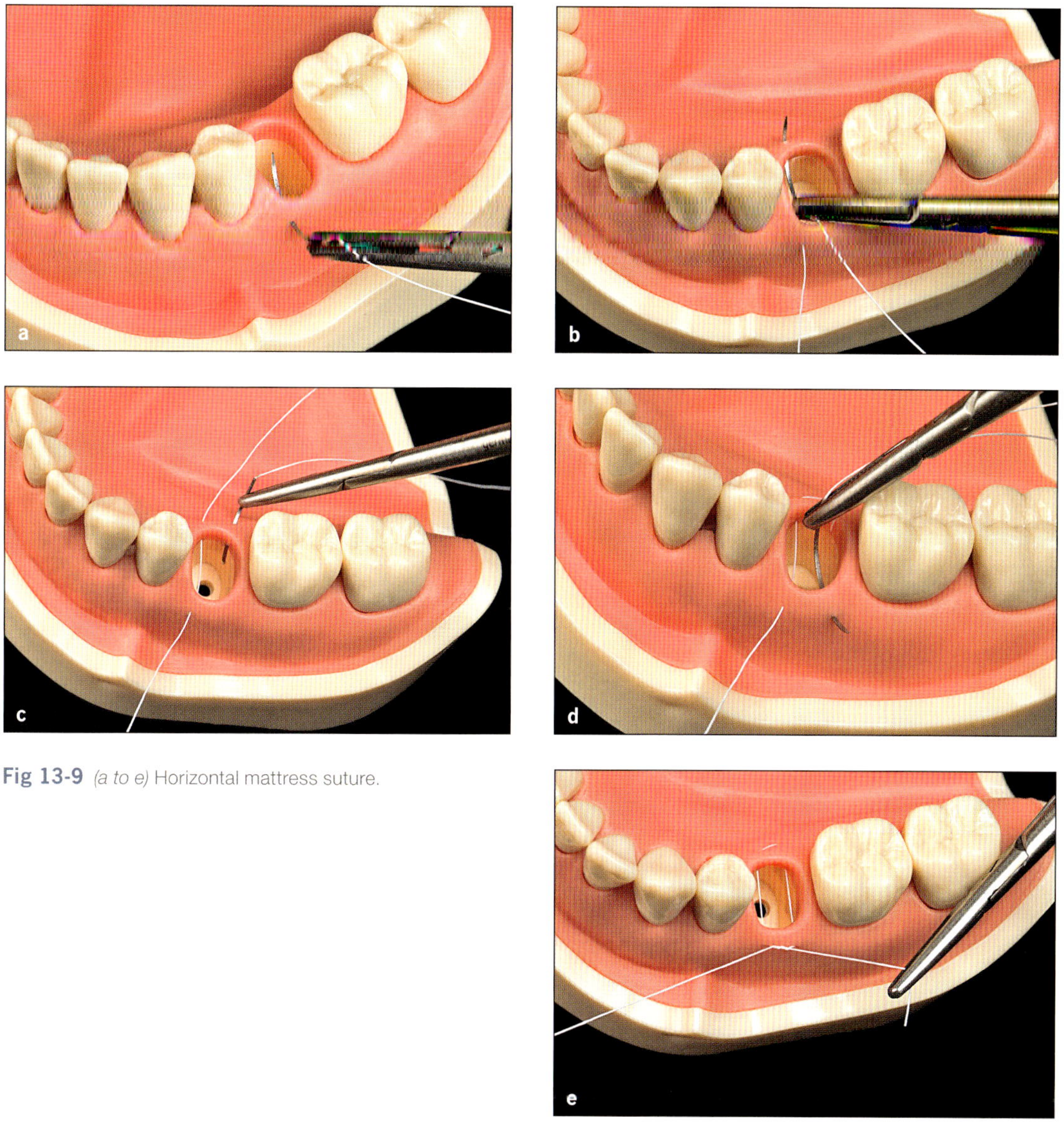

Fig 13-9 *(a to e)* Horizontal mattress suture.

cal flap is engaged. Continue distally by anchoring the flaps between the buccal and lingual sides until the entire span is secured. Once the initial point of entry is reached, pass the needle under the contact and secure (Fig 13-8e and Video 13-4).

Horizontal mattress suture

This suturing technique is preferred when muscular pull and subsequent flap contraction are expected. Therefore, it is highly advised for guided bone regeneration procedures such as ridge augmentation, for edentulous areas, as well for around teeth or implants. This is because the suture reduces flap tension, resulting in a more predictable primary closure and less tissue or flap necrosis.

Step-by-step technique

1. Pierce the external side of the buccal flap 3 to 4 mm from the flap margin (Fig 13-9a).
2. Pierce the internal side of the lingual tissue 3 to 4 mm from the lingual flap margin (Fig 13-9b).
3. Penetrate the external side of the lingual tissue 5 mm laterally from the second piercing (Fig 13-9c).
4. Pass the needle through the internal side of the buccal flap, and tie the free ends (Figs 13-9d and 13-9e and Video 13-5).

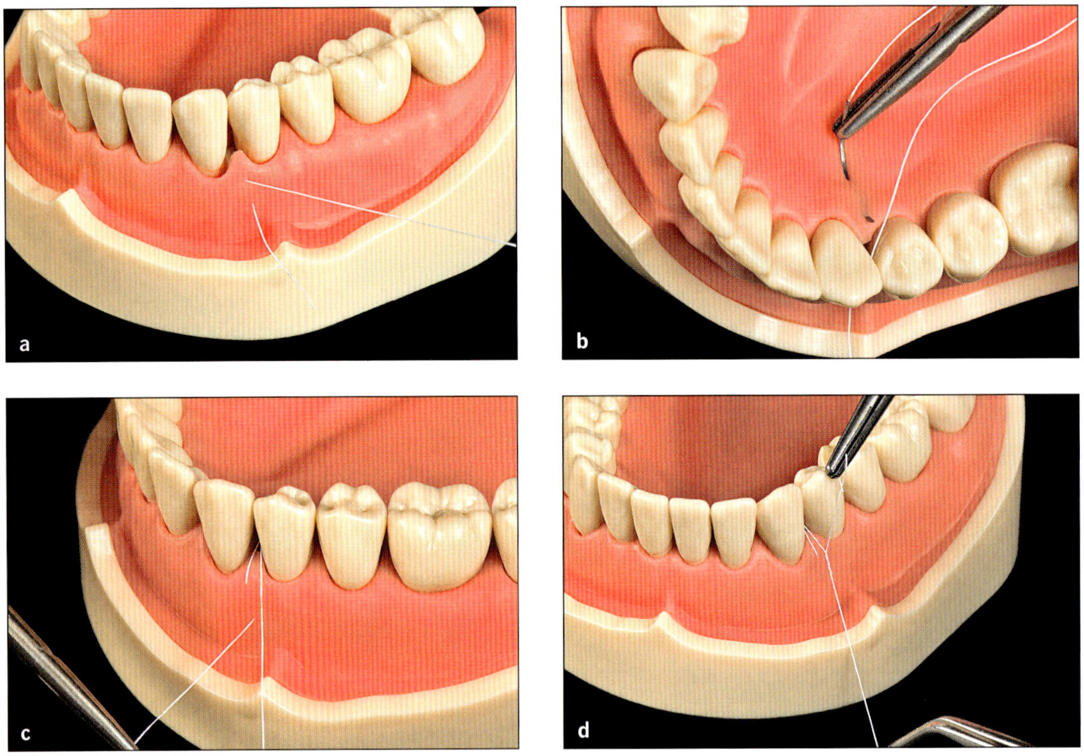

Fig 13-10 *(a to d)* Coronally advanced vertical mattress suture.

Coronally advanced vertical mattress suture

This suturing technique is commonly preferred for its ability to achieve precise flap and papilla positioning. It is commonly used in regenerative periodontal surgeries and guided tissue regeneration procedures.

Step-by-step technique

1. Pierce the buccal flap just above the mucogingival junction, anchoring the flap to the underlying periosteum. The needle should emerge from the center of the papilla 2 to 3 mm from the flap edge (Fig 13-10a).
2. Pass the needle through the contact area, and anchor the lingual tissue the same way, starting from the center of the lingual papilla 2 to 3 mm from the flap edges (Fig 13-10b).
3. Thread the needle through the interproximal contact, and tie and cut the suture on the buccal side, leaving 2 to 3 mm of suture material as a tail (Figs 13-10c and 13-10d).

Conclusion

Sutures play a significant role in the success or failure of the surgical procedure. Hence, proper material selection should be part of that success or failure. Several material properties are to be evaluated before proceeding with any suture, including resistance to traction, the least memory possible, knot safety, and decreased wicking that can compromise the wound healing process and interfere with proper flap adhesion. Several studies have been conducted to evaluate the bacterial response to suture materials. Studies show that significantly less bacterial colonization occurred around resorbable sutures removed at up to 21 days compared with nonresorbable suture material.[6–9]

Postsurgical Patient Management

Postsurgical management of the patient is just as important as the surgical procedure. It is imperative that the surgeon expresses to the patient a level of concern and reassurance regarding the patient's experience. In addition, verbal communication as well as detailed home care instructions should be provided to the patient about what is expected and what is considered normal postoperative sequelae. Patient instructions and expectations are detailed in the following sections.

Verbal communication

The possible intra- and postoperative complications that could arise as a result of the surgery should be discussed at the presurgical visit. These complications could include bleeding, swelling, infection, bruising, and altered nerve sensation.

Written consent and postoperative instructions

Obtaining written consent for all possible complications is of great importance. Consent forms should be unique for each patient as the amount of intra- and postoperative bleeding can differ significantly according to the local anatomy, type of flap reflection, dissection type, and any systemic conditions of the patient. Furthermore, a copy of this written consent should be sent home with the patient and kept by the front desk staff to help eliminate any future miscommunication.

Along with the consent forms, written postoperative instructions are essential to send home with the patient, especially if the patient has been sedated (Fig 13-11).

Follow-up phone call

Patients should be followed the night of surgery with a courtesy phone call, as early postoperative complications such as uncontrolled pain, bleeding, and hematoma formation could be detected quickly.

Bleeding (ecchymosis, petechiae, and hematoma)

When bleeding complications occur, it is very important to use the proper terminology in chart entries, as this will facilitate accurate follow-up and proper documentation: petechiae (< 2 mm in diameter), purpura (2 to 10 mm in diameter), and ecchymosis (> 10 mm in diameter).[8] The location of the bruising is mainly controlled by the anatomical site, but gravity can further explain bruising at distant locations (Fig 13-12).

The incidence of hemorrhagic occurrences could be lowered by properly designing the surgery, starting with an extensive review and update of the medical health history and anatomy, followed by proper flap elevation and limiting the extent of vertical incisions when possible. Healing of these occurrences usually goes through certain predictable color patterns. In the first 48 hours, soft tissue colors usually change from black to blue. By day 6, the tissues turn to a greenish color as a result of biliverdin. By day 9, yellowish-brownish discoloration usually develops, confirming the presence of subcutaneous bilirubin. In a typical situation, it takes about 2 to 3 weeks for the discoloration to subside completely.[11]

Swelling

Postoperative swelling can be intraoperatively controlled by proper flap suturing with adequate tension. Furthermore, 5 minutes of continuous pressure applied to the flap can establish proper hemostasis and reduce any blood collection below the flaps that could initiate hematoma formation and flap dehiscence.

Applying an ice pack in an extraoral manner can reduce the extraoral swelling and possible bruise formation as well as the patient's discomfort. Application of moist heat over the surgical site is recommended, as it will promote blood flow and increase the healing, but it should not be applied in the first 24 hours following surgery.

Paresthesia

A solid understanding of local anatomy is of great importance to prevent any accidental damage to vital sensory structures. When such loss of feeling occurs, patients should be assured that it may be the result of hematoma formation with local pressure to adjacent nerve structures. Proper follow-up and documentation should be done to monitor the degree of altered sensation and its subsequent resolution. Such assessment can be carried out using the nerve assessment tool found in Box 13-1.[10,12]

Oral rinses

Postoperative instructions include refraining temporarily from brushing the area of the surgical site and substituting with oral rinses. One of the popular mouthrinses is chlorhexidine gluconate 0.12% mouthwash. Care must

Postoperative Instructions and Information for Endodontic Surgery

- Take your medication(s) exactly as prescribed by your surgeon.
- Rinse with chlorhexidine in the morning and evening for 1 minute each and spit out. Do not use for more than 2 weeks because it may stain your teeth.
- A surgical dressing may be placed on the area to prevent food impaction and other trauma to the wound site. If it should break up or come off, do not panic. Should you swallow some of it, do not worry, it will not harm you.
- Swelling may occur. To minimize swelling, gently place an ice pack to the outside of your face for 15 minutes. Then remove it for 15 minutes. Repeat this routine for 2 hours.
- Oozing of blood from the surgical site will appear to be greatly exaggerated when it dissolves in the saliva. If there is bleeding and you cannot determine its origin, gently rinse your mouth with iced tea or ice water for ½ hour.
- Do not use a straw, as the suction effect may break up your blood clot.
- Sleep on two pillows or with your head slightly raised on the night of the surgical procedure.
- On the day after surgery and for the following week, rinse your mouth three or four times a day with room-temperature water to promote healing and to help keep the area clean.
- You may rinse with warm salt water several times a day using no more than ½ teaspoon of salt in a tall glass of body-temperature water.
- Do not spit; gently expel liquids from your mouth after rinsing/brushing.
- You may eat any food of your choice following surgery. However, you will be more comfortable if you avoid hard foods, chew in nonsurgical areas, and eat a generally semisoft diet. Drink plenty of liquids, especially juices and water. A high-protein diet is desirable (milk, eggs, cottage cheese, yogurt, and ground beef). A high-protein supplement can be used, such as Instant Breakfast or Ensure.
- Plan for minimal activity for the first 24 hours following surgery. Try to rest as much as possible during the day and get plenty of sleep the night after the surgery. This will minimize pain and swelling.
- Smoking: The less you smoke, the faster you will heal. Avoid smoking as much as you possibly can.

Cautions

- Avoid chewing on the side where the surgery was performed.
- Avoid brushing the surgical area.
- Avoid applying tongue or cheek pressure to the surgical site.
- Avoid eating very spicy or salty foods, drinking alcoholic beverages, drinking thermally hot liquids, or eating thermally hot foods.
- Do not be alarmed if one of the following occurs:
  a. Slight bleeding or swelling
  b. Discomfort in the surgical area
  c. You develop a "taste" or odor in the area
  d. The dressing breaks up or falls off
  e. There is tooth tenderness
  f. You see or feel threads in the surgical area; it is the suture material
- Do not hesitate to call your dentist or visit the hospital emergency room if you experience any of the following:
  a. Excessive bleeding
  b. Discomfort not controlled by the prescribed medication
  c. Any unfavorable reactions to the medication
  d. Fever, excessive swelling, or difficulty breathing

Fig 13-11 Sample postoperative instructions to send home with the patient.

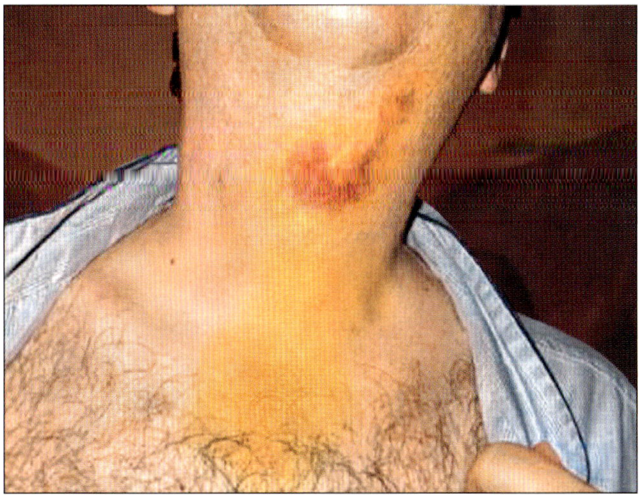

Fig 13-12 Ecchymosis extending to the pectoralis muscle after removal of a maxillary bone cyst. (Reprinted from Greenstein et al[10] with permission.)

Box 13-1 Tests to determine the extent of nerve injury

1. Light touch test: A soft brush is applied to the lip, and the patient is asked in which direction the stimulus was applied.
2. Pain test: A 27-gauge needle can be used to determine whether the patient perceives pain.
3. Two-point discrimination test: Calipers are opened progressively at 2-mm increments until the patient is able to discriminate the caliper ends as two separate points of contact.
4. Ice or a heated mirror handle (430) can be used to determine whether the patient is able to discriminate between hot and cold.

be taken to inform the patients about the temporary altered taste sensation associated with this product. The extrinsic staining of teeth should be addressed with the possible need for supragingival debridement and removal of stain. Additionally, early wound healing may be affected by this product due to the inhibitory effect of fibroblasts, so its use should be limited.

Pain management

Intraoperative pain control starts with proper selection of long- or short-acting local anesthesia. This could also be accompanied with the use of oral or intravenous sedation medications. For postoperative pain control and medications used to manage postoperative pain, see chapter 16.

Postsurgical antibiotics

There are two indications for the use of antibiotics: to treat an active infection or to prevent an infection. The treatment approach is different for each indication. For use of antibiotics in surgical endodontics, see chapter 16.

Supportive therapy

Supportive therapy includes a proper diet (eg, soups and soft foods), plenty of fluid intake, and a restriction of normal activities following the surgical procedure. In addition, it is necessary for all patients to restrict their activity during the 6 to 8 hours immediately following surgery, when rest and application of ice are necessary. Patients can return to work the day after surgery if their job does not require strenuous activity. Any activity that significantly raises the blood pressure, such as running or any strenuous form of exercise, should be avoided for 2 to 3 days after surgery. This is to prevent dislodgment of clots in the severed microvessels due to increased hydrostatic pressure. A progressive return to normal activities can occur 1 week following surgery.

Suture removal

The clinician may use his or her discretion as to when to remove the sutures. However, it should be realized that when the sutures are loose, they do not serve any additional purpose and become a source for plaque collection. The majority of sutures should be removed when local tissue edema subsides and sutures become loose. When removing sutures, a transient bacteremia can be expected. For this reason, the use of an oral disinfecting agent such as a chlorhexidine gluconate mouthrinse should be used or can be applied to the gingival tissue at the site of each suture entering the tissue.[13] The clinician should take care to cut the suture material at the tissue level, thus preventing contaminated material from being pulled through the soft tissue (Videos 13-6 and 13-7).

If the patient has questionable healing at the time of suture removal, a re-evaluation of the wound should be done in 7 to 10 days. However, if healing is within normal limits, the patient can be scheduled for a recall at 3 to 12 months.

References

1. Perez M, Fernandez I, Marquez D, Bretana RM. Use of N-butyl-2-cyanoacrylate in oral surgery: Biological and clinical evaluation. Artif Organs 2000;24:241–243.
2. Yücel EA, Oral O, Olgaç V, Oral CK. Effects of fibrin glue on wound healing in the oral cavity. J Dent 2003;31:569–575.
3. Hutchens LH. Periodontal suturing: A review of needles, materials and techniques. Postgrad Dent 1995;2:1–15
4. Griffin TJ, Hur Y, Bu J. Basic suture techniques for oral mucosa. Clin Adv Periodontics 2011;1:221–231.
5. Silverstein LH. Principles of Dental Suturing: The Complete Guide to Surgical Closure. Mahwah, NJ: Montage Media, 1999.
6. Banche G, Roana J, Mandras N, et al. Microbial adherence on various intraoral suture materials in patients undergoing dental surgery. J Oral Maxillofac Surg 2007;65:1503–1507.
7. Gazivoda D, Pelemiš D, Vujašković G. A clinical study on the influence of suturing material on oral wound healing. Vojnosanit Pregl 2015;72:765–769.
8. Chu CC, Williams DF. Effects of physical configuration and chemical structure of suture materials on bacterial adhesion: A possible link to wound infection. Am J Surg 1984;147:197–204.
9. Grigg TR, Liewehr FR, Patton WR, Buxton TB, McPherson JC. Effect of the wicking behavior of multifilament sutures. J Endod 2004;30:649–652.
10. Greenstein G, Cavallaro J, Romanos G, Tarnow D. Clinical recommendations for avoiding and managing surgical complications associated with implant dentistry: A review. J Periodontol 2008;79:1317–1329.
11. Family Practice Notebook. Purpura. http://www.fpnotebook.com/HemeOnc/Derm/Prpr.htm. Accessed 12 January 2017.
12. Hegedus F, Diecidue RJ. Trigeminal nerve injuries after mandibular implant placement—Practical knowledge for clinicians. Int J Oral Maxillofac Implants 2006;21:111–116.
13. Brown AR, Papasian CJ, Shultz P, Theisen FC, Shultz RE. Bacteremia and intraoral suture removal: Can an antimicrobial rinse help? J Am Dent Assoc 1998;129:1455–1461.

Chapter Fourteen

Wound Healing

Kathryn A. Jurosky

Wound healing is a complex series of overlapping and interrelated events essential for repairing injured tissues in the oral environment and elsewhere in the body. There is an overarching impression that oral wounds heal more rapidly and with less scarring than similar wounds in skin. Understanding why this perception of rapid oral healing is accurate begins with a foundational knowledge of general wound healing in the dermis and a recognition of the circumstances that negatively affect overall healing. Appreciating the phenotypic differences of the reparative cell—the fibroblast—and its crucial role in resolving inflammation quickly is key to understanding the accelerated healing seen in the mouth. The specifics of wound healing following endodontic surgery rest upon an understanding of these concepts. The purpose of this chapter is to review general wound healing concepts in skin prior to an in-depth exploration of wound healing following periradicular surgery.

General Wound Healing in Skin

For ease of description, the wound healing events in skin are discussed in phases, although there are truly no discrete phases.[1,2] A normal sequence of wound healing begins with phase I: hemostasis and inflammation, which is then followed by phase II: proliferation, and phase III: maturation and remodeling. It is important to keep in mind that there are many factors, both local and systemic, that may negatively affect the healing process.

Phase I: Hemostasis and inflammation

Healing in skin begins as soon as tissue injury and bleeding occur. The body's first reaction is to stem the flow of blood at the site of injury through hemostasis, beginning with an initial short-lived vasoconstriction followed by clot formation. Fibrin clot formation results as both the intrinsic and extrinsic clotting cascades produce intravascular and extravascular clotting. The intrinsic cascade is initiated when blood contacts exposed collagen, while the extrinsic cascade is initiated by the release of thromboplastin during tissue injury.[2] The clots that form serve as reservoirs of chemoattractants, including cytokines and growth factors, and provide a scaffolding for cell migration.[3] Examples of factors released by the clot include platelet-derived growth factor (PDGF), transforming growth factor beta (TGF-β), fibroblast growth factor (FGF), and epidermal growth factor (EGF).[1,2]

Complicating the understanding of the inflammatory process is the fact that individual cytokines and growth factors can have multiple influences on cell recruitment. For instance, the cytokine interleukin-6 (IL-6) is made by endothelial cells during acute inflammation and causes the chemoattraction of polymorphonuclear leukocytes (PMNs). Once the PMNs arrive, they produce a soluble IL-6 receptor, which causes the endothelial cells to switch their signaling to attract monocytes and T lymphocytes to clear PMNs initially attracted by IL-6 from the area through apoptosis.[4]

Many growth factors have multiple functions. For example, PDGF is chemotactic for fibroblasts and affects fibroblast mitosis,[2] and FGF affects both re-epithelialization and angiogenesis.[2,3] TGF-β is key to numerous healing events, facilitating PMN and macrophage migration, fibroblast mitosis, and extracellular matrix synthesis.[2,3,5]

As hemostasis is established, the inflammatory process ensues. PMNs are the first inflammatory cells to migrate to the injury in response to the release of cytokines and growth factors from the fibrin clot, usually arriving within 6 to 8 hours.[1,2,6] PMNs have the important task of cleansing the wound site by phagocytizing bacteria and tissue debris, thereby preventing infection. PMNs are the predominant cell in the wound site between 24 and 48 hours.[2] As bacterial contamination and tissue debris are removed, the number of PMNs drops precipitously by 72 hours.

As the need for PMNs drops in the wound site, the number of macrophages grows, and inflammation transitions to its late phase, with macrophages becoming the dominant cell between days 3 and 4.[2,6] These macrophages are primarily derived from circulating monocytes, which differentiate after leaving the blood vessels.[2,5] Macrophages are efficient at phagocytizing PMNs and other cells, continuing to clean up the wound while also producing growth factors.[1,2,6] Once the dead and dying cells are removed, the late inflammatory phase winds down, and the macrophage differentiates into the reparative cell responsible for directing most of the proliferative phase of healing, including fibroblast proliferation, smooth muscle formation, and angiogenesis.[6] Factors produced by the macrophage affecting wound healing include: TGF, cytokines, IL-1, tumor necrosis factor, and PDGF, among others.[2,6] The importance of the macrophage in this process cannot be overestimated.

Lymphocytes also migrate to the injury site, though the exact functions of T lymphocytes involved in wound healing are not completely understood.[1] Some T cells are thought to impair wound healing (T-suppressor-cytotoxic cells), while other T cells are thought to have positive effects (T-helper cells).[7,8] An interesting T-cell group shown to have an effect on wound healing is the dendritic epidermal T cell (DETC), which helps maintain normal tissue healing and repair through immunoregulation. DETCs produce various growth factors, chemokines, and cytokines that defend against pathogens and regulate inflammation.[1] A lack of skin DETCs in mice has been shown to cause delay in wound closure.[1,9]

Phase II: Proliferation

The proliferative phase of healing commonly overlaps with the late inflammatory phase and may last up to 4 weeks.[2,6] During proliferation, fibroblasts migrate, collagen and extracellular matrix form, and angiogenesis occurs. The important relationship between epithelialization and connective tissue healing is clearly demonstrated in the proliferative phase. Re-epithelialization takes place as epithelial cells migrate from the wound edges across the existing fibrin scaffolding. Once contact of epithelial cells is established, the initial tentative wound seal is formed, and connective tissue healing can begin. Early epithelial cell migration is seen within 24 hours, and a thin epithelial bridge across the wound is evident within 48 to 72 hours.[2,6]

Once the epithelial seal forms, fibroblasts and endothelial cells in the connective tissue proliferate, creating the environment for angiogenesis and collagen production. Within 5 to 7 days, fibroblasts are depositing Type III and Type I collagen.[2] Fibroblasts also produce glycosaminoglycans and proteoglycans, components of the extracellular matrix. Angiogenesis requires extracellular matrix to induce the migration and mitosis of endothelial cells. FGF and vascular endothelial growth factor help regulate angiogenesis.[2] The interdependence between fibroplasia (collagen production) and angiogenesis continues through the proliferative phase.

Phase III: Maturation and remodeling

Remodeling of the newly formed tissues involves continuous reorganization of collagen, beginning approximately 3 weeks after injury when collagen production reaches its peak, and may continue for years.[2] During the remodeling process, the overall collagen volume remains approximately the same, as fibers and bundles degrade and re-form in equilibrium, reorienting themselves to be similar to those of the surrounding tissues.[6] Collagen degradation occurs by specific metalloproteinases (interstitial collagenases, gelatinases, and stromelysins) that are activated and inhibited in carefully regulated ways.[6] The abundant neovascularization produced during the proliferative phase also reduces and reorganizes. Myofibroblasts, a variation of the fibroblast, cause the overall wound to contract.[1,2] In the epidermis and dermis, maximum wound tensile strength is achieved approximately 3 months after injury, reaching 80% of the original tissue strength.[2]

Local and Systemic Factors Affecting Wound Healing

In the normal course of healing, multiple checks and balances exist to limit untoward outcomes. However, it is important to keep in mind that numerous factors impact overall wound healing in a negative way. The following review is not exhaustive but addresses commonly encountered influences that adversely affect healing.[1,6] Local factors include tissue hypoxia and infection. Systemic factors include age, sex, diseases, obesity, medications, alcoholism, smoking, and malnutrition.

Local factors

Hypoxia initially stimulates repair in the early wound; however, prolonged hypoxia delays healing.[10] Oxygen is required to fuel cell metabolism and adenosine triphosphate (ATP) energy production. The formation of reactive oxygen species, such as superoxide ions and hydrogen peroxide, used by phagocytes in oxidative killing depends on adequate oxygen tension levels.[10,11] Oxygen is also necessary in the hydroxylation of lysine and proline during collagen synthesis, so the overall rate and stability of collagen production is inhibited by hypoxia.[12]

Infection delays wound healing.[6] Low levels of bacterial contamination and tissue debris in the early wound site help attract phagocytic leukocytes; however, prolonged infection and endotoxin production elevates proinflammatory cytokine levels, resulting in chronic infection.[1] When inflammation persists, matrix metalloproteinases (MMPs), the family of enzymes active in normal tissue turnover, degrade the extracellular matrix at a higher rate, damaging the tissue.[1,13] It has also been shown that long-standing biofilms shield bacteria from phagocytosis and may explain why antibiotics are sometimes ineffective.[13]

Systemic factors

Aging is considered a risk factor for delayed healing.[1,5,6] Age-related changes are evident in nearly every aspect of healing, including hindered inflammatory responses, altered macrophage phagocytic capability, delayed re-epithelialization, and reduced collagen synthesis and angiogenesis.[1,7] Exercise has been shown to improve age-related delays in wound healing in skin by reducing proinflammatory cytokines.[14]

An individual's sex plays a role in both oral mucosal wound healing and dermal wound healing in different ways. Testosterone found in the saliva is a potent anti-inflammatory agent and explains the faster healing observed in mucosal wounds in men compared with women.[5] In skin, wounds heal more quickly in women than in men.[5]

Diseases that impair vascular flow and tissue perfusion predispose a wound site to inadequate oxygenation and delayed healing.[6,10,12] Diabetes in particular compromises healing in a multitude of ways, resulting in an overall decreased host immune response and tissue hypoxia.[10] Hyperglycemia creates free radicals that damage tissues and reduces the chemotaxis of leukocytes, explaining delays in early wound healing.[12,15] Fibroblast and epidermal cell function as well as angiogenesis are compromised.[12] MMPs show increased activity favoring tissue destruction in diabetic patients.[16] The most important factor affecting healing in diabetic patients is maintenance of normal glucose levels.[17] Surgical procedures on diabetic patients require close follow-up for untoward complications.

Obesity is on the rise, and in 2013 the American Medical Association made a controversial decision to classify it as a disease.[18] Because adipose tissue secretes bioactive adipokines that impact the immune and inflammatory responses, researchers consider adipose tissue an endocrine organ.[19–21] Impaired peripheral blood mononuclear cell function, decreased lymphocyte proliferation, and altered peripheral cytokine levels are seen with obesity.[1] Weight loss has been shown to resolve these immune system changes.[21] Conversely, patients who are cachectic and thin often have poor oxygenation and nutritional status, which also compromises healing.[6]

Medications can alter wound repair.[6] Antiresorptive agents as well as radiation treatment can cause adverse responses to surgical procedures, including osteonecrosis of the jaw. Bisphosphonates and other bone-strengthening drugs used to treat osteoporosis and some malignancies occasionally produce a rare and dangerous reaction in the maxilla and mandible called *bisphosphonate-associated osteonecrosis of the jaw* (BONJ). Patients on intravenous (IV) antiresorptive therapies for greater than 2 years, especially those on formulations containing nitrogen, are at the greatest risk for developing BONJ.[22] Patients on oral bisphosphonates have a significantly lower risk. The exact mechanism for this osteonecrosis is still unknown but may be related to the fact that bisphosphonates inhibit angiogenesis and osteoclast function.[22] Endodontic surgical procedures present an increased risk for the development of BONJ in patients with a history of IV bisphosphonate use, and these procedures should be avoided.[22]

Chemotherapeutic agents and other immunosuppressive drugs can negatively impact wound healing.[6] Fibroblasts are profoundly affected by chemotherapeutic drugs.[15] Immunosuppressant drugs such as systemic steroids inhibit many of the pathways necessary for wound healing. Systemic glucocorticoids suppress fibroblast proliferation and collagen synthesis, resulting in incomplete granulation tissue formation and reduced wound contraction.[15] Steroids are known to increase the risk of infection.

The short-term use of systemic nonsteroidal anti-inflammatory drugs (NSAIDs) has little effect on wound healing. However, some animal studies have shown that the long-term use of ibuprofen delays early epithelialization, decreases fibroblast production, reduces wound contraction, and inhibits angiogenesis.[23–26] Most patients planning surgical procedures cease or reduce their NSAID use prior to their procedures, reducing this concern.

Alcohol consumption (acute, moderate, chronic, and excessive) impairs host defenses.[27] Alcohol induces specific changes in immune cell functions, causing a higher incidence of infection and prolonged healing.[27] Acute alcohol consumption has been shown to cause significant impairment by reducing early wound angiogenesis up to 61%.[28]

Smoking causes obvious health risks and chronic diseases including vascular disease, heart disease, lung disease, and various cancers. The components in cigarettes and their smoke create many deleterious effects, with tissue hypoxia considered the major mechanism impairing wound healing.[29] Nicotine induces vasoconstriction and tissue ischemia. Carbon monoxide fumes contribute to tissue hypoxia because of the molecules' higher binding affinity to hemoglobin than oxygen.[29] Because tobacco smoke impairs white blood cell migration, suppresses lymphocyte function, and reduces fibroblast migration/synthesis, it results in an increase in acute and chronic infections following surgical procedures.[29] Impaired healing has been reported with implant placement in patients who smoke.[30] Surgical treatment planning decisions should be carefully considered in these patients.

Malnutrition hinders the immune system, resulting in lower resistance to infection and compromised healing.[1,15,17] Protein, carbohydrates, and fats provide the necessary energy for healing to take place. All stages of wound healing require protein to help form collagen, the most abundant protein in the body.[6,30] Protein is essential for fibroblast proliferation, angiogenesis, and tissue remodeling.[6,15,17] Protein-calorie insufficiency, the most common form of malnutrition, affects healing by decreasing wound tensile strength, T-cell function, and phagocytic activity.[17] Complement and antibody levels are also reduced with inadequate protein intake.[17]

Supplements of arginine and glutamine have been shown to have beneficial effects on healing in some studies.[1,17] Deficiencies in vitamins A and C as well as reduced zinc and iron levels can impair healing.[15] Improved nutritional status in adults preoperatively and following surgery has been shown to correlate with enhanced wound healing.[17,31]

Fibroblast Phenotypes

The fibroblast is a connective tissue cell found throughout the body that is responsible for the formation of proteins (including collagen) and ground substance necessary for connective tissue production. The fibroblast is capable of differentiating into other cell types and plays an important role in wound healing.

The oversimplified term *fibroblast* encompasses a complex group of cells with varied phenotypes. Phenotypes may differ based on anatomical location. Even within the same tissue, there are distinctions between fibroblasts in the papillary layer of the lamina propria versus those in the reticular layer.[32] Oral and dermal fibroblasts are of different phenotypes, secreting different growth factors and extracellular matrix, and have been shown to respond differently to the same growth factors.[32,33]

The various phases of wound healing are also associated with different fibroblast phenotypes. The fibroblast of the inflammatory phase is derived from circulating monocytes, whereas the fibroblast of the proliferative phase is derived from the wound bed.[32] During the maturation phase of wound healing, fibroblasts are under mechanical stress and are influenced by PDGF, causing them to differentiate into myofibroblasts.[32]

Oral Fibroblasts and Healing

Rapid, nearly scarless healing occurs in the oral mucosa compared with equivalent wounds in skin. This is attributed in great part to the phenotypic differences in oral fibroblasts and the speed with which inflammation in oral wounds resolves. Interestingly, the oral mucosal fibroblast phenotype is most similar to the fibroblast isolated from fetal dermis, which heals without inflammation and scarring.[34–36] Wound healing in the oral mucosa proceeds quickly, with faster clearance of inflammation, resulting in less scar formation compared with adult skin.[32–36] This has been demonstrated both clinically and histologically.[35,36]

Rapid resolution of inflammation has a profound effect on reducing scar formation. TGF-β1 and TGF-β2 are key factors causing scarring and are primarily produced by inflammatory cells. Because inflammation clears more quickly in oral wounds than in skin, the presence of TGF-β was fleeting in oral wounds and elevated in skin wounds for up to 60 days in the pig model, resulting in scarless oral healing.[35] The overall inflammatory response in the oral mucosa is less severe than in skin, in part due to the cytokines, growth factors, and peptides in saliva that promote earlier epithelialization of the wound, especially EGF and salivary histatin.[33,36,37] In addition to the significant effect of early resolution of inflammation, Wong et al[36] have shown the prolonged accumulation of tenascin C (TN-C) in oral wounds. TN-C is a molecule expressed in scarless fetal healing, which modulates cell adhesion to the extracellular matrix, suppressing scar formation.[36]

Enoch et al[34] evaluated oral mucosal fibroblasts and skin-matched fibroblasts in tissue cultures from the same patients and found that oral fibroblasts demonstrated the ability to migrate and repopulate the wound space faster than skin. This faster cell migration was the result of the oral fibroblasts' ability to reorganize the extracellular matrix more rapidly by producing more mixed MMP-2 and fewer MMP inhibitors.[34]

Endodontic Surgical Wound Healing

The most common type of endodontic surgery in clinical practice today is periradicular surgery, involving full mucoperiosteal flap reflection to gain access to radicular tissues to eliminate etiologies of endodontic origin. For many years, endodontists relied on literature from other specialties such as oral surgery and periodontics to guide endodontic surgical practices. Most oral surgical and periodontal surgical procedures in the early 1990s involved the removal of diseased soft and osseous tissues and relied on healing by secondary intention. By comparison, endodontic surgeons endeavored to gain access to radicular tissues while maintaining the existing healthy tissues, striving for healing by primary intention. Though the endodontist's surgical repertoire has continued to evolve, the fundamental concepts involved in periradicular surgical access remain relevant.[38]

As a response to this void in the endodontic literature, a series of wound healing studies focusing on endodontic surgical access procedures was conducted at Baylor College of Dentistry.[39–41] These studies sought to clarify the early wound healing events in the periodontium to the incisional, dissectional, and excisional wounds of periradicular surgery. These investigations involved the incision and reflection of full mucoperiosteal flaps and the creation of excisional osseous defects in the maxillae and mandibles of mature rhesus monkeys. The surgical sites were irrigated frequently with sterile, physiologic saline. Flaps were reapproximated after 15 minutes and secured with interrupted sutures. Following wound closure, the tissues were compressed for 3 minutes by applying firm finger pressure against saline-soaked gauze over the surgical site. Responses to the surgical procedures were evaluated at 1, 2, 3, 4, 14, and 28 days. Block sections of the surgical sites were fixed, demineralized, and prepared for histologic examination. The results provided a chronologic sequence of tissue responses to periradicular surgery. These studies did not involve root-end resection but rather focused on surgical access techniques. Evidence-based best practices for endodontic surgical access to periradicular tissues were established through these investigations.

Types of tissues wounded

A simple but profound definition of a wound is "an injury which causes disruption of the anatomical continuity and/or function of living tissues resulting in cell injury and death."[42] Following injury, healing depends on the *type of tissue wounded* as well as the *type of wound the tissue receives*.[43,44]

The endodontist who has working knowledge of the various tissues involved in periradicular surgery and their individual responses to wounding can create the most predictable surgical outcomes. The tissues involved in periradicular surgery are the mucoperiosteal tissues (gingiva, alveolar mucosa, palatal mucosa, and underlying periosteum), the periradicular tissues (bone, gingival ligament, and periodontal ligament [PDL]), and the radicular tissues (cementum and dentin). Each of these tissues responds differently to the wounds it sustains. For an in-depth review of these tissues, please refer to chapter 2.

Types of wounds

Gaining access to radicular tissues for endodontic surgical procedures results in the creation of different types of intentional surgical wounds: *(1)* the *incisional wound*, forming the perimeter of the flap using a scalpel; *(2)* the more imprecise blunt *dissectional wound*, where the mucoperiosteal tissues are separated from the cortical bone during flap reflection with the periosteal elevator; and *(3)* the osseous *excisional wound*, prepared with a high-speed handpiece and a rotary bur, removing periradicular and radicular tissues. Understanding these wounds and their responses leads to better surgical planning.

Types of healing

Wounds heal by primary intention or by secondary intention. *Primary intention* healing occurs when wound edges are closely reapproximated and there is minimal intervening clot or coagulum. Healing by primary intention results in the restoration of the normal architecture, microanatomy, and function of the wounded tissue, known as *regeneration*.[43,44] Incisional wound edges, when well approximated, usually heal rapidly by primary intention. *Secondary intention* healing occurs when wound edges are not closely approximated following surgery, as in the excisional wound, and a thick clot or coagulum is present, resulting in the formation of large amounts of granulation tissue. In this case, healing is delayed and *repair* ensues.[43,44] During the biologic process of repair, the architecture, microanatomy, and function of the injured tissues are not fully restored. Scar formation may also occur.[45]

Terminology

Reattachment refers to the reunion of viable retained epithelial and/or connective tissue from respective wound edges. Reattachment results in earlier wound healing than new attachment.[46–48] *New attachment* occurs when one wound edge contributes to the initial attachment, as when flapped tissues create attachment with the denuded surface of the root or cortical bone.[42]

Granulomatous tissue is a connective tissue dominated by inflammatory cells and inflammatory infiltrate, whereas *granulation tissue* contains predominantly fibroblasts and is highly vascular. The transition from a granulomatous tissue to granulation tissue signals the successful progression of connective tissue healing.[42]

Sharpey fibers are collagen fibers embedded in bone or cementum.[49,50] They include fibers of the mucosal lamina propria and gingiva that are embedded into cortical bone, as well as fibers from the PDL inserted into cementum and alveolar bone proper.[42]

Phases of wound healing

Endodontic wound healing, much like general wound healing, is a complex series of overlapping events and for descriptive purposes is explained as follows:

- *Phase I*: Hemostasis and inflammation
- *Phase II*: Epithelial healing
- *Phase III*: Connective tissue healing
- *Phase IV*: Maturation and remodeling

Given the importance of epithelialization and its impact on connective tissue healing, the proliferative phase described in general wound healing has been broken down into separate epithelial and connective tissue descriptions. The incisional wound heals most rapidly and embodies most of the wound healing concepts, so the following discussion begins with the incisional wound. This provides the basis for additional comments regarding the dissectional and excisional wounds.

The Incisional Wound

Phase I: Hemostasis and inflammation

When initiating the incision with a scalpel, damage to the microvasculature of the mucoperiosteal tissues occurs. As a result of this damage, clotting cascades are activated to effect hemostasis. Both intrinsic and extrinsic pathways are responsible for the conversion of fibrinogen into fibrin, facilitating the formation of intravascular and extravascular clots.[43,51,52]

Within hours of the formation of a thin clot, the fibrin strands contract and are oriented parallel to the plane of the wound.[43,53] These thin strands establish the first fragile attachment of the wound edges and provide the initial migratory pathways for inflammatory cells and later for reparative cells.[52,54] When hemostasis is not established quickly and a large coagulum forms in the wound site, healing is delayed. Disorganized fibrin strands entangled with excess serum and formed blood elements (erythrocytes, leukocytes, and platelets) act as a barrier and must be resorbed before healing can progress.[44,55] A thin clot greatly enhances the healing process (Fig 14-1).

Inflammation is defined as "the response of all living tissues to all forms of injury, which involves vascular, humoral, and cellular reactions at the injury site and prepares the site for healing."[56] This seemingly simple statement belies the complex, interrelated systems with feedback mechanisms involved, including the amine, kinin, complement, fibrinolytic, arachidonic acid, lysosomal, lymphatic, and mononuclear phagocytic systems, among others.[57–59] All tissues respond to injury with inflammation; however, the scale of the inflammatory response varies based on the severity of the injury. Thankfully, the checks and balances between these systems usually result in a self-limiting process.[42,57,58]

In the early wound, inflammatory mediators cause hemodynamic changes, including vasodilation, increased blood volume (engorgement), decreased rate of blood flow, and leakage of the microvasculature along with the aggregation of erythrocytes.[42] The vasoactive amines, histamine (contained in mast cells and basophils), and serotonin (5-hydroxytryptamine found in platelets) cause contraction of the endothelial cells, affecting the permeability of the microvasculature. In the postcapillary venules, this produces an outflow of exudate.[42] As engorgement occurs, the leukocytes move to the periphery (*margination*),[6] and the red blood cells cluster centrally (*sludging*), clinging together in a *rouleaux*. The leukocytes begin adhering to the endothelial cells (*pavementing*) as they prepare to pass through the vascular walls between the cell junctions (*emigration*), migrating to the wound site by amoeboid action (*diapedesis*).[6,56,57] This process follows chemotactic gradients. PMNs, macrophages, basophils, and plasma membranes are some of the endogenous chemoattractants that drive this process. Exogenous chemoattractants include microorganisms.[56,57]

Overall, inflammation clears more quickly in oral wounds and is less severe than in the dermis, as discussed earlier. Rapid resolution of inflammation creates an environment for healing by clearing the way for the ingress of reparative cells. PMNs respond early and are seen in the wound site within hours of injury.[6] They are responsible for phagocytizing microorganisms and tissue debris, keeping infection at bay.[42,57] These neutrophils have a short life span in the extravascular environment and are unable to replicate.[57] Their numbers usually decline between 24 and 48 hours.[42,59] Although PMNs are the initial scavengers, they do not affect the qualitative or temporal course of healing of the wound.[60]

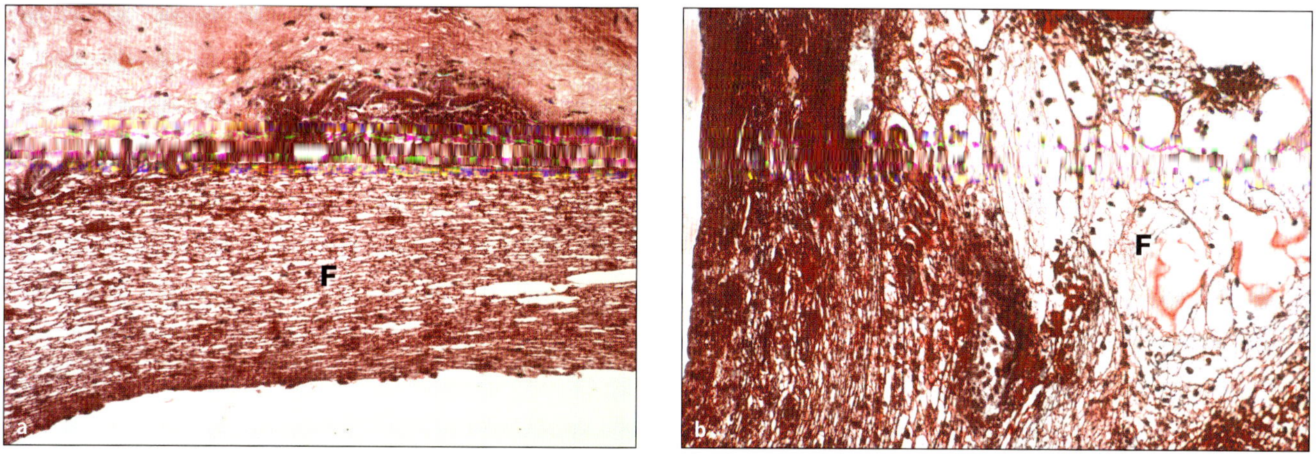

Fig 14-1 A thin clot enhances healing. *(a)* A thin fibrin clot 24 hours after flap reflection in the dissectional wound. Fibrin strands (F) are oriented parallel to the plane of the wound, providing migratory pathways for inflammatory and reparative cells (hematoxylin-eosin [h&e] stain; magnification ×66). *(b)* Thick coagulum 24 hours after flap reflection in a vertical incision. Haphazardly spaced fibrin strands (F) delay wound healing (h&e stain; magnification ×66).

The late inflammatory response is dominated by the macrophage, which is seen earlier in oral wounds than in skin. Macrophages in the oral wound site are derived from circulating plasma monocytes and are the predominant cell within 12 hours.[61,62] In contrast to the PMN, the life span of the macrophage can be months or longer, and it is capable of replicating.[57] This highly effective scavenger is responsible for phagocytizing neutrophils and is more effective at phagocytosis than the PMN.[57] The macrophage has been called the "supervisor of the reconstruction of damaged tissues."[42] Because the macrophage triggers humoral and cell-mediated immune responses and controls the extent of the inflammatory response, it creates an environment conducive to connective tissue healing.[42] In this environment, the macrophage stimulates undifferentiated ectomesenchymal cells and fibroblasts to migrate and synthesize collagen and ground substance, resulting in revascularization of the wound site.[56] The macrophage is essential to the qualitative and temporal healing of the wound.[60]

Phase II: Epithelial healing

"The key to rapid wound healing is early epithelialization of the incisional wound surface."[56] This statement summarizes the foundational concept that epithelial healing is essential for connective tissue healing.[63] Establishment of an epithelial seal enhances connective tissue healing, which in turn enhances epithelial maturation. The key event of epithelialization occurs early in oral wounds in part due to cytokines and growth factors present in saliva.[33,36]

This process of epithelialization begins with *epithelial streaming*. Mobilization of epithelial cells is caused by two distinct consequences of tissue injury—a deficiency of tissue and damage to cells—and both stimulate mitosis.[63] As the desmosomal attachments loosen between the basal cells and the suprabasal prickle cells in the epithelial layer, these cells dedifferentiate, gaining amoeboid movement and phagocytic capabilities.[43,44,52,53,62] Mitosis occurs in the stationary cells of the wound margin and not the advancing edges.[63] This monolayer of advancing cells begins migrating by *contact guidance*, following the predetermined routes of the fibrin strands, moving toward the center of the wound and dissecting between the fibrin clot and the surface coagulum.[42] The cells stop migrating when *contact inhibition* occurs, and there is cell-to-cell contact on all sides.[42] Interestingly, streaming begins with the unflapped wound edge rather than the flapped wound edge.[39] Ruben et al[52] reported that oral epithelial monolayers were capable of migrating 0.5 to 1 mm in 24 hours in alveolar mucosa. The Baylor study evaluating incisional wound healing supports this finding, showing epithelial streaming from the unflapped wound edge within 24 hours.[39] Epithelial streaming occurred more rapidly from the unflapped edge in all incisions except the intrasulcular incision, where the rate of streaming was about the same from both wound edges.[39] In some incision samples in the Baylor studies, the epithelium was seen migrating to different depths along the wound edges into the connective tissue, similar to descriptions by Ordman and Gillman.[39,63]

An *epithelial seal* is established when epithelial cells from both wound edges come in contact with each other. Once the epithelial seal becomes a few cell layers thick, it is called an *epithelial bridge*, and its cells begin to differentiate again, undergoing rapid mitosis to re-form the layers of the epithelium.[42] The Baylor study showed

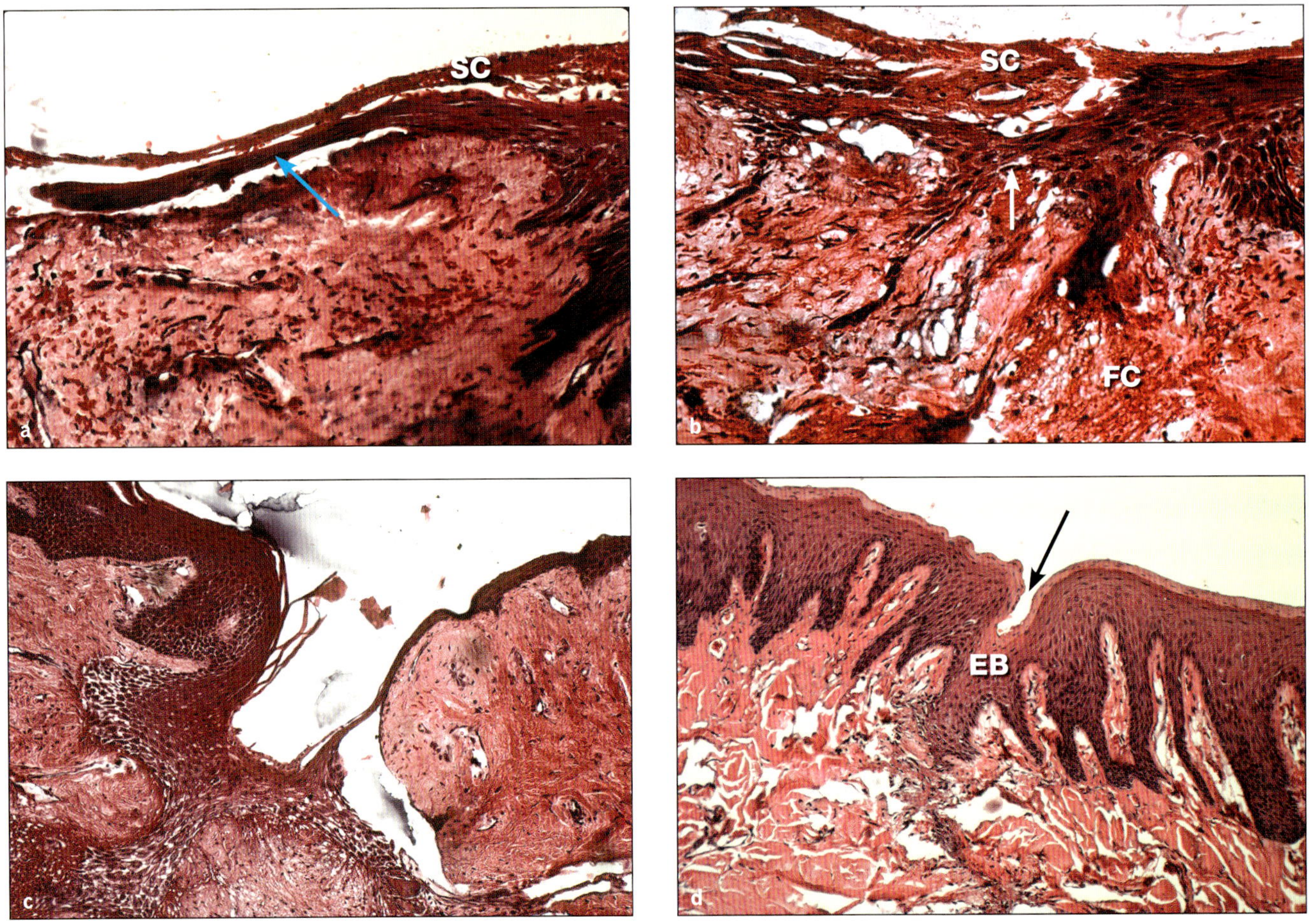

Fig 14-2 Epithelial healing. *(a)* Epithelial streaming *(arrow)* from the unflapped wound edge in the vertical incision 2 days after surgery. Remnants of the surface coagulum (SC) are seen above the epithelium (h&e stain; magnification ×66). *(b)* A multilayer epithelial seal *(arrow)* in the vertical incision 2 days after surgery. Surface coagulum (SC) is evident above the seal, and the fibrin clot (FC) is seen below (h&e stain; magnification ×66). *(c)* Epithelial bridging across the vertical incision 3 days after surgery. Epithelial cell downgrowth into the incision has occurred, but identifiable layers of the epithelium have not yet formed (h&e stain; magnification ×33). *(d)* Epithelial barrier (EB) formation in the vertical incision 3 days after surgery. Identifiable layers of the stratified squamous epithelium are evident. Note the epithelial invagination in the incision path *(arrow)* (h&e stain; magnification ×33).

the epithelial seal present as early as 24 to 48 hours and epithelial bridging as early as 48 hours.[39] Mittleman et al[59] showed epithelial seal formation between 21 and 28 hours in human volunteers. As discussed earlier, the PMN was the prominent inflammatory cell at 24 hours and was significantly reduced by 48 hours. This reduction in PMNs was facilitated in part by the formation of the epithelial seal/bridge, which decreased the access of bacteria from the oral environment to the wound site, reducing the inflammatory mediators attracting PMNs to the area.

The *epithelial barrier* develops as epithelial cells mature into identifiable layers of stratified squamous epithelium. A well-established, multilayered epithelial barrier prevents the entry of oral irritants, inhibits fluid and nutrient loss, and increases wound strength.[52,55,56] Once this barrier is formed, connective tissue healing progresses quickly. There is significant interplay between epithelial healing and connective tissue healing. In the studies conducted at Baylor, the epithelial barrier occurred within 48 to 72 hours[39] (Fig 14-2). Mittleman et al[59] showed epithelial barrier formation in oral mucoperiosteal tissues of human volunteers as early as 36 hours after wounding.

Phase III: Connective tissue healing

As mentioned earlier, the progression of connective tissue healing is directly related to the formation of the epithelial seal and the maturation of the epithelial barrier.[39,63] With protection from the epithelial barrier, microorganisms are kept at bay, and the tissues remain hydrated and the nutrients contained. In this environment, macrophages release factors that mobilize fibroblasts from undifferentiated ectomesenchymal cells in the perivascular tissues around the wound site[44,62,64] (Fig 14-3).

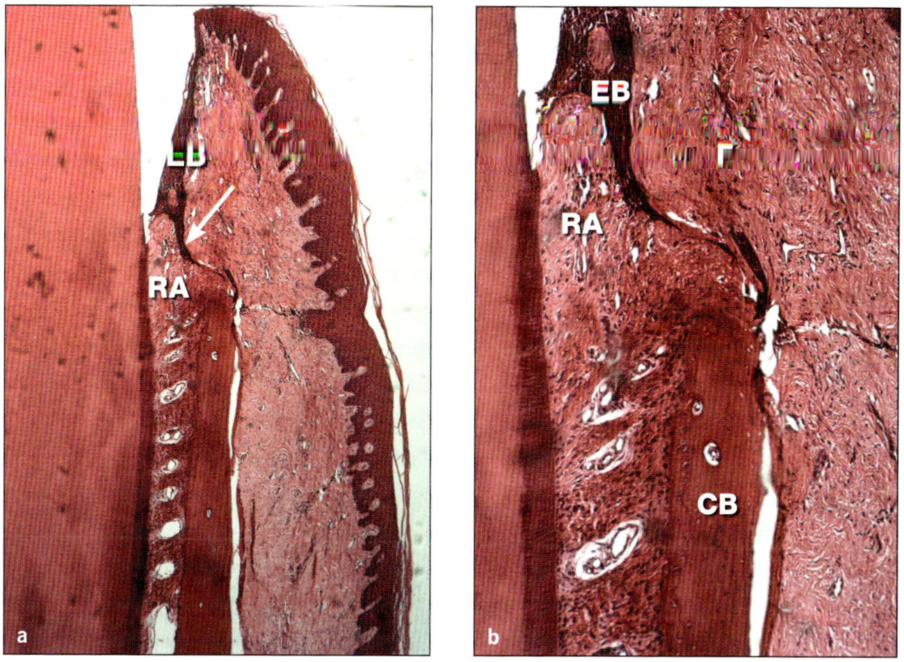

Fig 14-3 Connective tissue healing. *(a)* Viable root-attached tissues (RA; epithelium and connective tissue) in the intrasulcular incision 4 days after surgery. An epithelial barrier (EB) has formed. The *arrow* shows the incision path (h&e stain; magnification ×13). *(b)* There is no evidence of apical epithelial migration along the root surface. Both wound edges—root-attached tissues (RA) and flapped tissues (F)—contributed to the formation of the epithelial barrier (EB). Note the slight artefactual separation from the root. CB, crestal bone (h&e stain; magnification ×33). (Reprinted from Harrison[56] with permission.)

Fibroplasia and angiogenesis

Fibroblasts and undifferentiated ectomesenchymal cells synthesize ground substance (glycosaminoglycans and glycoproteins) and thin, delicate, first-formed Type III collagen (reticulin). The Baylor study showed reticular fiber formation 2 days following surgery and within 24 hours of epithelial seal/bridge formation.[39] This is remarkable, and given the limits of the light microscope, it is likely that collagen is produced even earlier than was visible.[39] As fibroblasts generate extracellular Type I collagen, macrophages are stimulated to produce angiogenesis factors. These factors induce endothelial cells and smooth muscle cells to migrate to the area.[43,54] The early neovascularization that results is haphazardly organized and is found on the periphery of the wound site.[52] The transition to revascularization depends on the maturation of the endothelial cells, which in turn depends on the production of collagen by fibroblasts.[52,56] This interdependent relationship between angiogenesis, fibroplasia (production of collagen), and revascularization proceeds from the periphery of the wound site toward the center, determining the qualitative and temporal progression of connective tissue healing[60,65] (Fig 14-4).

As macrophages decline and fibroblasts become the dominant cell in the wound site, the transition from a granulomatous tissue (of inflammatory cells and infiltrate) to a granulation tissue (of fibroblasts and high vascularity) has occurred.[54] This progression indicates successful connective tissue healing.[42] As the granulation tissue organizes and collagen aggregates, it becomes more fibrous. Concurrently, the ground substance is also undergoing a process of gelation.[52] At this point the wound site contains a high number of fibroblasts and less dense collagen fibers compared with the surrounding tissues.[42]

Phase IV: Maturation and remodeling

The beginning of the maturation and remodeling phase is signaled by the decreasing numbers of fibroblasts and a reduction in vascularity in the connective tissue.[42] During this phase, more collagen synthesis than degradation is occurring as the granulation tissue transitions to fibrous connective tissue. The overall volume of collagen in the wound site stays about the same during this transition.[66] The highly soluble newer collagen fibers simultaneously deaggregate (depolymerize) and reaggregate (repolymer-

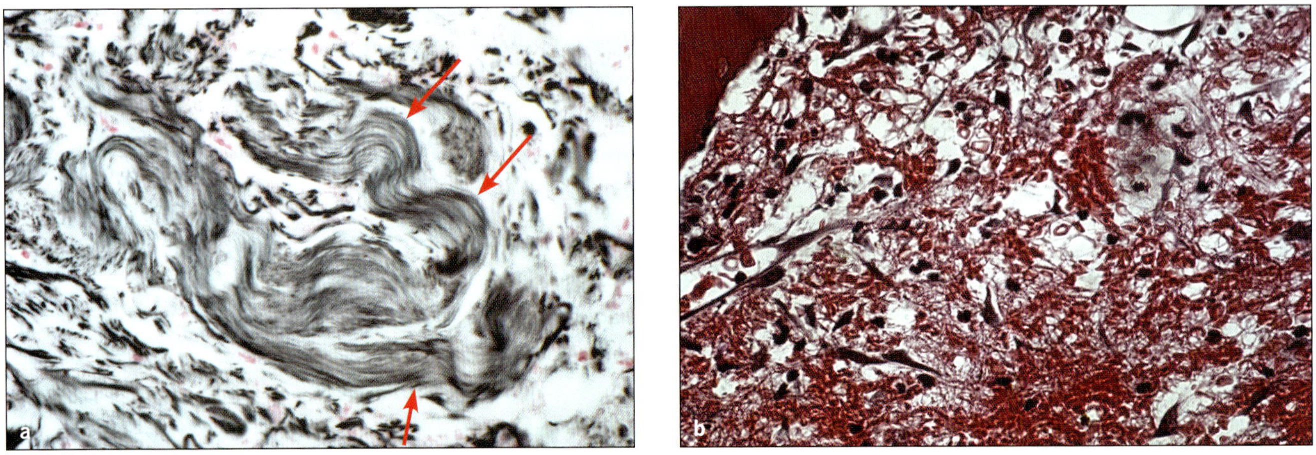

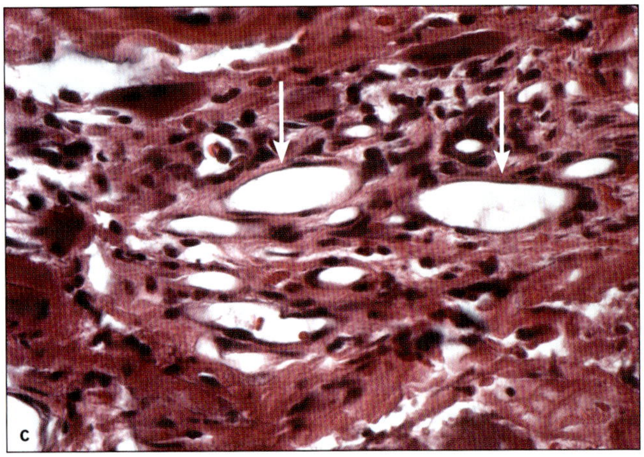

Fig 14-4 Fibroplasia and angiogenesis. *(a)* Early Type III (reticular) collagen visible 2 days after surgery. Type III collagen *(arrows)* forms prior to Type I collagen (reticulin stain; magnification ×132). (Reprinted from Harrison[56] with permission.) *(b)* As fibroblasts and undifferentiated ectomesenchymal cells enter the coagulum, granulomatous tissue transitions to granulation tissue (h&e stain; magnification ×132). *(c)* As the clot organizes and collagen molecules are released extracellularly, angiogenesis proceeds from the periphery toward the center of the wound. Note the neovascularization *(arrows)* present at 2 days (h&e stain; magnification ×132).

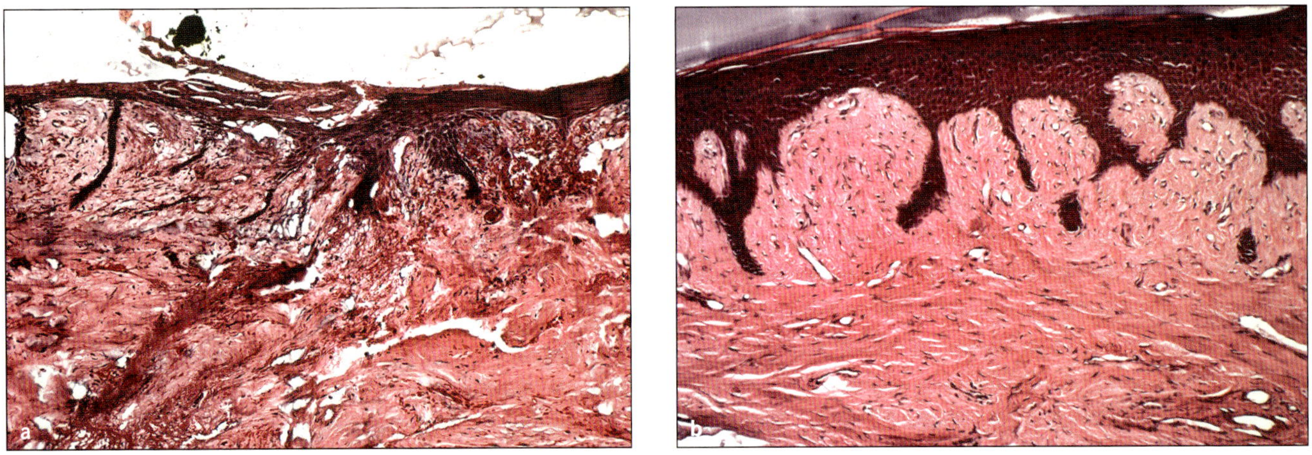

Fig 14-5 Maturation and remodeling of epithelium and connective tissue. *(a)* Incision 2 days after surgery showing a newly formed epithelial seal (h&e stain; magnification ×33). *(b)* Incision 28 days after surgery with excellent healing of epithelium and connective tissue (h&e stain; magnification ×33).

ize), changing in orientation from parallel to the plane of the wound to more like that of the surrounding tissues.[62,66] There is a progression toward greater fiber strength through the crosslinking, along with an increase in fiber size and decrease in fiber solubility.[53,62] This process slows to the normal remodeling rate in the lamina propria as the tissue architecture and number of fibroblasts approaches that of the surrounding tissue[56] (Fig 14-5).

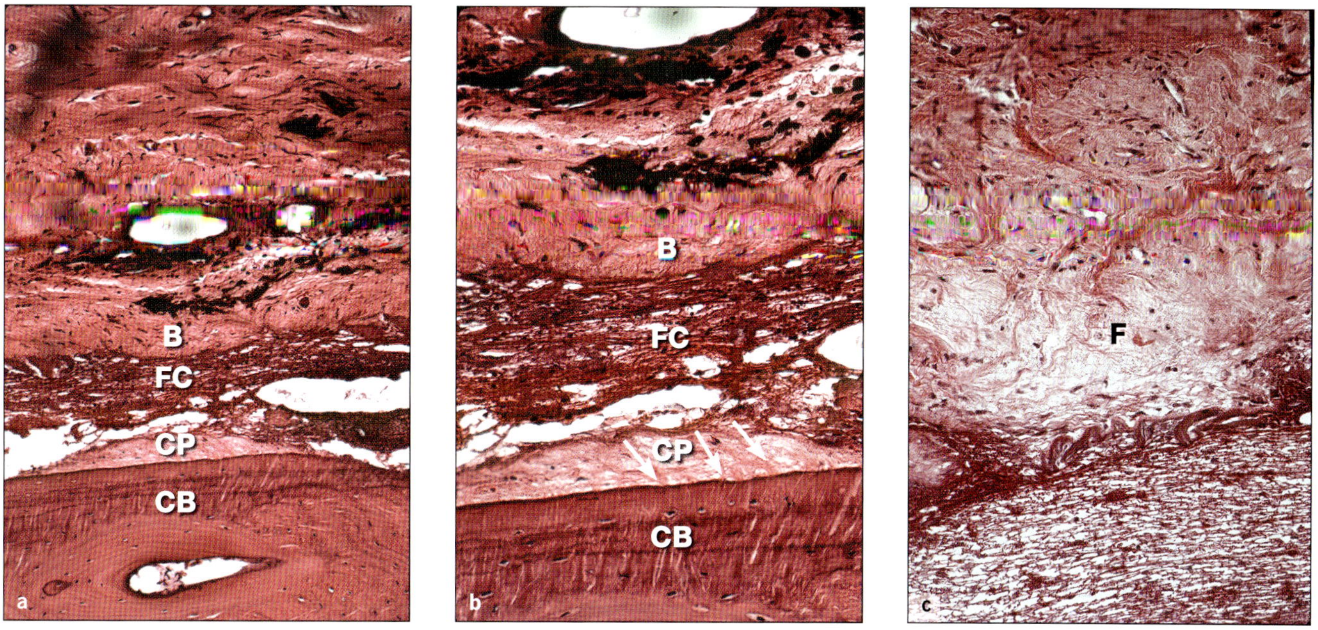

Fig 14-6 The periosteum does not survive flap reflection. *(a)* The periosteum is destroyed within 24 hours of flap elevation as seen in this dissectional wound. A thin fibrin clot (FC) separates the base (B) of the flap with its depolymerized collagen from the cortical bone (CB). Depolymerized cortical retained periosteal tissues (CP) remain on the bone surface (h&e stain; magnification ×33). *(b)* A closer view of the CP with depolymerized collagen and intact Sharpey fiber attachments *(arrows)* to vital CB. Surface lamellae under CP contain vital osteocytes (h&e stain; magnification ×66). *(c)* The base of the flap 2 days after surgery showing that the periosteum did not survive. Cells of the osteogenic layer of the periosteum were destroyed, and collagen of the fibrous layer (F) became depolymerized (h&e stain; magnification ×66).

Oral wounds scar less frequently than skin wounds. However, when wound edges are not well approximated, an intraoral scar may form. The exact cause of scar formation is unclear, but it has been postulated that low oxygen tension in a larger collagen mass may induce a higher collagen polymerization rate than normal.[67] Another theory is that mature scar collagen binds less water, making it resistant to degradation and depolymerization.[68]

The Dissectional Wound

The dissectional wound is created using a periosteal elevator to separate the full mucoperiosteal flap from the cortical bone to gain access to the periradicular tissues. The healing of the dissectional wound is rapid, but it is slower than that of the incisional wound. Unlike the incisional wound, which has two wound edges of similar tissues contributing to healing, the dissectional wound edges are of dissimilar tissues, with one wound edge—the lamina propria of the base of the flap—contributing to healing without help from the second wound edge, the denuded cortical bone.[69] During flap reflection, mechanical forces are applied in an imprecise way, creating damage to both the flap and the cortical bone.

The periosteum does not survive the forces of flap reflection.[40] The cells of the osteogenic layer (cambium layer) no longer exist after flap reflection, and the fibrous layer remains microscopically identifiable as a mass of depolymerized collagen. The Baylor study showed that the periosteum on the base of the flap was destroyed within 24 hours of flap elevation.[40] Other researchers have noted this lack of periosteum following flap reflection.[70–73] The Baylor study also showed the periosteum re-forming by day 14; by day 28, the periosteum appeared normal with osteogenic and fibrous layers[40,70,71] (Fig 14-6).

The imprecise blunt dissection of the flap leaves unpredictable amounts of tissue remnants on the cortical plate. The cells of the osteogenic layer do not survive in these cortical retained periosteal tissues, and the collagen becomes depolymerized, though it remains attached to the cortical bone associated with Sharpey fibers.[40]

The presence of opposing depolymerized collagen masses (the base of the reflected flap and cortical retained periosteal tissues), is thought to contribute to the rapid

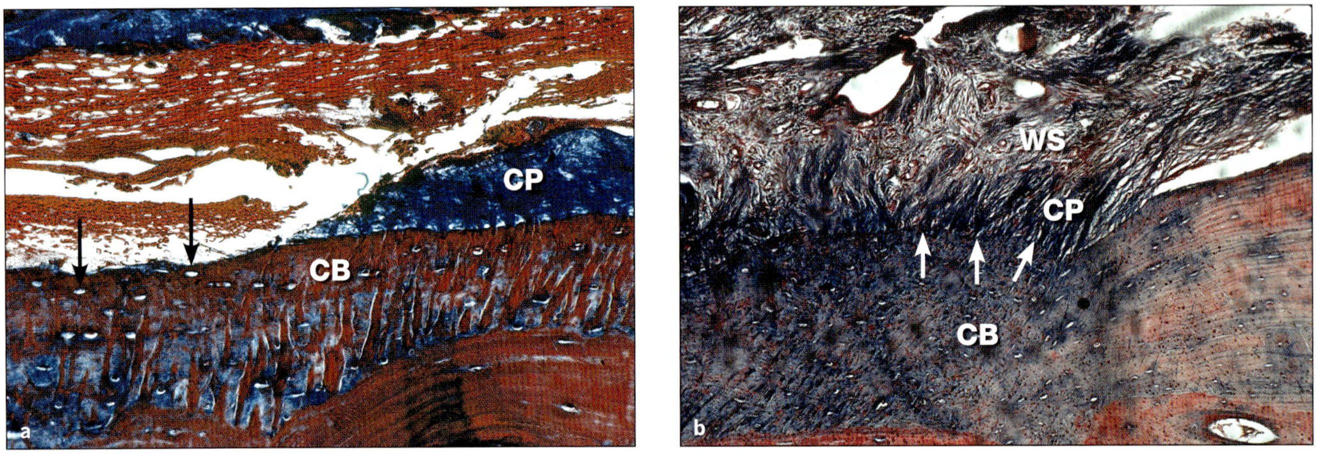

Fig 14-7 Protective role of cortical retained periosteal tissues. *(a)* Cortical bone (CB) below cortical retained periosteal tissues (CP) contains vital osteocytes. In areas where CP are absent, lacunae lack osteocytes *(arrows)* (Masson trichrome stain; magnification ×66). (Reprinted from Harrison[56] with permission). *(b)* CB with CP 14 days after surgery. Collagen in the wound site (WS) is repolymerizing with collagen of the CP associated with Sharpey fibers *(arrows)* (Masson trichrome stain; magnification ×33).

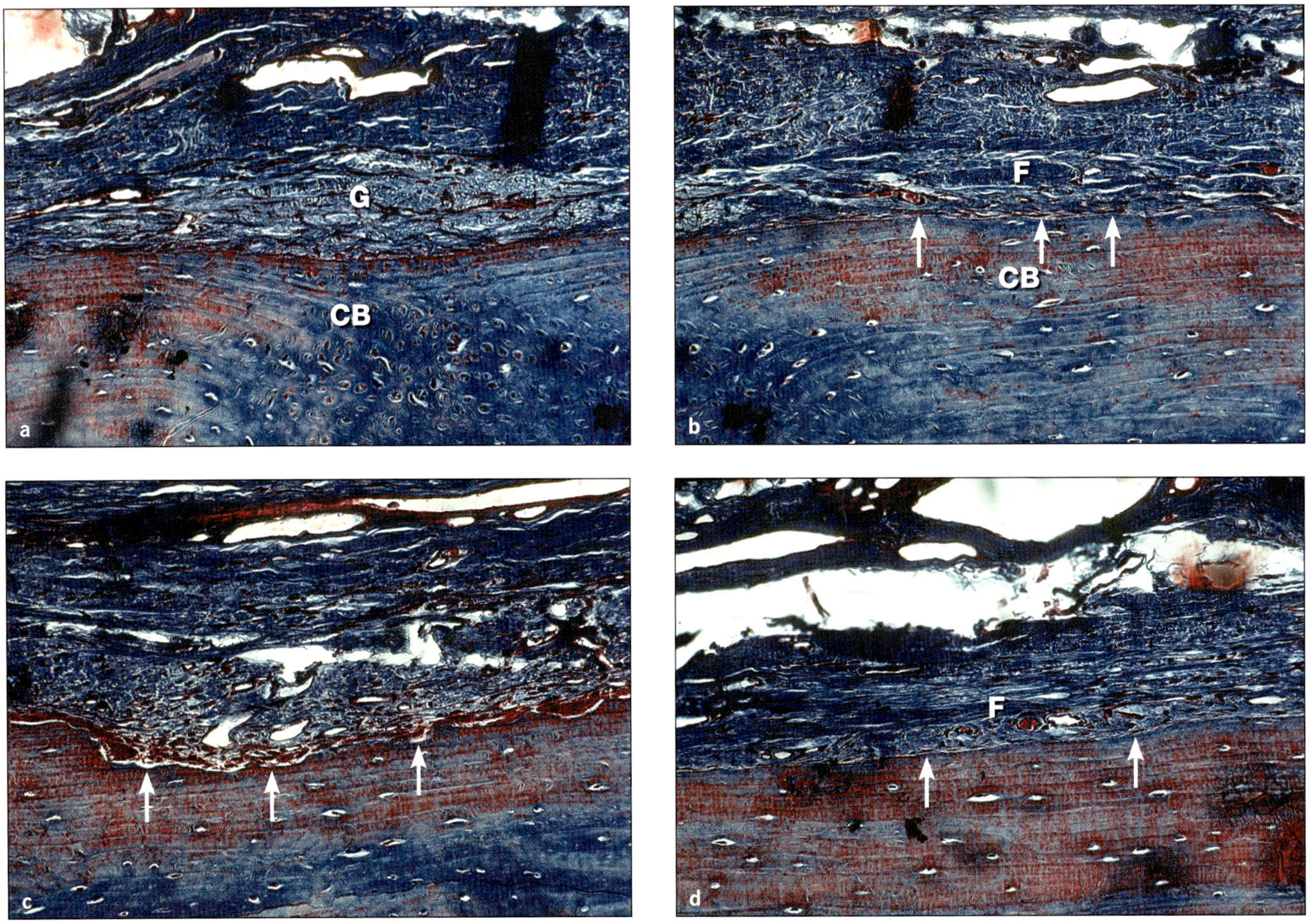

Fig 14-8 Re-formation of the periosteum. *(a)* Granulation tissue (G) in the wound site organizes. CB, cortical bone. *(b)* The osteogenic (cellular) layer of the periosteum *(arrows)* re-establishes itself adjacent to the CB and may be several cell layers thick. The outer fibrous layer (F) matures. *(c)* Osteoclastic activity *(arrows)* removes necrotic surface lamellae, exposing collagen for new attachment. Osteoblastic activity may follow osteoclastic activity in some areas. *(d)* Collagen of the fibrous layer (F) matures, and the cellularity of the osteogenic layer *(arrows)* decreases. (All parts 28-day dissectional wound stained with Masson trichrome stain; magnification ×66.)

reattachment of flapped tissues to bone rather than new attachment, in areas where these retained fibers occur.[40] Researchers Klein and Weiss[66] showed that under appropriate conditions, collagen may depolymerize into subunits, remain in the wound site, and then rapidly reaggregate to form new collagen.[48] This likely explains the rapid reattachment of the base of the flap to existing Sharpey fibers without the intervening osteoclastic and osteoblastic activity required to establish new attachment (Fig 14-7).

Interestingly, cortical retained periosteal tissues provide some sort of a protective role against osteoclastic activity and surface bone necrosis. Osteocytes are noted in the surface lamellae underneath cortical retained periosteal tissues.[40] In areas without cortical retained periosteal tissues, essentially a denuded cortical plate, the lacunae were empty, suggesting surface lamellar necrosis.[40]

Osteoclastic and osteoblastic activity along the periosteal surface of the cortical plate was not observed until 14 days following surgery.[40] When observed, this activity was limited, irregular, and delayed and was never seen where cortical retained periosteal tissues existed.[40] It is postulated that the delay in osteoclastic and osteoblastic activity resulted because the cells of the osteogenic layer of the periosteum were completely disrupted with flap elevation and required time to re-form. Also, the clot under the base of the flap required time to transition to granulation tissue before osteoclastic and osteoblastic activity was seen.[40] Given the minimal amount of resorption and repair evident on the cortical plate, it is likely that the purpose of this activity is to access collagen for new attachment.[56] In support of the Baylor studies, Craig and Harrison[70] and Creel[71] also showed limited osteoclastic activity at 14 days (Fig 14-8).

Evidence of Type III collagen formation in the dissectional wound at 2 days is significant.[40] The matrix provided by Type III collagen helps in the formation of Type I collagen. As previously discussed, extracellular collagen produced ahead of microvessel formation triggers macrophages to produce angiogenesis factors, which in turn stimulates smooth muscle cells and endothelial cells to migrate, resulting in angiogenesis.[69] The interplay between collagen production and revascularization clearly contributes to early wound healing. The Baylor studies showed advanced healing in the dissectional wound by the fourth postsurgical day,[40] with nearly complete healing by day 14 and remodeling and maturation continuing through day 28.[40,70,71]

The Excisional Wound

In the third Baylor study,[41] the excisional bony defect was examined as a separate entity, and root structures were not involved. This allowed concentration on osseous wound healing without introducing other variables. Postsurgical observation periods of 1 to 4 days, 14 days, and 28 days proved fruitful for evaluating the soft tissue incisional and dissectional wounds; however, key biologic events in osseous wound healing occurred between days 4 and 14 and were not evaluated in this study.[39,40,41]

When an excisional defect is created using a rotary instrument in a high-speed handpiece, wound edges cannot be reapproximated because the tissues have been intentionally removed. As a result, the wound heals by secondary intention. A disorganized coagulum with widely spaced fibrin strands fills the defect. This haphazard accumulation of fibrin strands, erythrocytes, tissue debris, and scattered inflammatory cells provides an initial barrier to healing rather than migratory pathways for the inflammatory and reparative cells.[41] Within 2 to 4 days of the initial wounding, granulation tissue emanating from the exposed endosteal tissues (and also from the PDL when root-end resection is involved) occurs.[56] By day 3, inflammatory cells (PMNs and macrophages) and reparative cells (undifferentiated ectomesenchymal cells, fibroblasts, and fibroblast-like cells) are seen migrating into the coagulum from the deeper internal periphery endosteal tissues. Occasionally, cells are contributed from the overlying mucoperiosteal tissues. Cortical and trabecular (cancellous) bone of the wound edges appeared devitalized and without osteocytes in the peripheral lacunae.[41] Endosteal tissues continue proliferating into the coagulum on day 4 from the deeper, internal intertrabecular spaces. Inflammatory and reparative cells precede the proliferating endosteal tissues with additional inflammatory and reparative cells entering from the overlying mucoperiosteal tissues. Healing proceeds from the periphery of the defect centrally and from the deeper internal surface toward the external location of the previous cortical plate[41] (Fig 14-9).

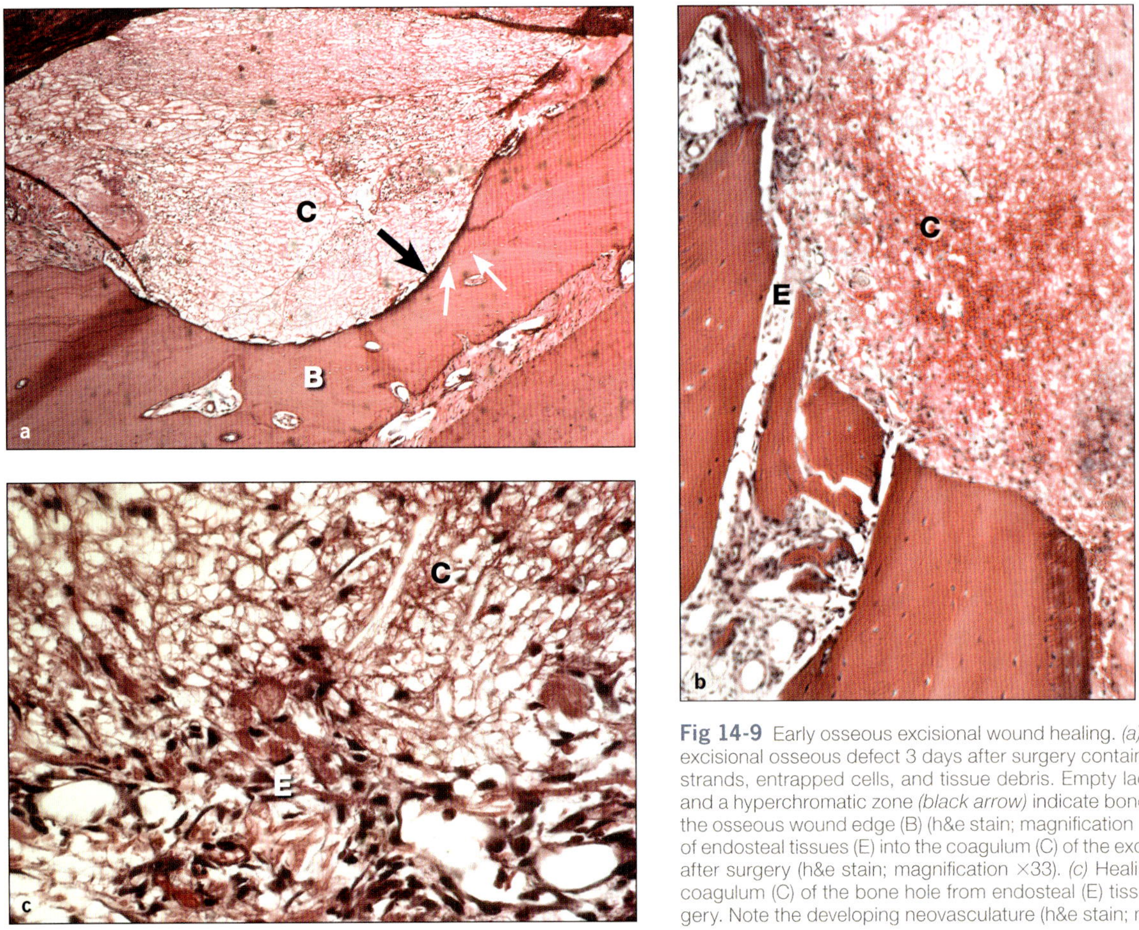

Fig 14-9 Early osseous excisional wound healing. *(a)* Coagulum (C) in the excisional osseous defect 3 days after surgery contains disorganized fibrin strands, entrapped cells, and tissue debris. Empty lacunae *(white arrows)* and a hyperchromatic zone *(black arrow)* indicate bone devitalization along the osseous wound edge (B) (h&e stain; magnification ×13). *(b)* Proliferation of endosteal tissues (E) into the coagulum (C) of the excisional defect 4 days after surgery (h&e stain; magnification ×33). *(c)* Healing front entering the coagulum (C) of the bone hole from endosteal (E) tissues 4 days after surgery. Note the developing neovasculature (h&e stain; magnification ×132).

By day 14, multiple woven bone trabeculae filled nearly four-fifths of the excisional defect. Woven bone was seen forming by direct appositional growth onto the devitalized cortical and trabecular bone of the wound edge in all 14- and 28-day specimens.[41] Spatz similarly noticed this lack of resorption prior to apposition of new bone on excisional defects in the mandibles of dogs.[74] Superficial new woven bone trabeculae were in contact with a dense band of cellular connective tissue separating the excisional wound from the mucoperiosteal tissues. This connective tissue band is referred to as the *delimiting membrane*.[41] This has been identified as the early re-forming periosteum by other investigators[70,73] (Fig 14-10).

By day 28, the woven bone trabeculae were more mature and coalescing, occupying slightly more area than the endosteal tissues. The re-forming periosteum plays an active role in repair of the cortical plate, with cells similar to the osteogenic layer of the periosteum depositing osteoid on the outer periosteal surface of the trabeculae.[41] This was interpreted as the beginning of the re-formation of the cortical plate.[41,73] Within 16 to 20 weeks, maturation and remodeling of bone in the excisional defect was complete[56] (Fig 14-11).

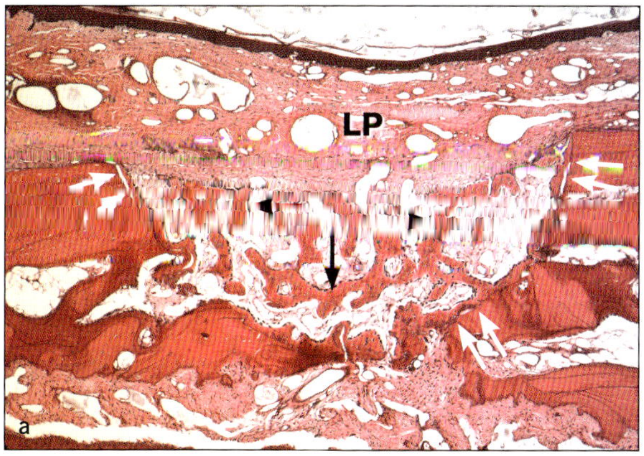

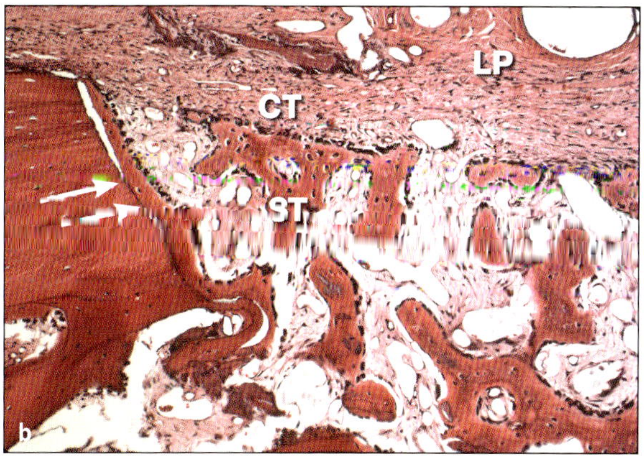

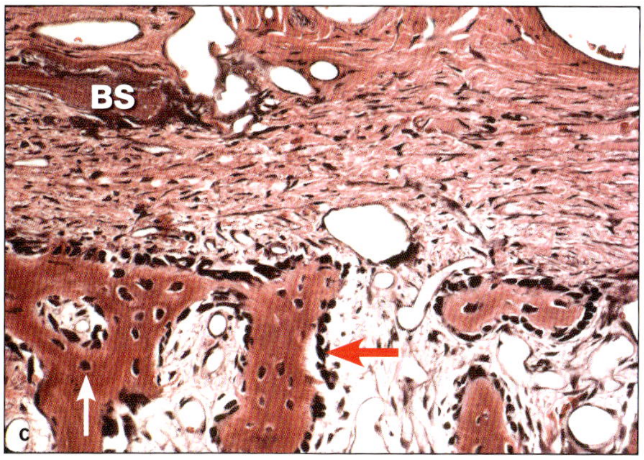

Fig 14-10 Osseous excisional wound healing at 14 days. *(a)* Coagulum has been replaced by endosteal tissue and new bone 14 days after surgery. Woven bone trabeculae *(black arrows)* are seen within the endosteal tissue. Appositional bone growth *(white arrows)* is seen on devitalized cortical bone of the wound edge. LP, lamina propria of the alveolar mucosa (h&e stain; magnification ×13). *(b)* The surface trabeculae (ST) are in contact with connective tissue (CT) of the re-forming periosteum. The *arrows* indicate appositional bone growth (h&e stain; magnification ×33). *(c)* Large osteocytes *(white arrow)* occupy lacunae, and active osteoblasts *(red arrow)* surround the new trabeculae. BS, bone sliver (h&e stain; magnification ×66).

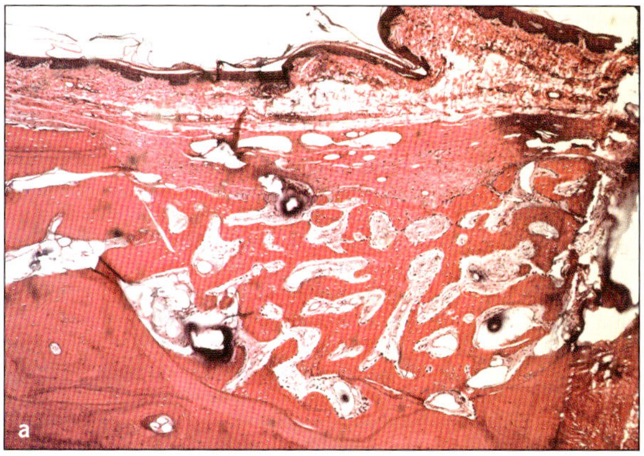

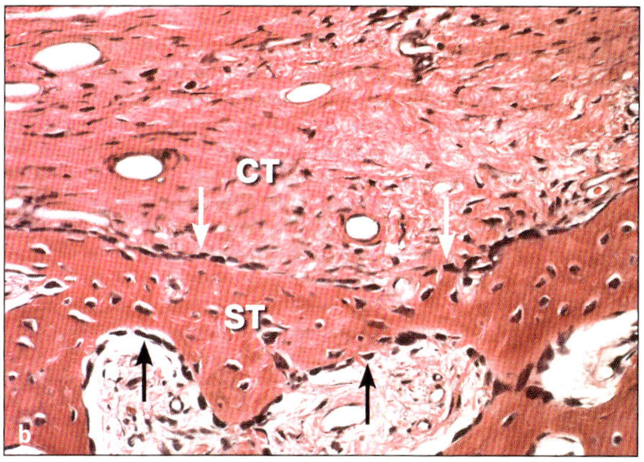

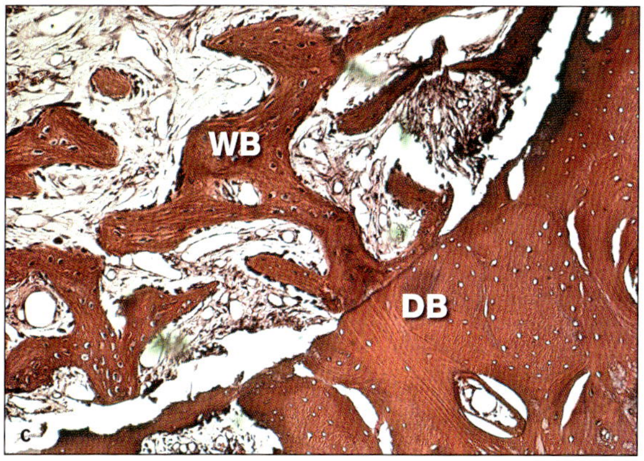

Fig 14-11 Osseous excisional wound healing at 28 days. *(a)* Woven bone trabeculae are coarser, fill more of the defect, and are bordered by fewer active osteoblasts than at 14 days (h&e stain; magnification ×13). *(b)* The surface trabeculae (ST) have coalesced and are in contact with the fibrous connective tissue (CT) of the re-forming periosteum. Cells are depositing osteoid on the outer periosteal surface *(white arrows)* of the trabeculae and on the inner endosteal surface *(black arrows)* (h&e stain; magnification ×66). *(c)* Maturing woven bone attached to devitalized bone (DB) at 28 days. Note the absence of osteocytes in the lacunae of devitalized bone (h&e stain; magnification ×33).

Dentoalveolar Healing

A discussion of wound healing would not be complete without including details of apical dentoalveolar healing. Additional studies at Baylor and elsewhere have helped to illuminate this process.[70,75,76]

The pluripotent cells of the PDL and the endosteum contribute to healing in the area of the resected root end.[70,75] Alveolar healing primarily results from endosteal-derived tissues.[70,75] The re-establishment of apical attachment apparatus or dentoalveolar healing results from PDL-derived tissues.[70]

Craig and Harrison resected root ends in the dog model, demonstrating the formation of granulation tissue originating from the PDL by 4 days and encapsulating the root end by 8 days.[70] Cementum deposition on resected root ends in the control group was seen at 16 days, though functional apical attachment apparatus had not re-formed at 45 days.[70] In this study, the experimental group, with resected root ends demineralized with citric acid, showed significantly earlier cementogenesis by 12 days, with more than 50% of the resected surface covered with cementum by 16 days, and overall earlier dentoalveolar healing completed by 45 days.[70] This is likely explained by the removal of the smear layer on the resected root ends with citric acid, exposing cementogenesis-inducing collagen in the dentin and cementum.[70] This supports the demineralization of resected root ends with citric acid during periradicular surgery.[70]

The process of re-establishing the PDL begins as woven bone trabeculae form near the encapsulating granulation tissue of the resected root end. Osteoblasts deposit osteoid on the side of the trabeculae closest to the granulation tissue between 30 and 45 days after root-end resection.[70] This induces the osteogenic activity of the functioning PDL.[70]

As alveolar healing progresses in these excisional sites, new woven bone is deposited directly on devitalized trabecular and cortical bone on the periphery of the defect without osteoclastic activity, similar to that seen in the earlier Baylor studies.[40,41] Woven bone trabeculae fill the excisional site beginning deep and internal to the defect, progressing externally toward the level of the preexisting cortical plate.[40,41,70] Re-establishment of the functional periosteum occurred with contact of the newly formed woven bone trabeculae to the delimiting membrane. Between 30 and 45 days, the cortical plate forms and remodels.[70] Other studies in monkeys have demonstrated nearly complete regeneration of the cortical plate and repair of the apical periodontium by 16 weeks.[75,76]

Research Observations and Their Clinical Implications

Incisional wound[39]

- Healing responses of the mucoperiosteal tissues to incisional wounding in periradicular tissues are remarkably fast.
- The intrasulcular incision leaves a thin layer of vital tissues attached to the supracrestal root surfaces. This root-attached connective tissue and epithelium are often not clinically visible.
- With close flap reapproximation and the formation of a thin fibrin clot in the wound site, apical epithelial downgrowth along the root surface does not occur if the vitality of the root-attached tissues is maintained during periradicular surgery. Loss of soft tissue attachment levels following periradicular surgery is preventable.
- In the presence of root-attached tissues, the temporal and qualitative wound healing in the intrasulcular incision is essentially the same as that of other incisional wounds evaluated in the study.
- Vitality of root-attached tissues can be predictably maintained by *(1)* initiating the flap in the vertical incision in the attached gingiva using an undermining elevation to reflect the flap; *(2)* avoiding curettage of the supracrestal root surfaces; and *(3)* preventing dehydration of these tissues with frequent irrigation.
- Preservation of root-attached epithelium promotes rapid epithelial seal formation. Preservation of root-attached connective tissue enhances connective tissue reattachment rather than new attachment.
- In the vertical incisions of full mucoperiosteal flaps, epithelial closure occurs rapidly, with a multilayer epithelial seal established at 24 to 48 hours and epithelial barrier formation occurring between 48 and 72 hours.

Dissectional wound[40]

- The elevated periosteum is destroyed by the reflective forces of dissectional wounding. The cells of the osteogenic (cambium) layer do not survive flap reflection, and the collagen of the fibrous layer becomes depolymerized but remains a microscopically identifiable structure at the base of the flapped tissues during the early phases of wound healing (Fig 14-12).
- Cortical retained periosteal tissues remain on the cortical surface in unpredictable amounts after flap reflection. Periosteal cells of the osteogenic layer do not survive in the cortical retained tissues, and the collagen becomes depolymerized but remains attached to the cortical bone associated with Sharpey fibers.

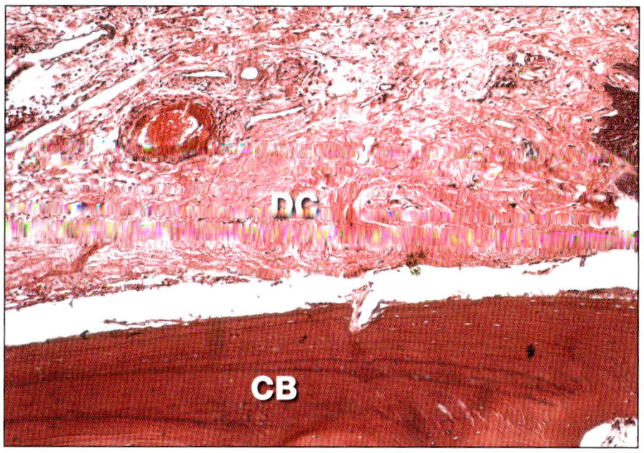

Fig 14-12 The periosteum does not survive flap reflection but remains a microscopically discernable band of depolymerized collagen (DC) at the base of the flap. CB, cortical bone (h&e stain; magnification ×33).

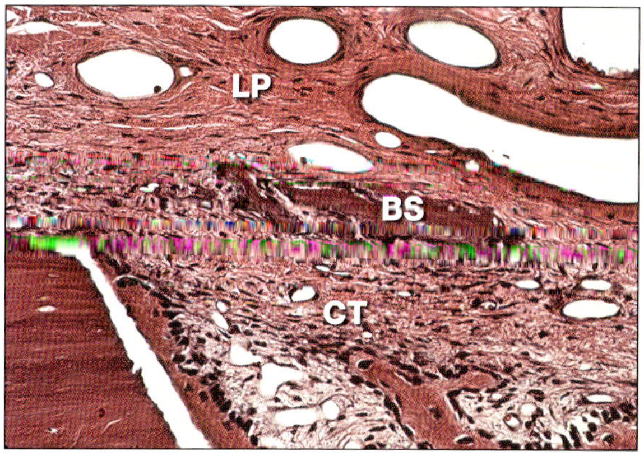

Fig 14-13 Bone sliver (BS) 14 days after surgery. Bone slivers dislodged from the cortical surface by the periosteal elevator during flap elevation are well tolerated in the flap. LP, lamina propria; CT, newly forming periosteum (h&e stain; magnification ×66).

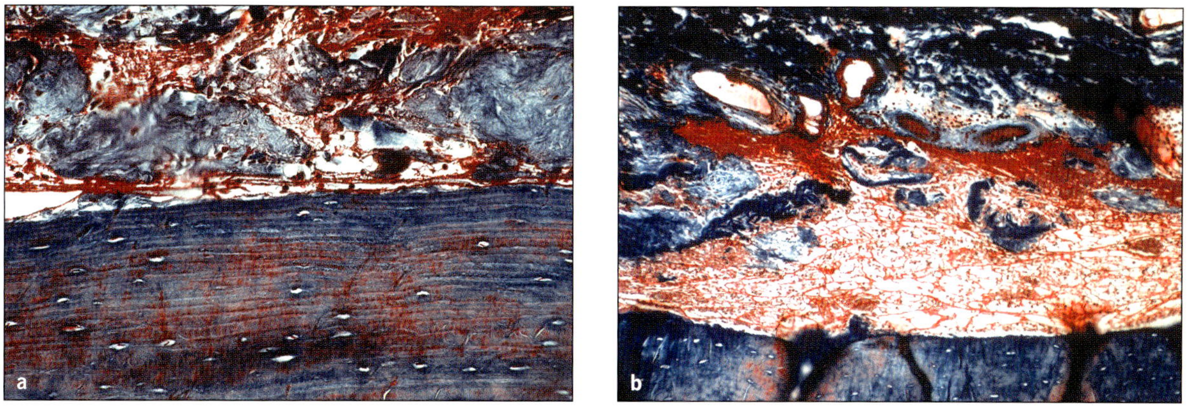

Fig 14-14 Importance of compression. *(a)* A well-compressed, thin fibrin clot with parallel fibrin strands provides migratory pathways for inflammatory and reparative cells (Masson trichrome stain; magnification ×66). *(b)* A thick clot or coagulum with widely spaced, haphazard fibrin strands delays wound healing (Masson trichrome stain; magnification ×33).

- Cortical retained periosteal tissues apparently exert some protective influence, which prevents necrosis of surface lamellae in underlying cortical bone.
- Crestal bone osteoclastic activity occurs following reflection of full mucoperiosteal flaps. However, osteoblastic repair occurs, and crestal bone height is not altered.
- Reflective forces exerted with a periosteal elevator cause dislodgement of bony slivers from the surface of cortical bone that may become embedded in the base of the flapped tissue. When this occurs, these bony slivers seem well tolerated (Fig 14-13).

Osseous excisional wound[41]

- Coagulum filling the bony defects is replaced by granulation tissue originating from endosteal tissues.
- Cortical and trabecular bone forming the wound edges of the excisional defect is devitalized and without osteocytes in the lacunae. This peripheral devitalization is likely the result of penetrating the interdental cortical plate with a #10 round bur.
- Within the osseous defect, new bone is deposited on devitalized bone without evidence of preceding osteoclastic activity.
- Fourteen days postsurgery, woven bone trabeculae occupy most of the defect with the more superficial trabeculae in direct contact with the thick band of dense fibrous connective tissue, the early re-forming periosteum.
- At 28 days, woven bone trabeculae are more mature, and a functioning periosteum is now active in repairing the cortical plate.
- The periosteum does not function in cortical bone repair until the excisional wound is nearly filled with woven bone trabeculae.

Clinical Applications

- Compression of the flap following suture placement helps create a thin fibrin clot, which enhances early wound healing (Fig 14-14).

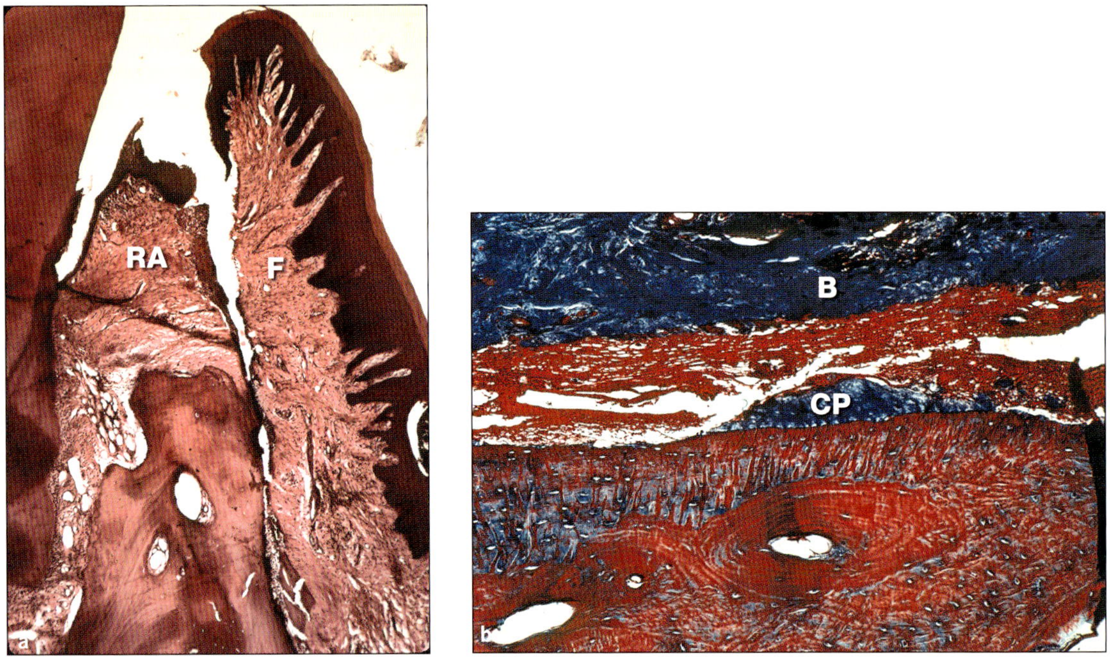

Fig 14-15 Importance of the preservation of attached tissues. *(a)* Root-attached epithelium and connective tissues (RA) and flapped tissues (F) of the intrasulcular incision 1 day following surgery. Artefactual separation along the incisional line permits clear visualization of these two wound edges, both of which contribute to healing (h&e stain; magnification ×13). (Courtesy of Dr D. C. Loth, Fort Worth, Texas.) *(b)* Cortical retained periosteal tissues (CP) in the dissectional wound 2 days after surgery. Two wound edges—the CP and the base of the flap (B)—contribute to reattachment, resulting in earlier wound healing (Masson trichrome stain; magnification ×33).

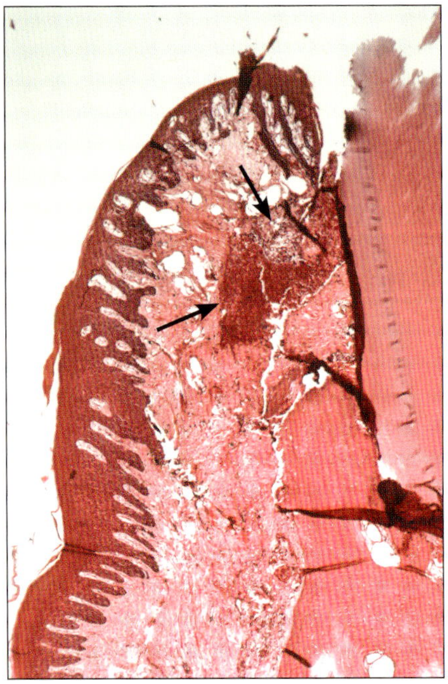

Fig 14-16 Inflammatory cells and tissue breakdown in the marginal gingiva *(arrows)* 2 days following surgery. This damage was produced by an improper reflection technique in the fragile marginal gingiva (h&e stain; magnification ×13).

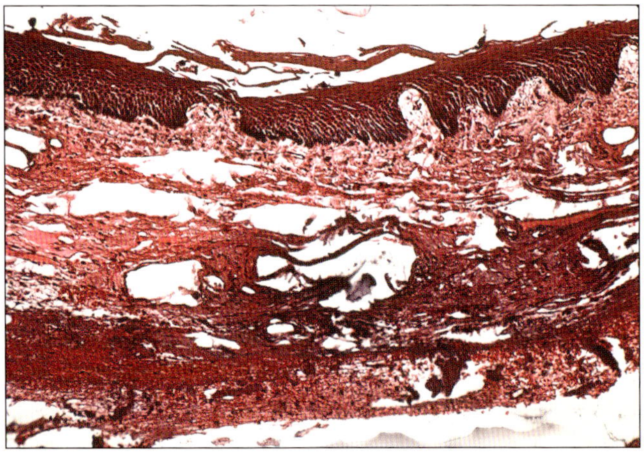

Fig 14-17 Inflammatory cells and general tissue breakdown 2 days following surgery. A Minnesota retractor impinged on the alveolar mucosa, resulting in this tissue damage (h&e stain; magnification ×33).

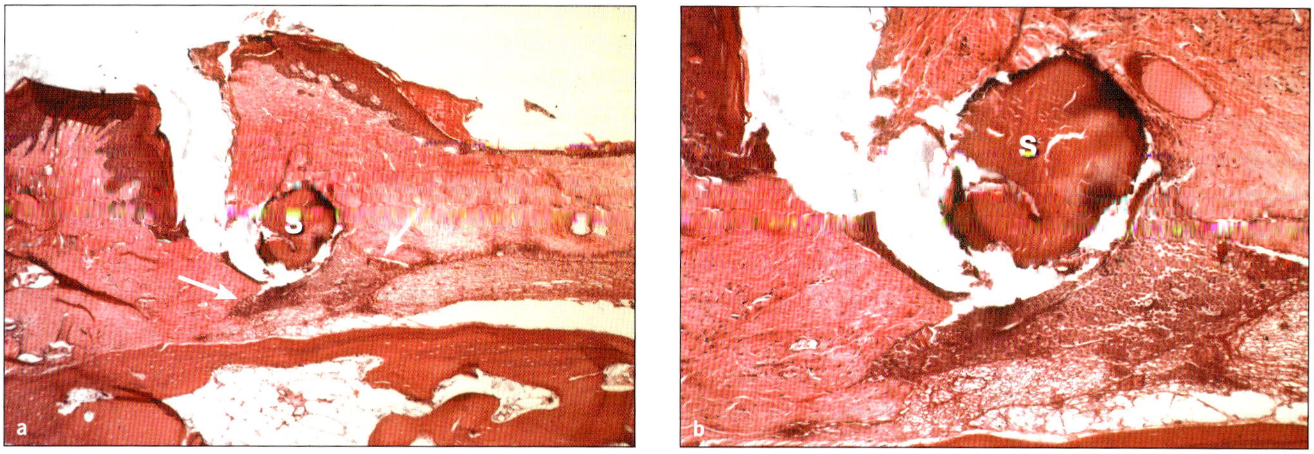

Fig 14-18 Suture tract showing inflammation. *(a)* Inflammation *(arrows)* on the apical side of the suture tract 1 day following surgery. Suture (S) material acts as a foreign body until removed (h&e stain; magnification ×13). *(b)* A closer view of inflammation associated with a suture (h&e stain; magnification ×33).

- Preservation of root-attached epithelium and connective tissue and cortical retained periosteal tissues aids in early reattachment. Bleeding "tissue tags" should not be curetted away. These retained fibers can be preserved with frequent hydration using sterile physiologic saline during surgical procedures (Fig 14-15).
- Avoid reflective damage to fragile marginal gingiva by initiating flap reflection in the attached gingiva of the vertical incision, using the undermining elevation technique for flap reflection (Fig 14-16).
- Avoid retraction force damage to tissues by ensuring that retractors do not impinge on alveolar mucosa or other tissues during surgical procedures (Fig 14-17).
- When creating the excisional wound, damage to osseous tissues from frictional heat can be minimized by using round burs at high speed with water or saline coolant, while performing a superficial shaving or brush stroke technique with minimal hand pressure.[41]
- Consider early suture removal at 5 days. The gingival sulcus and the interdental gingiva (col) were highly inflamed in many tissue samples.[39–41] Sutures add an additional foreign body to an already inflamed area (Fig 14-18).

Future Healing: Tissue Engineering and Regenerative Therapy

Concepts and techniques used in periodontal regenerative therapy offer possibilities for enhancing and advancing endodontic surgical procedures. Regenerative techniques will benefit both surgical as well as nonsurgical endodontic procedures. Successful regenerative therapy requires three components: *(1)* a source of precursor stem cells (PDL stem cells, dental papilla stem cells, pulpal stem cells, etc), *(2)* the presence of biologic mediators, and *(3)* appropriate scaffolding/matrices (collagen, dentin, synthetic materials like mineral trioxide aggregate [MTA], hydrogel, bone replacement grafts, etc).[77–79] Manipulating these variables to regenerate tissues of the periodontium is a reality in dentistry today and an active area of research.

Although there are numerous biologic mediators with various influences on regenerative healing, this review discusses two well-studied, long-standing, safe-to-use classifications of biologic mediators: enamel matrix derivatives (EMDs) and PDGF. These products are commercially available as Emdogain Gel (Straumann) and Gem-21 (Osteohealth), respectively. Clinicians should be aware that these mediators have short half-lives and that the regenerative events they induce occur after they are gone.[78] Bone morphogenetic proteins have demonstrated mixed results, including healing with ankylosis and root resorption, and are not discussed here.[80] Platelet-rich plasma requires centrifugation of a patient's own blood, resulting in a high concentration of biologic growth factors and cytokines that likely enhances wound healing.[81] However, both promising and contradictory results indicate that its use requires further study, so it is not discussed here.

Matrices and scaffolding including bone replacement grafts and barrier membranes have been thoroughly discussed in the periodontal literature by Kao et al[78] and nicely summarized in an endodontic review article by Bashutski and Wang.[82] The reader is referred to these works for more information. Biologically active matrices and graft materials can interplay with biologic mediators, furthering the complexity of tissue engineering. An interesting recent case report details the first 3D-printed bioresorbable polymer scaffold used to treat a case of aggressive periodontitis.[83] Though the 3D matrix failed at 14 months, it highlights the ingenuity being applied to regenerative periodontal therapies.

Enamel matrix derivatives

EMDs have garnered much attention since the original works published by Lars Hammarstrom[84,85] demonstrated true histologic regeneration of periodontal tissues with their use.[86,87] The major component of EMD, harvested from developing porcine teeth, is the protein amelogenin,[84,86] which is secreted by Hertwig epithelial root sheath during tooth development.[78,84,85,88,89] Amelogenin was originally thought to be enamel specific, but it is now known to have a broader spectrum. Amelogenin is responsible for the differentiation of periodontal tissues, including cementum, PDL, and alveolar bone, as well as an increase in PDL cell activity.[84,85] EMD stimulates the differentiation of mesenchymal cells, including osteoblasts.[78,89] Lesser components in EMD include other enamel matrix proteins, such as enamelins, tuftelin, amelin, and ameloblastin.[88] Emdogain Gel, containing amelogenin as the primary active component,[90] has been used safely for over 20 years.[87,91]

Two outstanding review articles in the periodontal literature on EMDs summarize the actions, physiology, and uses of EMD.[86,87] EMDs mitigate the inflammatory response by reducing the production of interleukins and by increasing the ability of PMNs to clear bacteria and tissue debris from the wound site.[86] EMDs have also been shown to promote wound healing by stimulating fibroplasia, extracellular matrix production, and angiogenesis.[86] A recent in vivo study showed that EMD promotes postsurgical healing of the mucosal incisional wound during the proliferative phase of healing.[90] EMDs diminish osteoclast activity and promote osteoblast growth,[89] favoring new bone formation over resorption.[86]

Platelet-derived growth factor

PDGF has also been extensively investigated since the first study more than 25 years ago demonstrated periodontal regeneration in both hard and soft tissues using a combination of PDGF and insulinlike growth factor.[92,93] PDGF is a potent mitogenic and chemotactic factor for mesenchymal cells[78] and stimulates the periodontal regeneration of bone, cementum, and PDL.[78,82,92–96] PGDF-BB is the best of the PDGF isomers in promoting collagen synthesis.[96] PDGF-BB alone or in combination with other growth factors is a strong mitogenic and chemotactic agent for cells of the PDL and alveolar bone.[92,94,96] The safety and efficacy of recombinant human PDGF-BB (rhPDGF-BB) has been well established.[95]

A plethora of studies in the periodontal literature support the many regenerative capacities of EMD and PDGF-BB. Long-term clinical improvements for patients have been seen with both of these biologic mediators when combined with periodontal surgical procedures to treat intrabony defects, supra-alveolar defects, and recession. There is also interest in combining these mediators with other therapies for addressing peri-implantitis.

Periodontal uses

The combination of EMDs and bone grafting materials has been effective in treating intrabony defects.[87,97] A new liquid EMD carrier system, Osteogain (Straumann), has been developed specifically for use with bone grafting materials in an effort to improve the adsorption of EMD to various available grafting materials.[87] Studies are currently underway with this system. Similarly, intrabony defects and class II furcation defects have been successfully regenerated with the combination of rhPDGF-BB and a bone allograft.[94]

When treating supra-alveolar periodontal defects, better regenerative results occur if EMD is used with flap techniques.[87,98] Gingival recession defects are improved when either EMDs or rhPDGF-BBs are combined with coronally advanced flap and/or connective tissue graft procedures.[85,95] Soft tissue height, thickness, and keratinization are all enhanced with their use.[85,95,99]

In a clinical study of 51 cases with peri-implantitis and recession around implants, EMD was used in combination with PDGF, bone grafting materials, and connective tissue grafts with successful results.[100,101] Further controlled studies are needed[87] to clarify the effects of EMD on peri-implantitis.[87] PDGF combined with insulinlike growth factor accelerated and enhanced osseointegration of titanium implants, demonstrating its potential for implant site development.[102] A case report of a large defect successfully grafted with bone allograft and PDGF after an extraction of a tooth in preparation for implant placement supports the use of PDGF in implant site preparation.[81,103]

Endodontic uses

In the endodontic literature, regenerative procedures using EMDs and PDGFs are taking shape through research and case reports. Creating treatment protocols that strive for the "triad of tissue engineering,"[77] including the availability of pluripotent cells, specific growth factors, and scaffolding, will enhance regenerative outcomes.

EMDs have been used in vital pulp therapy as pulp capping agents,[104] with particular success in combination with MTA,[105] inducing hard tissue formation where applied.[104] Laboratory-produced recombinant amelogenin has been used as an apexification agent in necrotic teeth, demonstrating pulpal regeneration.[106] rhPDGF-BB has also been successfully used to promote continued root maturation in a necrotic immature molar.[107] In cases where regenerative therapy of this type is indicated, procedures should be developed that move away from largely disinfection-based protocols to those that will support regeneration.[77,108]

Given the regenerative abilities demonstrated by EMDs and PDGFs, it is interesting to think about how biologic mediators might improve endodontic surgical outcomes. Earlier establishment of new cementum, a functional PDL, and new alveolar bone following root-end resection might improve surgical success rates. An in vitro study of root-end filling materials showed substantial amounts of EMD adhering to dentin and composite resin but not to amalgam or intermediate restorative material.[109] Further studies exploring the adherence of EMD or PDGF to MTA root-end fillings would be of interest.

Iatrogenic repairs following perforation, stripping, or apical transportation errors might be enhanced by the use of EMD or PDGF-BB. Difficult-to-heal lesions of endodontic origin might benefit from the use of these mediators in combination with scaffolding materials and membranes. Developmental anomalies such as deep palatogingival grooves on maxillary lateral incisors have been treated successfully through combined surgical therapy with EMD.[110] Placement of EMD under full mucoperiosteal flaps prior to wound closure has been shown to accelerate healing and might prove helpful in compromised patients.[90] It is interesting to note that EMD has been used successfully to treat other non-oral, hard-to-heal wounds such as venous leg ulcers, diabetic foot ulcers, and other skin lesions under the proprietary name Xelma (Mölnlycke Health Care).[86] In the same manner, PDGF-BB is also used for the treatment of cutaneous ulcers in the legs of diabetic patients.[94] EMDs and PDGFs deserve more investigation and attention in the endodontic literature in terms of surgical applications and other nonsurgical endodontic uses.

Dedication

A special debt of gratitude goes to John W. Harrison, DMD, MS, to whom I am ever grateful for the countless hours we shared over a teaching microscope.

References

1. Guo S, DiPietro LA. Factors affecting wound healing. J Dent Res 2010;89:219–229.
2. Mercandetti M. Wound healing and repair: Overview, types of wound healing, categories of wound healing. Medscape. http://emedicine.medscape.com/article/1298129-overview. Last updated 12 March 2015, accessed 13 June 2016.
3. Rozenfeld H. A clinical review of wound healing. Dentistry IQ. http://www.dentistryiq.com/articles/2012/06/a-clinical-review-of-wound-healing.html. Accessed 13 June 2016.
4. Scheller J, Chalaris A, Schmidt-Arras D, Rose-John S. The pro- and anti-inflammatory properties of the cytokine interleukin-6. Biochim Biophys Acta 2011;1813:878–888.
5. Engeland CG, Bosch JA, Cacioppo JT, Marucha PT. Mucosal wound healing: The roles of age and sex. Arch Surg 2011;141:1193–1197.
6. Enoch S, Leaper DJ. Basic science of wound healing. Surgery (Oxford) 2005; 23:37–42.
7. Swift ME, Burns AL, Gray KL, DiPietro LA. Age-related alterations in the inflammatory response to dermal injury. J Invest Dermatol 2001;117:1027–1035.
8. Barbul A, Shawe T, Rotter SM, Efron JE, Wasserkrug HL, Badawy SB. Wound healing in nude mice: A study on the regulatory role of lymphocytes in fibroplasia. Surgery 1989;105:764–769.
9. Mills RE, Taylor KR, Podshivalova K, Mckay DB, Jameson JM. Defects in skin T cell function contribute to delayed wound repair in rapamycin-treated mice. J Immunol 2008;181:3974–3983.
10. Bishop A. Role of oxygen in wound healing. J Wound Care 2008;17:399–402.
11. Kanta J. The role of hydrogen peroxide and other reactive oxygen species in wound healing. Acta Medica (Hradec Kralove) 2011;54(3):97–101.
12. Mathieu D, Linke JC, Wattel F. Non-healing wounds. In: Mathieu D (ed). Handbook on Hyperbaric Medicine. Dordrecht, Nl: Springer, 2006:401–427.
13. Edwards R, Harding KG. Bacteria and wound healing. Curr Opin Infect Dis 2004;17:91–96.
14. Emery CF, Kiecolt-Glaser JK, Glaser R, Malarkey WB, Frid DJ. Exercise accelerates wound healing among healthy older adults: A preliminary investigation. J Gerontol A Biol Sci Med Sci 2005;60:1432–1436.
15. Franz MG, Steed DL, Robson MC. Optimizing healing of the acute wound by minimizing complications. Curr Probl Surg 2007;44:691–763.
16. Sorsa T, Tjäderhane L, Salo T. Matrix metalloproteinases (MMPs) in oral diseases. Oral Dis 2004;10:311–318.
17. Arnold M, Barbul A. Nutrition and wound healing. Plast Reconstr Surg 2006;117 (7 suppl):42S–58S.
18. Pollack A. A.M.A recognizes obesity as a disease. The New York Times. http://www.nytimes.com/2013/06/19/business/ama-recognizes-obesity-as-a-disease.html. Published on 18 June 2013, accessed on 13 January 2017.
19. Pierpont YN, Dinh TP, Salas RE, et al. Obesity and surgical wound healing: A current review. ISRN Obes 2014;2014:1–13.
20. Kershaw EE, Flier JS. Adipose tissue as an endocrine organ. J Clin Endocrinol Metabolism 2004;89:2548–2556.
21. Greenberg AS, Obin MS. Obesity and the role of adipose tissue in inflammation and metabolism. Am J Clin Nutr 2006;83(2, suppl):461S–465S.
22. Goodell GG. Bisphosphonate-associated osteonecrosis of the jaw. Endod: Colleagues Excellence 2012;(2):1–8.
23. Dong Y-L, Fleming RYD, Yan TZ, Herndon DN, Waymack JP. Effect of ibuprofen on the inflammatory response to surgical wounds. J Trauma 1993;35:340–343.
24. Krischak G, Augat P, Claes L, Kinzl L, Beck A. The effects of non-steroidal anti-inflammatory drug application on incisional wound healing in rats. J Wound Care 2007;16:76–78.
25. Monnier Y, Zaric J, Ruegg C. Inhibition of angiogenesis by non-steroidal anti-inflammatory drugs: from the bench to the bedside and back. Curr Drug Targets Inflamm Allergy 2005;4:31–38.

26. Jones MK, Wang H, Peskar BM, et al. Inhibition of angiogenesis by nonsteroidal anti-inflammatory drugs: Insight into mechanisms and implications for cancer growth and healing. Nat Med 1999;5:1418–1423.
27. Szabo G, Mandrekar P. A recent perspective on alcohol, immunity, and host defense. Alcohol Clin Exper Res 2009;33:220–232.
28. Radek KA, Kovacs EJ, Gallo RL, Dipietro LA. Acute ethanol exposure disrupts VEGF receptor cell signaling in endothelial cells. Am J Physiol Heart Circ Physiol 2008;295:H174–H184.
29. Ahn C, Mulligan P, Salcido RS. Smoking-the bane of wound healing. Adv Skin Wound Care;2008;21:227–236.
30. Levin L, Schwartz-Arad D. The effect of cigarette smoking on dental implants and related surgery. Implant Dent 2005;14:357–363.
31. Posthauer ME. The role of nutrition in wound care. Adv Skin Wound Care 2012;25:62–63.
32. Rodemann HP, Rennekampff HO. Functional diversity of fibroblasts. In: Mueller MM, Fusenig NE (eds). Tumor-Associated Fibroblasts and Their Matrix. Dordrecht, NL: Springer, 2011: 23–36.
33. Lee H-G, Eun HC. Differences between fibroblasts cultured from oral mucosa and normal skin: Implication to wound healing. J Dermatol Sci 1999;21:176–182.
34. Enoch S, Peake MA, Wall I, et al. 'Young' oral fibroblasts are geno/phenotypically distinct. J Dent Res 2010;89:1407–1413.
35. Mak K, Manji A, Gallant-Behm C. Scarless healing of oral mucosa is characterized by faster resolution of inflammation and control of myofibroblast action compared to skin wounds in the red duroc pig model. J Dermatol Sci 2009;56:168–180.
36. Wong JW, Gallant-Behm C, Wiebe C, et al. Wound healing in oral mucosa results in reduced scar formation as compared with skin: Evidence from the red duroc pig model and humans. Wound Repair Regen 2009;17:717–729.
37. Brand HS, Veerman EC. Saliva and wound healing. Chin J Dent Res 2013;16: 7–12.
38. Polimeni G, Xiropaidis AV, Wikesjo UME. Biology and principles of periodontal wound healing/regeneration. Periodontol 2000 2006;41:30–47.
39. Harrison JW, Jurosky KA. Wound healing in the tissues of the periodontium following periradicular surgery. I. The incisional wound. J Endod 1991;17:425–435.
40. Harrison JW, Jurosky KA. Wound healing in the tissues of the periodontium following periradicular surgery. II. The dissectional wound. J Endod 1991;17:544–552.
41. Harrison JW, Jurosky KA. Wound healing in the tissues of the periodontium following periradicular surgery. III. The osseous excisional wound. J Endod 1992; 18:76–81.
42. Harrison JW. Healing of surgical wounds in oral mucoperiosteal tissues. J Endod 1991;17:401–408.
43. Krawczyk WS. Wound healing in the oral cavity. In: Shaw JH, Sweeney EA, Cappuccino CC (eds). Textbook of Oral Biology. Philadelphia: Saunders, 1978: 937–54.
44. Melcher AH. Healing of wounds in the peridontium. In: Melcher AH, Bowen WH (eds). Biology of the Periodontium. London: Academic, 1969:499–529.
45. American Academy of Periodontology. Glossary of periodontic terms. J Periodontol 1986;57(suppl):10–25.
46. Bowers GM, Granet M, Stevens M, et al. Histologic evaluation of new attachment in humans: A preliminary report. J Periodontol 1985;56:381–396.
47. Levine HL. Periodontal flap surgery with gingival fiber retention. J Periodontol 1972;43:91–98.
48. Levine HL, Stahl SS. Repair following periodontal flap surgery with the retention of gingival fibers. J Periodontol 1972;43:99–103.
49. Quigley MD. Perforating Sharpey's fibers of the periodontal ligament and bone. Ala J Med Sci 1970;7:336–342.
50. Quain J. Elements of Anatomy, ed 6. London: Longman, Green & Co, 1856.
51. Langley LL, Telford IR, Christensen JB. Dynamic anatomy and physiology. In: Dynamic Anatomy and Physiology, ed 5. New York: McGraw-Hill, 1980:394–414.
52. Ruben MP, Smukler H, Schulman SM, Kon S, Bloom AA. Healing of periodontal surgical wounds. In: Goldman HM, Cohen DW (eds). Periodontal Therapy, ed 5. St Louis: Mosby, 1980:640–754.
53. Ordman LN, Gillman T. Studies in the Healing of Cutaneous Wounds. Part III. A critical comparison in the pig of the healing of surgical incisions closed with sutures or adhesive tape based on tensile strength and clinical and histologic criteria. Arch Surg 1966;93:911–928.
54. Hunt TK, Knighton DR, Thakral KK, Goodson WH, Andrews WS. Studies on inflammation and wound healing: angiogenesis and collagen synthesis stimulated in vivo by resident and activated wound macrophages. Surgery 1984;96:48–54.
55. Hiatt WH, Stallard RE, Butler ED, Badgett B. Repair following mucoperiosteal flap surgery with full gingival retention. J Periodontol 1968;39(1):11–16.
56. Harrison JW. Surgical wound healing. In: Gutmann JL, Harrison JW. Surgical Endodontics. Boston: Blackwell Scientific, 1991:300–337.
57. Trowbridge HO, Emling RC. Inflammation: A Review of the Process, ed 5. Chicago: Quintessence, 1997.
58. Ryan GB, Majno, G. Acute inflammation. A review. Am J Pathol 1977;86:183–276.
59. Mittleman HR, Toto PD, Sicher H, Wentz FM. Healing in the human attached gingiva. Periodontics 1964;2:106–114.
60. McGrath MH, Emery JM. The effect of inhibition of angiogenesis in granulation tissue on wound healing and the fibroblast. Ann Plast Surg 1985;15(2):105–122.
61. Nathan CF, Murray HW, Cohn ZA. The macrophage as an effector cell. N Engl J Med 1980;303:622–626.
62. Sciubba JJ, Waterhouse JP, Meyer J. A fine structural comparison of the healing of incisional wounds of mucosa and skin. J Oral Pathol Med 1978;7:214–227.
63. Ordman LJ, Gillman T. Studies in the healing of cutaneous wounds. I. The healing of incisions through the skin of pigs. Arch Surg 1966;93:857–882.
64. Boucek RJ. Factors affecting wound healing. Otolaryngol Clin North Am 1984; 17:243–264.
65. Hunt TK, Andrews WS, Halliday B. Coagulation and macrophage stimulation of angiogenesis and wound healing. In: Dineen P, Hildick-Smith G (eds). The Surgical Wound. Philadelphia: Lea & Febiger, 1981:1–18.
66. Klein LR, Weiss PH. Induced connective tissue metabolism in vivo: Reutilization of preexisting collagen. Proc Natl Acad Sci U S A 1966;56:277–284.
67. Knighton DR, Silver IA, Hunt TK. Regulation of wound healing angiogenesis-effect of oxygen gradients and inspired oxygen concentration. Surgery 1981;90:262–270.
68. Chvapil M, Koopman CF. Scar formation: Physiology and pathological states. Otolaryngol Clin North Am 1984;17:243–264.
69. Nobuto T, Tokioka T, Limai H, Suwa F, Ohta Y, Yamaoka A. Microvascularization of gingival wound healing using corrosion casts. J Periodontol 1987;58:240–246.
70. Craig KR, Harrison JW. Wound healing following demineralization of resected root ends in periradicular surgery. J Endod 1993;19:339–347.
71. Creel DC. Histologic Evaluation of Fibrin Adhesives in Endodontic Surgical Wound Closure [thesis]. Dallas: Baylor College of Dentistry, 1990.
72. Klingsberg J, Butcher EO. Epithelial function in periodontal repair in the rat. J Periodontol 1963;34:315–321.
73. Melcher AH, Irving JT. The healing mechanism in artificially created circumscribed defects in the femora of albino rats. Bone Joint J 1962;44:928–936.
74. Spatz S. Early reaction in bone following the use of burs rotating at conventional and ultra speeds. Oral Surg Oral Med Oral Pathol 1965;19:808–816.
75. Corcoran JF, Sieraski SM, Ellison RL. Osseous healing kinetics after apicoectomy in monkeys: II. A quantitative histological appraisal. J Endod 1985;11:269–274.
76. Sieraski SM, Corcoran JF. Osseous healing kinetics after apicoectomy in monkeys: I. An isodensitometric interpretation of radiographic images. J Endod 1984; 10:233–239.
77. Hargreaves KM, Diogenes A, Teixeira FB. Treatment options: Biological basis of regenerative endodontic procedures. J Endod 2013;39:30S–43S.
78. Kao RT, Murakami S, Beirne OR. The use of biologic mediators and tissue engineering in dentistry. Periodontol 2000 2009;50:127–153.
79. Kao RT, Takei HH, Cochran DL, Nevins ML. Periodontal regeneration and reconstructive surgery. In: Newman MG, Takei HH, Klokkevold PR, Carranza FA (eds). Carranza's Clinical Periodontology, ed 12. St Louis: Saunders, 2015:610–620.
80. Ripamonti U, Heliotis M, van den Heever B, Reddi AH. Bone morphogenetic proteins induce periodontal regeneration in the baboon (Papio ursinus). J Periodontal Res 1994;29:439–445.
81. Albanese A, Licata ME, Polizzi B, Campisi G. Platelet-rich plasma (PRP) in dental and oral surgery from the wound healing to bone regeneration. Immun Ageing 2013;10:23.
82. Bashutski JD, Wang H-L. Periodontal and endodontic regeneration. J Endod 2009;35:321–328.
83. Rasperini G, Pilipchuk SP, Flanagan CL, et al. 3D-printed bioresorbable scaffold for periodontal repair. J Dental Res 2015;94(suppl, 9):153S–157S.
84. Hammarström L. The role of enamel matrix proteins in the development of cementum and periodontal tissues. Ciba Found Symp 1997:246–260.
85. Hammarstrom L, Heijl L, Gestrelius S. Periodontal regeneration in a buccal dehiscence model in monkeys after application of enamel matrix proteins. J Clin Periodontol 1997;24:669–677.
86. Miron RJ, Dard M, Weinreb M. Enamel matrix derivative, inflammation and soft tissue wound healing. J Periodontal Res 2015;50:555–569.
87. Miron RJ, Sculean A, Cochran DL, et al. Twenty years of enamel matrix derivative: The past, the present and the future. J Clin Periodontol 2016;43:668–683.
88. Kaida H, Hamachi T, Anan H, Maeda K. Wound healing process of injured pulp tissues with emdogain gel. J Endod 2008;34:26–30.
89. Jiang J, Safavi K, Spangberg L, Zhu Q. Enamel matrix derivative prolongs primary osteoblast growth. J Endod 2001;27:110–112.

90. Maymon-Gil T, Weinberg E, Nemcovsky C, Weinreb M. Enamel matrix derivative promotes healing of a surgical wound in the rat oral mucosa. J Periodontol 2016;87:601–609.
91. Zetterstrom O, Andersson C, Eriksson L, et al. Clinical safety of enamel matrix derivative (EMDOGAINR) in the treatment of periodontal defects. J Clin Periodontol 1997;24:697–704.
92. Lynch SE, Williams RC, Polson AM, et al. A combination of platelet derived and insulin-like growth factors enhances periodontal regeneration. J Clin Periodontol 1989;16:545–548.
93. Lynch SE, Castilla GRD, Williams RC, et al. The effects of short term application of a combination of platelet-derived and insulin-like growth factors on periodontal wound healing. J Periodontol 1991;62:458–467.
94. Nevins M, Camelo M, Nevins ML, Schenk RK, Lynch SE. Periodontal regeneration in humans using recombinant human platelet-derived growth factor-BB (rhPDGF-BB) and allogenic bone. J Periodontol 2003;74:1282–1292.
95. Nevins M, Giannobile WV, Mcguire MK, et al. Platelet-derived growth factor stimulates bone fill and rate of attachment level gain: Results of a large multicenter randomized controlled trial. J Periodontol 2005;76:2205–2215.
96. Dereka XE, Markopoulou CE, Vrotsos IA. Role of growth factors on periodontal repair. Growth Factors 2006;24:260–267.
97. Matarasso M, Iorio-Siciliano V, Blasi A, Ramaglia L, Salvi GE, Sculean A. Enamel matrix derivative and bone grafts for periodontal regeneration of intrabony defects. A systematic review and meta-analysis. Clin Oral Invest 2015;19:1581–1593.
98. Di Tullio M, Femminella B, Pilloni A, et al. Treatment of supra-alveolar-ype defects by a simplified papilla preservation technique for access flap surgery with or without enamel matrix proteins. J Periodontol 2013;84:1100–1110.
99. Cairo F, Nieri M, Pagliaro U. Efficacy of periodontal plastic surgery procedures in the treatment of localized facial gingival recessions. A systematic review. J Clin Periodontol 2014;41(suppl 15):44S–62S.
100. Chong CH, Carnes DL, Moritz AJ, et al. Human periodontal fibroblast response to enamel matrix derivative, amelogenin, and platelet-derived growth factor-BB. J Periodontol 2006;77:1242–1252.
101. Froum SJ, Froum SH, Rosen PS. Successful management of peri-implantitis with a regenerative approach: A consecutive series of 51 treated implants with 3- to 7.5-year follow-up. Int J Periodontics Restorative Dent 2012;32:10–20.
102. Lynch SE, Buser D, Hernandez RA, et al. Effects of the platelet-derived growth factor/insulin-like growth factor-I combination on bone regeneration around titanium dental implants. Results of a pilot study in beagle dogs. J Periodontol 1991;62:710–716.
103. Lin S, Mayer Y. Treatment of a large periradicular lesion of endodontic origin around a dental implant with enamel matrix protein derivative. J Periodontol 2007;78:2385–2388.
104. Ishizaki N, Matsumoto K, Kimura Y, Wang X, Yamashita A. Histopathological study of dental pulp tissue capped with enamel matrix derivative. J Endod 2003;29:176–179.
105. Min KS, Yang SH, Kim EC. The combined effect of mineral trioxide aggregate and enamel matrix derivative on odontoblastic differentiation in human dental pulp cells. J Endod 2009;35:847–851.
106. Mounir MM, Matar MA, Lei Y, Snead ML. Recombinant amelogenin protein induces apical closure and pulp regeneration in open-apex, nonvital permanent canine teeth. J Endod 2016;42:402–412.
107. Zhujiang A, Kim SG. Regenerative endodontic treatment of an immature necrotic molar with arrested root development by using recombinant human platelet-derived growth factor: A case report. J Endod 2016;42:72–75.
108. Galler KM, D'Souza RN, Federlin M, et al. Dentin conditioning codetermines cell fate in regenerative endodontics. J Endod 2011;37:1536–1541.
109. Safavi K, Kazemi R, Watkins D. Adherence of enamel matrix derivatives on root-end filling materials. J Endod 1999;25:710–712.
110. Castelo-Baz P, Ramos-Barbosa I, Martín-Biedma B, Dablanca-Blanco AB, Varela-Patiño P, Blanco-Carrión J. Combined endodontic-periodontal treatment of a palatogingival groove. J Endod 2015;41:1918–1922.

Chapter Fifteen

Adjunctive Procedures

Mahmoud Torabinejad, Tord Lundgren, Dimitris N. Tatakis, Mohamed I. Fayad

Adjunctive surgical procedures are those that are required to repair defects that occur in root or furcation areas as a result of either procedural accidents or pathologic processes. As discussed in chapter 5, performing root canal treatment can result in mishaps and accidents. The procedural accidents include ledge formation, root perforation, separated instruments, and underfilled or overfilled canals. Most of these accidents can be corrected nonsurgically. However, when nonsurgical correction of these accidents is not feasible or practical, periapical surgery is indicated. Surgical management of some of these mishaps is discussed in chapter 5.

Traumatic injuries that result in horizontal fractures may require a surgical approach to retain the remaining root of a tooth. Pathologic processes may also cause root defects that may need surgical intervention. These include caries, periodontal lesions, external resorption, and perforating internal resorption.

The purpose of this chapter is to discuss the etiology, treatment, and prognosis of perforations and resorptions and describe root resection, hemisection, tooth replantation, and transplantation. In addition, crown lengthening and graft materials used for some of these procedures are discussed.

Management of Perforations

Crown perforation

Regardless of tooth type, the pulp chamber is usually located in the center of the anatomical crown. Lack of attention to the degree of axial inclination of a tooth in relation to adjacent teeth and to alveolar bone during access preparation can result in either gouging or perforation of the crown or the root at various levels (Fig 15-1). The location and size of the perforation during access are important factors in the treatment of crown perforations. If the defect is located at or above the height of the crestal bone, it can be easily repaired with restorative materials such as amalgam, glass ionomer, or composite (Fig 15-2). The prognosis for this type of perforation is favorable.[1,2] When the defect is close to the crestal bone, it should be externalized by either orthodontic root extrusion or crown lengthening procedures. Orthodontic root extrusion is generally the procedure of choice for teeth in the esthetic zone.[3–5] Surgical crown lengthening is considered when esthetics are not an issue or when adjacent teeth require surgical periodontal therapy. After externalizing the defect, a full-coverage crown extending apical to the defect can be constructed.

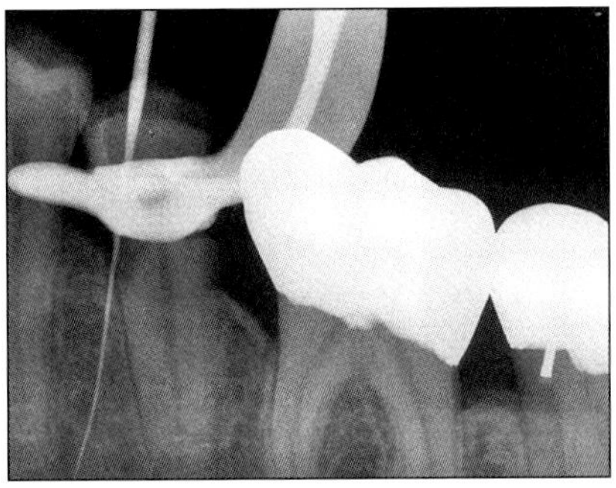

Fig 15-1 Lack of attention to the degree of axial inclination of a mandibular second premolar in relation to the alveolar bone during access preparation has resulted in a perforation of the crown at the cementoenamel junction.

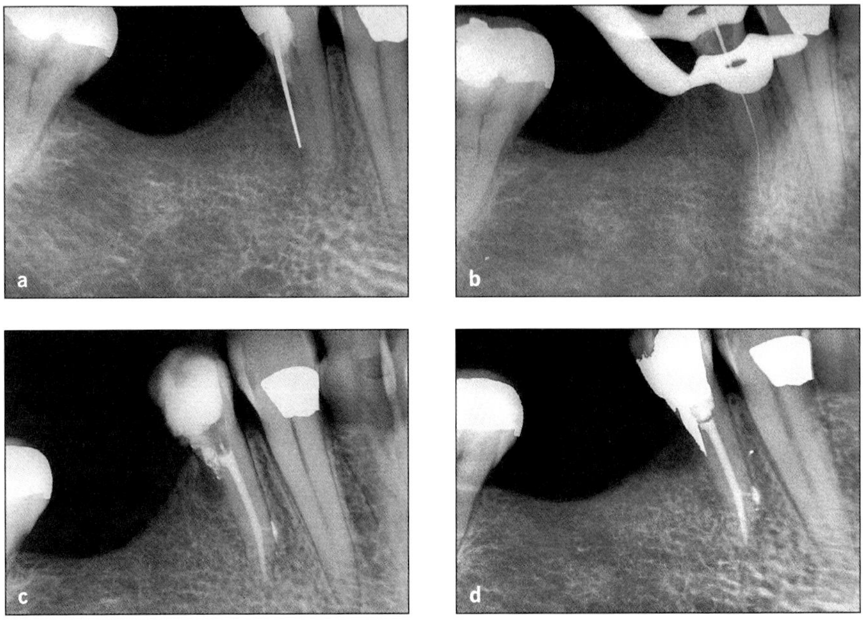

Fig 15-2 *(a)* Preoperative radiograph of a mandibular premolar with coronal root perforation. *(b)* Radiograph taken after removal of a silver point from the perforation site and locating of the root canal. *(c)* Postoperative radiograph after completion of root canal treatment. *(d)* Postoperative radiograph after repair of the coronal perforation with amalgam.

Furcation perforation

Maxillary and mandibular molar teeth with calcified pulp chambers have the greatest potential for furcation perforations. When a perforation occurs in these teeth, the defect should be repaired internally with a nonsurgical approach (Fig 15-3). Surgical procedures are reserved for instances when nonsurgical repair is not a treatment option or the attempted nonsurgical repair has been unsuccessful. When surgery is indicated, after raising a buccal mucoperiosteal flap, the furcation is curetted completely and the defect is repaired. It is critical to preserve the coronal bone during the surgery to avoid development of a periodontal defect (Fig 15-4). In cases where the coronal bone is removed or absent, placement of a resorbable membrane will help prevent development of a periodontal defect. In an animal study, Dean et al[6] reported excellent healing when the perforation was repaired surgically and the defect site was filled with decalcified freeze-dried bone or blood covered with a periodontal membrane. Poor results were reported when only the perforation was repaired and the other two procedures were not performed. If the perforation is not repairable or accessible by a surgical approach, hemisection, bicuspidization, root amputation, or tooth replantation should be considered. The prognosis for surgically treated teeth is guarded because of the increased technical difficulty associated with restorative procedures and demanding oral hygiene requirements. The remaining roots are prone to caries, periodontal disease, and vertical root fracture.

Root perforations

Root perforations usually start with a ledge formation. The major causes of ledge formation include inadequate straight-line access into the canal, inadequate irrigation or lubrication, excessive enlargement of a curved canal with files, and packing debris in the apical portion of the canal. Once created, ledged canals are difficult to manage. If the ledge cannot be negotiated, cleaning and shaping of the existing canal space is completed at the new working length, and the canal is obturated to the new length. The prognosis for a root canal–treated tooth with a ledge depends on the amount of debris left in the uninstrumented and unfilled portion of the canal. Many ledges can be corrected nonsurgically. However, there are situations in which the ledge can only be corrected through a surgical approach. The surgery consists of raising a soft tissue flap, performing an osteotomy, removing the root apical to the ledge formation, and sealing the apical portion of the remaining root (Fig 15-5).

Root perforation can occur at different levels during cleaning and shaping of the root canal systems. Root perforation can be apical, midroot, or coronal.

Apical root perforation

Instrumentation of the canal beyond the apical constriction results in apical root perforation. Establishing a new working length, creating an apical seal, and obturating the apical portion of the canal with MTA to its new working

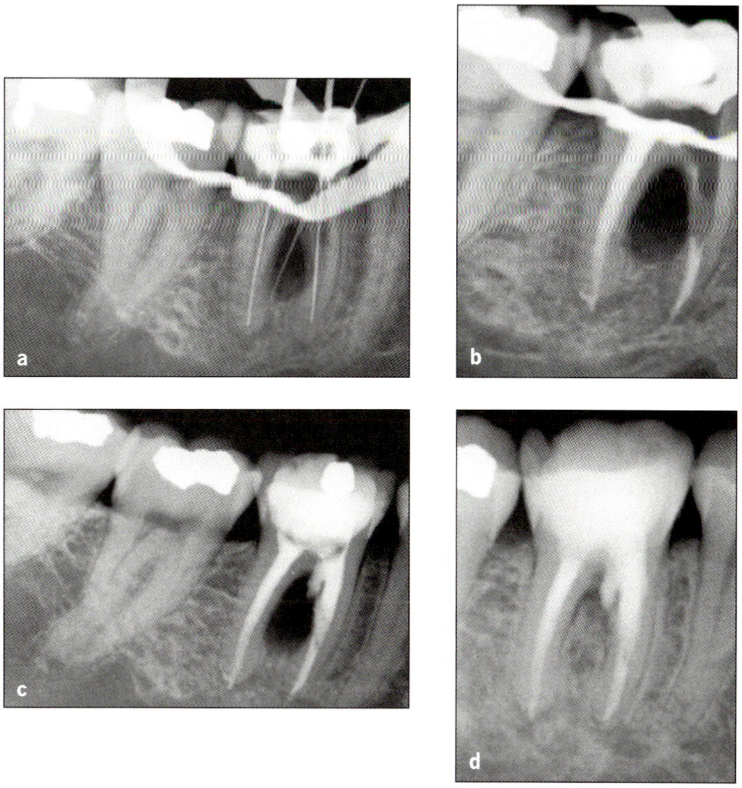

Fig 15-3 *(a)* Preoperative radiograph of a mandibular molar with a furcation perforation and a large furcal lesion. *(b)* Postoperative radiograph of the tooth after root canal treatment. *(c)* Postoperative radiograph of the tooth after repair of the perforation with mineral trioxide aggregate (MTA). *(d)* Postoperative radiograph 9 months after treatment showing excellent healing. The tooth had no clinical symptoms and no abnormal periodontal pockets.

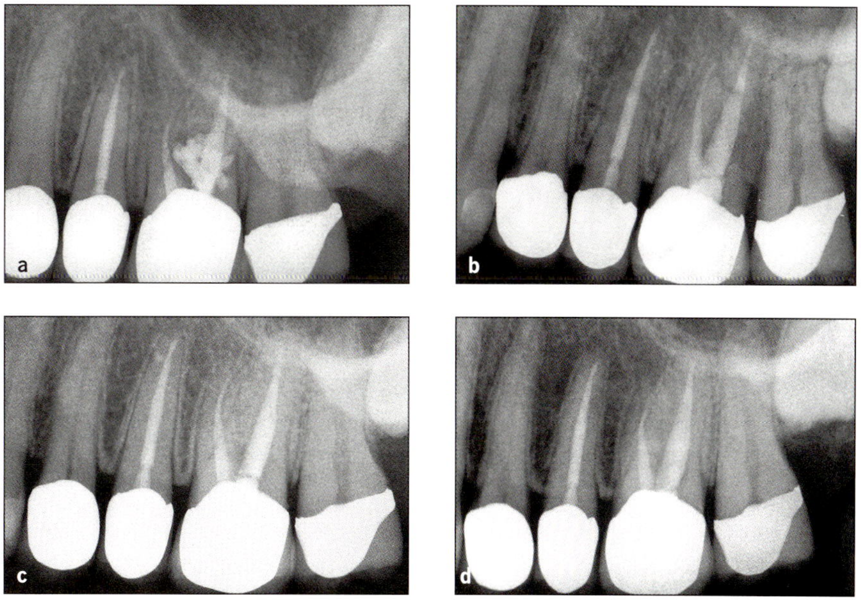

Fig 15-4 *(a)* Preoperative radiograph of a maxillary first molar with a furcation perforation and a large amount of gutta-percha extruded in the furcation. *(b)* Postoperative radiograph of the tooth after raising a buccal mucoperiosteal flap, preserving the coronal bone, curetting the furcation, and repairing the defect with MTA. *(c)* Postoperative radiograph of the tooth after 1 year. *(d)* Postoperative radiograph of the tooth after 3 years.

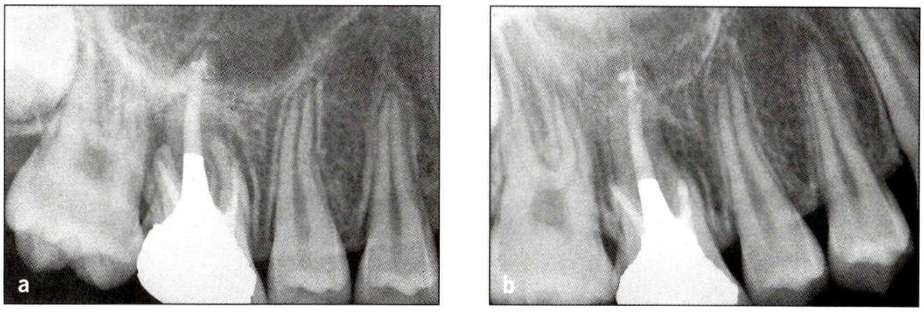

Fig 15-5 *(a)* Preoperative radiograph of a maxillary first molar with inadequate root canal treatment in the distobuccal root and ledge formation in the mesiobuccal root. *(b)* Postoperative radiograph after surgery to correct these inadequacies.

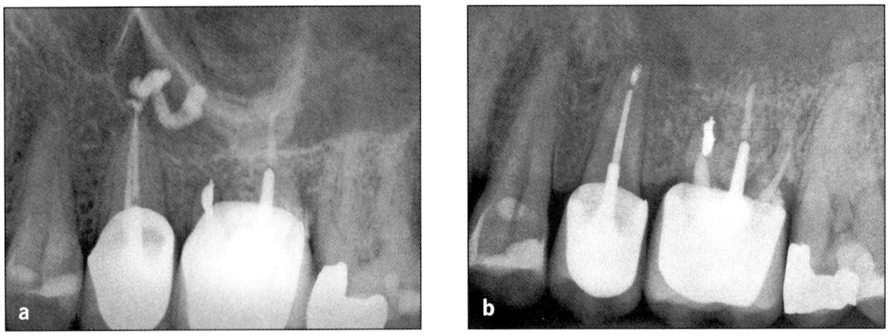

Fig 15-6 *(a)* Preoperative radiograph of a maxillary second premolar with an overfill into the maxillary sinus. *(b)* Postoperative radiograph after surgery to remove the overfill and placement of MTA as a root-end filling material.

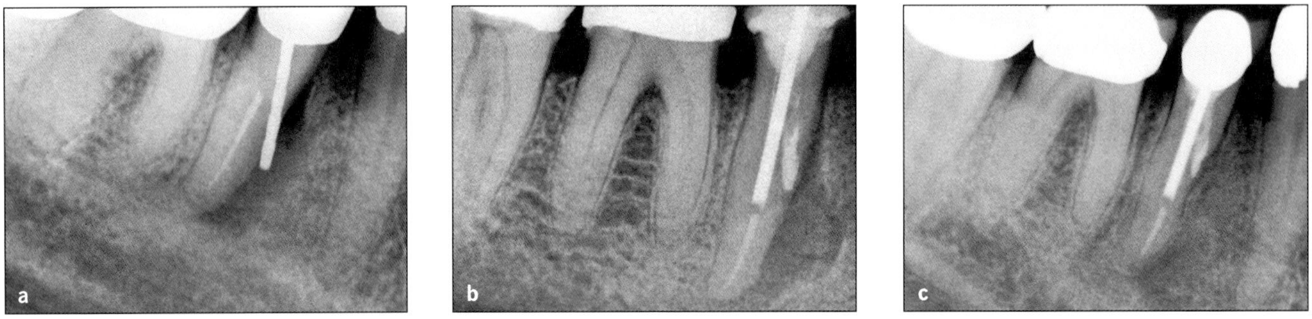

Fig 15-7 *(a)* Preoperative radiograph of a mandibular premolar with midroot post perforation. *(b)* Postoperative radiograph after root canal treatment, placement of a post in the canal, and repair of the perforation with MTA. *(c)* Postoperative radiograph 3 years later showing resolution of the lateral lesion. The tooth had no clinical symptoms. (Courtesy of Dr Noah Chivian, West Orange, New Jersey.)

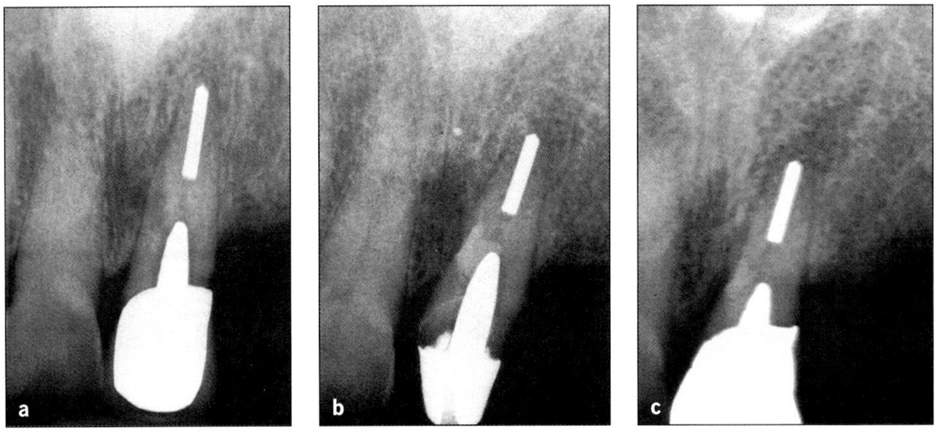

Fig 15-8 *(a)* Preoperative radiograph of a maxillary lateral incisor with coronal post perforation. *(b)* Postoperative radiograph after rotation of the tooth in its socket and repair of the mesiolingual perforation with MTA. *(c)* Postoperative radiograph 5 years after treatment showing complete healing. The tooth had no clinical symptoms and was an abutment for a partial denture.

length usually results in good outcomes. If unsuccessful, sealing of the apex by surgical approach should be considered. The surgery consists of raising a soft tissue flap, performing an osteotomy, and sealing the apical portion of the root (Fig 15-6).

Midroot perforation

The inability to maintain canal curvature is the major cause of lateral root perforation. The treatment of lateral root perforation consists of negotiating the original canal anatomy and obturation of the entire root canal system (Fig 15-7). If unsuccessful, the operator should concentrate on cleaning, shaping, and obturating the coronal segment of the canal, establishing a new working length confined to the root. Like ledge formation, the prognosis of lateral perforation depends mainly on the amount of remaining undebrided and unfilled canal. When nonsurgical treatment of midroot perforations is not possible or fails, surgical treatment should be attempted. Corrective surgery consists of raising a soft tissue flap, performing an osteotomy, and sealing the midroot perforation.

Coronal root perforations

Coronal root perforations occur during access preparation when the operator tries to locate canal orifices, or during coronal flaring when the operator uses rotary instruments

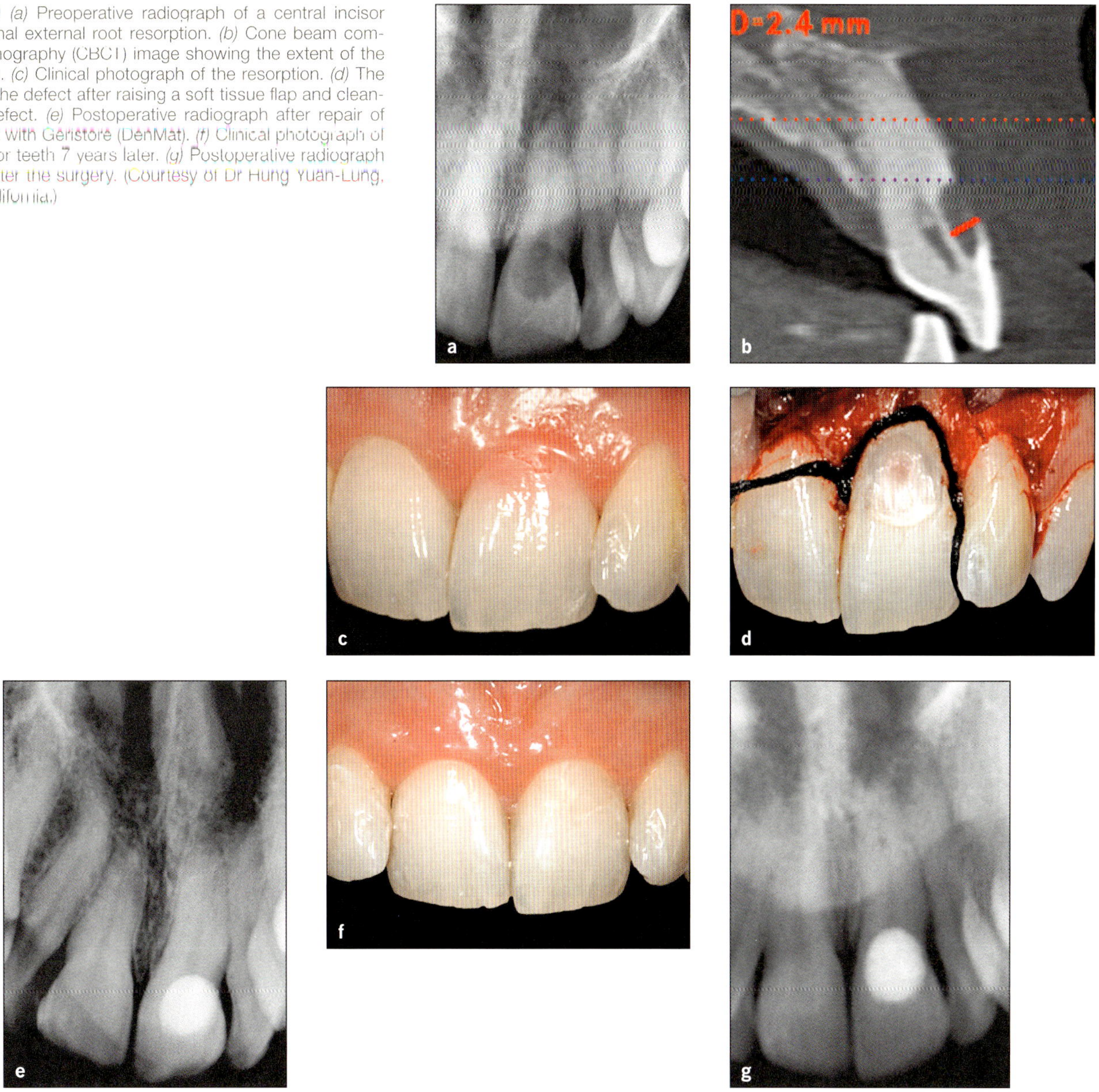

Fig 15-9 *(a)* Preoperative radiograph of a central incisor with coronal external root resorption. *(b)* Cone beam computed tomography (CBCT) image showing the extent of the resorption. *(c)* Clinical photograph of the resorption. *(d)* The extent of the defect after raising a soft tissue flap and cleaning the defect. *(e)* Postoperative radiograph after repair of the defect with Geristore (DenMat). *(f)* Clinical photograph of the anterior teeth 7 years later. *(g)* Postoperative radiograph 7 years after the surgery. (Courtesy of Dr Hung Yuan-Lung, Chino, California.)

such as Gates-Glidden drills or Peeso reamers. They can also occur during post space preparation (Fig 15-8).

Management of Resorptive Defects

Resorptive root defects are either internal or external. Internal resorptive defects are usually treated nonsurgically. Depending on the etiology, location, and extent of external root resorption, different treatment options are available. The location and the extent of the defect in relationship to the canal space determine the treatment. If the external root resorption defect does not penetrate into the pulp canal space, it can be cleaned and repaired after raising a soft tissue flap and locating the defect (Fig 15-9). The type of restorative material used to repair these defects depends on their location in relationship with the crestal bone. If the defect communicates with the oral cavity and presents a cosmetic concern for the patient, a composite resin or glass-ionomer material can be used to repair the defect (Fig 15-10). The use of MTA in these cases is contraindicated. MTA is the material of choice if the defect is in an area where esthetics are not an issue and the defect is below the crestal bone, which prevents any communication with the oral cavity (Fig 15-11). When the resorptive defects are approached surgically, a

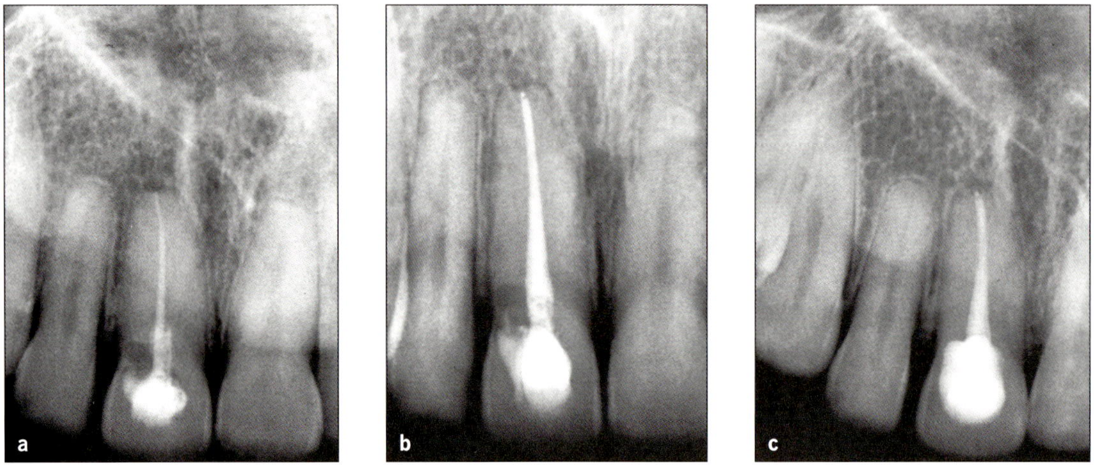

Fig 15-10 *(a)* Preoperative radiograph of a central incisor with coronal root resorption and inadequate root canal treatment. *(b)* Radiograph after retreatment. *(c)* Postoperative radiograph after repair of the perforation with Geristore.

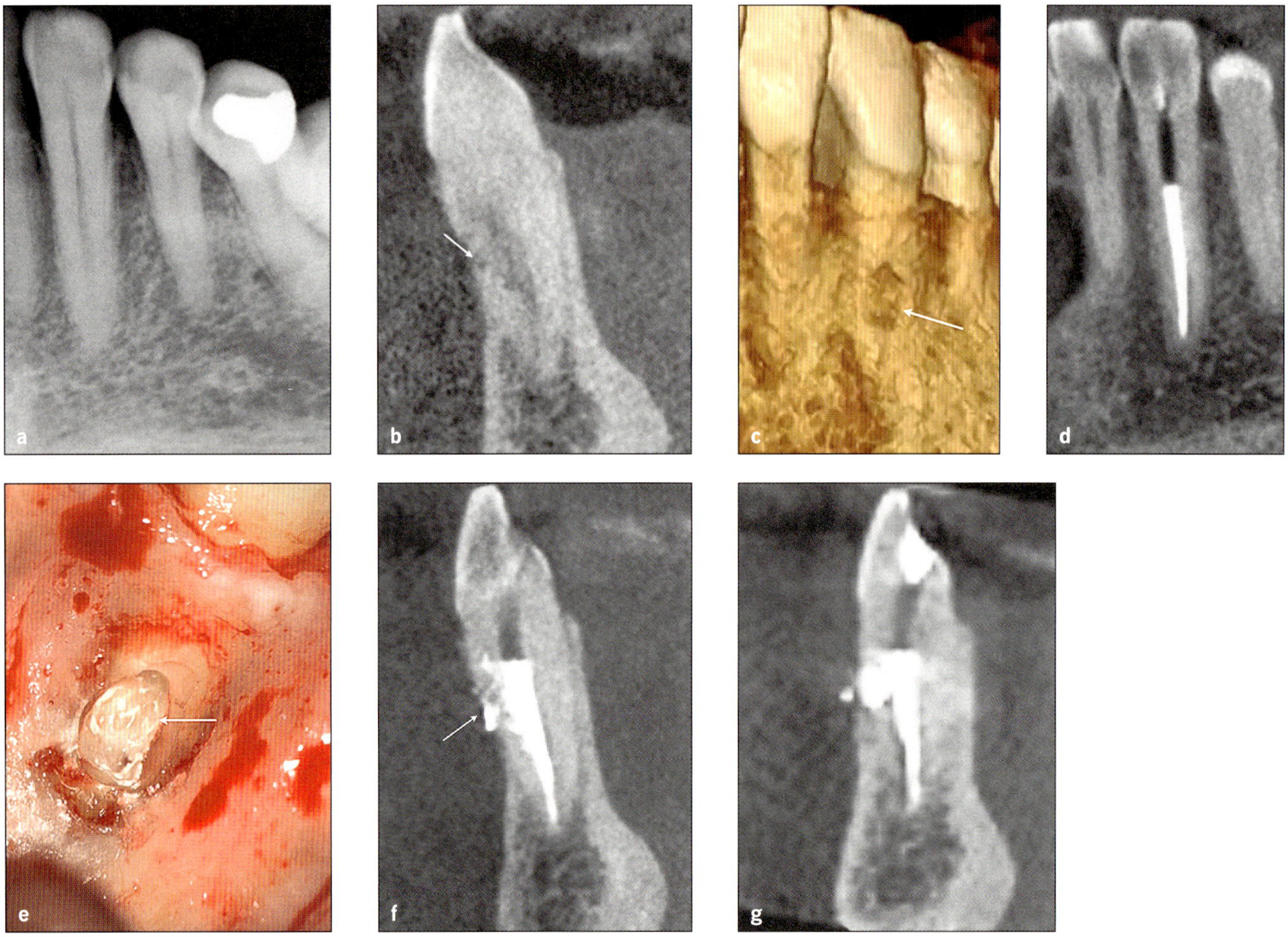

Fig 15-11 *(a)* Preoperative radiograph of a mandibular canine with midroot external resorption. *(b)* CBCT image showing the extent of the resorption *(arrow)*. *(c)* Another CBCT image showing the buccal resorption *(arrow)*. *(d)* Postoperative radiograph after root canal treatment. *(e)* The extent of the defect *(arrow)* after raising a soft tissue flap and cleaning the defect. *(f)* Postoperative CBCT image after repair of the defect *(arrow)*. *(g)* Postoperative CBCT image 18 months after surgery.

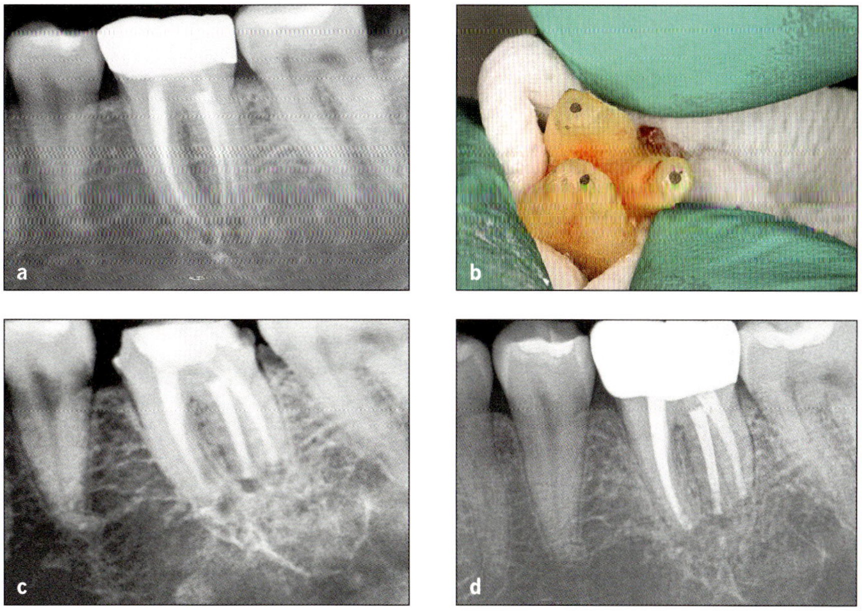

Fig 15-12 *(a)* Preoperative radiograph of a mandibular first molar with completed root canal treatment. CBCT examinations showed the presence of two separate distal roots and two mesial roots that joined at the apex. *(b)* Photograph of the extracted tooth after root-end resection, root end preparation, and placement of MTA as a root-end filling material. *(c)* Immediate postoperative radiograph after tooth replantation. *(d)* Postoperative radiograph 1 year later showing complete healing. A crown has been placed as a permanent restoration, and the tooth had no clinical symptoms at this time. (Courtesy of Dr Tory Silvestrin, Loma Linda, California.)

full-thickness flap is reflected, the defect site is enlarged for visualization, and the defect is curetted and prepared for placement of MTA. If there is no bone covering the root surface coronal to the defect, a periodontal regenerative procedure may also be performed in conjunction with the corrective surgical procedure. Periodontal pocketing caused by external resorptive defects can be treated by crown lengthening or orthodontic root extrusion.

The location of the defect on the surface of the root is another factor that affects treatment. Lesions located on the buccal aspect of the root are easier to treat. However, if the lesion is located on the distal or lingual aspect of the root, it is difficult to visualize and get the proper access needed for correction by surgical approach. In these situations, internal repair with MTA, tooth replantation, root resection, or hemisection can be treatment options to retain the tooth (Video 15-1).

When an external root resorptive defect communicates with the root canal system or an internal resorptive defect has perforated to the external root surface, both nonsurgical and surgical treatment modalities are required. In these situations, root canal treatment should be performed first, and in a subsequent visit the external portion of the perforation defect can be repaired surgically. As with situations in which the external root resorption defect does not communicate with the root canal space, the repair material is selected based on whether the defect communicates with the oral cavity or is located below the crestal bone. When the defect communicates with the oral cavity, the use of MTA is contraindicated. MTA is the material of choice if the defect is in an area where esthetics are not an issue and the defect is below the crestal bone. When it is difficult to adequately clean, dry, and obturate the root canal system, a combination of surgery and root canal treatment can be performed after raising a soft tissue flap; locating the defect; completing the cleaning, drying, and obturation of the canal space; and finally repairing the defect with the appropriate material.

Tooth Replantation

Tooth replantation is the reinsertion of a tooth into its own alveolus after the tooth has been extracted for the purpose of performing root-end surgery or repairing a root defect in the hand out of the socket.[7] Tooth replantation is indicated when there is no other treatment alternative to maintain a tooth. This procedure is mainly indicated when an apical surgery is contraindicated due to patient medical conditions, the proximity of critical anatomical structures such as the mental foramen or mandibular canal to the surgical site, and/or the presence of thick cortical bone.[8] Intentional replantation is contraindicated for teeth that are badly broken down, have inadequate bony support, and are difficult to extract. After obtaining anesthesia and without raising a flap, the tooth is extracted atraumatically with minimal damage to the periodontium. The deficiencies are corrected outside of the mouth, and then the tooth is reinserted into its original socket. The tooth should be kept in moist gauze during the operation out of the bony socket (Video 15-2).

Tooth replantation has a long history in dentistry.[8] When properly planned and executed, intentional replantation has been shown to be quite successful in providing patients with additional years of service (Fig 15-12). In a systematic review and meta-analysis, Torabinejad et al[8] compared the survival of intentionally replanted teeth

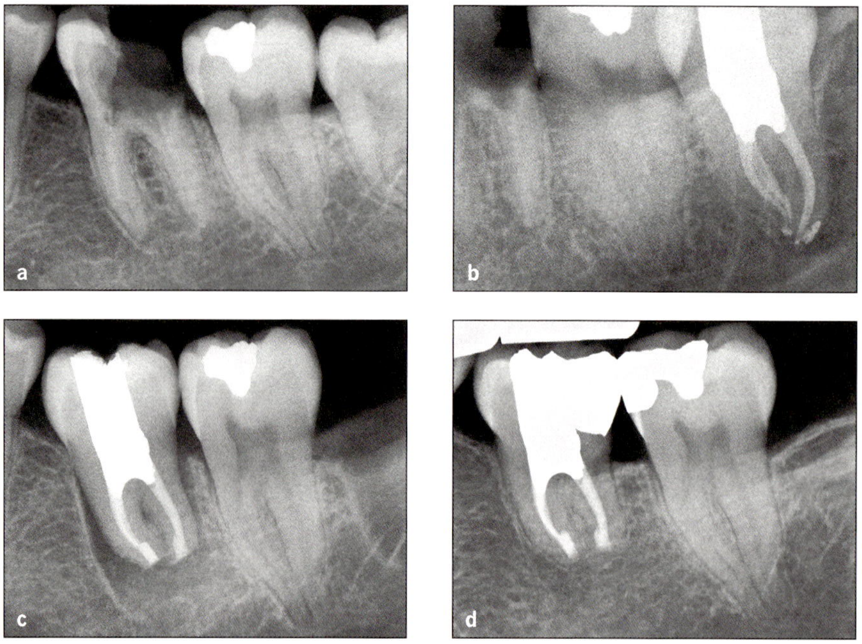

Fig 15-13 *(a)* Preoperative radiograph of a nonrestorable mandibular first molar with incomplete root canal treatment. Radiographic and clinical examinations showed the presence of an intact third molar suitable for transplantation. *(b)* Postoperative radiograph after completion of root canal treatment on the third molar. *(c)* Immediate postoperative radiograph after tooth transplantation. *(d)* Postoperative radiograph 9 years later showing the excellent condition of this tooth. The tooth had no clinical symptoms at this time.

with that of implant-supported single crowns. Meta-analysis of current data revealed a weighted mean survival of 88% (95% confidence interval, 81%–94%) for intentionally replanted teeth, with a root resorption rate of 11% for these cases.

Transplantation

Transplantation or autotransplantation is defined by extraction of an erupted, embedded, or impacted tooth from one part of the mouth into an extraction site or surgically prepared recipient site within the same individual.[7] Transplantation of a tooth has long been an acceptable treatment and is indicated for either a nonsalvageable or missing tooth.[9–11] It is contraindicated if the transplanted tooth is badly broken down, has inadequate bony support, is difficult to extract, or does not fit the recipient site. Ideally, root canal treatment should be performed on the tooth that is going to be transplanted. After extracting the unsalvageable tooth and preparing the socket for transplantation of a new tooth, the new tooth is extracted atraumatically with minimal damage to the periodontium. Its roots are resected, and Class I root-end cavity preparations are prepared and filled with a root-end filling material outside of the mouth. The tooth is then replanted into its new socket (Fig 15-13). During tooth transplantation, the tooth must be kept in moist gauze to prevent dehydration and necrosis of the periodontal ligament (PDL). When appropriately indicated and performed, transplanted teeth have a good prognosis[11] (Video 15-3). Ankylosis and resorption are the most common problems for this procedure.

Management of Periodontal Defects

Root resection

Root resection is the complete or partial removal of one or more roots from a multirooted tooth, before or after endodontic therapy. It is usually performed in maxillary molars but can also be performed in mandibular molars.[12]

Indications

The indications for root resection include the presence of severe bone loss in a periodontally involved root; severe furcation involvement not amenable to other surgical treatment options; root proximity unfavorable for other periodontal treatment options; untreatable roots with a separated instrument, perforations, caries, resorption, or vertical root fracture; and calcified canals in a multirooted tooth.

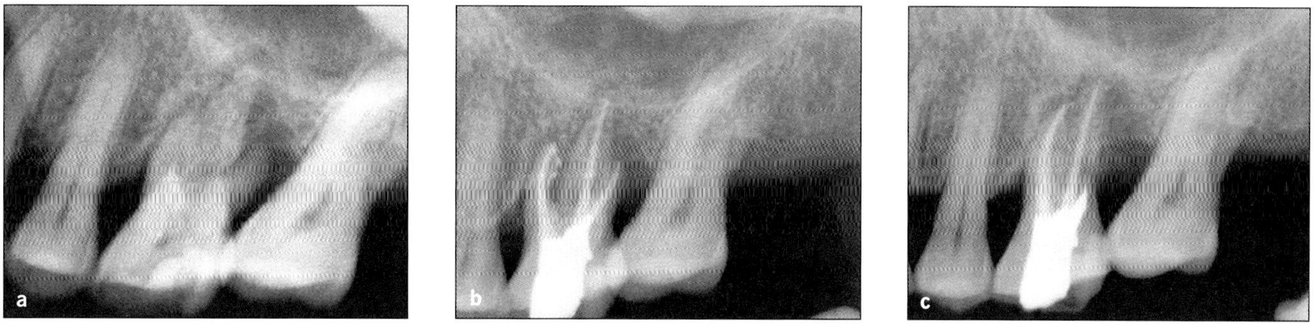

Fig 15-14 *(a)* Preoperative radiograph of a maxillary first molar with severe periodontal pockets around its distal root. *(b)* Postoperative radiograph following root canal treatment on the mesial and palatal roots and placement of amalgam in the orifice of the distal root. *(c)* Postoperative radiograph after distobuccal root amputation.

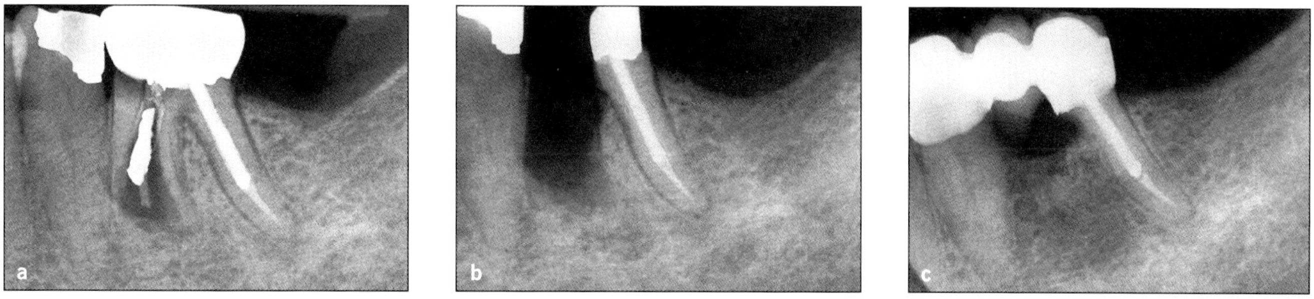

Fig 15-15 *(a)* Preoperative radiograph of a mandibular first molar with cracked mesial roots and a distal root with root canal treatment and a post. *(b)* Immediate postoperative radiograph after hemisection. *(c)* Postoperative radiograph 1 year later showing the distal root being used as a partial denture abutment. No radiographic pathosis is noted.

Contraindications

The contraindications for root resection are insufficient bony support for the remaining root or roots, the presence of fused roots, a long root trunk (apical furcation location), the inability to establish a favorable postoperative restorative margin, and poor patient home care.

Procedures

After raising a flap, root resection is performed by making a horizontal cut to separate the root from the crown. The crown remains intact, and the remaining stump is gradually resected to the buccal aspect of the root, resulting in good anatomical contour and access for good hygiene maintenance by the patient (Fig 15-14 and Video 15-4). The prognosis for root resection has been reported as good by some but only fair by others.[12]

Hemisection

Hemisection is the surgical division of a multirooted tooth into two segments. It is usually performed in mandibular molars and in rare occasions in maxillary molars. The indications and contraindications for hemisection are similar to those for root resection.[13–17]

Procedures

After raising a flap, hemisection is usually carried out by making a vertical cut through the crown into the furcation. In mandibular molars, the tooth is sectioned buccolingually through the bifurcation. In maxillary molars, the tooth is sectioned mesiodistally through the furcation. This action results in complete division of the tooth into two segments. The initial cut should be made close to the unsalvageable root. The unsalvageable root and its coronal segment are then removed. The anatomical crown of the remaining root(s) should then be carefully prepared to provide good, smooth margins for the prosthetic crown and adequate access for good hygiene by the patient, without any ledges left on the retained root (Fig 15-15 and Video 15-5).

Prognosis

The prognosis of teeth that have had root amputation or hemisection varies, with most studies reporting excellent long-term outcomes with failure rates under 15%, while some studies report failure rates of approximately 30%.[14,15] Major factors affecting the long-term success of these procedures include case selection and the patient's oral hygiene. In terms of case selection, increased failure rates have been reported for molars that have less than 50% bony support on the roots remaining after the procedure[17] and molars that are the lone terminal abutment for a fixed prosthesis.[16] Proper case selection and thorough maintenance protocols are critical in achieving a high long-term success rate.[14,17]

Crown lengthening

Periodontal health is essential for the long-term success of any dental treatment. However, proper periodontal assessment and management is critical in cases of multidisciplinary treatment, such as when periodontal-restorative interactions are present. A typical example of a periodontal-restorative interaction is the determination of where the margins of the restoration should be placed relative to the position of soft and hard periodontal tissues. Although clinicians often prefer supragingival margin placement because it facilitates preparation work, impression making, cleansing, detection of secondary caries, and maintenance of a healthy periodontium,[18–24] many instances (eg, subgingival caries, tooth fracture, root perforation, short clinical crown, tooth hypersensitivity, or esthetic demands) may dictate subgingival restoration margin placement. Restorations with subgingival margins may have destructive effects on the periodontium supporting not only the restored tooth itself but also the adjacent teeth; these negative consequences can include persistent gingival inflammation, increased attachment loss, greater bone loss, and in some cases gingival enlargement.[19–31]

The term *biologic width* was coined by Cohen[32] (1962) based on an investigation by Gargiulo et al,[33] who reported on the proportional relationship between the alveolar bone crest, connective tissue attachment (1.07 mm), epithelial attachment (0.97 mm), and gingival sulcus (0.69 mm). A significant finding of this study was the high variability of the junctional epithelium length and the relative stability of the connective tissue attachment length. Others have confirmed these findings.[27] This dimensional stability implies that the biologic width must be respected and preserved when restorations are placed subgingivally.

Regarding restorative margin location, evidence suggests that its position relative to the alveolar bone crest is more critical than its position relative to the free gingival margin.[34] Therefore, the clinician must determine the location of the osseous crest and the dentogingival attachment dimension for each tooth treatment-planned to receive subgingival restoration margins in order to assess the available distance from the anticipated restoration margin. Knowing where the planned restorative margin will be placed, and having obtained the aforementioned anatomical measurements, the clinician can determine the possible need for crown lengthening.

Crown lengthening surgery (CLS) is a procedure that may include resection of soft, hard (bone), or both tissues to create a longer clinical crown and to reestablish the proper biologic width dimensions around the tooth of interest. The reestablishment of the dentogingival junction at a more apical root level accommodates the junctional epithelium and the connective tissue attachment, thus helping to maintain healthy long-term periodontal conditions.[35–38]

In certain cases, an alternative to the surgical technique might be orthodontic extrusion (see below), which oftentimes will also require subsequent CLS.[39,40]

Indications

The indications for CLS stem from the need to have adequate exposure of the clinical crown, access for restorative margin preparation, and proper restoration margin placement relative to the alveolar crest. Therefore, CLS may be indicated for teeth with a short clinical crown (eg, because of altered passive eruption), teeth with a shortened crown (eg, due to fracture or extensive caries, resorption, or iatrogenic perforation), and teeth with caries or fractures that extend subgingivally.[41,42] More specifically, in cases where restorative treatment is planned, CLS is typically indicated whenever it is anticipated that the final restorative margin will be located less than 3 mm from the alveolar bone crest.

Contraindications

CLS is contraindicated for patients in whom periodontal surgery is contraindicated for medical reasons. In addition, it is contraindicated for teeth that have short or compromised roots, because the postsurgical crown-to-root ratio will be unfavorable, and for teeth with inadequate periodontal support. If the desired crown length increase could result in exposure of a tooth furcation, or if the anticipated alveolar bone reduction could result in close proximity to vital anatomical structures (eg, mental nerve, maxillary sinus, ascending ramus), CLS is contraindicated. Furthermore, CLS is contraindicated for single teeth in the esthetic zone, because significant apical displacement of the gingival margin of only one tooth will create esthetic complications.[42]

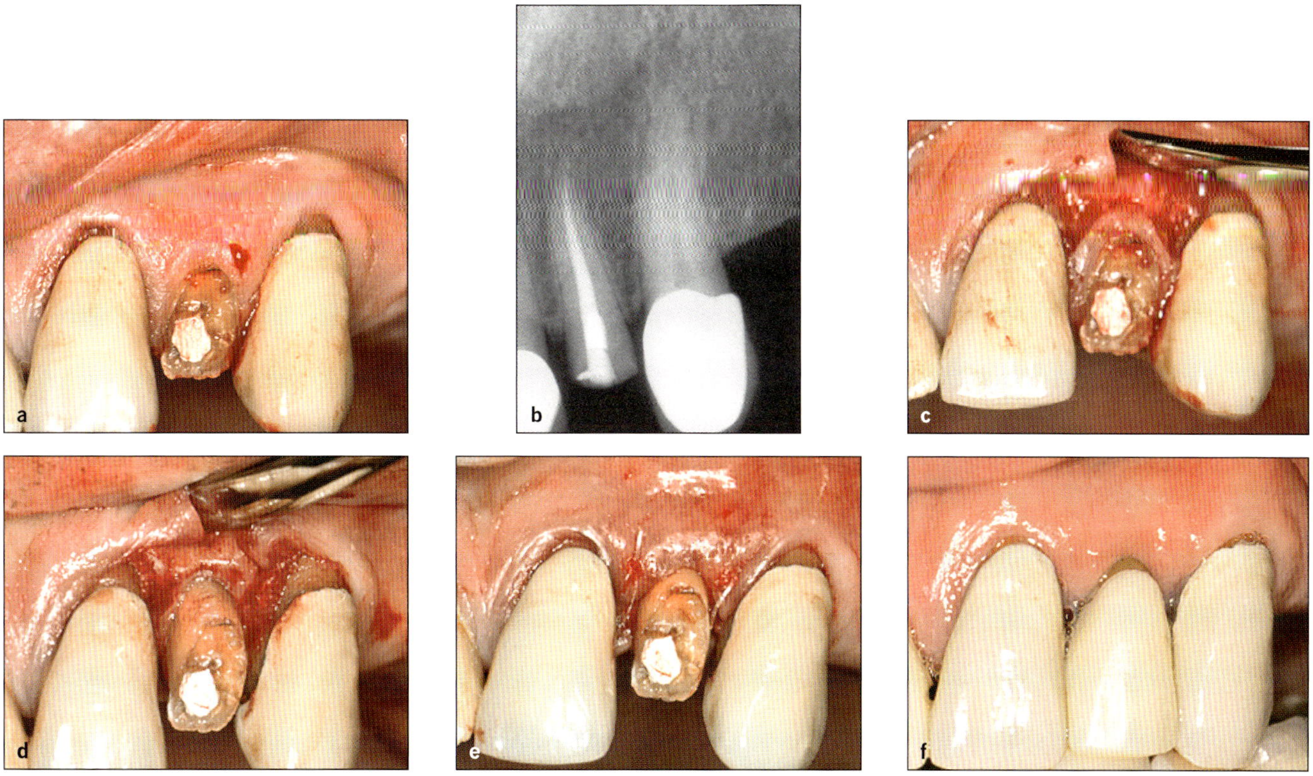

Fig 15-16 *(a)* Clinical appearance of a tooth requiring CLS. *(b)* A radiograph of the same tooth showing the presence of adequate root canal treatment. *(c)* A full-thickness flap is elevated after a submarginal incision is performed. *(d)* Soft (gingivectomy) and hard (ostectomy) tissues are removed. *(e)* Flaps are sutured. Note the increase in supragingival tooth structure compared with *a*. *(f)* Provisional restoration in place 2 months after surgery.

Procedures

CLS is typically accomplished by either gingivectomy or an apically positioned flap (APF) with or without osseous resection[26] (Fig 15-16). The choice of surgical technique is dictated by anatomical, esthetic, and restorative factors. In preparation for CLS, the clinician should review several aspects of the case related to both the patient and the specific tooth, including the medical history, clinical and radiographic periodontal examination, occlusion, tooth root anatomy, tooth size and shape, crown-to-root ratio, soft tissue biotype (thick vs thin), keratinized tissue width, alveolar crest position and contour, tooth crown and gingival display during rest, speech, and smile (relation with lip line). Ideally, provisional restorations should be in place prior to CLS; alternatively, a stent that identifies the anticipated or desired restoration margin location will help the surgeon perform adequate hard and/or soft tissue reduction to properly accommodate the definitive restorations.

Thorough consideration of the parameters listed above will allow the clinician to correctly choose the most appropriate surgical technique and execute the needed CLS adequately. In terms of postsurgical supracrestal tooth structure, approximately 7 to 9 mm are needed for re-establishment of the epithelial and connective tissue attachment and for allowance of sufficient tooth structure for adequate support of the planned restoration (Fig 15-17). In this context, it is important to consider biologic width differences between individuals and between teeth within the same patient.[26,43,44]

When periodontal surgical treatment is considered, baseline healthy tissue conditions are important. Therefore, it is often necessary to review with the patient oral hygiene instructions and to complete any needed nonsurgical periodontal therapy prior to performing CLS. Successful CLS is facilitated by preparative interdisciplinary treatment, such as root canal therapy, post preparation, and provisional restoration (Video 15-6).

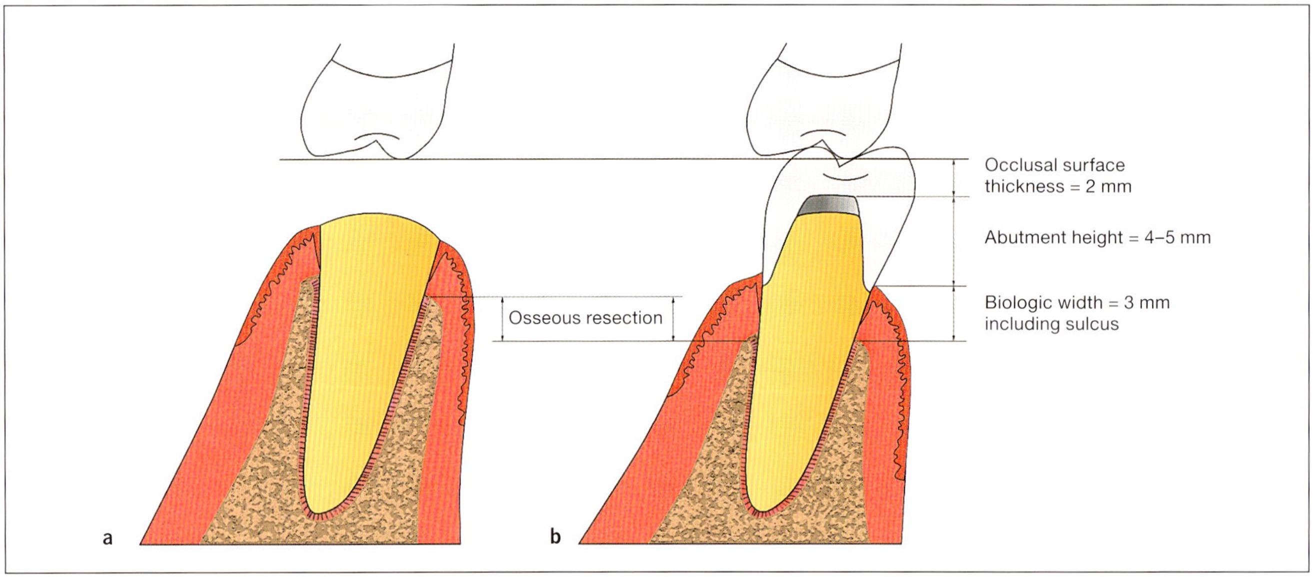

Fig 15-17 *(a)* Diagram of a tooth with an inadequate clinical crown. *(b)* Diagram after osseous resection and gingivectomy to allow for adequate biologic width, abutment height, and occlusal clearance for placement of a crown.

Prognosis

According to a recent systematic review, the available literature on CLS performed for restorative reasons includes studies that have only limited follow-up, most only up to 6 months' duration.[43] The reported results suggest that, within this relatively short time period, the treated teeth are successfully restored and maintained; however, after CLS it is possible that the soft tissue margin may exhibit significant rebound, especially during the first 3 months after CLS.[45] These findings suggest that it is best not to place definitive restorations on CLS-treated teeth earlier than 3 months postoperatively.[45] A recent long-term retrospective study of 245 endodontically treated teeth that had undergone CLS and prosthodontic treatment reported a mean tooth survival of 98%, 96%, and 83% at 3, 5, and 10 years posttreatment, respectively.[46] Fifty percent of the teeth lost (or deemed hopeless) during follow-up were lost because of advanced caries or vertical root fracture, while the remaining were lost for other reasons (eg, furcation involvement, mobility, sinus tract).[46] The crown-to-root ratio and restoration margin position relative to the gingival margin were reported as the major determinants of tooth loss.[46]

CLS is often done in conjunction with other procedures (endodontic, restorative, etc) with the combined goal of improving tooth retention while providing proper functional, esthetic, and restorative outcomes. The combined time, effort, and cost required for the various procedures should be considered vis-à-vis the prognosis to reach a sound decision whether it is reasonable to opt for CLS or choose instead other treatment choices (eg, tooth extraction and replacement by a fixed or removable partial denture or a dental implant).

Root extrusion

Performing CLS is associated with several complications. They include reduced alveolar bone for the treated tooth as well as the adjacent teeth. Removing bone not only reduces the alveolar support for the treated tooth, but it also increases the crown-to-root ratio and increases the clinical crown, which may result in esthetic issues in the anterior region of the mouth. An alternative to CLS is orthodontic extrusion or forced eruption. In 1973, Heithersay proposed the use of orthodontic forced eruption for teeth with horizontal cervical root fracture.[47] This action results in movement of the root in a vertical direction and exposes the coronal root for preparation and restoration of the tooth. Ingber suggested forced eruption for the treatment of isolated one- and two-wall infrabony osseous defects, nonrestorable teeth, and soft tissue cosmetic deformities.[48–50] Simon popularized the use of orthodontic forced eruption in endodontically treated teeth with inadequate crown structure.[51–54]

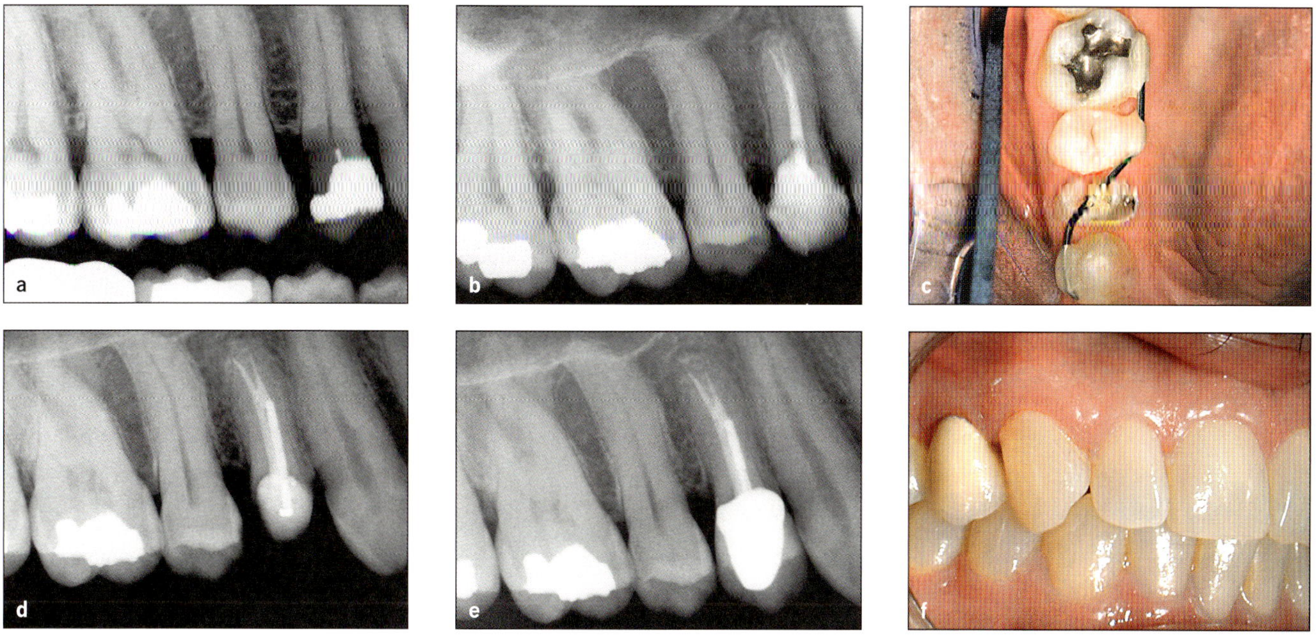

Fig 15-18 *(a)* Preoperative radiograph of a maxillary first premolar with an inadequate clinical crown for restoration. *(b)* Radiograph showing completed root canal treatment on this tooth. *(c)* Clinical photograph of placement of the extrusion apparatus to extrude the tooth orthodontically. *(d)* Postoperative radiograph after extrusion of this tooth. *(e)* Postoperative radiograph after root canal treatment, extrusion, and placement of a crown 15 months after completion of the procedures. *(f)* Clinical photograph of the restored tooth showing excellent results. (Courtesy of Dr Manouchehr Pouresmail, Paso Robles, California.)

Indications and contraindications

Root extrusion is indicated in any tooth with a cervical root defect that involves or extends below the crestal bone (0 to 4 mm).[54] These defects include horizontal crown or root fractures, decay, resorption, and accidental perforations. The contraindications for root extrusion are short roots, insufficient space to extrude the root, and periodontal disease.[54]

Procedures

The procedures involved in root extrusion depend on the presence or absence of adequate coronal tooth structure. When there is enough tooth structure after root canal treatment, brackets are placed on the incisal third of the crown of the target tooth and the adjacent teeth. Vertical force is applied to the target tooth by placing elastic bands on the adjacent teeth and connecting them to the endodontically treated tooth with inadequate coronal structure. When there is not enough coronal tooth structure after root canal treatment, a temporary post is made from a paper clip and cemented in the coronal half to two-thirds of the root with intermediate restorative material. After cementing a horizontal wire on the adjacent teeth, vertical force is applied to the target tooth by placing elastic bands from the paper clip in the root canal–treated tooth to the horizontal wire. During this noninvasive approach, the tooth is extruded using light extrusion forces and anchorage from the adjacent teeth. As a result, the entire periodontal attachment apparatus will move coronally, along with the tooth. This procedure may take 2 to 4 weeks. After accomplishing adequate extrusion, the tooth must be stabilized for at least 2 months before a definitive restoration is placed[54] (Fig 15-18). Because of the coronal movement of the supporting tissues, subsequent CLS (bone removal) might still be necessary.[55] Orthodontic treatment can also be performed in combination with fiberotomy to induce rapid extrusion; in such instances, the marginal bone level will mostly stay in the original position.[55] Gingival recession and undesired attachment loss are possible after this treatment approach.[40]

The disadvantages of orthodontic root extrusion include esthetic issues during the procedure, the time required to accomplish ideal results, and surgical fiberotomy following root extrusion. Because of these issues, surgical extrusion (Fig 15-19) of teeth that might otherwise be considered unrestorable has been suggested as an alternative to CLS and orthodontic extrusion.[56] The surgical extrusion concept is based on information from the dental trauma literature regarding extrusive luxation. This procedure does not have the disadvantages of orthodontic root extrusion. A histologic study compared orthodontic extrusion with surgical extrusion in a dog model and reported transient resorption and eventual repair in both groups.[57]

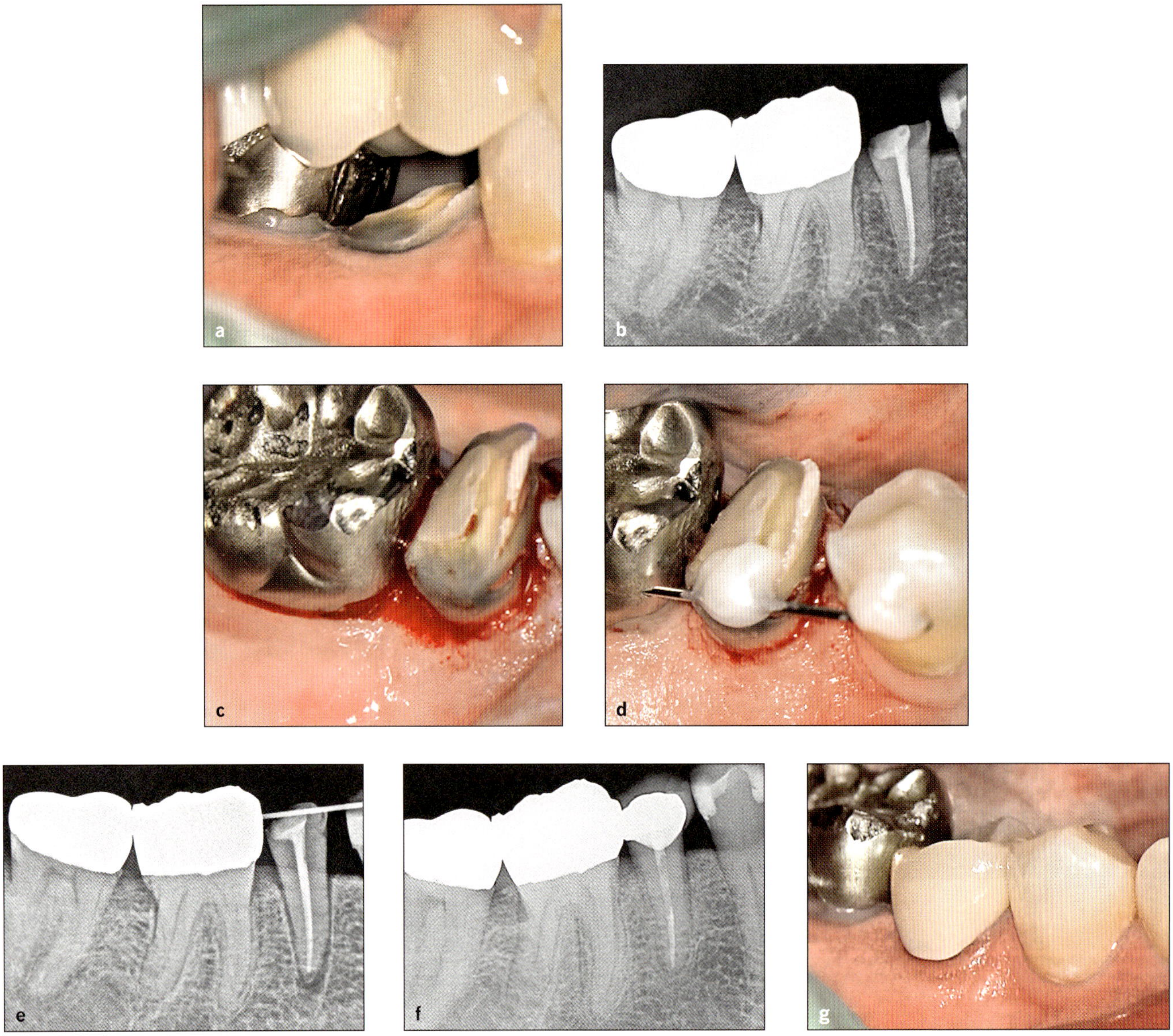

Fig 15-19 *(a)* Preoperative photograph of a mandibular second premolar with an inadequate clinical crown for restoration. *(b)* Radiograph showing that this tooth has adequate root canal treatment. *(c)* Clinical photograph of this tooth after surgical extrusion. *(d)* Clinical photograph of this tooth being splinted to its adjacent teeth. *(e)* Postoperative radiograph after extrusion and splinting of this tooth. *(f)* Postoperative radiograph after root canal treatment, extrusion, and placement of a crown 18 months after completion of the procedures. *(g)* Clinical photograph of this tooth restored with a crown 18 months after surgical extrusion. (Courtesy of Dr Rajiv Patel, Flower Mound, Texas.)

Regenerative Techniques and Guided Bone Regeneration in Endodontic Surgery

The main objective of periapical surgery is to create an optimal environment for periapical tissue regeneration. The outcome of periapical surgery can be affected by several factors, among which the size and location of the periapical bone loss are thought to be the most considerable, together with bacterial factors. In large periapical defects, lesions will often be filled with fibrous connective tissues. The ingrowth of nonosteogenic tissues and the downgrowth of the epithelial tissue along the root surface can result in repair. *Repair* is defined as the formation of new cells and structures that differ from the original cells and structures instead of achieving the expected regeneration. *Regeneration* is defined as the reproduction or reconstruction of the lost tissues and restoration of various functions of the damaged tissues and organs. The principal functions of regenerative techniques (RTs) in periapical surgery are *(1)* to improve the regenerative healing process by excluding the undesired proliferation of connective tissue and oral epithelium into the defect, and *(2)* to maintain space below the membrane to allow cells of the PDL and trabecular bone to regenerate.

Deng et al[58] performed a meta-analysis to evaluate the effect of RTs on periapical surgery using different protocols for different lesion types. It was concluded that both the isolated use of bone-replacement analogs and the combination of membranes and bone-replacement analogs can improve the outcome of periapical surgery. The use of RTs for through-and-through and large lesions was recommended.

RTs and guided bone regeneration (GBR) have been proposed as adjuncts to periapical surgery. The amount and location of bone adjacent to the root structures affect the prognosis of periradicular surgery. Kim and Kratchman[59] propose a six-category classification system to assist in predicting surgical prognosis and determining the need for bone grafting and barrier techniques. Class A (no lesion), class B (small periapical lesion), and class C (large periapical lesion without periodontal communication) all represent situations that are favorable for healing without supplemental grafting or barriers. Class D (similar to class C with independent periodontal pocketing), class E (endodontic-periodontal communication to the apex), and class F (apical lesion with complete loss of buccal bone) represent situations with a more guarded prognosis and usually require concurrent use of bone grafting and barrier techniques.

Apicomarginal defects and periapical lesions 15 mm or larger have been determined to negatively impact surgical outcomes. An apicomarginal defect[60] or a localized bony defect distinguished by a total deficiency of alveolar bone over the entire root length has a significant adverse effect on the outcome, reducing the rate of complete healing by approximately 20% or more when compared to teeth with an isolated endodontic-only lesion.[61–63] Figure 15-20 illustrates the case of an apicomarginal defect related to the maxillary right first molar that presented for apical surgery.

The presence of a periradicular lesion 15 mm or greater in diameter also has been linked to a poorer prognosis.[61] Advanced periodontitis with deep pocket formation has been associated with chronic periradicular inflammation after endodontic surgery and subsequent failure of the root-end surgery.[64] The cause of failure has been identified as ingrowth of nonosteogenic tissues into the periradicular surgical site and downgrowth of epithelial tissue along the root surface. Successful treatment may depend more on controlling epithelial proliferation than root-end management. Guided tissue regeneration techniques have been advocated for use in such cases.[65,66] Video 15-7 shows an example of the utilization of endodontic surgery and GBR in a molar with a furcation perforation and a large periodontal defect. Figure 15-21 illustrates a large cystic lesion with sinus perforation that presented for apical surgery.

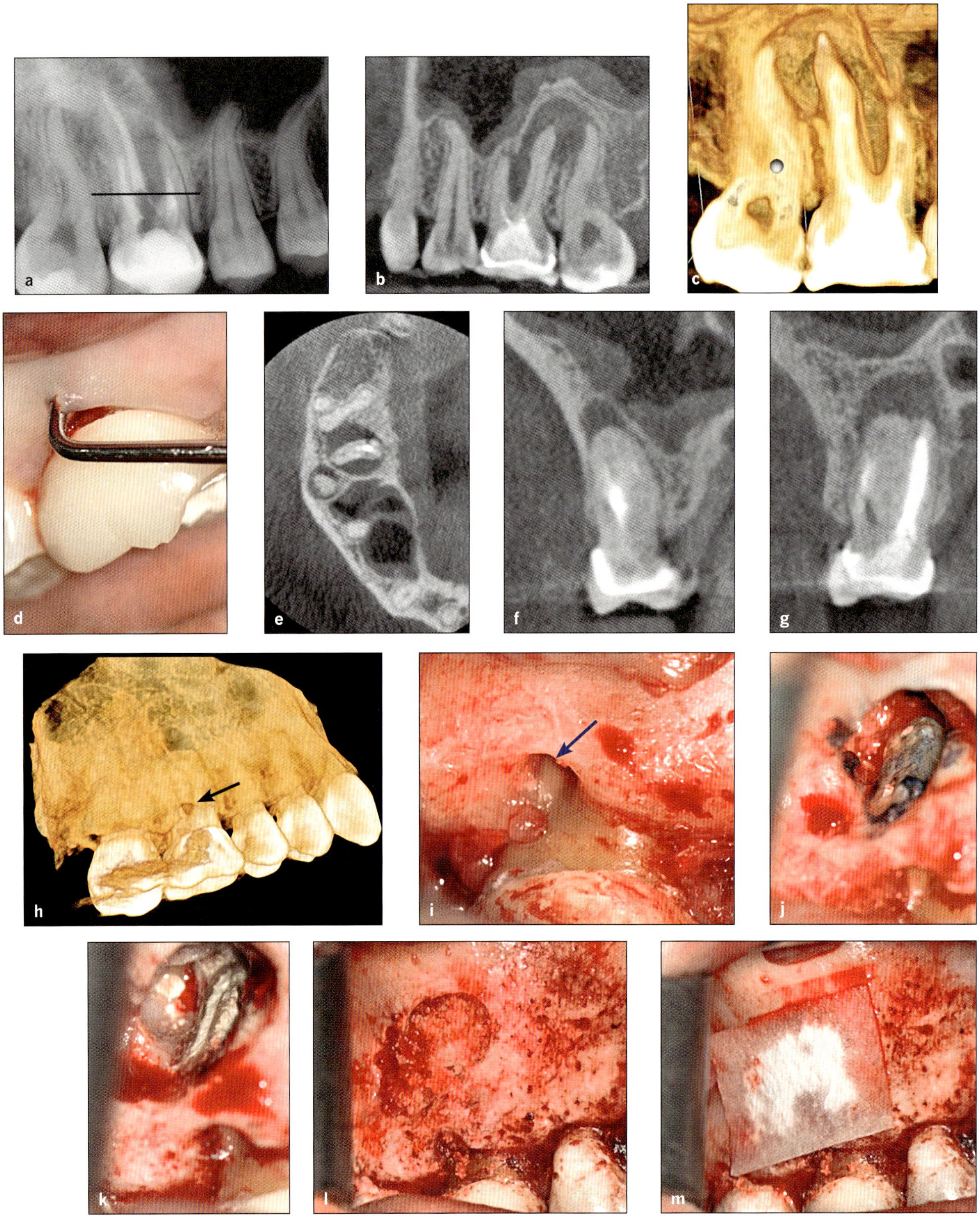

Fig 15-20 *(a)* Periapical radiograph of a maxillary first molar that was referred for periapical surgery. A nonsurgical retreatment attempt was performed prior to periapical microsurgery, but the mesiobuccal canal was blocked. The *black line* in *a* corresponds to the level of the axial view in *e*. *(b)* Sagittal view demonstrating the extent of the periapical defect. *(c)* Three-dimensional (3D) rendering of the periapical defect. *(d)* Clinical photograph demonstrating the endodontic-periodontal communication. *(e)* Axial view of the mesiobuccal, distobuccal, and palatal roots. Note the fused distal and palatal roots. *(f and g)* Coronal views of the mesiobuccal root and the fused distal-palatal roots. *(h)* 3D rendering demonstrating the periodontal defect *(black arrow)*. *(i)* After full-thickness flap reflection, the periodontal defect was determined to communicate with the periapical defect *(blue arrow)*. *(j)* Root resection of the fused distal-palatal roots prior to ultrasonic preparation. *(k)* MTA root-end filling of the ultrasonically prepared distal and palatal preparation. *(l)* Periodontal and periapical defects grafted with Puros allograft material (Zimmer). *(m)* Grafted defect covered with a CopiOs membrane (Zimmer). →

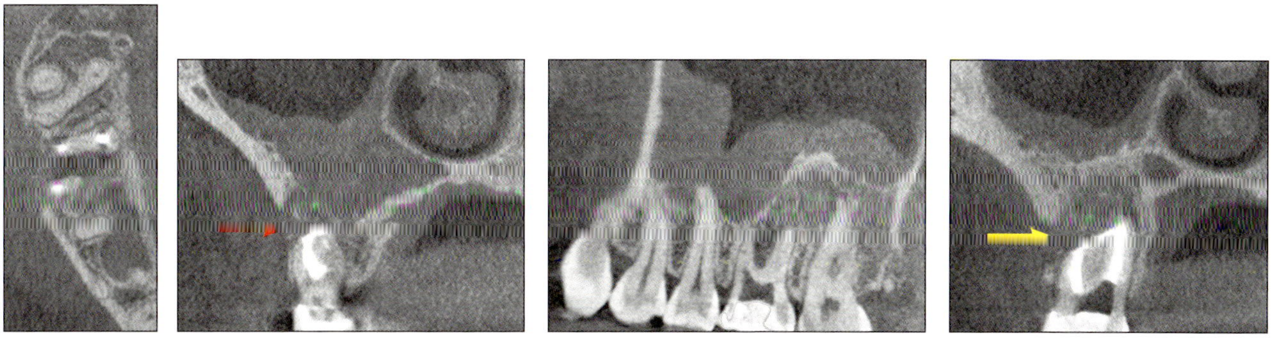

n

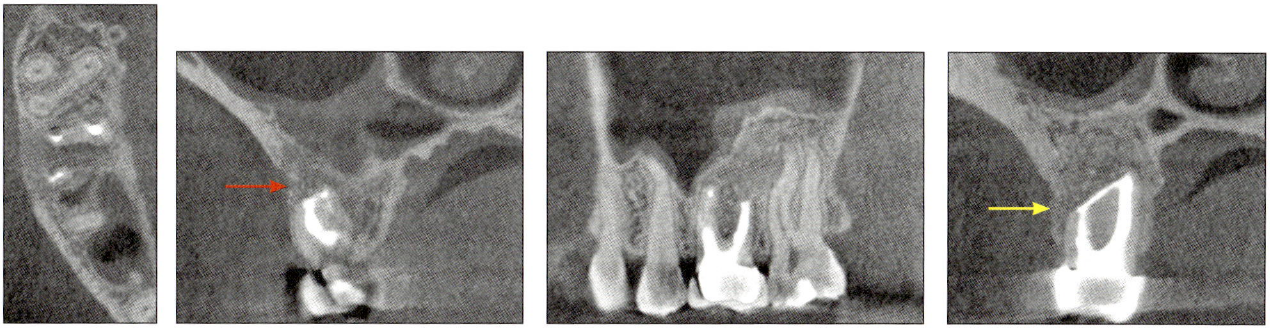

o

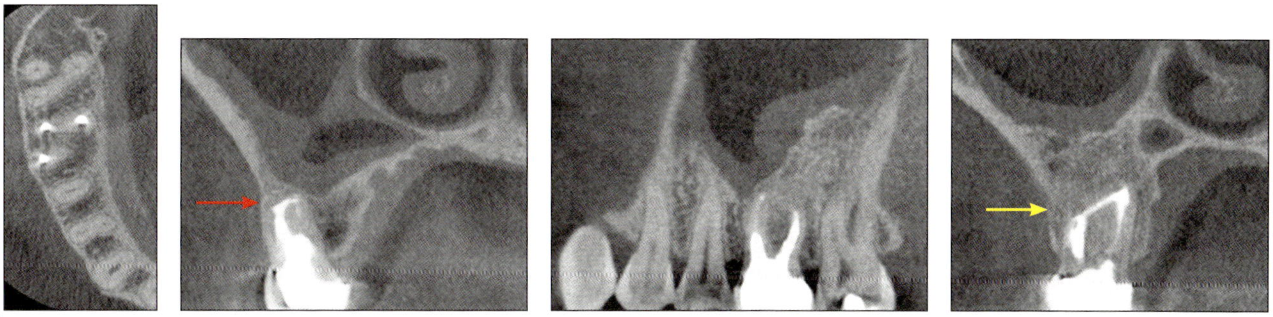

p

Fig 15-20 *(cont) (n)* Immediate postsurgical CBCT scan images. Note the buccal defect *(red and yellow arrows)*. *(o)* Six-month recall CBCT scan images. Note the initial regeneration of the defect, including the buccal cortical plate. *(p)* One-year recall CBCT scan images demonstrating complete remodeling of the defect and the buccal plate *(red and yellow arrows)*.

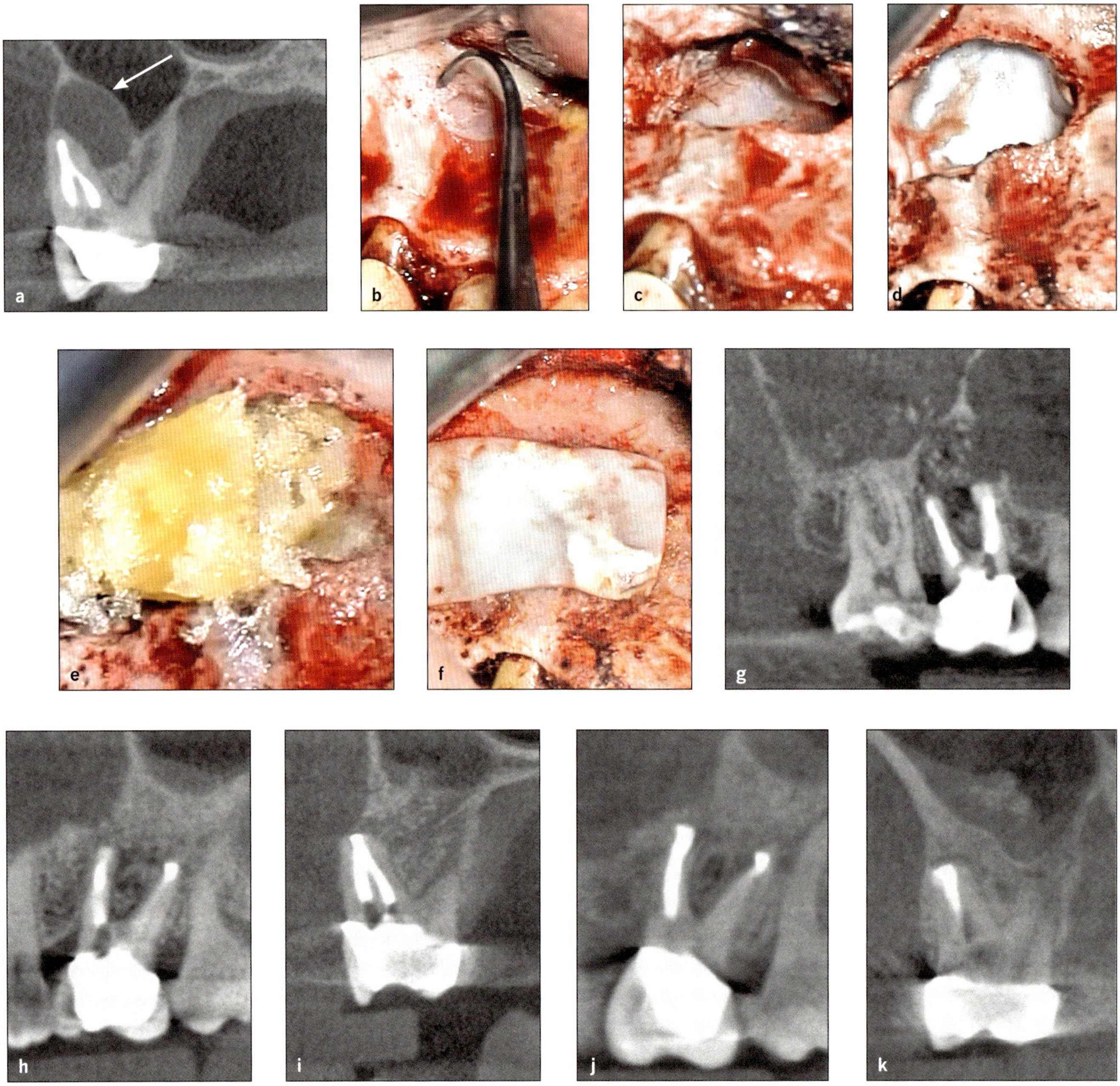

Fig 15-21 *(a)* Coronal view of the mesiobuccal root of a maxillary right first molar that presented for periapical surgery. Note the low-density lesion causing thinning of the lateral wall of the maxillary sinus *(white arrow)*. *(b)* Clinical photograph demonstrating the porous and thin cortical plate that coincides with a periapical cyst. *(c)* Clinical photograph after degranulation of the lesion demonstrating the maxillary sinus exposure. The vascularity of the sinus and bony spicule can be noted. *(d)* The sinus perforation was covered with a CopiOs membrane. *(e)* Periapical defects grafted with Puros allograft material. *(f)* Grafted defect covered with a CopiOs membrane. *(g)* Immediate postoperative CBCT scan. *(h and i)* Sagittal and coronal CBCT views at the 1-year recall. *(j and k)* Sagittal and coronal CBCT views at the 2-year recall.

Table 15-1 Types of membranes

Membrane type	Trade name (manufacturer)
Resorbable membranes	
Collagen	CopiOs Pericardium Membrane (Zimmer)
Polylactic acid	Biomend (Zimmer)
Polylactic acid, polyglycolic acid, and trimethylene carbonate	Bio-Gide (Osteohealth)
Laminar bone	Bicon Resorbable Collagen Membrane (Bicon)
Nonresorbable membranes	
Polytetrafluoroethylene	Guidor (Guidor) Atrisorb (CollaGenex) Resolut (WL Gore) Lambone (Pacific Coast Tissues Bank) Gore-Tex (WL Gore) TefGen FD (Lifecore Biomedical) Bicon Barrier Membrane (Bicon) Cytoflex (Unicare Biomedical)

Principles of GBR

The basic principle of guided tissue and bone regeneration is the different rate at which different types of cells repopulate during healing. The soft tissue cells are considerably more motile than the hard tissue cells, and therefore they tend to migrate into the wound more quickly during healing. A barrier interposed between the gingival tissue and the exposed root surfaces and supporting alveolar bone prevents colonization of the exposed root surface by gingival cells. This encourages selective repopulation of the root surface by PDL cells. The use of a resorbable barrier theoretically would allow PDL cells and other cells with osteogenic potential to repopulate the defect, resulting in new connective tissue attachment and bone formation. Dahlin et al[67,68] demonstrated that in monkeys, a significant increase in osseous healing occurs when membranes are used in through-and-through bone defects in periradicular surgery of the maxillary lateral incisors. The use of resorbable guided tissue regeneration (GTR) membranes in endodontic surgery with buccal apicomarginal-type defects also has been shown to enhance regeneration of the periodontium and surrounding bone in dogs.[69] This type of matrix barrier promoted greater amounts of connective tissue and alveolar bone and minimized the formation of junctional epithelium.

Several case reports have discussed the use of GTR techniques in conjunction with endodontic surgery.[70–82] These studies largely have reported favorable outcomes in cases involving large periradicular lesions, through-and-through bone defects, and repair of a surgical perforation or loss of the buccal cortical plate adjacent to the root.

Pecora et al[83] compared the healing of 20 large periradicular defects (greater than 10-mm diameter) with and without the use of a resorbable membrane. They reported that at 12 months after surgery, the sites in which membranes had been used had better healing and that the quality and quantity of the regenerated bone was superior. One study evaluated periradicular and periodontal healing in cases involving apicomarginal defects when GTR (Bio-Oss and Bio-Gide membrane, Osteohealth) was performed in conjunction with periradicular surgery. At 12 months after surgery, 86% of cases were considered healed clinically and radiographically. It was concluded that GTR should be considered as an adjunct to periradicular surgery in cases of apicomarginal defects.[84] However, when a standard apical osteotomy is performed and the buccal bone over the remainder of the root is intact, use of a resorbable membrane has no beneficial effect on healing.[85]

Several different types of membranes are available. They can be grouped into two broad categories: nonresorbable and resorbable (Table 15-1). Resorbable membranes are generally better suited for endodontic uses because a second surgical procedure is not required to remove the membrane.

Table 15-2 Bone graft materials

Graft type	Description	Product (manufacturer)
Autogenous graft	From patient's own body (chin, ramus, iliac crest)	NA
Allograft	Demineralized freeze-dried human bone or freeze-dried human bone	Puros (Zimmer) enCore (Osteogenics Biomedical) MTF DeMin Bone (Dentsply) Dynagraft (GenSci) Opteform (Exactech) Osteofil (Regeneration Technologies) Grafton (Osteotech)
Xenograft	Inorganic bovine bone particles	Bio-Oss (Osteohealth) OsteoGraf (Dentsply)
Ceramic and synthetic grafts	Bioactive glass	PerioGlas (NovaBone)
	Calcium sulfate	CapSet (Lifecore Biomedical)
	Calcium phosphate/hydroxyapatite	OsteoSet (Wright Medical Technology) Bioplant HTR (Kerr) Biogran (Biomet 3i) Norian SRS (Synthes) NovaBone-C/M (NovaBone)
Bioactive proteins (growth factors)	Bone morphogenetic proteins	Infuse (Medtronic)
Combination graft	Allograft, xenograft, or ceramic/synthetic grafts plus bioactive protein	PepGen P-15 (Dentsply)

NA, not applicable.

Membranes frequently require support so that the membrane does not collapse into the defect itself. Support for the membrane may be provided by using either a titanium-tented membrane or a graft material. Graft materials have two main functions: *(1)* to act as a mechanical substructure that supports the membrane and the overlying soft tissues, and *(2)* to serve as a biologic component that enhances bone formation. Bone graft materials (Table 15-2) can be categorized as osteoconductive or osteoinductive. An osteoconductive material provides a framework into which bone can grow. The pore size of the material is similar to that of normal bone, and the material eventually is absorbed and remodeled. An osteoinductive material stimulates the production of new bone cells such that healing occurs more quickly. The bone morphogenetic protein family has been investigated extensively for use in this role. A combination of osteoconductive and osteoinductive materials also can be used for bone grafts.

Indications for RTs and GBR

- Large lesions > 10 mm
- Through-and-through lesions
- Apicomarginal defects

If GTR techniques are to be used during periradicular surgery, a resorbable membrane should be chosen and a protocol followed (see Video 15-7).

Technique

1. The membrane is extended to cover 2 to 3 mm of bone peripheral to the margins of the crypt; it should be supported with a bone substitute graft material so that it does not collapse into the crypt or onto underlying tooth structures.
2. Tissue closure techniques should ensure total tissue coverage of the membrane. The traditional postoperative compression is eliminated, because this would collapse the membrane onto the underlying structures.

Smoking is contraindicated with GTR techniques because it has consistently been shown to adversely affect the outcome.[86–89]

The use of GTR techniques raises several additional issues that should be discussed with the patient before surgery. These include the cost of the additional material, the origin of the material (synthetic, animal, or human), the need to manage the wound for a longer period, and potential postoperative complications related specifically to these techniques and materials. Discussion of the composition of the materials to be used is very important, because some patients may have concerns based on religious or ethical grounds. The surgeon must discuss all the ramifications of using these materials with the patient before beginning the procedure, because it is not always possible to predict before surgery when grafting materials may be needed.

References

1. Lemon RR. Furcation perforation management: Classic and new concepts. In: Hardin JF (ed). Clark's Clinical Dentistry. Philadelphia: JB Lippincott, 1990:1–15.
2. Lemon RR. Nonsurgical repair of perforation defects. Internal matrix concept. Dent Clin North Am 1992;36:439–457.
3. Simon JH, Kelly WH, Gordon DG, Ericksen GW. Extrusion of endodontically treated teeth. J Am Dent Assoc 1978;97:17–23.
4. Lemon RR. Simplified esthetic root extrusion techniques. Oral Surg Oral Med Oral Pathol 1982;54:93–99.
5. Suprabha BS, Kundabala M, Subraya M, Kancherla P. Reattachment and orthodontic extrusion in the management of an incisor crown-root fracture: A case report. J Clin Pediatr Dent 2006;30:211–214.
6. Dean JW, Lenox RA, Lucas FL, Culley WL, Himel VT. Evaluation of a combined surgical repair and guided tissue regeneration technique to treat recent root canal perforations. J Endod 1997;23:525–532.
7. American Association of Endodontists. An Annotated Glossary of Terms Used in Endodontics, ed 8. Chicago: American Association of Endodontists, 2015.
8. Torabinejad M, Dinsbach N, Turman M, Handysides R, Bahjri K, White S. Survival of intentionally replanted teeth and implant-supported single crowns: A systemic review. J Endod 2015;41:992–998.
9. Miller HM. Transplantation: A case report. J Am Dent Assoc 1950;40:237.
10. Tsukiboshi M. Autogenous tooth transplantation: A reevaluation. Int J Periodontics Restorative Dent 1993;13:120–149.
11. Andreasen JO, Paulsen HU, Yu Z, Bayer T, Schwartz O. A long-term study of 370 autotransplanted premolars. Part II. Tooth survival and pulp healing subsequent to transplantation. Eur J Orthod 1990;12:14–24.
12. Langer B, Stein S, Wagenberg B. An evaluation of root resections. A ten-year study. J Periodontol 1981;52:719–722.
13. Green EN. Hemisection and root amputation. J Am Dent Assoc 1986;112:511–518.
14. Carnevale G, Di Febo G, Tonelli MP, Marin C, Fuzzi M. A retrospective analysis of the periodontal-prosthetic treatment of molars with interradicular lesions. Int J Periodontics Restorative Dent 1991;11:189–205.
15. Basten CH, Ammons WF Jr, Persson R. Long-term evaluation of root-resected molars: A retrospective study. Int J Periodontics Restorative Dent 1996;16:206–219.
16. Fugazzotto PA. A comparison of the success of root resected molars and molar position implants in function in a private practice: Results of up to 15-plus years. J Periodontol 2001;72:1113–1123.
17. Park SY, Shin SY, Yang SM, Kye SB. Factors influencing the outcome of root-resection therapy in molars: A 10-year retrospective study. J Periodontol 2009;80:32–40.
18. Silness J. Periodontal conditions in patients treated with dental bridges. II. The influence of full and partial crowns on plaque accumulation, development of gingivitis and pocket formation. J Periodontal Res 1970;5:219–224.
19. Bader JD, Rozier RG, McFall WT, Ramsey DL. Effect of crown margins on periodontal conditions in regularly attending patients. J Prosthet Dent 1991;65:75–79.
20. Bader JD, Rozier RG, McFall WT. The effect of crown receipt on measures of gingival status. J Dent Res 1991;70:1386–1389.
21. Newcomb G. The relationship between the location of subgingival crown margins and gingival inflammation. J Periodontol 1974;45:151–154.
22. Silness J. Periodontal conditions in patients treated with dental bridges. III. The relationship between location of the crown margin and the periodontal condition. J Periodontal Res 1970;5:225–229.
23. Orkin DA, Reddy J, Bradshaw D. The relationship of the position of crown margins to gingival health. J Prosthet Dent 1987;57:421–424.
24. Renggli H, Regolati B. Gingival inflammation and plaque accumulation by well adapted supragingival and sub-gingival proximal restorations. Helv Odontol Acta 1972;16:99–101.
25. Block PL. Restorative margins and periodontal health: A new look at an old perspective. J Prosthet Dent 1987;57:683–689.
26. Maynard JG, Wilson RD. Physiologic dimensions of the periodontium significant to restorative dentists. J Periodontol 1979;50:170–174.
27. Vacek JS, Gher ME, Assad DA, Richardson AC, Giambarresi LI. The dimensions of the human dentogingival junction. Int J Periodontics Restorative Dent 1994;14:155–165.
28. Gunay, H. Seeger A, Tschernitchek H, Geurtsen W. Placement of the preparation line and periodontal health—A prospective 2 year clinical study. Int J Periodontics Restorative Dent 2000;20:171–181.
29. Tarnow DP, Magner AW, Fletcher P. The effect of the distance from the contact point to the crest of bone on the presence or absence of the interproximal dental papilla. J Periodontol 1992;63:995–996.
30. de Waal H, Castellucci G. The importance of restorative margin placement to the biologic width and periodontal health. Part II. Int J Periodontics Restorative Dent 1994;14:70–83.
31. Valderhaug J. A 15-year clinical evaluation of fixed prosthodontics. Act Odontol Scan 1991;49:35–40.
32. Ingber JS, Rose LF, Coslet JG. The "biologic width"—A concept in periodontics and restorative dentistry. Alpha Omegan 1977;70:62–65.
33. Gargiulo A, Wentz F, Orban B. Dimensions and relations of the dentogingival junction in humans. J Periodontol 1961;32:261–267.
34. Simeone P, Leofreddi G, Kois JC. Managing severe periodontal esthetic challenges: The restorative-surgical connection. Int J Periodontics Restorative Dent 2016;36:83–93.
35. van der Velden U. Regeneration of the interdental soft tissues following denudation procedures. J Clin Periodontol 1982;9:455–459.
36. Carnevale G, Sterrantino SF, Di Febo G. Soft and hard tissue wound healing following tooth preparation to the alveolar crest. Int J Periodontics Restorative Dent 1983;3(6):36–53.
37. Oakley E, Rhyu IC, Karatzas S, Gandini-Santiago L, Nevins M, Caton J. Formation of the biologic width following crown lengthening in nonhuman primates. Int J Periodontics Restorative Dent 1999;19:529–541.
38. Davarpanah M, Jansen CE, Vidjak FM, Etienne D, Kebir M, Martinez H. Restorative and periodontal considerations of short clinical crowns. Int. J Periodontics Restorative Dent 1998;18:424–433.
39. Hohlt WF. Orthodontic crown lengthening. J Indiana Dent Assoc 1992;71(6):24–27.
40. Berglundh T, Marinello CP, Lindhe J, Thilander B, Liljenberg B. Periodontal tissue reactions to orthodontic extrusion. An experimental study in the dog. J Clin Periodontol 1991;18:330–336.
41. Rosenberg ES, Garber DA, Evlan C. Tooth lengthening procedures. Compend Contin Educ Dent 1980;1:161–172.
42. Becker W, Ochsenbein C, Becker BE. Crown lengthening: The periodontal-restorative connection. Compend Contin Educ Dent 1998;19:239–246.
43. Fugazzotto P. Periodontal restorative interrelationships: The isolated restoration. J Am Dent Assoc 1985;110:915–917.
44. Smukler H, Chaibi M. Periodontal and dental considerations in clinical crown extension: A rational basis for treatment. Int J Periodontics Restorative Dent 1997;17:464–477.
45. Pilalas I, Tsalikis L, Tatakis DN. Pre-restorative crown lengthening surgery outcomes: A systematic review. J Clin Periodontol 2016;43:1094–1108.
46. Moghaddam AS, Radafshar G, Taramsari M, Darabi F. Long-term survival rate of teeth receiving multidisciplinary endodontic, periodontal and prosthodontic treatments. J Oral Rehabil 2014;41:236–242.
47. Heithersay GS. Combined endodontic-orthodontic treatment of transverse root fractures in the region of the alveolar crest. Oral Surg Oral Med Oral Pathol 1973;36:404–415.
48. Ingber JS. Forced eruption. I. A method of treating isolated one and two wall infrabony osseous defects-rationale and case report. J Periodontol 1974;45:199–206.
49. Ingber JS. Forced eruption: Part II. A method of treating non-restorable teeth: Periodontal and restorative considerations. J Periodontol 1976;47:203–216.
50. Ingber JS. Forced eruption: Alteration of soft tissue cosmetic deformities. Int J Periodontics Restorative Dent 1989;9:416–425.
51. Simon JH. Vertical movement of endodontically treated roots. In: Cohen S, Burns RC (eds). Pathways of the Pulp, ed 1. St. Louis: Mosby, 1976.

52. Simon JH, Kelly WH, Gordon DG, Ericksen GW. Extrusion of endodontically treated teeth. J Am Dent Assoc 1978;97:17–23.
53. Lythgoe JR, Torabinejad M, Simon JH. Extrusion techniques for the general dentist. J Acad Gen Dent 1980;28:42–49.
54. Simon JH. Root extrusion. Rationale and techniques. Dent Clin North Am 1984; 28:909–921.
55. Pontoriero R, Celenza F Jr, Ricci G, Carnevale G. Rapid extrusion with fiber resection: A combined orthodontic-periodontic treatment modality. Int J Periodontics Restorative Dent 1987;7(5):30–43.
56. Chien M, Patel R. Immediate surgical extrusion. In: Schwartz RS, Canakapalli V (eds). Best Practices in Endodontics: A Desk Reference. Chicago: Quintessence, 2015:275–281.
57. Kim SH, Tramontina VA, Ramos CM, Prado AM, Passanezi E, Greghi SL. Experimental surgical and orthodontic extrusion of teeth in dogs. Int J Periodontics Restorative Dent 2009;29:435–443
58. Deng Y, Zhu X, Yang J, Jiang H, Yan P. The effect of regeneration techniques on periapical surgery with different protocols for different lesion types: A meta-analysis. J Oral Maxillofac Surg 2016;74:239–246
59. Kim S, Kratchman S. Modern endodontic surgery concepts and practice: A review. J Endod 2006;32:601–623.
60. Dietrich T, Zunker P, Dietrich D, Bernimoulin JP. Apicomarginal defects in periradicular surgery: Classification and diagnostic aspects. Oral Surg Oral Med Oral Pathol Oral Radiol Endod 2002;94:233–239.
61. Hirsch JM, Ahlström U, Henrikson PA, Heyden G, Peterson LE. Periapical surgery, Int J Oral Surg 1979;8:173–185.
62. Kim E, Song JS, Jung IY, Lee SJ, Kim S. Prospective clinical study evaluating endodontic microsurgery outcomes for cases with lesions of endodontic origin compared with cases with lesions of combined periodontal-endodontic origin. J Endod 2008;34:546–551.
63. Skoglund A, Persson G. A follow-up study of apicoectomized teeth with total loss of the buccal bone plate. Oral Surg Oral Med Oral Pathol 1985;59:78–81.
64. Rud J, Andreasen JO, Jensen JF. A multivariate analysis of the influence of various factors upon healing after endodontic surgery. Int J Oral Surg 1972;1:258–271.
65. Goyal B, Tewari S, Duhan J, Sehgal PK. Comparative evaluation of platelet-rich plasma and guided tissue regeneration membrane in the healing of apicomarginal defects: A clinical study. J Endod 2011;37:773–780.
66. Tsesis I, Rosen E, Tamse A, Taschieri S, Del Fabbro M. Effect of guided tissue regeneration on the outcome of surgical endodontic treatment: A systematic review and meta-analysis. J Endod 2011;37:1039–1045.
67. Dahlin C, Gottlow J, Linde A, Nyman S. Healing of maxillary and mandibular bone defects using a membrane technique: An experimental study in monkeys. Scand J Plast Reconstr Surg Hand Surg 1990;24:13–19.
68. Dahlin C, Linde A, Gottlow J, Nyman S. Healing of bone defects by guided tissue regeneration. Plast Reconstr Surg 1988;81:672–676.
69. Douthitt JC, Gutmann JL, Witherspoon DE. Histologic assessment of healing after the use of a bioresorbable membrane in the management of buccal bone loss concomitant with periradicular surgery. J Endod 2001;27:404–410.
70. Abramowitz PN, Rankow H, Trope M. Multidisciplinary approach to apical surgery in conjunction with the loss of buccal cortical plate. Oral Surg Oral Med Oral Pathol 1994;77:502–506.
71. Artzi Z, Wasersprung N, Weinreb M, Steigmann M, Prasad HS, Tsesis I. Effect of guided tissue regeneration on newly formed bone and cementum in periapical tissue healing after endodontic surgery: An in vivo study in the cat. J Endod 2012;38:163–169.
72. Brugnami F, Mellonig JT. Treatment of a large periapical lesion with loss of labial cortical plate using GTR: A case report. Int J Periodontics Restorative Dent 1999;19:243–249.
73. Danesh-Meyer MJ. Guided tissue regeneration in the management of severe periodontal-endodontic lesions. N Z Dent J 1999;95(419):7–10.
74. Duggins LD, Clay JR, Himel VT, Dean JW. A combined endodontic retrofill and periodontal guided tissue regeneration technique for the repair of molar endodontic furcation perforations: Report of a case. Quintessence Int 1994;25:109–114.
75. Kellert M, Chalfin H, Solomon C. Guided tissue regeneration: An adjunct to endodontic surgery. J Am Dent Assoc 1994;125:1229–1233.
76. Mastromihalis N, Goldstein S, Greenberg M, Friedman S. Applications for guided bone regeneration in endodontic surgery. N Y State Dent J 1999;65:30–32.
77. Pompa DG. Guided tissue repair of complete buccal dehiscences associated with periapical defects: A clinical retrospective study. J Am Dent Assoc 1997;128:989–997.
78. Rankow HJ, Krasner PR. Endodontic applications of guided tissue regeneration in endodontic surgery. Oral Health 1996;86:33–40.
79. Taschieri S, Corbella S, Tsesis I, Bortolin M, Del Fabbro M. Effect of guided tissue regeneration on the outcome of surgical endodontic treatment of through-and-through lesions: A retrospective study at 4-year follow-up. Oral Maxillofac Surg 2011;15:153–159.
80. Tseng CC, Harn WM, Chen YH, Huang CC, Yuan K, Huang PH. A new approach to the treatment of true-combined endodontic-periodontic lesions by the guided tissue regeneration technique. J Endod 1996;22:693–696.
81. Uchin RA. Use of a bioresorbable guided tissue membrane at an adjunct to bony regeneration in cases requiring endodontic surgical intervention. J Endod 1996;22:94–96.
82. Zubery Y, Kozlovsky A. Two approaches to the treatment of true combined periodontal-endodontal lesions. J Endod 1993;19:414–416.
83. Pecora G, Kim S, Celletti R, Davarpanah M. The guided tissue regeneration principle in endodontic surgery: One-year postoperative results of large periapical lesions. Int Endod J 1995;28:41–46.
84. Dietrich T, Zunker P, Dietrich D, Bernimoulin JP. Periapical and periodontal healing after osseous grafting and guided tissue regeneration treatment of apicomarginal defects in periradicular surgery: Results after 12 months. Oral Surg Oral Med Oral Pathol Oral Radiol Endod 2003;95:474–482.
85. Garrett K, Kerr M, Hartwell G, O'Sullivan S, Mayer P. The effect of a bioresorbable matrix barrier in endodontic surgery on the rate of periapical healing: An in vivo study. J Endod 2002;28:503–506.
86. Bowers GM, Schallhorn RG, McClain PK, Morrison GM, Morgan R, Reynolds MA. Factors influencing the outcome of regenerative therapy in mandibular Class II furcations: Part I. J Periodontol 2003;74:1255–1268.
87. Machtei EE, Oettinger-Barak O, Peled M. Guided tissue regeneration in smokers: Effect of aggressive anti-infective therapy in Class II furcation defects. J Periodontol 2003;74:579–584.
88. Trombelli L, Kim CK, Zimmerman GJ, Wikesjo UM. Retrospective analysis of factors related to clinical outcome of guided tissue regeneration procedures in intrabony defects. J Clin Periodontol 1997;24:366–371.
89. Trombelli L, Scabbia A. Healing response of gingival recession defects following guided tissue regeneration procedures in smokers and non-smokers. J Clin Periodontol 1997;24:529–533.

Chapter Sixteen

Pharmacology in Surgical Endodontics

Karl Keiser

The drugs used as adjuncts to endodontic surgery include anxiolytics, analgesics, antibiotics, and local anesthetics. Chapter 8 already provided a very thorough discussion of local anesthetics, so this chapter covers the science of preoperative anxiolytics and pre- and postoperative analgesics and antibiotics. The indications, pharmacodynamics (what the drug does to the body), and pharmacokinetics (what the body does to the drug) of each drug are reviewed, along with recommended dosages, efficacy, and toxicology.

Anxiolytics

Indications

The words *root canal* have long been associated with a painful and unpleasant experience in spite of advances in local anesthesia and endodontic technique. Add the word *surgery*, and the potential exists for a very anxious patient. It is generally accepted that the higher the level of preoperative anxiety, the higher the pain level reported by the patient after a noxious stimulus.[1–4] Preoperative anxiety not only makes the patient more difficult to manage, but it can actually lead to the patient remembering the experience as negative, even as much as 18 months after the procedure.[5] Therefore, it is essential that the clinician do as much as practical to identify and reduce patient anxiety. While a caring chairside manner is helpful,[6] sometimes pharmacologic assistance is needed, although risk management dictates that only those patients who are truly in need of pharmacologic anxiolysis should be considered before medications are prescribed or dispensed. Risk management also dictates that the providing clinician be well trained in enteral conscious sedation, that appropriate monitoring equipment be utilized, and that reversal agents be readily available. The entire dental team should be well coached in emergency preparedness.[7]

In order to identify patients in need of anxiety-reducing medications, the clinician may consider using a simple questionnaire, such as a version of the Modified Dental Anxiety Scale,[8] along with taking a careful dental history at the evaluation appointment.

Choice of drugs

Benzodiazepines

Mechanism of action. As a class, benzodiazepines act to decrease anxiety by binding to inhibitory neurotransmitter receptors in the central nervous system (CNS) that are directly activated by the amino acid gamma-aminobutyric acid (GABA). Other effects include muscle relaxation, anterograde amnesia, and anticonvulsant activity. Respiratory depression is not typically seen with hypnotic doses in normal patients, unless they have ingested another CNS depressant, most commonly alcohol.[9]

Several benzodiazepines are available for oral administration; those most studied for use in dental procedures are diazepam (trade name Valium [Roche]) and triazolam (Halcion [Pharmacia]). Because of its short half-life (2.9 hours),[9] triazolam is ideally suited for endodontic surgery. Compared with oral diazepam, oral triazolam was found to provide significantly better reduction in anxiety with fewer side effects in a randomized clinical trial of 79 nonsurgical endodontic patients.[10] In an oral surgery model (third molar extractions), oral triazolam was as effective as intravenous diazepam, with less psychomotor impairment and better ambulatory function.[11] Oral triazolam has also been shown to have an effect on medical patients' total pain experience, including reduction of fear and decreased memory of the procedure as painful.[12]

Pharmacokinetics. Benzodiazepines are completely absorbed and are primarily metabolized by microsomal enzymes in the liver (most notably the cytochrome P450, CYP3A4) and excreted in the urine after glucuronidation. Both diazepam and triazolam have active metabolites, but the major metabolite of triazolam (α-hydroxytriazolam) is short acting.

Benzodiazepines have high lipid-water distribution coefficients, and this suggests the possibility of absorption through oral mucous membranes. In fact, the bioavailability and peak plasma concentration of triazolam have been shown to be significantly increased by sublingual administration, with peak plasma concentration occurring at 1.22 hours.[13] This is likely due to increased absorption and avoidance of first-pass metabolism in the liver. In a randomized clinical trial with an oral surgery model, sublingual triazolam provided greater anxiolysis and less overall pain perception than oral triazolam due to increased plasma concentrations.[14]

Patients should be cautioned against taking any oral benzodiazepine with grapefruit juice. Grapefruit juice contains furanocoumarins that have been shown to inhibit the activity of CYP3A4 and thus slow the breakdown of these drugs.[15–17] Ingesting the juice along with a benzodiazepine will therefore increase systemic exposure to the drug and prolong its effects.

Caution should also be exercised in using benzodiazepines in the elderly and in those patients with liver disease due to prolonged effects. HIV-positive individuals who are taking antiretroviral drugs including protease inhibitors may see a doubling of plasma concentration of triazolam and increased duration due to inhibition of CYP3A4.[18] Triazolam is contraindicated in pregnant women due to potential teratogenicity and should be avoided during breastfeeding, as it does cross into breast milk and newborns are less able to metabolize benzodiazepines.[9]

Dosing: Triazolam. Triazolam was developed as a soporific agent for patients with insomnia, with a recommended dosage of 0.25 mg, not to exceed 0.5 mg. In a placebo-controlled randomized clinical trial, 0.125 mg, 0.25 mg, and 0.5 mg oral triazolam were compared prior to impacted third molar surgery. The 0.25-mg dose provided more consistent anxiolysis than the 0.125-mg dose and better patient cooperation than the 0.5-mg dose.[11]

A sublingual dose of 0.25 mg can be given 1 hour prior to the procedure with the patient in the operatory. Continuous monitoring of blood oxygen saturation, heart rate, and respiratory rate should be initiated at this time. Blood pressure should be monitored at 5-minute intervals (this can be automated). At about 45 minutes, the patient can be reassessed, and if further sedation is indicated, additional triazolam can be given sublingually. To avoid oversedation, the clinician may consider the addition of nitrous oxide instead of extra triazolam (see below). For an excellent review of multidose enteral sedation, see Dionne et al.[7]

Reversal agent. Released for use in 1991, flumazenil (Romazicon [Roche]) is an imidazobenzodiazepine that antagonizes the actions of benzodiazepines by competitively inhibiting binding at the GABA-benzodiazepine receptor complex.[9] It is available for intravenous administration (the starting dose is 0.2 mg); it is ineffective as an oral agent due to extensive first-pass hepatic metabolism. Administration by way of intramuscular, subcutaneous, and sublingual routes was successful in reversing respiratory depression in dogs,[19] but these have not been extensively studied in humans.

The half-life of flumazenil is approximately 1 hour, so there is a possibility of resedation. Should this occur, repeated doses of 0.1 mg can be given at 20-minute intervals.

Nitrous oxide

Mechanism of action. Nitrous oxide (N_2O), was synthesized by Joseph Priestley in 1776; its potential as an anesthetic agent was brought to the attention of the public by the dentist Horace Wells in 1844, when he had one of

his own teeth extracted painlessly while under the influence of the gas.[20] It is now widely known for its analgesic, anxiolytic, and anesthetic properties. Its mechanism(s) of action, however, remain unclear. Animal studies suggest that the antinociceptive properties of N_2O are mediated by the release of endogenous opioids, specifically dynorphin and methionine enkephalin.[21] The anxiolytic effects of N_2O are thought to be related to a benzodiazepine-like mechanism via GABA receptors.[22] As an anesthetic, N_2O by itself would require concentrations that would create hypoxia; therefore, it is typically used during general anesthesia to reduce the minimum alveolar concentration of a second inhalation agent and to enhance analgesia.[23]

Pharmacokinetics. N_2O has very low solubility in blood and adipose tissues, so it equilibrates swiftly and enters the brain quickly for a rapid onset of action. It has very little effect on cardiovascular and respiratory function, and its potency is increased with concomitant administration of other sedatives; therefore, a lower concentration may suffice. This is especially true in the elderly.[24]

Almost no biotransformation of N_2O occurs after inhalation; it is eliminated in expired gases, making it an ideal agent in an outpatient setting. An added benefit during triazolam sedation is the increase in blood oxygen saturation, and it has also been shown to prevent gagging during dental procedures.[25,26]

Dosing and precautions. Because of its rapid onset, patients can be easily titrated to a desired level of anxiolysis. Starting with 30% N_2O/70% oxygen allows the patient to begin to appreciate its effects; then, if necessary, the concentration can be increased to 50% N_2O/50% oxygen. Because it is given at high concentrations, abruptly discontinuing N_2O can lead to diffusion hypoxia, as the expired gas dilutes available oxygen in the alveoli. This can be prevented by providing 100% oxygen near the end of the procedure.[24] N_2O should not be used in patients with severe chronic obstructive pulmonary diseases (COPD) such as severe chronic bronchitis or severe emphysema. If used in patients with mild to moderate COPD, the flow rate should be reduced to 3 L/minute, and a doubling of the induction and recovery times are likely.[27] Recent middle/inner ear surgery and retinal surgery are contraindications to the use of N_2O due to the possibility of expansion of damaging gas bubbles.[24]

Training and record keeping

As previously mentioned, it is imperative that the clinician who employs enteral conscious sedation in the practice of endodontic surgery receive the proper training and licensing and transfer the appropriate information to his or her staff. The dental board of each state has specific regulations regarding the education and training necessary prior to the provision of oral sedation in the clinical setting. The practitioner is referred to his or her respective state board for detailed information.

It is also critically important to create a time-oriented sedation record for each patient procedure. The requirements may vary from state to state but should minimally include:

- Baseline vital signs, including height and weight
- Review of medical history with complete American Society of Anesthesiologists Classification, airway classification, drug allergies, and any medications that the patient may be taking
- Attachment of the patient to monitors
- Administration of oral sedative in the dental chair; dosage and time
- N_2O administration, if used; include maximum dose, duration start and stop time, and clearance with 100% oxygen
- Local anesthesia administration
- Periodic vital signs (blood pressure, pulse, oxygen saturation, and respiratory rate); check state regulations for required intervals
- How the patient tolerated the procedure and instructions given
- Clinician's name and all staff present

This record should be clear to anyone who reads it as to what was done, when it was done, and who was present at the time.

Analgesics

Indications

Predicting which patients will experience pain following endodontic surgery, and the intensity of that pain, can be challenging. Several studies have attempted to quantify the prevalence and degree of pain following endodontic surgery and to identify predisposing factors; however, great variation exists in the procedures, the way pain is assessed and reported, as well as in the use of perioperative medications. Isolated studies have suggested increased postoperative pain reports in females,[28,29] in patients who smoke tobacco with poor oral hygiene,[30] in patients with a previous acute apical abscess,[31] and in longer-duration surgeries on multiple teeth.[32] While there is no consensus as to predisposing factors, there is general agreement that postoperative pain following endodontic surgery is most likely to occur the evening following the procedure and may persist for the first 24 to 48 hours.[28–38]

Thus, it is appropriate to consider the use of analgesics in the immediate postoperative period.

Choice of drugs

Nonsteroidal anti-inflammatory drugs (NSAIDs)

Mechanism of action. The anti-inflammatory, antipyretic, and analgesic actions of NSAIDs are thought to be mediated by their ability to inhibit the action of the cyclooxygenase enzymes responsible for the formation of proinflammatory prostaglandins. Sir John Vane is credited with this discovery,[39] in part for which he received the Nobel Prize in Medicine in 1982.

Two isoforms of cyclooxygenase are found in humans, labeled COX-1 and COX-2. COX-1 is constitutively expressed in most cells and catalyzes the formation of prostaglandins that perform many homeostatic functions, including maintenance of the stomach lining, blood flow in the kidneys, and platelet function. COX-2 is inducible by soluble factors such as cytokines, growth factors, and endotoxin and is found primarily at sites of inflammation.[40] NSAIDs that more selectively block the action of COX-1 (such as aspirin) are more likely to cause gastrointestinal side effects, so NSAIDs that are relatively COX-2 selective have been developed. Unfortunately, these were associated with negative cardiac effects, probably due to increased platelet aggregation, and two such drugs—rofecoxib (Vioxx [Merck]) and valdecoxib (Bextra [Pfizer])—have been withdrawn from the market. Celecoxib (Celebrex [Pfizer]) is a COX-2 selective NSAID that is currently available but carries clear labeling about its cardiovascular risk profile.

Several relatively nonselective oral NSAIDs have been evaluated for the treatment of acute pain.[41] Ibuprofen (Motrin [Johnson & Johnson], Advil [Pfizer], and others) and naproxen (Aleve [Bayer], Naprosyn [RPG LS], and others) are the most commonly prescribed NSAIDs in the United States; diclofenac (Voltaren [GlaxoSmithKline] and others) is most commonly prescribed in the United Kingdom.[42] Because of their high COX-1 selectivity and resultant inhibition of platelet activity and increased bleeding, ketoprofen and aspirin are not considered here as appropriate postsurgical analgesics.

Efficacy. A recent overview of 39 Cochrane reviews of randomized, placebo-controlled trials of analgesic efficacy in acute postoperative pain was published by Moore et al in 2015.[43] Comparisons were made using the NNT, the number of patients needed to treat in order to see one additional patient with at least 50% pain reduction compared with placebo. The ideal NNT is 1.0. For NSAIDs currently available in the United States, ibuprofen alone in a fast-acting formulation and ibuprofen in combination with acetaminophen had lower NNTs than naproxen, acetaminophen, and the acetaminophen/opioid combinations (Table 16-1). Additionally, the combination of ibuprofen 400 mg and acetaminophen 1,000 mg provided long-lasting analgesia, with a mean time to remedication of over 8 hours. The combination of ibuprofen and acetaminophen has also been shown to be more effective than either drug alone in an impacted third molar model[44] as well as in the treatment of postendodontic pain.[45]

A recent review of clinical trials comparing fast-acting formulations of ibuprofen with traditional formulations not only showed more rapid absorption and faster initial pain reduction but also suggested longer-lasting analgesia, perhaps due to the prevention of central sensitization.[46]

Pharmacokinetics. In general, NSAIDs have high bioavailability, as they are well absorbed after oral administration with low hepatic clearance.[47] All available NSAIDs are highly bound to plasma proteins and should be used with caution in patients who are taking other medications that are protein bound.[48] An example would be warfarin (Coumadin [Bristol-Myers Squibb]). If a patient is on warfarin and is given ibuprofen, a portion of the warfarin will be displaced from plasma proteins, and its available effective concentration will be increased, leading to increased bleeding.

The half-life of ibuprofen is approximately 2 hours.[42] Mean maximum plasma concentration of fast-acting formulations is reached in 31 to 48 minutes compared with 100 minutes for standard formulations.[46]

Adverse effects/precautions. Because they block the formation of compounds that have a significant role in homeostasis, NSAIDs have the potential to cause a broad range of side effects. These include gastrointestinal complications, renal toxicity, and cardiovascular events. Because they may cause fluid retention, there may also be an exacerbation of hypertension.[42] While these are more likely to occur with long-term use of NSAIDs, in 2014 the US Food and Drug Administration strengthened its warning of potential heart attack and stroke associated with *all* NSAIDs and noted that this could happen as early as the first few weeks of use.[49] They also noted an increased risk with higher doses. Therefore, it is incumbent upon the clinician to use the smallest effective dose with the shortest duration.

NSAIDs should not be used during pregnancy, in patients with known hypersensitivity reactions to NSAIDs or aspirin, in patients with active peptic ulcer disease, or in patients taking anticoagulants. They should be used with caution in patients with asthma, patients with hepatic or renal impairment, and in women who are breastfeeding.[50]

Table 16-1 Analgesics and analgesic combinations listed in descending order of efficacy, based on the NNT

Drug	Dose (mg)	Study participants (n)	NNT	95% confidence interval
Ibuprofen + acetaminophen	400 + 1,000	543	1.5	1.4–1.7
	200 + 500	808	1.6	1.5–1.8
Acetaminophen + oxycodone	1,000 + 10	289	1.8	1.6–2.2
Ibuprofen fast acting	400	1,364	2.1	1.9–2.3
	200	828	2.1	1.9–2.4
Naproxen/naproxen sodium	500/550	784	2.7	2.3–3.3
Acetaminophen	975/1,000	3,232	3.6	3.2–4.1
Acetaminophen + codeine	600/650 + 60	1,413	3.9	3.3–4.7

NNT represents the number of patients that need to be treated with the analgesic for one patient to experience at least 50% pain reduction over 4 to 6 hours in single-dose, randomized, placebo-controlled trials, deemed reliable by the Cochrane Collaboration. The ideal NNT is 1.0. The 95% confidence interval gives the range within which one can be 95% certain contains the mean NNT. (Adapted from Moore et al.[43])

Patients who are taking daily aspirin for its cardioprotective effects should be advised to take the aspirin at least 2 hours before taking ibuprofen, due to ibuprofen's ability to block the binding site of aspirin at the active site of the cyclooxygenase enzyme.[51]

Dosing. As suggested by Table 16-1, recommended dosages are as follows:

- Ibuprofen 400 mg + acetaminophen 1,000 mg every 6 to 8 hours when increased pain is anticipated
- Ibuprofen 200 mg + acetaminophen 500 mg every 4 to 6 hours, or fast-acting ibuprofen 400 mg every 4 to 6 hours, when mild pain is anticipated

Acetaminophen

Mechanism of action/efficacy. Acetaminophen (Tylenol [Johnson & Johnson]), or paracetamol, has been used in medicine since 1893 and has fallen in and out of favor since then. It is currently the most commonly used analgesic worldwide[52] and is recommended by the World Health Organization as a first step in the treatment of all pain conditions.[53] In spite of its widespread use for many years, the mechanism of action of acetaminophen remains unclear. It is becoming generally accepted that it inhibits both COX-1 and especially COX-2 (hence the fewer gastrointestinal side effects), and interestingly, its analgesic effects are reduced by inhibitors of serotonergic, opioid, and cannabinoid systems.[54] Compared with other NSAIDs, however, acetaminophen has weak anti-inflammatory activity.

As can be seen in Table 16-1, the efficacy of acetaminophen alone is not as good as typical NSAIDs (evidenced by higher NNTs), but in combination with ibuprofen, it outperforms even opioid combinations.[43]

Pharmacokinetics. Acetaminophen is widely distributed throughout the body and undergoes very little plasma protein binding. It has a half-life of approximately 2 hours and undergoes extensive conjugation with glucuronic and sulfuric acids (and to a lesser extent cysteine) in the liver, followed by excretion in the urine.[48] A small portion of acetaminophen is hydroxylated by the cytochrome P450 CYP2E1 to form the hepatotoxic metabolite N-acetyl-benzoquinoneimine (NAPQI). NAPQI is normally detoxified by reaction with sulfhydryl groups in glutathione; however, in the presence of large amounts of NAPQI following overdosage of acetaminophen, glutathione levels are depleted, and hepatic necrosis can result.[48]

Adverse effects/precautions. Acetaminophen is generally very well tolerated at therapeutic dosages. The most notable adverse effect is hepatotoxicity, as previously mentioned. Overdose of acetaminophen is the leading cause of acute liver failure in the United States and United Kingdom.[54] Accordingly, the FDA has asked manufacturers to limit the amount of acetaminophen to 325 mg per capsule in prescription drug combination products such as Tylenol with codeine.[55] Patients should be advised to be aware of the acetaminophen content of other over-the-counter medication combinations they may be taking, such as sinus or cold preparations, so as not to exceed the maximum recommended daily dose of 4,000 mg.

The risk of hepatotoxicity is thought to be increased with chronic alcohol abuse due to the increased activity of CYP2E1, which is also partly responsible for the metabolism of ethanol.[56] However, a randomized, placebo-controlled trial of newly abstinent alcoholics showed no elevation in serum markers of hepatic injury when taking 4,000 mg of acetaminophen for 5 days.[57]

Acetaminophen is classified as pregnancy category B and can be safely used in all trimesters.[58] Concerns have recently been raised about a possibly causal link between acetaminophen use during pregnancy and autism spectrum disorder (for review, see Andrade[59]); the safest treatment plan would call for endodontic surgery after delivery.

Dosing. Acetaminophen 1,000 mg every 6 hours may be expected to provide some pain relief after oral surgery, but results could vary. The most predictable pain relief is obtained when 1,000 mg acetaminophen is combined with 400 mg ibuprofen. For patients who cannot take NSAIDs, 1,000 mg acetaminophen can be combined with an opiate for more predictable outcomes.[43]

Opioid analgesics

Mechanism of action/efficacy. Opiates are a group of over 20 natural alkaloids derived from opium and an assortment of semisynthetic congeners.[60] Unlike the anti-inflammatory actions of NSAIDs, opiates act to decrease pain perception by binding to receptors for endogenous ligands that are located on neurons involved in pain-modulating descending pathways.[61] Their value as analgesics, and in the treatment of dysentery, has been appreciated for millennia; however, their use is limited by a variety of adverse effects and the potential for addiction. Oral opiates typically used in the treatment of pain after oral surgery include codeine, hydrocodone, and oxycodone.[43] Several studies using a third molar extraction model have been performed to evaluate the analgesic effects of these drugs; their efficacy in descending order is oxycodone, hydrocodone, and codeine.[43,62,63]

In 2014, the Drug Enforcement Administration rescheduled combination products containing hydrocodone and oxycodone from schedule III to schedule II to combat potential abuse of these drugs. This has resulted in a dramatic increase in the prescription of codeine-containing analgesic combinations.[64]

Pharmacokinetics. Codeine achieves most of its analgesic effects primarily through its transformation to morphine by the cytochrome P450 isozyme CYP2D6. Morphine is then further metabolized to the active compound morphine-6-glucuronide and the inactive morphine-3-glucuronide.[65] Codeine is also metabolized to another active form, codeine-6-glucuronide.[66] Hydrocodone is a prodrug; its analgesic activity is conferred by metabolism via CYP2D6 to the active form, hydromorphone.[67] Oxycodone is primarily metabolized by CYP3A to the inactive moiety noroxycodone.[68]

This information can be used to predict drug-drug interactions with other drugs that are metabolized by or inhibit the activity of these two CYP isozymes. Some examples that may be seen in endodontic patients include fluoxetine (Prozac [Eli Lilly], Sarafem [Eli Lilly]), paroxetine (Paxil [GlaxoSmithKline]), terbinafine (Lamisil [Novartis]), clarithromycin (Biaxin [AbbVie]), diltiazem (Cardizem [Valeant]), fluconazole (Diflucan [Pfizer]), and verapamil (Calan [Pfizer]).[65]

Dosing. Recommended dosages are as follows:

- 10 mg oxycodone with 650 mg acetaminophen for severe pain
- 5 to 10 mg hydrocodone with 650 mg acetaminophen for moderate to severe pain
- 60 mg codeine with 650 mg acetaminophen for moderate pain

Adverse effects/precautions. Opiates have the potential to produce a wide variety of untoward effects, including respiratory depression, nausea, itching, constipation, dizziness, urinary retention, and hypotension.[60]

Because opiates are metabolized by the liver, they should be used with caution in patients with hepatic disease due to increased bioavailability after oral administration.[69] Patients with renal disease may experience increased effects of codeine due to the accumulation of the active metabolite, morphine-6-glucuronide.[60] Negative effects on respiration may be exacerbated by opiates in patients taking other respiratory depressants and in patients with compromised respiratory function, such as those with emphysema.[60] Opioids also produce euphoria in many patients, providing the incentive for abuse, especially in young adults.[70]

Given the host of possible adverse effects, and the recent awareness of the efficacy of ibuprofen/acetaminophen combinations, the clinician would do well to develop the routine practice of avoiding opioid analgesics unless the patient cannot tolerate NSAIDs.

Timing of analgesic administration

The medical literature is replete with papers evaluating the efficacy of preemptive analgesia in attenuating postoperative pain following surgical procedures. This concept was proposed as early as 1913,[71] and advances in neuroscience have provided the theoretical basis that preoperative pain, the afferent barrage of input to the CNS during surgery, and the inflammation that occurs postoperatively all contribute to the hyperexcitability of central components of the pain-processing pathways (for an excellent review, see Katz et al[72]).

While the concept seems plausible, the reports of efficacy vary greatly. A review of the literature by Ong et al[73] evaluated five types of preoperative analgesic interventions: epidural anesthesia, wound infiltration with local anesthetics, N-methyl-D-aspartic acid (NMDA) receptor antagonists, NSAIDs, and opioid analgesics. The outcome measures analyzed were postoperative pain intensity, analgesic consumption, and time to first analgesic consumption. The relevant findings were that preemptive local anesthesia (always provided in endodontic surgery) and preemptive NSAID administration both improved time to first analgesic consumption and total analgesic consumption but did not improve reported postoperative pain. There was also variability depending on the type of surgery provided.

A recent meta-analysis of randomized clinical trials evaluating the effects of preemptive NSAIDs before the surgical removal of third molars under local anesthesia could not show a reduction in postoperative pain; however, the authors noted that there was significant variability in the methodologies of the included studies and called for more careful clinical trials in this area.[74]

Given that the literature is equivocal, if an NSAID or NSAID/acetaminophen analgesic is going to be recommended to the patient following endodontic surgery, having him or her take it 1 hour before the procedure would do no harm and has the potential to have a positive impact on the overall pain experience.

Corticosteroids

Mechanism of action/efficacy

Corticosteroids are steroid hormones released from the adrenal glands in response to stress. Receptors for corticosteroids are found on nearly every cell type, and therefore their actions are wide-ranging. Once bound to the receptor, the steroid-receptor complex has the potential to block several inflammatory pathways both by inducing the transcription of anti-inflammatory proteins and by blocking the transcription of proinflammatory proteins.[75] Because they modulate the immune response, they have been used in the treatment of a variety of inflammatory disorders since the 1940s.[76]

Several studies have evaluated corticosteroids for their potential to prevent pain after nonsurgical endodontic treatment[77–83]; however, there are few randomized, controlled trials examining the possible benefits of these steroids following surgical endodontic therapy. Lin et al[84] found both an NSAID (etodolac 600 mg 2 hours preoperatively and 1 and 2 days after surgery) and a corticosteroid (dexamethasone 8 mg 2 hours preoperatively and 4 mg at days 1 and 2) to be effective at reducing pain after root-end surgery compared with placebo; however, the two drugs were not directly compared.

The third molar surgery model has been used in many studies to evaluate the efficacy of corticosteroids in the prevention of postsurgical pain and swelling. A systematic review by Herrera-Briones et al[85] concluded that preoperative administration of corticosteroids significantly reduces swelling and trismus, and to a lesser extent, pain, following extraction of impacted third molars. In general, parenteral administration was more effective than oral delivery of the drugs. A randomized clinical trial by Grossi et al[86] compared no medication to 4 and 8 mg dexamethasone injected into the buccal vestibule in patients having *one* impacted mandibular third molar removed (most studies using this model have multiple extractions per patient). This model is perhaps closer to the trauma caused by endodontic root-end surgery. Postoperative swelling was significantly reduced in both steroid groups, with no difference between the 4-mg and 8-mg dosages. Postoperative pain was not significantly reduced by the dexamethasone.

In 50% of the studies regarding pain and swelling after endodontic surgery reviewed by Garcia et al,[33] swelling was a factor in patient discomfort for the first 1 to 2 days following the procedure. A single dose of 4 mg dexamethasone injected in the buccal vestibule after administration of local anesthesia and prior to surgery would likely help those patients.

Adverse effects/precautions

Side effects of administered corticosteroids are diverse, ranging from hypertension, hyperglycemia, adrenal insufficiency, and increased risk of infections to cataracts and osteoporosis; however, these are typically associated with long-term use.[75] Corticosteroids are contraindicated in patients with active or incompletely resolved tuberculosis, active viral or fungal infections, and primary glaucoma.[87] Caution should be exercised and medical consultation considered for patients with Cushing syndrome, myasthenia gravis, poorly controlled hypertension or Type I diabetes, renal insufficiency, or peptic ulcers as well as in pregnant patients.[87]

Given that corticosteroids are immunosuppressants, there is some concern that antibiotics should be given concomitantly to avoid postoperative infection. As pointed out by Hargreaves et al,[88] several studies on the use of steroids in conjunction with endodontic procedures in teeth with necrotic pulps and apical periodontitis showed no need for perioperative antibiotics, and there was no association between steroid use and postoperative infections compared with control groups. This was also noted by Sisk and Bonnington in patients following removal of impacted third molars.[89] In the otherwise healthy patient, there does not appear to be a need for antibiotics because of the administration of corticosteroids.

Box 16-1 Cardiac conditions for which antibiotic prophylaxis is recommended

- Prosthetic cardiac valve or cardiac valve repair with prosthetic material
- Previous infective endocarditis
- Congenital heart disease (CHD)
  - Unrepaired cyanotic CHD, including palliative shunts and conduits
  - Completely repaired congenital heart defect with prosthetic material or device, whether placed by surgery or by catheter intervention, during the first 6 months after the procedure
  - Repaired CHD with residual defects at the site or adjacent to the site of a prosthetic patch or prosthetic device
- Cardiac transplantation recipients who develop cardiac valvulopathy

Adapted from Wilson et al.[101]

Antibiotics

Antibiotic stewardship

Prior to considering specific indications for antibiotic therapy before or after endodontic surgery, one must consider the potential abuse of these life-saving drugs. Preceding the introduction of antimicrobials into clinical practice, infectious diseases were the leading cause of morbidity and mortality in the general population.[90] A return to those times via the development of antibiotic-resistant microbes would be disastrous. In his Nobel lecture on December 11, 1945, Sir Alexander Fleming sounded a warning when he noted that it is "not difficult to make microbes resistant to penicillin."[91] Unfortunately, along with an increase in bacterial resistance to antibiotics, there has been a concomitant *decrease* in the discovery of new antibiotics. In fact, from the 1980s to the early 2000s, approval of novel antibiotics decreased by 90%.[92] In 2016, the World Health Organization issued a call for the development of a global action plan to increase awareness of the devastating consequences of microbial resistance and the need for aggressive antibiotic stewardship.[93]

These represent global concerns; local concerns include the possibility of adverse reactions to antibiotics, including life-threatening anaphylaxis. Additionally, clinicians would find themselves in an indefensible position if a patient had an adverse reaction to an antibiotic that was not necessary.

Indications for antibiotics

True indications for the use of antibiotics in an otherwise healthy patient are signs and symptoms of systemic involvement. These include body temperature above 101°F or below 96.8°F, heart rate above 90 beats per minute, respiratory rate above 20 breaths per minute, malaise, rapidly progressive swelling, or cellulitis.[94,95] If these signs or symptoms develop after root-end surgery, then antibiotics should be prescribed. Preoperative use of antibiotics in otherwise healthy patients has not been shown to reduce postoperative infection[96,97] or to enhance long-term healing after endodontic surgery.[98,99]

This discussion is limited to the otherwise healthy patient. There are certain patient populations in which prophylactic antibiotics are indicated and patients for whom perioperative antibiotics should be considered.

Antibiotic prophylaxis

Infective endocarditis

Antibiotic prophylaxis is recommended by the American Heart Association for the prevention of infective endocarditis in patients who are undergoing procedures likely to cause bacteremia and who have a defined cardiac condition. Endodontic surgery is highly likely to cause bacteremia.[100] Cardiac conditions recommended for prophylaxis are listed in Box 16-1.[101] Recommended antibiotic regimens are shown in Box 5-1.[101]

Late prosthetic joint infection

The guidelines for antibiotic prophylaxis in patients undergoing dental procedures who have prosthetic joints are less clear. In 2012, a panel of experts representing the American Academy of Orthopedic Surgeons (AAOS) and the American Dental Association (ADA) undertook a systematic review of the literature and the following year published a clinical practice guideline to address the question of whether patients with prosthetic joints should receive antibiotic prophylaxis prior to dental procedures.[102] With regard to the use of systemic antibiotics, it was recommended that "The practitioner might consider discontinuing the practice of routinely prescribing prophylactic antibiotics for patients with hip and knee prosthetic joint implants undergoing dental procedures."

This was updated in 2014 by a panel of experts convened by the ADA Council on Scientific Affairs in an attempt to clarify the previous guidelines.[103] In the update, four additional studies were reviewed that assessed the relationship between dental procedures likely to produce bacteremia ("high-risk dental procedures") and the development of late prosthetic joint infection (LPJI) of the knee or hip. Three of the four studies showed no relationship between dental procedures and LPJI; the fourth actually showed dental procedures to have a protective effect. Based on its updated review, the 2014 panel gave the following clinical recommendation: "In general, for patients with prosthetic joint implants, prophylactic antibiotics are *not* recommended prior to dental procedures to prevent prosthetic joint infections." They go on to say, however, that "the individual patient's circumstances and preferences should be considered when deciding whether to prescribe prophylactic antibiotics prior to dental procedures." This includes a history of joint replacement with complications, in which case consultation with the patient and his or her orthopedic surgeon should be considered before prescribing prophylactic antibiotics. In such cases, the orthopedic surgeon should take responsibility for the choice of antibiotic and dosage.

For patients who have been identified as needing antibiotic prophylaxis for *any* reason and who are on an existing antibiotic regimen (or who have been on antibiotics within the past 10 days), a different antibiotic should be prescribed for prophylaxis due to the likely presence of newly resistant microorganisms.[101]

Antibiotic considerations for medically compromised patients

HIV-positive patients

In general, patients infected with HIV have not been found to be more susceptible to post–oral surgical infection.[104,105] Patients whose viral load is greater than 30,000 copies/mL[106] or whose CD4+ T-lymphocyte count is less than 200 cells/μL[107] are at higher risk for infection, and perioperative antibiotic therapy should be considered.

Patients with diabetes mellitus

The American Diabetes Association suggests that diabetes may be considered well-controlled if the patient's glycosylated hemoglobin (A1C) is 7% or less. Such patients are not at higher risk for postsurgical infections and do not require antibiotic coverage.[108] Diabetic patients whose disease process is not well-controlled are thought to be more prone to infections and may benefit from antibiotics.[109,110]

Immunosuppressed patients

Reduction of a patient's defensive capacity due to pharmacologic immunosuppression may require the use of antibiotics in the pre- and postsurgical period. Examples include chemotherapeutic agents, long-term corticosteroids, and antirejection drugs following organ transplantation.[110,111]

Patients taking antiresorptive drugs

Patients who are taking antiresorptive drugs for the management of metabolic and metastatic disease of the bone are at some risk for developing antiresorptive agent–induced osteonecrosis of the jaws (ARONJ), especially after dental trauma.[112] An executive summary of recommendations for the management of care for dental patients receiving antiresorptive medications from the ADA Council on Scientific Affairs advises that the same strategies be employed for patients undergoing endodontic surgical procedures as those undergoing any oral and maxillofacial surgical procedures. These include a conservative surgical technique with primary closure, use of a chlorhexidine mouthrinse before and after surgery until the site has healed, and systemic antibiotics beginning 1 day before and continuing 3 to 7 days following surgery.[113]

A medical consultation is always recommended prior to endodontic surgery in medically compromised patients and should include consideration of the potential use of antibiotics. If indicated, antibiotics should be given 2 hours before surgery and continued up to 5 days.[114,115]

General principles of antibiotic dosing

The goal of antibiotic therapy is to assist the temporarily overwhelmed defense mechanisms of the body in controlling pathogenic microorganisms. Because each oral infection is a distinct interaction between the individual host and the causative agents, it is difficult to establish concrete unit dosages, dosing intervals, and duration for relevant antibiotics. According to Pallasch,[116] however, the following general principles can be applied:

- Start with a loading dose that is higher than the maintenance dose.
- Achieve blood levels of the antibiotic that are two to eight times the minimal inhibitory concentration.
- Maintain those levels with frequent dosing intervals.
- Terminate therapy when the infection has resolved.

Patients should be monitored daily to assess their progress. Additionally, if a postsurgical infection occurs with fluctuant area, it should be drained in order to allow penetration of the antibiotic.

Choice of antibiotic/dosing

Beta-lactams

This group shares a beta-lactam ring in their molecular structure and includes penicillin and its derivatives and the cephalosporin and carbapenem classes of antibiotics. Beta-lactam antibiotics exert their bactericidal effect by inhibiting a group of enzymes that are involved in the cross-linking of peptidoglycan during bacterial cell wall synthesis, resulting in cell death due to osmotic instability or autolysis.[117]

Penicillin. Discovered serendipitously in discarded culture plates by Sir Alexander Fleming in 1928, penicillin is a naturally occurring antibiotic synthesized by the fungus *Penicillium chrysogenum*. Its congener, penicillin-VK, is well absorbed after oral administration and widely distributed. It is rapidly eliminated by the kidneys, with a serum half-life of 30 minutes.[118] Most of the bacteria associated with endodontic infections are susceptible to penicillin, and it remains an appropriate first choice for postsurgical infections.[119–123] Because of its short half-life, penicillin-VK should be administered frequently. Adult dosage typically involves a loading dose of 1,000 mg, followed by 500 mg every 4 to 6 hours.[118]

Amoxicillin. First synthesized in 1964, amoxicillin is a semisynthetic penicillin that has a broader spectrum of antibacterial activity than penicillin.[124] It is rapidly absorbed and reaches peak plasma concentration in about 2 hours after oral administration, with a serum half-life of about 1 hour. It is primarily excreted in the urine in an active form. Amoxicillin is also a valid choice for postsurgical infections; however, like penicillin-VK, it is susceptible to inactivation by bacteria that produce beta-lactamase enzymes. Research aimed at finding microorganisms that produce inhibitors of beta-lactamase resulted in the discovery of clavulanic acid, a product of *Streptococcus clavuligerus*. In 1981, the combination of amoxicillin and clavulanic acid was brought to market in the United Kingdom as Augmentin (GlaxoSmithKline).[125] Augmentin has been shown to be effective against microbes isolated from endodontic and dentoalveolar infections.[119,120,122] Adult dosage calls for a loading dose of 1,000 mg, followed by 500 mg every 8 hours.

Cephalosporins. The first cephalosporins were isolated in 1948 from the fungus *Cephalosporium acremonuim* found near a sewer outlet on the coast of Sardinia.[118] While third and fourth generations have activity against gram-positive cocci and gram-negative bacilli, they are also susceptible to beta-lactamase and offer no advantage over the other beta-lactams and would not be considered a drug of first choice for postendodontic surgical infections. For patients allergic to penicillin, cephalosporins have been proposed as an alternative for prophylaxis against infective endocarditis.[101] There is some concern about cross-reactivity between penicillin and cephalosporins (it has been estimated at 10%), but recent findings suggest that the likelihood is about 1%.[126]

Lincosamides

This class of antibiotics originates from lincomycin, a naturally occurring antibiotic isolated from the bacterium *Streptococcus lincolnensis* found in a soil sample in Lincoln, Nebraska. It includes lincomycin, clindamycin, and pirlimycin. Of the three, clindamycin has relevance in the treatment of odontogenic infections.

Clindamycin. Clindamycin is almost completely absorbed after oral administration and reaches peak plasma concentrations within an hour, regardless of the presence of food in the stomach, with a plasma half-life of approximately 3 hours. Inactivation of clindamycin occurs by metabolism to N-demethylclindamycin and clindamycin sulfoxide in the liver; excretion occurs in urine and bile.[127] It exerts its antibacterial activity by binding to the 50S subunit of bacterial ribosomes and thus prevents protein synthesis. Clindamycin has activity against many aerobic, anaerobic, and beta-lactamase–producing bacteria and would be a good choice for postsurgical infections.[120,128,129] Adult dosage is a 600-mg loading dose followed by 300 mg every 6 hours.

A historical concern with the use of oral clindamycin has been the overgrowth of *Clostridium difficile* in the colon and the development of pseudomembranous colitis. A review of the literature shows that the antibiotic-associated occurrence of *C difficile* infection is rare in outpatient settings, and clindamycin poses no greater risk than amoxicillin.[130]

Macrolides

The first commercially available macrolide, erythromycin, was isolated from *Streptomyces erythrus* in the 1950s. Macrolides act by reversibly binding to the 50S ribosomal subunit of susceptible bacteria and preventing protein synthesis and are primarily bacteriostatic. Because erythromycin is not well tolerated and has poor activity against anaerobes associated with odontogenic infection, particularly *Fusobacterium*, it would not be an appropriate choice for postsurgical infections.[131] The semisynthetic derivatives azithromycin and clarithromycin have a broader spectrum of antimicrobial activity and are better tolerated, but the emergence of macrolide-resistant microbes limits the use of these agents to patients who cannot tolerate more suitable antibiotics.

Nitroimidazoles

The nitroimidazoles are derivatives of azomycin, an antiprotozoal compound isolated from extracts of *Streptomyces* spp in 1955. Metronidazole, a synthetic derivative, was found by accident to have antibacterial activity when a patient being treated for trichomonad vaginitis was also cured of a bacterial gingivitis.[132] It is completely absorbed after oral administration and has a plasma half-life of about 8 hours. A disulfram-like effect has been reported, and patients should be cautioned against consuming alcohol along with this antibiotic.

Metronidazole is effective against many anaerobic bacteria, including *Bacteroides*, but is ineffective against aerobic and facultatively anaerobic bacteria; thus, it is not a good choice for odontogenic infections when used alone.[133] It has been recommended in combination with amoxicillin for the treatment of periodontal infections[134] and may be considered for patients who are not responding to a beta-lactam antibiotic during postsurgical infection. A better choice would be to switch to either clindamycin or Augmentin.

Conclusion

Hopefully the reader has found this chapter to be a useful tool when considering the use of adjunctive drugs for endodontic surgery patients. Because of the ever-changing landscape of commercial pharmacology, it would be wise to remain vigilant of new developments via the published medical literature. Helpful websites include the following:

- PubMed of the US National Library of Medicine: https://www.ncbi.nlm.nih.gov/pubmed
- Cochrane Database of Systematic Reviews: http://www.cochranelibrary.com/cochrane-database-of-systematic-reviews/

References

1. Maggirias J, Locker D. Psychological factors and perceptions of pain associated with dental treatment. Community Dent Oral Epidemiol 2002;30:151–159.
2. Klages U, Ulusoy O, Kianifard S, Wehrbein H. Dental trait anxiety and pain sensitivity as predictors of expected and experienced pain in stressful dental procedures. Eur J Oral Sci 2004;112:477–483.
3. Peters ML. Emotional and cognitive influences on pain experience. Mod Trends Pharmacopsychiatri 2015;30:138–152.
4. Janssen SA, Arntz A. Anxiety and pain: Attentional and endorphinergic influences. Pain 1996;66:145–50.
5. Gedney JJ, Logan H, Baron RS. Predictors of short-term and long-term memory of sensory and affective dimensions of pain. J Pain 2003;4(2):47–55.
6. Jepsen CH. Chairside manner. Where clinical dentistry meets behavioral science. Dentistry 1987;7(3):7–12.
7. Dionne RA, Yagiela JA, Coté CJ, et al. Balancing efficacy and safety in the use of oral sedation in dental outpatients. J Am Dent Assoc 2006;137:502–513.
8. Humphris GM, Morrison T, Lindsay SJ. The Modified Dental Anxiety Scale: Validation and United Kingdom norms. Community Dent Health 1995;12:143–150.
9. Hobbs W, Rall T, Verdoorn T. Hypnotics and sedatives: ethanol, In: Hardman J, Limbard LE, eds. Goodman and Gilman's The Pharmacological Basis of Therapeutics, ed 9. New York: McGraw-Hill, 1996:362–373.
10. Ehrich DG, Lundgren JP, Dionne RA, Nicoll BK, Hutter JW. Comparison of triazolam, diazepam, and placebo as outpatient oral premedication for endodontic patients. J Endod 1997;23:181–184.
11. Kaufman E, Hargreaves KM, Dionne RA. Comparison of oral triazolam and nitrous oxide with placebo and intravenous diazepam for outpatient premedication. Oral Surg Oral Med Oral Pathol 1993;75:156–164.
12. Fabian TJ, Schwartzman DS, Ujhelyi MR, et al. Decreasing pain and anxiety associated with patient-activated atrial shock: A placebo-controlled study of adjunctive sedation with oral triazolam. J Cardiovasc Electrophysiol 2006;17:391–395.
13. Scavone JM, Greenblatt DJ, Friedman H, Shader RI. Enhanced bioavailability of triazolam following sublingual versus oral administration. J Clin Pharmacol 1986;26:208–210.
14. Berthold CW, Dionne RA, Corey SE. Comparison of sublingually and orally administered triazolam for premedication before oral surgery. Oral Surg Oral Med Oral Pathol Oral Radiol Endod 1997;84:119–124.
15. Paine MF, Widmer WW, Hart HL, et al. A furanocoumarin-free grapefruit juice establishes furanocoumarins as the mediators of the grapefruit juice-felodipine interaction. Am J Clin Nutr 2006;83:1097–1105 [erratum 2006 Jul;84:264].
16. Lilja JJ, Kivistö KT, Backman JT, Neuvonen PJ. Effect of grapefruit juice dose on grapefruit juice-triazolam interaction: Repeated consumption prolongs triazolam half-life. Eur J Clin Pharmacol 2000;56:411–415.
17. Hukkinen SK, Varhe A, Olkkola KT, Neuvonen PJ. Plasma concentrations of triazolam are increased by concomitant ingestion of grapefruit juice. Clin Pharmacol Ther 1995;58:127–131.
18. Greenblatt DJ, von Moltke LL, Harmatz JS, et al. Differential impairment of triazolam and zolpidem clearance by ritonavir. J Acquir Immune Defic Syndr 2000;24:129–136.
19. Heniff MS, Moore GP, Trout A, Cordell WH, Nelson DR. Comparison of routes of flumazenil administration to reverse midazolam-induced respiratory depression in a canine model. Acad Emerg Med 1997;4:1115–1118.
20. Kennedy S, Longnecker D. History and principles of anesthesiology. In: Hardman J, Limbard LE, eds. Goodman and Gilman's The Pharmacological Basis of Therapeutics, ed 9. New York: McGraw-Hill, 1996:295–306.
21. Emmanouil DE, Dickens AS, Heckert RW, et al. Nitrous oxide-antinociception is mediated by opioid receptors and nitric oxide in the periaqueductal gray region of the midbrain. Eur Neuropsychopharmacol 2008;18:194–199.
22. Emmanouil DE, Quock RM. Advances in understanding the actions of nitrous oxide. Anesth Prog 2007;54:9–18.
23. Hornbein TF, Eger EI 2nd, Winter PM, Smith G, Wetstone D, Smith KH. The minimum alveolar concentration of nitrous oxide in man. Anesth Analg 1982;61:553–556.
24. Becker DE, Rosenberg M. Nitrous oxide and the inhalation anesthetics. Anesth Prog 2008;55(4):124–130.
25. Packer ME, Joarder C, Lall BA. The use of relative analgesia in the prosthetic treatment of the 'gagging' patient. Dent Update 2005;32:544–550.
26. Chidiac JJ, Chamseddine L, Bellos G. Gagging prevention using nitrous oxide or table salt: A comparative pilot study. Int J Prosthodont 2001;14:364–366.
27. Vichitvejpaisal P, Joshi GP, Liu J, White PF. Effect of severity of pulmonary disease on nitrous oxide washin and washout characteristics. J Med Assoc Thai 1997;80:378–383.
28. Christiansen R, Kirkevang LL, Hørsted-Bindslev P, Wenzel A. Patient discomfort following periapical surgery. Oral Surg Oral Med Oral Pathol Oral Radiol Endod 2008;105:245–250.
29. Iqbal MK, Kratchman SI, Guess GM, Karabucak B, Kim S. Microscopic periradicular surgery: Perioperative predictors for postoperative clinical outcomes and quality of life assessment. J Endod 2007;33:239–244.
30. García B, Penarrocha M, Martí E, Gay-Escodad C, von Arx T. Pain and swelling after periapical surgery related to oral hygiene and smoking. Oral Surg Oral Med Oral Pathol Oral Radiol Endod 2007;104:271–276.
31. Seymour RA, Meechan JG, Blair GS. Postoperative pain after apicoectomy. A clinical investigation. Int Endod J 1986;19:242–247.
32. Penarrocha M, Garcia B, Marti E, Balaguer J. Pain and inflammation after periapical surgery in 60 patients. J Oral Maxillofac Surg 2006;64:429–433.
33. García B, Larrazabal C, Peñarrocha M, Peñarrocha M. Pain and swelling in periapical surgery. A literature update. Med Oral Patol Oral Cir Bucal 2008;13(11):E726–E729.

34. Del Fabbro M, Ceresoli V, Lolato A, Taschieri S. Effect of platelet concentrate on quality of life after periradicular surgery: A randomized clinical study. J Endod 2012;38:733–739.
35. Chong BS, Pitt Ford TR. Postoperative pain after root-end resection and filling. Oral Surg Oral Med Oral Pathol Oral Radiol Endod 2005;100:762–766.
36. Tsesis I, Fuss Z, Lin S, Tilinger G, Peled M. Analysis of postoperative symptoms following surgical endodontic treatment. Quintessence Int 2003;34:756–760.
37. Kvist T, Reit C. Results of endodontic retreatment: A randomized clinical study comparing surgical and nonsurgical procedures. J Endod 1999;25:814–817.
38. Peñarrocha-Diago M, Maestre-Ferrín L, Peñarrocha-Oltra D, Gay-Escoda C, von-Arx T, Peñarrocha-Diago M. Pain and swelling after periapical surgery related to the hemostatic agent used: anesthetic solution with vasoconstrictor or aluminum chloride. Med Oral Patol Oral Cir Bucal 2012;17(4):e594–e600.
39. Vane JR. Inhibition of prostaglandin synthesis as a mechanism of action for aspirin-like drugs. Nat New Biol 1971;231(25):232–235.
40. Smith WL. Prostanoid biosynthesis and mechanisms of action. Am J Physiol 1992;263(2 pt 2):F181–F191.
41. Richards D. The Oxford Pain Group League table of analgesic efficacy. Evid Based Dent 2004;5:22–23.
42. Conaghan PG. A turbulent decade for NSAIDs: Update on current concepts of classification, epidemiology, comparative efficacy, and toxicity. Rheumatol Int 2012;32:1491–1502.
43. Moore RA, Derry S, Aldington D, Wiffen PJ. Single dose oral analgesics for acute postoperative pain in adults—An overview of Cochrane reviews. Cochrane Database Syst Rev 2015;(9):CD008659.
44. Mehlisch DR, Aspley S, Daniels SE, Southerden KA, Christensen KS. A single-tablet fixed-dose combination of racemic ibuprofen/paracetamol in the management of moderate to severe postoperative dental pain in adult and adolescent patients: A multicenter, two-stage, randomized, double-blind, parallel-group, placebo-controlled, factorial study. Clin Ther 2010;32:1033–1049.
45. Menhinick KA, Gutmann JL, Regan JD, Taylor SE, Buschang PH. The efficacy of pain control following nonsurgical root canal treatment using ibuprofen or a combination of ibuprofen and acetaminophen in a randomized, double-blind, placebo-controlled study. Int Endod J 2004;37:531–541.
46. Moore RA, Derry S, Straube S, Ireson-Paine J, Wiffen PJ. Faster, higher, stronger? Evidence for formulation and efficacy for ibuprofen in acute pain. Pain 2014; 155:14–21.
47. Day RO, Graham GG, Williams KM. Pharmacokinetics of non-steroidal anti-inflammatory drugs. Baillieres Clin Rheumatol 1988;2:363–393.
48. Insel P. Analgesic-antipyretic and anti-inflammatory agents and drugs employed in the treatment of gout. In: Hardman J, Limbard LE, eds. Goodman and Gilman's The Pharmacological Basis of Therapeutics, ed 9. New York: McGraw-Hill, 1996:617–639.
49. US Food & Drug Administration. FDA Drug Safety Communication: FDA strengthens warning that non-aspirin nonsteroidal anti-inflammatory drugs (NSAIDs) can cause heart attacks or strokes. http://www.fda.gov/Drugs/DrugSafety/ucm451800.htm. Published 9 July 2015, accessed 17 January 2017.
50. Bushra R, Aslam N. An overview of clinical pharmacology of Ibuprofen. Oman Med J 2010;25(3):155–161.
51. Catella-Lawson F, Reilly MP, Kapoor SC, et al. Cyclooxygenase inhibitors and the antiplatelet effects of aspirin. N Engl J Med 2001;345:1809–1817.
52. Ennis ZN, Dideriksen D, Vaegter HB, Handberg G, Pottegård A. Acetaminophen for chronic pain: A systematic review on efficacy. Basic Clin Pharmacol Toxicol 2016;118:184–189.
53. World Health Organization. WHO's cancer pain ladder for adults. www.who.int/cancer/palliative/painladder/en/. Accessed 17 January 2017.
54. Graham GG, Davies MJ, Day RO, Mohamudally A, Scott KF. The modern pharmacology of paracetamol: therapeutic actions, mechanism of action, metabolism, toxicity and recent pharmacological findings. Inflammopharmacology 2013;21: 201–232.
55. US Food & Drug Administration. Acetaminophen information. www.fda.gov/acetaminophen. Last updated 13 April 2016, accessed 17 January 2017.
56. Zakhari S. Overview: How is alcohol metabolized by the body? National Institute on Alcohol Abuse and Alcoholism. http://pubs.niaaa.nih.gov/publications/arh294/245-255.htm. Accessed 17 January 2017.
57. Dart RC, Green JL, Kuffner EK, Heard K, Sproule B, Brands B. The effects of paracetamol (acetaminophen) on hepatic tests in patients who chronically abuse alcohol—A randomized study. Aliment Pharmacol Ther 2010;32:478–486.
58. Servey J, Chang J. Over-the-counter medications in pregnancy. Am Fam Physician 2014;90:548–555.
59. Andrade C. Use of acetaminophen (paracetamol) during pregnancy and the risk of attention-deficit/hyperactivity disorder in the offspring. J Clin Psychiatry 2016; 77(3):e312–e314.
60. Reisine T, Pasternak G. Opioid analgesics and antagonists. In: Hardman J, Limbard LE, eds. Goodman and Gilman's The Pharmacological Basis of Therapeutics, ed 9. New York: McGraw-Hill, 1996:521–556.
61. Al-Hasani R, Bruchas MR. Molecular mechanisms of opioid receptor-dependent signaling and behavior. Anesthesiology 2011;115:1363–1381.
62. Forbes JA, Bates JA, Edquist IA, et al. Evaluation of two opioid-acetaminophen combinations and placebo in postoperative oral surgery pain. Pharmacotherapy 1994;14:139–146.
63. Litkowski LJ, Christensen SE, Adamson DN, Van Dyke T, Han SH, Newman KB. Analgesic efficacy and tolerability of oxycodone 5 mg/ibuprofen 400 mg compared with those of oxycodone 5 mg/acetaminophen 325 mg and hydrocodone 7.5 mg/acetaminophen 500 mg in patients with moderate to severe postoperative pain: A randomized, double-blind, placebo-controlled, single-dose, parallel-group study in a dental pain model. Clin Ther 2005;27:418–429.
64. Seago S, Hayek A, Pruszynski J, Newman MG. Change in prescription habits after federal rescheduling of hydrocodone combination products. Proc (Bayl Univ Med Cent) 2016;29:268–270.
65. Overholser BR, Foster DR. Opioid pharmacokinetic drug-drug interactions. Am J Manag Care 2011;17(11, suppl):276S–287S.
66. Vree TB, van Dongen RT, Koopman-Kimenai PM. Codeine analgesia is due to codeine-6-glucuronide, not morphine. Int J Clin Pract 2000;54:395–398.
67. Hutchinson MR, Menelaou A, Foster DJ, Coller JK, Somogyi AA. CYP2D6 and CYP3A4 involvement in the primary oxidative metabolism of hydrocodone by human liver microsomes. Br J Clin Pharmacol 2004;57:287–297.
68. Smith HS. Opioid metabolism. Mayo Clin Proc 2009;84:613–624.
69. Soleimanpour H, Safari S, Shahsavari Nia K, Sanaie S, Alavian SM. Opioid drugs in patients with liver disease: A systematic review. Hepat Mon 2016;16(4):e32636.
70. Drazdowski TK. A systematic review of the motivations for the non-medical use of prescription drugs in young adults. Drug Alcohol Depend 2016;162:3–25.
71. Crile G. The kinetic theory of shock and is prevention through anoci-assosication (shockless operation). Lancet 1913;185:7–16.
72. Katz J, Clarke H, Seltzer Z. Review article: Preventive analgesia: Quo vadimus? Anesth Analg 2011;113:1242–1253 [erratum 2011;113:1475].
73. Ong CK, Lirk P, Seymour RA, Jenkins BJ. The efficacy of preemptive analgesia for acute postoperative pain management: A meta-analysis. Anesth Analg 2005; 100:757–773.
74. Costa FW, Esses DF, de Barros Silva PG, et al. Does the preemptive use of oral nonsteroidal anti-inflammatory drugs reduce postoperative pain in surgical removal of third molars? A meta-analysis of randomized clinical trials. Anesth Prog 2015;62(2):57–63.
75. Rhen T, Cidlowski JA. Antiinflammatory action of glucocorticoids—New mechanisms for old drugs. N Engl J Med 2005;353:1711–1723.
76. Cruz-Topete D, Cidlowski JA. One hormone, two actions: Anti- and pro-inflammatory effects of glucocorticoids. Neuroimmunomodulation 2015;22:20–32.
77. Marshall JG, Walton RE. The effect of intramuscular injection of steroid on post-treatment endodontic pain. J Endod 1984;10:584–588.
78. Krasner P, Jackson E. Management of posttreatment endodontic pain with oral dexamethasone: A double-blind study. Oral Surg Oral Med Oral Pathol 1986; 62:187–190.
79. Liesinger A, Marshall FJ, Marshall JG. Effect of variable doses of dexamethasone on posttreatment endodontic pain. J Endod 1993;19:35–39.
80. Mehrvarzfar P, Shababi B, Sayyad R, Fallahdoost A, Kheradpir K. Effect of supraperiosteal injection of dexamethasone on postoperative pain. Aust Endod J 2008;34:25–29.
81. Pochapski MT, Santos FA, de Andrade ED, Sydney GB. Effect of pretreatment dexamethasone on postendodontic pain. Oral Surg Oral Med Oral Pathol Oral Radiol Endod 2009;108:790–795.
82. Jalalzadeh SM, Mamavi A, Shahriari S, Santos FA, Pochapski MT. Effect of pretreatment prednisolone on postendodontic pain: A double-blind parallel-randomized clinical trial. J Endod 2010;36:978–981.
83. Shantiaee Y, Mahjour F, Dianat O. Efficacy comparison of periapical infiltration injection of dexamethasone, morphine and placebo for postoperative endodontic pain. Int Dent J 2012;62(2):74–78.
84. Lin S, Levin L, Emodi O, Abu El-Naaj I, Peled M. Etodolac versus dexamethasone effect in reduction of postoperative symptoms following surgical endodontic treatment: A double-blind study. Oral Surg Oral Med Oral Pathol Oral Radiol Endod 2006;101:814–817.
85. Herrera-Briones FJ, Prados Sánchez E, Reyes Botella C, Vallecillo Capilla M. Update on the use of corticosteroids in third molar surgery: Systematic review of the literature. Oral Surg Oral Med Oral Pathol Oral Radiol 2013;116(5):e342–e351.
86. Grossi GB, Maiorana C, Garramone RA, et al. Effect of submucosal injection of dexamethasone on postoperative discomfort after third molar surgery: A prospective study. J Oral Maxillofac Surg 2007;65:2218–2226.

87. Alexander RE, Throndson RR. A review of perioperative corticosteroid use in dentoalveolar surgery. Oral Surg Oral Med Oral Pathol Oral Radiol Endod 2000; 90:406–415.
88. Hargreaves KM, Reader A, Nusstein JM, Marshall JG, Gibbs JL. Pharmacologic management of endodontic pain. In: Ingle JI, Bakland L, Baumgartner JC (eds). Ingle's Endodontics, ed 6. Hamilton, Ontario: BC Decker, 2008:713–736.
89. Sisk AL, Bonnington GJ. Evaluation of methylprednisolone and flurbiprofen for inhibition of the postoperative inflammatory response. Oral Surg Oral Med Oral Pathol [illegible]
90. Aminov R. History of antimicrobial drug discovery—Major classes and health impact [epub ahead of print 5 October 2016]. Biochem Pharmacol doi:10.1016/j.bcp.2016.10.001.
91. Fleming A. Penicillin. In: Nobel Foundation. Nobel Lectures: Physiology or Medicine, 1942–1962. Amsterdam: Elsevier, 1964:83–93.
92. Luepke KH, Suda KJ, Boucher H, et al. Past, present, and future of antibacterial economics: Increasing bacterial resistance, limited antibiotic pipeline, and societal implications. Pharmacotherapy 2017;37:71–84.
93. Goff DA, Kullar R, Goldstein EJ, et al. A global call from five countries to collaborate in antibiotic stewardship: United we succeed, divided we might fail. Lancet Infect Dis 2017;17:e56–e63.
94. Mayo Clinic staff. Sepsis. Mayo Clinic Patient Care & Health Information: Diseases & Conditions. http://www.mayoclinic.org/diseases-conditions/sepsis/symptoms-causes/dxc-20169787. Last updated 16 January 2016, accessed 17 January 2017.
95. Baumgartner JC, Rosenberg PA, Hoen MM, Lin LM. Treatment of endodontic infections, cysts, and flare-ups. In: Ingle JI, Bakland L, Baumgartner JC (eds). Ingle's Endodontics, ed 6. Hamilton, Ontario: BC Decker, 2008:690–712.
96. Lindeboom JA, Frenken JW, Valkenburg P, van den Akker HP. The role of preoperative prophylactic antibiotic administration in periapical endodontic surgery: A randomized, prospective double-blind placebo-controlled study. Int Endod J 2005;38:877–881.
97. Moreno-Drada JA, García-Perdomo HA. Effectiveness of antimicrobial prophylaxis in preventing the spread of infection as a result of oral procedures: A systematic review and meta-analysis. J Oral Maxillofac Surg 2016;74:1313–1321.
98. von Arx T, Peñarrocha M, Jensen S. Prognostic factors in apical surgery with root-end filling: A meta-analysis. J Endod 2010;36:957–973.
99. von Arx T, Jensen SS, Hänni S. Clinical and radiographic assessment of various predictors for healing outcome 1 year after periapical surgery. J Endod 2007; 33:123–128.
100. Baumgartner JC, Heggers JP, Harrison JW. Incidence of bacteremias related to endodontic procedures. II. Surgical endodontics. J Endod 1977;3:399–402.
101. Wilson W, Taubert KA, Gewitz M, et al; American Heart Association. Prevention of infective endocarditis: Guidelines from the American Heart Association: A guideline from the American Heart Association Rheumatic Fever, Endocarditis and Kawasaki Disease Committee, Council on Cardiovascular Disease in the Young, and the Council on Clinical Cardiology, Council on Cardiovascular Surgery and Anesthesia, and the Quality of Care and Outcomes Research Interdisciplinary Working Group. J Am Dent Assoc 2008;139(suppl):3S–24S [erratum 2008; 139:253].
102. Rethman MP, Watters W 3rd, Abt E, et al; American Academy of Orthopaedic Surgeons; American Dental Association. The American Academy of Orthopaedic Surgeons and the American Dental Association clinical practice guideline on the prevention of orthopaedic implant infection in patients undergoing dental procedures. J Bone Joint Surg Am 2013;95:745–747.
103. Sollecito TP, Abt E, Lockhart PB, et al. The use of prophylactic antibiotics prior to dental procedures in patients with prosthetic joints: Evidence-based clinical practice guideline for dental practitioners—A report of the American Dental Association Council on Scientific Affairs. J Am Dent Assoc 2015;146:11–16.e8.
104. Robinson PG, Cooper H, Hatt J. Healing after dental extractions in men with HIV infection. Oral Surg Oral Med Oral Pathol 1992;74:426–430.
105. Porter SR, Scully C, Luker J. Complications of dental surgery in persons with HIV disease. Oral Surg Oral Med Oral Pathol 1993;75:165–167.
106. Horberg MA, Hurley LB, Klein DB, et al. Surgical outcomes in human immunodeficiency virus-infected patients in the era of highly active antiretroviral therapy. Arch Surg 2006;141:1238–1245.
107. Abalo A, Patassi A, James YE, Walla A, Sangare A, Dossim A. Risk factors for surgical wound infection in HIV-positive patients undergoing surgery for orthopaedic trauma. J Orthop Surg (Hong Kong) 2010;18:224–227.
108. McKenna SJ. Dental management of patients with diabetes. Dent Clin North Am 2006;50:591–606.
109. Peterson LJ. Antibiotic prophylaxis against wound infections in oral and maxillofacial surgery. J Oral Maxillofac Surg 1990;48:617–620.
110. Sancho-Puchades M, Herráez-Vilas JM, Berini-Aytés L, Gay-Escoda C. Antibiotic prophylaxis to prevent local infection in oral surgery: Use or abuse? Med Oral Patol Oral Cir Bucal 2009;14(1): E28–E33.
111. Guggenheimer J, Eghtesad B, Stock DJ. Dental management of the (solid) organ transplant patient. Oral Surg Oral Med Oral Pathol Oral Radiol Endod 2003;95: 383–389.
112. Uyanne J, Calhoun CC, Le AD. Antiresorptive drug-related osteonecrosis of the jaw. Dent Clin North Am 2014;[illegible].
113. Hellstein JW, Adler RA, Edwards B, et al; American Dental Association Council on Scientific Affairs Expert Panel on Antiresorptive Agents. Managing the care of patients receiving antiresorptive therapy for prevention and treatment of osteoporosis: Executive summary of recommendations from the American Dental Association Council on Scientific Affairs. J Am Dent Assoc 2011;142:1243–1251.
114. Paluzzi RG. Antimicrobial prophylaxis for surgery. Med Clin North Am 1993;77: 427–441.
115. Ren YF, Malmstrom HS. Effectiveness of antibiotic prophylaxis in third molar surgery: A meta-analysis of randomized controlled clinical trials. J Oral Maxillofac Surg 2007;65:1909–1921.
116. Pallasch TJ. Pharmacokinetic principles of antimicrobial therapy. Periodontol 2000 1996;10:5–11.
117. Kong KF, Schneper L, Mathee K. Beta-lactam antibiotics: From antibiosis to resistance and bacteriology. APMIS 2010;118:1–36.
118. Mandell G, Petri W. Antimicrobial agents. Penicillins, cephalosporins and other Beta-lactam antibiotics. In: Hardman J, Limbard LE, eds. Goodman and Gilman's The Pharmacological Basis of Therapeutics, ed 9. New York: McGraw-Hill, 1996: 987–1008.
119. Baumgartner JC, Xia T. Antibiotic susceptibility of bacteria associated with endodontic abscesses. J Endod 2003;29:44–47.
120. Kuriyama T, Williams DW, Yanagisawa M, et al., Antimicrobial susceptibility of 800 anaerobic isolates from patients with dentoalveolar infection to 13 oral antibiotics. Oral Microbiol Immunol 2007;22:285–288.
121. Lang PM, Jacinto RC, Dal Pizzol TS, Ferreira MB, Montagner F. Resistance profiles to antimicrobial agents in bacteria isolated from acute endodontic infections: Systematic review and meta-analysis. Int J Antimicrob Agents 2016;48:467–474.
122. Khemaleelakul S, Baumgartner JC, Pruksakorn S. Identification of bacteria in acute endodontic infections and their antimicrobial susceptibility. Oral Surg Oral Med Oral Pathol Oral Radiol Endod 2002;94:746–755.
123. Holmes CJ, Pellecchia R. Antimicrobial therapy in management of odontogenic infections in general dentistry. Dent Clin North Am 2016;60:497–507.
124. Rolinson GN, Geddes AM. The 50th anniversary of the discovery of 6-aminopenicillanic acid (6-APA). Int J Antimicrob Agents 2007;29:3–8.
125. Geddes AM, Klugman KP, Rolinson GN. Introduction: Historical perspective and development of amoxicillin/clavulanate. Int J Antimicrob Agents 2007;30(2 suppl):109S–112S.
126. Lee QU. Use of cephalosporins in patients with immediate penicillin hypersensitivity: Cross reactivity revisited. Hong Kong Med J 2014;20:428–436.
127. Kapusnik-Uner J, Sande M, Chambers H. Antimicrobial agents. Tetracyclines, chloramphenicol, erythromycin and miscellaneous antibacterial agents. In: Hardman J, Limbard LE, eds. Goodman and Gilman's The Pharmacological Basis of Therapeutics. New York: McGraw-Hill, 1996:1123–1153.
128. Kuriyama T, Karasawa T, Nakagawa K, Saiki Y, Yamamoto E, Nakamura S. Bacteriologic features and antimicrobial susceptibility in isolates from orofacial odontogenic infections. Oral Surg Oral Med Oral Pathol Oral Radiol Endod 2000;90: 600–608.
129. Tancawan AL, Pato MN, Abidin KZ, et al. Amoxicillin/clavulanic acid for the treatment of odontogenic infections: A randomised study comparing efficacy and tolerability versus clindamycin. Int J Dent 2015;2015:472470.
130. Brook I, Lewis MA, Sándor GK, Jeffcoat M, Samaranayake LP, Vera Rojas J. Clindamycin in dentistry: More than just effective prophylaxis for endocarditis? Oral Surg Oral Med Oral Pathol Oral Radiol Endod 2005;100:550–558.
131. Shweta, Prakash SK. Dental abscess: A microbiological review. Dent Res J (Isfahan) 2013;10:585–591.
132. Samuelson J. Why metronidazole is active against both bacteria and parasites. Antimicrob Agents Chemother 1999;43:1533–1541.
133. Tracy J, Webster L. Drugs used in the chemotherapy of protozoal infections. In: Hardman J, Limbard LE, eds. Goodman and Gilman's The Pharmacological Basis of Therapeutics, ed 9. New York: McGraw-Hill, 1996:987–1008.
134. Sgolastra F, Gatto R, Petrucci A, Monaco A. Effectiveness of systemic amoxicillin/metronidazole as adjunctive therapy to scaling and root planing in the treatment of chronic periodontitis: A systematic review and meta-analysis. J Periodontol 2012;83:1257–1269.

Chapter Seventeen

Outcomes of Endodontic Surgery

Thomas von Arx, Shane N. White

Retaining teeth that have been afflicted by inflammation or infection arising from disease of pulpal origin or trauma provides esthetics, comfort, and function for patients. Initial nonsurgical root canal treatment (NSRCT) and restoration aim to eliminate and permanently exclude bacteria from the root canal system. Sometimes, despite all best efforts, these goals may not be attained. Results from systematic reviews of the outcomes of nonsurgical retreatment and apical surgery, including modern apical microsurgery, suggest that the first-line treatment option after failure of initial NSRCT is nonsurgical retreatment.[1] Nonsurgical retreatment is noninvasive and generally effective, and it addresses intracanal bacteria throughout the entire root canal system, shows increased healing rates over time, and preserves root length.[2] Furthermore, apical surgery has better outcomes if it follows nonsurgical retreatment.[3]

However, a small proportion of nonsurgically re-treated cases will still not heal, likely because some bacteria were still not eliminated or because extracanal bacteria were present.[4] These cases are best addressed by modern apical microsurgery using microscopy, ultrasonic instruments, and current retrofilling materials such as mineral trioxide aggregate (MTA).[1,5] Apical surgery has the ability to address extracanal bacteria. Moreover, some unhealed NSRCT cases are not amenable to nonsurgical retreatment. Therefore, modern apical microsurgery will continue to have an important place in endodontics and tooth retention.

Apical surgery is the most widely used type of endodontic surgery and the primary focus of the endodontic surgical literature. However, it must be remembered that other endodontic surgical procedures can also benefit patients with persistent endodontic problems.[1] Intentional replantation remains a viable alternative to extraction. Autotransplantation has a place, particularly in growing patients with an appropriate donor tooth. Root amputation can be valuable when a severe problem is localized to a single root on an otherwise sound tooth.

The purposes of this chapter are to *(1)* introduce the place of endodontic surgery, *(2)* describe endodontic surgical outcome measures, *(3)* define follow-up times for postsurgical evaluation, *(4)* describe outcomes of apical surgery, *(5)* describe prognostic predictors of apical surgery, and *(6)* concisely summarize endodontic surgical outcomes.

Endodontic Surgical Outcome Measures

Stakeholders, patients, dentists, and third-party payers are deeply vested in surgical success, but perspectives may vary. Patient symptoms, clinical examination, and radiography have formed the basis for the measurement of endodontic surgical outcomes. Apical surgery principally involves three tissues: the root and its periodontal ligament, the alveolar bone, and the soft tissues (gingiva, papillae, and alveolar mucosa). Outcome measures should address all of these tissues. Additionally, the impact of surgery on patient-centered measures, including quality of life, pain, esthetics, and cost, must also be considered.

Clearly, the persistence of pain or other symptoms indicates failure, as do clinical findings indicative of inflammation or infection, such as tenderness to percussion or the presence of a sinus tract. Treated teeth must be without clinical signs and symptoms of reinfection. Traditionally, outcome assessment of apical surgery has been based on two-dimensional radiographic judgment of periapical healing with re-formation of an adequately sized periodontal ligament space at the cut root face and bone formation within the periapical bone defect. Radiographic examination must systematically include analyses of the periodontal ligament space, the continuity of the lamina dura, trabecular patterns, and bone density.[6]

Andreasen and Rud[7] related radiographic findings to histology following endodontic surgery. They characterized healing as a decrease in the extent of rarefaction and noted that persistent scar tissue was characterized by a decrease in the size of a lesion but without complete resolution. They also characterized persistent inflammation as a circular or semicircular radiographic rarefaction more than twice the width of the normal periodontal ligament space, which blends or funnels into the ligament space.

Molven et al[8] described a strategy for classifying endodontic surgical cases into four categories: complete healing, incomplete healing (scar tissue), uncertain healing, and unsatisfactory healing (failure). Their strategy uses reference radiographs and schematic diagrams. This classification system has satisfactory interobserver agreement and remains the most widely used system.

The idea has been advanced that favorable healing may be represented by the persistence of scar tissue or the radiographic appearance of increased width of the periodontal ligament space.[8–10] A study of 24 teeth that were originally classified as incomplete healing at 2 to 6 years postsurgery showed that over time, the vast majority continued to demonstrate a reduction in the size of the rarefaction.

This situation following apical surgery differs from that following NSRCT or nonsurgical retreatment where the apical pathology remains and must resolve itself before it can be replaced by bone. The very nature of apical surgery facilitates swift bone healing. Pathologic apical tissues and inflamed or infected tissues are removed; the crypt is small, surrounded by walls on all four sides, and with only a conservative buccal access. A blood clot forms, which can be quickly turned into bone, and the overlying soft tissue is well supported and stabilized using sutures, all creating a great scenario for healing.

When to Evaluate Healing

A follow-up period of 1 year has long been recommended for assessing endodontic surgery. Halse et al[11] determined that a 1-year follow-up will provide a valid diagnosis for the majority of cases; only a small number of uncertain cases will need additional follow-up. This finding is consistent with that of Burstein et al,[12] who determined that the size of the apical crypt generally decreases by 80% within 1 year. Some additional healing is expected after 1 year.[13] Indeed, late healing over the following decades is possible.[14] Unfortunately, a significant proportion of early successes may revert to failure over time.[2,5,15] Because apical surgery only addresses the apical part of an affected root, not the entire root canal system, it is possible that bacteria may migrate from untreated areas back to the root end. Therefore, a comprehensive 1-year endodontic evaluation including patient history, clinical examination, and radiography of teeth treated through endodontic surgery is required, but additional follow-up should be part of every subsequent comprehensive patient examination.

Apical Surgery Outcomes

This chapter primarily focuses on apical surgery because it is by far the most widely used procedure. Apical surgery is indicated when nonsurgical retreatment has not successfully resolved disease of pulpal origin, or when it is not practicable. With the introduction of microsurgical principles and techniques in the early 1990s, apical surgery was transformed from a traditional to a modern technique. When appraising data on apical surgery outcomes, one must consider the scientific quality of the study, the specific outcome measures used, and the technical procedures and materials used. Apical surgery outcome papers have generally been low-level case series studies; very few randomized clinical trials have been conducted.[16]

Traditional techniques

Hepworth and Friedman[3] provided a literature review of apical surgery studies published up to 1995. They distinguished between apical surgery studies with and without simultaneous orthograde treatment. They calculated weighted success rates of 81% for apical surgery with simultaneous nonsurgical endodontic treatment and just 59% without simultaneous nonsurgical treatment. They noted considerable variation in case selection, treatment procedures, and methodology among the included studies. They explained that many of the included studies already had limited clinical relevance due to subsequent improvements in surgical techniques. Therefore, this chapter focuses on the newer literature.

Newer literature

Apical surgery studies published in English since 1996 are summarized in two distinct tables. Studies where higher magnification (surgical microscope or endoscope) was used are summarized in Table 17-1, and studies without higher magnification are summarized in Table 17-2. Despite considerable variation, studies using higher magnification generally produced higher success rates. The success rates of studies using higher magnification ranged from 67% to 97%; only one study had a success rate below 70% (data of teeth without root-end filling excepted). In contrast, 12 of 36 studies without higher magnification had success rates below 70%, four studies had success rates below 50%, and one study had a success rate as low as 31%.

Tsesis et al[90] performed a meta-analysis of the modern apical surgical literature (magnification, root-end resection with minimal or no bevel, root-end cavity preparation with microtips, and root-end filling). The 1-year-plus success rate was 92%. The authors also reported that age, sex, tooth type, type of root-end filling material, and magnification method had no significant effect on success rates.

Comparison of traditional and modern techniques

Only a few clinical studies have compared the outcome of apical surgery using burs with those using ultrasonic microtips for root-end cavity preparation.[57,60,78,85] All of these studies were performed without higher magnification. Cases treated using microtips always had higher success rates than cases treated using burs (81% to 100% vs 65% to 91%, respectively). In three studies, the same root-end filling material was used in both preparation groups. However, Testori et al[60] filled cavities prepared using burs with amalgam and cavities prepared using microtips with SuperEBA; their outcome may have been influenced by the root-end filling material.

Tsesis et al[22] retrospectively compared the traditional root-end resection technique (a 45-degree bevel using a bur) with a modern technique (resection perpendicular to the long axis of the root using microtip preparation and microscopy). The complete healing rate after a follow-up period of at least 6 months was dramatically higher for cases treated using a modern technique (91%) than a traditional technique (44%).

Setzer et al[91] performed the first meta-analysis to compare traditional root-end surgery (TRS) and endodontic microsurgery (EMS). TRS included no or low magnification (up to 4×) and root-end preparation with burs; EMS used magnification of 10× and higher and microtips for root-end preparation. A total of 12 TRS studies (925 treated teeth) and 9 EMS studies (699 treated teeth) were analyzed. EMS had a pooled weighted success rate of 94%, significantly higher than the 59% success rate for TRS. The probability of success (relative risk ratio) for EMS was 1.6 times higher than that for TRS.

The same group published a second meta-analysis comparing EMS with and without high magnification.[92] They classified studies utilizing microinstruments but no visualization aids (or only loupes) as contemporary root-end surgery (CRS). In contrast, studies applying the surgical operating microscope or endoscope were defined as EMS. Higher magnification produced slightly higher success rates for EMS (94%) than for CRS (88%).

Tsesis et al[93] published a meta-analysis of 18 studies using modern surgical endodontic techniques. A 1-year success rate of 89% was reported. Success rates did not differ between operating microscopes and endoscopes, but both produced significantly higher success rates than loupes. Additionally, MTA resulted in significantly higher success rates than other retrofilling materials.

Comparison of two systematic reviews by Torabinejad et al[2,5] provides robust insight as to the superiority of modern endodontic surgical techniques. The 2009 surgery study of all eligible prior surgeries reported a 2- to 4-year success rate of 78% and a 4- to 6-year success rate of 72%. However, the 2015 study, limited to microsurgery, reported markedly superior 2- to 4-year and 4- to 6-year success rates of 90% and 84%, respectively. For microsurgery, the tooth survival rates were even higher, at 94% and 88% at 2 to 4 years and 4 to 6 years, respectively, indicating that teeth treated using microsurgery may still continue to be lost at low rates over time.

Modern surgical techniques are clearly superior to traditional techniques, and they should be universally adopted for endodontic surgery. However, it is also clear that even with the use of modern microsurgery, treated teeth tend to be lost at low rates over time.

Table 17-1 Outcome studies on apical surgery with higher magnification

Authors (year)	Study type (years when surgeries were done)	Follow-up	Magnification	REF material
Rud et al[17] (1997)	Cohort retrospective (1989–1992)	2–4 years	MSC	Retroplast (no microtips)
Rubinstein and Kim[19] (1999)	Cohort prospective (NA)	1 year	MSC	SuperEBA
Rubinstein and Kim[20] (2002)	Cohort prospective (NA)	5–7 years	MSC	SuperEBA
Taschieri et al[21] (2006)	RCT (2001–2003)	1 year	ESC Loupes	SuperEBA
Tsesis et al[22] (2006)	Clinical retrospective comparative study (2000–2002)	Minimum 6 months	MSC None (naked eye)	IRM IRM (no microtips)
Taschieri et al[23] (2007)	Cohort prospective (2001–2003)	1 year	ESC	SuperEBA
Von Arx et al[24] (2007)	Clinical prospective comparative study (2000–2003)	1 year	ESC	MTA (ProRoot) Retroplast (no microtips) SuperEBA
Kim et al[27] (2008)	Cohort prospective (2001–2005)	6 months–5 years	MSC	IRM, SuperEBA, or MTA (ProRoot)
Saunders[28] (2008)	Cohort prospective (2000–2006)	4 months–6 years (mean 18 months)	MSC	MTA (ProRoot)
Taschieri et al[29] (2008)	RCT (2001–2004)	2 years	ESC MSC	SuperEBA
Christiansen et al[30] (2009)	RCT (2005–2006)	1 year	MSC	MTA (ProRoot) None (only smoothing of existing RCF; no microtips)
Barone et al[32] (2010)	Cohort prospective (1998–2003)	4–10 years	MSC	Various
Von Arx et al[34] (2010)	Clinical prospective comparative study (2001–2007)	1 year	MSC and ESC	MTA (ProRoot) Retroplast (no microtips)
Song et al[36] (2011)	Cohort prospective (2001–2009)	1 year	MSC	MTA (ProRoot) or SuperEBA
Song et al[37] (2011)	Clinical comparative study (2004–2008)	1 year	MSC	MTA (ProRoot) SuperEBA IRM
Song et al[38] (2012)	RCT (2003–2010)	1 year	MSC	MTA (ProRoot) SuperEBA
Song et al[39] (2012)	Cohort prospective (2001–2005)	6–10 years	MSC	IRM, SuperEBA, or MTA (ProRoot)
Von Arx et al[26] (2012)	Clinical prospective comparative study (2000–2003)	5 years	ESC	MTA (ProRoot) Retroplast (no microtips) SuperEBA

➤Studies using a surgical microscope or endoscope, and ultrasonic microtips for root-end preparation, unless otherwise noted.
BC RRM, bioceramic root repair material; EBA, ethoxybenzoic acid; ESC, endoscope; IRM, intermediate restorative material; MSC, microscope; NA, not available; REF, root-end filling; RCF, root-canal filling; RCT, randomized controlled trial.

	N initial (teeth)	N follow-up (teeth)	Drop-out rate	Healing criteria	Success rate	Comments
	*909	*551	39%	Rud et al[18] (1972)	86%	*N refers to roots
	*170	*101	27%	Success = lamina dura restored or healed by scar; asymptomatic and functional	97%	*N refers to roots; long-term data presented in study Rubinstein and Kim[20] (2002)
	*91	*59	35%	Rud et al[18] (1972)	92%	*N refers to roots; includes only successful 1-year cases of study Rubinstein and Kim[19] (1999)
	43	39	9%	Molven et al[8,9] (1987,1996)	95%	$P = .08$; no molars treated
	37	32	14%		91%	
	NA	45	NA	Rud et al[18] (1972),	91%	$P < .0001$
	NA	43	NA	Molven et al[8] (1987)	44%	
	28	27	3%	Molven et al[9] (1996)	78%	Only resurgery cases included
	53	51	4%	Rud et al[18] (1972),	90%	$P > .05$; long-term data
	86	85	1%	Molven et al[8] (1987),	85%	presented in study
	55	55	0%	Zuolo et al[25] (2000)	76%	Von Arx et al[26] (2012)
	263	192	27%	Molven et al[8,9] (1987,1996)	95% for lesions of isolated endodontic origin, 78% for lesions of combined endodontic-periodontal origin	$P < .05$; data not available separately for REF material
	321	276	14%	Halse et al[6] (2002), Halse and Molven[10] (2004)	89%	NA
	50	41	18%	Molven et al[8,9] (1987,1996)	90%	$P = .1$
	63	59	6%		92%	
	26	25	4%	Rud et al[18] (1972),	97%	$P < .001$; long-term data
	26	21	19%	Molven et al[8,9] (1987,1996)	52%	presented in study Kruse et al[31] (2016)
	73	40	45%	Rud et al[18] (1972), Orstavik et al[33] (1986)	72%	NA
	178	173	3%	Rud et al[18] (1972),	91%	$P = .003$; long-term data pre-
	175	166	5%	Molven et al[8,9] (1987,1996)	80%	sented in study Von Arx et al[35] (2014)
	54	42	22%	Molven et al[8,9] (1987,1996)	93%	All cases were resurgery cases; data not available separately for REF material
	NA	214	NA	Molven et al[8,9] (1987,1996)	87%	$P = 0$
	NA	111	NA		86%	
	NA	102	NA		79%	
	130	90	31%	Molven et al[8,9] (1987,1996)	96%	$P = .5$
	130	102	22%		93%	
	172	104	40%	Molven et al[8,9] (1987,1996)	93%	Successful cases of study Kim et al[27] (2008); data not available separately for REF material
	53	44	17%	Rud et al[18] (1972),	*86%	Same material as in study Von
	86	77	11%	Molven et al[8] (1987),	75%	Arx et al[24] (2007); *significant
	55	49	11%	Zuolo et al[25] (2000)	*67%	difference

(cont)

Table 17-1 *(cont)* **Outcome studies on apical surgery with higher magnification**

Authors (year)	Study type (years when surgeries were done)	Follow-up	Magnification	REF material
Kreisler et al[40] (2013)	Cohort retrospective study (2009)	6–12 months (mean 8 months)	Loupes, MSC, or ESC	Various
Song et al[41] (2013)	Clinical prospective comparative study (2001–2011)	1–10 years	MSC	MTA (ProRoot)
				SuperEBA
				IRM
Li et al[42] (2014)	Cohort retrospective (2007–2010)	2 years	MSC	SuperEBA
Lui et al[43] (2014)	Cohort retrospective (1997–2003)	1–2 years	MSC	IRM or MTA (ProRoot)
Song et al[45] (2014)	Cohort retrospective (2004–2007)	1 year	MSC	IRM, SuperEBA, or MTA (ProRoot)
		4–8 years		
Tortorci et al[46] (2014)	Clinical retrospective comparative study (1985–1993)	5 years	MSC	MTA (ProRoot)
	Clinical retrospective comparative study (1993–2005)		None (naked eye)	Amalgam (burs)
Von Arx et al[35] (2014)	Clinical prospective comparative study (2001–2007)	5 years	MSC and ESC	MTA (ProRoot)
				Retroplast (no microtips)
Shinbori et al[47] (2015)	Cohort retrospective (2009–2013)	12–33 months	MSC	BC RRM (endosequence)
Tawil et al[48] (2015)	Cohort prospective (2009–2010)	1 year	MSC	MTA (ProRoot) or SuperEBA
		3 years		
Çalişkan et al[49] (2016)	Cohort prospective (2007–2013)	2–6 years	MSC	MTA (ProRoot)
Kruse et al[31] (2016)	RCT (2005–2006)	6 years	MSC	MTA (ProRoot)
				None (only smoothing of existing RCF; no microtips)

➤Studies using a surgical microscope or endoscope, and ultrasonic microtips for root-end preparation, unless otherwise noted.
BC RRM, bioceramic root repair material; EBA, ethoxybenzoic acid; ESC, endoscope; IRM, intermediate restorative material; MSC, microscope; NA, not available; REF, root-end filling; RCF, root-canal filling; RCT, randomized controlled trial.

N initial (teeth)	N follow-up (teeth)	Drop-out rate	Healing criteria	Success rate	Comments
NA	281	NA	Rud et al[18] (1972), Molven et al[0] (1987)	88%	Multicenter study
NA	150	NA	Molven et al[8,9] (1987,1996)	90%	$P > .05$
NA	186	NA		87%	
NA	8	NA		88%	
116	101	13%	Molven et al[8,9] (1987,1996)	93%	NA
243	93	62%	Rud et al[18] (1972), Friedman[44] (2005)	79%	Data not available separately for REF material
115	105	9%	Rud et al[18] (1972)	91%	Data not available separately for REF material
115	105	9%		88%	
NA	322	NA	Rud et al[18] (1972), Molven et al[8,9] (1987,1996)	96%	$P = .00214$
NA	217	NA		91%	
178	134	25%	Rud et al[18] (1972), Molven et al[8,9] (1987,1996)	93%	$P = .0003$; same material as in study Von Arx et al[34] (2010)
175	137	22%		77%	
113	113	0%	Rud et al[18] (1972), Molven et al[8,9] (1987,1996)	92%	All patients treated in an endodontic private practice
87	77	12%	Rud et al[18] (1972), Molven et al[8,9] (1987,1996)	95%	All patients treated in an endodontic private practice; data not available separately for REF material
87	73	16%		97%	
108	90	17%	Molven et al[8,9] (1987,1996)	80%	Only single-rooted anterior teeth
26	19	27%	Rud et al[18] (1972), Molven et al[8,9] (1987,1996)	84%	$P = .04$; same material as in study Christiansen et al[30] (2009)
26	20	23%		55%	

Table 17-2 Outcome studies on apical surgery without higher magnification

Authors (year)	Study type (years when surgeries were done)	Follow-up	Magnification	REF material
August[50] (1996)	Cohort retrospective (1969–1983)	11–24 years (mean 15 years)	None (naked eye)	Amalgam (no microtips)
Danin et al[51] (1996)	*Cohort prospective (NA)	1 year	NA	GIC (chem fill; no microtips)
Rud et al[52] (1996)	Cohort retrospective (1984)	8–9 years	NA	Retroplast (no microtips)
Rud et al[53] (1996)	Cohort prospective (1990–1992)	1 year	NA	Retroplast (no microtips)
Sumi et al[54] (1996)	Cohort retrospective (1992–1994)	6–36 months	NA	SuperEBA
Jansson et al[56] (1997)	Cohort prospective (1993)	11–16 months (mean 13 months)	NA	GIC (Ketac Silver; no microtips)
Bader and Lejeune[57] (1998)	Clinical prospective comparative study (1992–1993)	1 year	NA	IRM
				IRM (and treatment of exposed dentin with CO_2 laser)
				IRM (no microtips)
				IRM (no microtips and treatment of exposed dentin with CO_2 laser)
Kvist and Reit[58] (1999)	*Cohort prospective (1989–1992)	4 years	NA	Gutta-percha (no microtips)
Testori et al[60] (1999)	Cohort retrospective (1985–1994)	1–6 years (mean 5 years)	NA	Amalgam (no microtips)
				SuperEBA
Von Arx et al[61] (1998)	Cohort prospective (1992–1993)	1 year	None (naked eye)	SuperEBA
Zuolo et al[25] (2000)	Cohort prospective (1992–1993)	1–4 years	NA	IRM
Rahbaran et al[64] (2001)	Cohort retrospective (1990–1995)	Minimum 4 years	NA	Various (no microtips until 1993)
Rud et al[65] (2001)	Cohort prospective (1984–1997)	6 months–13 years	NA	Retroplast (no microtips)
Von Arx et al[66] (2001)	Cohort prospective (NA)	1 year	None (naked eye)	SuperEBA
Jensen et al[67] (2002)	RCT (1996–1999)	1 year	NA	Retroplast (no microtips)
				GIC (Chelon Silver; no microtips)
Chong et al[13] (2003)	RCT (NA)	1 year	NA	MTA
				IRM
		2 years		MTA
				IRM

➤Studies without a surgical microscope or endoscope; microtips were used for root-end preparation unless otherwise noted.
EBA, ethoxybenzoic acid; GIC, glass-ionomer cement; IRM, intermediate restorative material; NA, not available; REF, root-end filling; RCT, randomized controlled trial.

N initial (teeth)	N follow-up (teeth)	Drop-out rate	Healing criteria	Success rate	Comments
220	41	81%	Authors' own criteria	*63%	*Refers to 26 teeth (remaining tooth only had apicoectomy without root-end filling)
19	19	0%	Rud et al[18] (1972)	58%	*Data extracted from RCT comparing surgical and nonsurgical retreatment; no molars included
*34	33	3%	Rud et al[18] (1972)	97%	*First cases treated with Retroplast and showing complete healing after 1 year
*561	*351	37%	Rud et al[18] (1972)	82%	*N refers to roots
NA	157	NA	Amagasa et al[55] (1989)	92%	NA
NA	59	NA	Authors' own criteria	31%	Only single-rooted teeth included
80	NA	NA	Authors' own criteria	95%	NA
80	NA	NA		90%	
80	NA	NA		65%	
80	NA	NA		68%	
47	NA	NA	Reit and Gröndahl[59] (1983)	60%	*Data extracted from RCT comparing surgical and nonsurgical retreatment; only incisors and canines treated
NA	207 apices	NA	Rud et al[18] (1972)	68%	The total evaluated teeth was N = 181
NA	95 apices	NA		85%	
50	43	14%	Zetterqvist et al[62] (1991), Jesslén et al[63] (1995)	82%	NA
114	102	11%	Molven et al[8,9] (1987, 1996)	91%	All cases treated in private practice
NA	83	NA	Authors' own criteria	37%	Only data extracted from patients treated in the endodontic unit
639	520	19%	Rud et al[18] (1972)	92%	Only mandibular molars included; cases considered healed after 6–18 months were no longer recalled and were transferred from early recall to final healing
56	55	2%	Zetterqvist et al[62] (1991), Jesslén et al[63] (1995)	88%	Only molars included
67	60	10%	Rud et al[18] (1972)	73%	$P < .001$; long-term data of cases treated with Retroplast presented in study Yazdi et al[68] (2007)
67	62	8%		31%	
NA	64	NA	Molven et al[8] (1987)	84%	$P > .05$; initial study sample N = 183
NA	58	NA		76%	
NA	47	NA		92%	
NA	39	NA		87%	

(cont)

Table 17-2 (cont) Outcome studies on apical surgery without higher magnification

Authors (year)	Study type (years when surgeries were done)	Follow-up	Magnification	REF material
Maddalone and Gagliani[69] (2003)	Cohort prospective (NA)	3 years	Loupes (×4)	SuperEBA
Schwartz-Arad et al[70] (2003)	Cohort prospective (1994–1999)	6–45 months (mean 11 months)	NA	Amalgam or IRM (no microtips)
Wesson and Gale[71] (2003)	Cohort prospective (1974–1995)	5 years	None (naked eye)	Amalgam (no microtips)
Sahlin Platt and Wannfors[72] (2004)	Clinical prospective comparative study (NA)	1 year	NA	Compomer (Dyract AP; no microtips) GIC (Ketac Silver; no microtips)
Wang et al[74] (2004)	Cohort prospective (NA)	4–8 years	Loupes	Various
Gagliani et al[75] (2005)	Cohort prospective (1995–1996)	5 years	Loupes (×4.5)	SuperEBA
Lindeboom et al[76] (2005)	RCT (NA)	1 year	Loupes (×3.5)	MTA (ProRoot) IRM
Taschieri et al[77] (2005)	Cohort prospective (NA)	1 year	Loupes (×3.4)	SuperEBA
De Lange et al[78] (2007)	RCT (NA)	1 year	None (naked eye)	IRM
Peñarrocha et al[79] (2007)	Cohort prospective (NA)	1–10 years (mean 28 months)	NA	Amalgam
Wälivaara et al[81] (2007)	Cohort prospective (2002)	12–19 months	NA	IRM
Yazdi et al[68] (2007)	Cohort prospective (1996–1999)	7–9 years (mean 8 years)	NA	Retroplast (no microtips)
García et al[82] (2008)	Cohort prospective (1999–2004)	1 year	Loupes (×2.6)	Amalgam
Martí et al[83] (2008)	Cohort prospective (1999–2004)	1 year	Loupes (×2.6)	Amalgam
Ortega Sánchez et al[84] (2009)	Cohort prospective (2004–2005)	12–19 months (mean 14 months)	NA	Amalgam
Shearer and McManners[85] (2009)	RCT (NA)	6 months	NA	Zinc oxide/eugenol cement (Kalzinol)
Wälivaara et al[86] (2009)	RCT (NA)	12–38 months (mean 16 months)	Loupes	IRM Gutta-percha/AHplus
Wälivaara et al[87] (2011)	RCT (2006–2008)	12–21 months (mean 13 months)	Loupes	IRM SuperEBA
Villa-Machado et al[88] (2013)	Cohort retrospective (1995–2011)	1–16 years (mean 5 years)	Not specified	Various
Kurt et al[89] (2014)	RCT (NA)	1 year	Loupes	MTA

➤Studies without a surgical microscope or endoscope; microtips were used for root-end preparation unless otherwise noted.
EBA, ethoxybenzoic acid; GIC, glass-ionomer cement; IRM, intermediate restorative material; NA, not available; REF, root-end filling; RCT, randomized controlled trial.

N initial (teeth)	N follow-up (teeth)	Drop-out rate	Healing criteria	Success rate	Comments
128	120	6%	Molven et al[8,9] (1987,1996)	93%	NA
262	122	53%	NA	56%	NA
1,007	790	22%	Rud et al[18] (1972)	57%	Only molars were included
18	18	0%	Molven et al[73] (1991)	89%	Significant difference; only incisors and canines included
16	16	0%		44%	
155	94	39%	Rud et al[18] (1972), Orstavik et al[33] (1986)	74%	NA
194	168	13%	Rud et al[18] (1972)	78%	NA
50	50	0%	Rud et al[18] (1972), Molven et al[8] (1987)	92%	$P > .05$; no molars treated
50	50	0%		86%	
50	46	8%	Rud et al[18] (1972), Molven et al[8,9] (1987, 1996)	91%	NA
399	290	27%	Rud et al[18] (1972)	81% (microtip); 71% (bur)	$P = .06$; randomization per root-end preparation technique (microtip vs bur)
333	NA	NA	Von Arx and Kurt[80] (1999)	72%	NA
56	55	2%	Rud et al[18] (1972)	80%	NA
87	60	31%	Rud et al[18] (1972)	78%	Partially same material (Retroplast cases) as in study Jensen et al[67] (2002)
NA	106	NA	Von Arx and Kurt[80] (1999)	75%	Only maxillary premolars and molars included
NA	88	NA	Von Arx and Kurt[80] (1999)	67%	Only mandibular molars included
NA	30	NA	Von Arx et al[61] (1998)	73%	NA
50	47	6%	Authors' own criteria	100% (microtip); 91% (bur)	Randomization per root-end preparation technique (microtip vs bur); only maxillary anterior teeth included
77	69	10%	Rud et al[18] (1972), Molven et al[8,9] (1987,1996)	85%	$P = .5$
83	78	6%		90%	
99	96	3%	Rud et al[18] (1972), Molven et al[8,9] (1987,1996)	91%	$P = .1$
107	98	8%		82%	
271	171	37%	Friedman[44] (2005), Barone et al[32] (2010)	84%	NA
20	20	0%	Zetterqvist et al[62] (1991), Jesslén et al[63] (1995)	75% with preoperative CBCT	Study sample consisted only of maxillary first molars
20	19	5%		74% with preoperative conventional radiography	

Long-term studies

Few studies published from 1996 to 2016 have prospectively documented long-term outcomes (5+ years) of apical surgery through a standardized observation period[26,35,31,71,75] (see Tables 17-1 and 17-2). One of these used a traditional technique.[71] Another did not use high magnification and included many resurgery cases.[75] Many other so-called long-term studies include patients with a vast range of follow-up times, from several months to several years, thus representing varying healing periods.[27,28,32,49,50,60,65,68,74,79,88]

Von Arx et al,[26] using a modern technique, followed up their modern apical surgery cases at 1 and 5 years. Success rates for all materials (including MTA, Retroplast [Retroplast Trading], and SuperEBA [Bosworth]) decreased from 1 to 5 years (90%, 85%, 76% and 86%, 75%, and 67%, respectively). MTA had proportionally fewer late failures than Retroplast or SuperEBA. Similar trends were observed in a subsequent study with larger samples of MTA- and Retroplast-treated teeth.[35] Success rates for MTA and Retroplast were 91% and 80% at 1 year and 93% and 77% at 5 years, respectively.

Kruse et al[31] invited all patients who participated in a 1-year follow-up for a 6-year postoperative examination. Of the 26 teeth that were treated initially with MTA, one failed due to root fracture in less than a year.[30] The other 25 cases were examined at 1 year, and 19 were examined at 6 years, of which 16 were judged to be successful. If the early failure is ignored, 1-year and 6-year success rates of 100% and 84% can be calculated. If the early failure is included, the 1-year and 6-year success rates become 96% and 80%, respectively. In either case, the confidence intervals would have been wide because almost a quarter of the patients were lost to follow-up and the sample size was small. Although some cases failed over time, several others progressed from incomplete healing (scar tissue) to complete healing over time, both ratings being categorized as success. The same study reported considerably lower success rates for teeth treated using simple resections, leaving gutta-percha in place instead of receiving MTA retrofillings.

It can be concluded that long-term surgical results are good, particularly when MTA retrofillings are used.

Short-term versus long-term results

Most clinicians evaluate the outcome of apical surgery after 1 year using a clinical and radiographic reexamination. Data collected at 1 year has been generally considered to be predictive of future trends. However, long-term outcomes are less favorable than those presented in short-term studies.[5,39] Some studies have reported long-term follow-up only for cases classified as successful at the short-term follow-up, effectively ignoring or censoring early failures and thus not providing valid data describing the inception cohort.[20,39,41,45,52,53] Such studies can be helpful in understanding the rate of additional failures over specific time periods. However, a more useful approach would be to provide Kaplan-Meier analyses or life tables. Unfortunately, this approach remains absent from the dental surgical literature. Hence, the authors review the following literature but must appreciate the limitations of the data.

Rubinstein and Kim[20] recalled patients with cases that had been considered to have healed within 1 year of the surgery 5 to 7 years later. Of 59 reexamined roots, 92% remained healed at the long-term follow-up.

Yazdi et al[68] reported that a total of 95% of the roots classified as (radiographically) completely healed at the 1-year follow-up were also judged as completely healed at the final examination at least 5 years after apical surgery (mean long-term follow-up of 8 years). Moreover, 60% of the roots classified as uncertain healing at 1 year demonstrated complete or incomplete healing at the final examination, while the remaining 40% remained unchanged or were classified as unsatisfactory.

From 6 to 10 years after apical surgery, Song et al[39] recalled 172 cases that were determined to have had successful outcomes at the short-term follow-up. Of 104 cases that attended the long-term follow-up, 97 cases were included in the successful group (91 with complete healing and 6 with incomplete healing). The overall maintained success rate was 93%.

Song et al[45] evaluated the change in outcome by comparing 1-year results with long-term results (4 to 8 years) after apical surgery. Cases classified as completely healed at 1 year remained so in 93% of patients at the long-term follow-up. Incompletely healed and uncertain cases at 1 year showed varied change patterns at the long-term reexamination. All cases considered unsatisfactory at 1 year were also judged to be unsatisfactory at long-term follow-up.

In a clinical study of two different root-end preparation and filling techniques, von Arx et al[35] compared 1- and 5-year outcomes. Most cases treated with MTA or Retroplast that were considered healed at 1 year remained so after 5 years (97% and 91%, respectively). In contrast, only 24% of Retroplast-treated teeth that had been rated as not healed after 1 year were classified as healed after 5 years, compared with 54% of MTA-treated teeth. MTA produced twice as much late healing as Retroplast.

Kruse et al[31] reported that 80% of cases treated with MTA and assessed as successful after 1 year remained successful at the reexamination 6 years after apical surgery. The failed cases (n = 3) were lost because of vertical root fractures.

To summarize all of this data, a successful 1-year follow-up diagnosis is reasonably suggestive of the long-term prognosis for most cases. However, caution should be exercised when comparing short-term and long-term success rates or when applying general findings to individual cases.[26,35]

Soft tissue healing outcomes

Apical surgery involves the incision and the elevation of a mucoperiosteal flap to gain access to the surgical site. Consequently, scarring of the incised tissues, gingival recession, and changes in probing depth or level of clinical attachment may occur. However, few clinical reports have documented the soft tissue outcome following apical surgery. In patients with high smile lines, scarring and recession might have a considerable impact on gingival and mucosal esthetics.

Gingival and mucosal scarring

Chindia and Valderhaug[94] described more noticeable scarring for semilunar incisions within the alveolar mucosa than for intrasulcular incisions with trapezoidal releasing incisions, but follow-up time was just 6 months. Using a visual scoring system, von Arx et al[95] evaluated scarring 1 year after apical surgery for 72 cases. Gingiva and mucosa both showed no scarring in 33% of the cases; mild scarring in 60% and 47% of the cases, respectively; and severe scarring in 7% and 19% of the cases, respectively. The much higher rate of severe scarring of the alveolar mucosa compared with the gingiva might be explained by alveolar mucosa being much more mobile than attached gingiva. Although the intrasulcular incision (ISI) and the papilla base incision never produced substantial scarring of the gingiva, 10% of submarginal incisions (SMI) did. Additionally, Kreisler et al[96] observed more unfavorable scar formation in SMI-treated sites than ISI-treated sites at 6-month follow-up.[96]

Gingival recession

Von Arx et al[97] reported a mean recession of 0.4 mm with a standard deviation (SD) of 0.7 mm at buccal sites for ISI reexamined 1 year after apical surgery. In contrast, SMI essentially produced no change, with a tiny gain of 0.05 mm (SD 0.7 mm). Kreisler et al[96] also observed slight gingival recession of 0.2 mm (SD 0.4 mm) 6 months after apical surgery for ISI-treated teeth. This corresponded to a decrease in probing depths at the same ISI sites. When visually assessing the level of the midfacial gingiva in 70 anterior maxillary treated teeth, von Arx et al[98] reported no significant changes between presurgical and 1-year clinical photographs.

Papillary recession

To prevent shrinkage of the interdental papilla after apical surgery and the occurrence of "black triangles," the papilla base incision (PBI) was proposed.[99,100] Using a split tooth experimental design, Velvart et al[101] evaluated the behavior of the papilla by using the PBI on one side of the treated tooth and the ISI on the other side. At the 1-year follow-up, papilla height was fully maintained at the PBI sites but reduced by 1 mm at the ISI sites. Taschieri et al[102] reported no statistically significant shrinkage of the papilla 6 months after apical surgery in a nonrandomized study. They compared ISI (0.4-mm loss of mesial papilla, 0.5-mm loss of distal papilla) with PBI (0.2-mm loss of mesial papilla, 0.1-mm loss of distal papilla). The authors speculated that if the palatal aspect of the papilla were to remain in situ, no long-term loss of papilla height would occur even when using the ISI technique.[102] Kreisler et al[96] also observed neither loss of papilla height nor opening of interproximal spaces 6 months after apical surgery when comparing ISI and SMI. Similarly, von Arx et al[98] found no significant changes of papillary height regardless of the incision technique when visually assessing preoperative and 1-year follow-up clinical photographs of 70 treated anterior maxillary teeth. In summary, papillary recession is generally not problematic following careful surgery.

Changes in probing depth and attachment level

Jansson et al[56] reported a mean loss in the clinical attachment level of 0.3 mm (SD 0.7 mm) 1 year after apical surgery of anterior and premolar teeth (ISI), but periodontal pocket depth remained stable (mean change of 0.08 mm, SD 0.07 mm). Kreisler et al[96] observed no significant changes in the periodontal probing depths and clinical attachment levels within a follow-up period of 6 months except at buccal sites in the ISI group. Mean probing depth significantly diminished from 3.0 mm (SD 1.2 mm) preoperatively to 2.6 mm (SD 0.8 mm) at follow-up. A 5-year longitudinal study of 186 treated teeth revealed a significant change of the clinical attachment level (loss of 0.2 mm) within the first year after surgery but no further change between 1 and 5 years after surgery.[103] In conclusion, changes in probing depth and attachment level are small and appear to stabilize within a year of surgery.

Quality of life and patient-centered outcomes

The study of endodontic quality-of-life issues and endodontic patient-centered outcomes is still in its infancy.[104] However, patients are universally concerned about cost, appearance or esthetics, comfort, and disability, whether of mastication or life function, including incapacity for work or sport. Fortunately, some helpful data on quality of life and patient-centered outcomes of endodontic surgery exists. Soft tissue outcomes directly influence appearance and esthetics; these have been reviewed above. Dentists must consider patient-based and psychosocial impacts of apical surgery.

Kvist and Reit[105] compared postoperative discomfort in surgical and nonsurgical retreatment. In 95 patients, the mode of retreatment was randomly assigned, and patients were asked to record their degree of pain and swelling during the first week after treatment using a visual analog scale (VAS). Significantly more patients reported discomfort after apical surgery than after nonsurgical retreatment. During the first postoperative week, 11 patients (all from the surgical group) reported having been absent from work at some time, mainly due to swelling and discoloration of the skin.

Tsesis et al[106] evaluated pain and swelling after apical surgery in 82 patients who had received oral dexamethasone preoperatively and 2 days postoperatively. At 1 day after surgery, 76% of the patients were completely free of pain. Interestingly, patients with preoperative pain were more likely to report postoperative pain. In 65% of the patients, no swelling was observed.

Tsesis et al[107] assessed patient experience after apical surgery, comparing traditional surgical techniques with modern microsurgical techniques. Patients were given a questionnaire to fill out daily for 7 days postoperatively using a five-point scale. Patients in the modern technique group reported significantly less postoperative pain but more difficulties in function (mouth opening, mastication, and ability to speak) than patients in the traditional technique group. Patients in both groups reported that postoperative symptoms were maximal within the first 3 days after surgery. After this, symptoms generally subsided.

Payer et al[108] evaluated the effect of low-level laser therapy (LLLT) on the postoperative course of apical surgery. Surgical cases (72 in total) were randomly allocated to LLLT-test, LLLT-placebo, and control groups. The test and placebo groups did not differ with respect to postoperative pain. None of the patients suffered from more than minor or moderate pain. The maximal postoperative pain was experienced 1 day after surgery. The vast majority of patients (97%) suffered only from minor swelling without postoperative bleeding, inflammation, or dehiscence.

Peñarrocha et al[109] evaluated the postoperative course after apical surgery in 60 patients. Patients recorded pain and swelling using a descriptive four-point scale over a period of 7 days. Maximum pain was noted after 2 days, but at this point, two-thirds of the patients reported either no pain or only mild pain. Likewise, swelling similarly peaked on the second postoperative day, with two-thirds of the patients presenting with moderate swelling. Swelling correlated with the duration of surgery and the number of treated teeth.

García et al[110] evaluated pain and swelling after apical surgery in 102 patients. Patients recorded scores for pain and swelling at 2, 6, and 12 hours after surgery and daily thereafter for 1 week. In general, low levels of pain were experienced for the first 48 hours, after which pain continuously subsided. Moderate swelling peaked on the second postoperative day. Patients with poor oral hygiene experienced more pain and swelling than patients with good oral hygiene. Smokers reported more pain than nonsmokers.

Iqbal et al[111] reported data from a self-assessment questionnaire completed by 199 patients after apical surgery. Data were collected during a period of 2 weeks postoperatively. Overall, the patients described little postsurgical pain; however, variability was noted. A majority of the patients (67%) rated apical surgery as more pleasant than expected and found it to be less painful (48%) or the same (38%) as NSRCT.

Christiansen et al[112] assessed patient discomfort after apical surgery from 3 hours postsurgically until the day of suture removal. Pooled VAS data from all patients showed that pain peaked 3 hours postoperatively and that swelling peaked 1 day after surgery. Importantly, patients experienced little pain and only moderate swelling. Neither pain nor swelling correlated with the duration of the surgery. Patients' overall perception of postoperative discomfort was influenced by oral awareness (86%), swelling (71%), compromised chewing ability (43%), pain (36%), and difficulty with mouth opening (21%).

Del Fabbro et al[113] evaluated postoperative pain, functional limitations, and other symptoms for 7 days after apical surgery using daily questionnaires and VAS. Pain, swelling, and impairments to chewing and phonetics peaked in the first 2 days postoperatively. Postsurgical bleeding was not a concern, but some patients complained about bad taste or breath. Sleeping was not affected very much, and all patients had returned to work 4 days postoperatively. All study parameters had returned to normal (VAS 0) by 6 days postoperatively.

Georgelin-Gurgel et al[114] monitored heart rate and systolic and diastolic blood pressure during apical surgery in 30 healthy patients. Patients scored their anxiety before treatment and reported pain, stress, and discomfort experienced during care. Heart rate increased and was highest during periradicular curettage, whereas systolic blood pressure was highest before local anesthesia. The mean VAS scores (0 to 10 scale) were low: stress (2.5), discomfort (1.0), and pain (0.8). The level of stress experienced during surgery was correlated to the level of anticipated anxiety.

Kim and Solomon[115] found endodontic microsurgery to be more cost-effective than other treatment options; however, their findings were generally based on comparisons of short-term microsurgical success rates with longer-term survival rates of the alternatives. It has been suggested that patients may sometimes inappropriately choose apical surgery over nonsurgical retreatment to avoid the costs of restoration replacement.[116] Apical surgery tends to result in larger indirect costs than nonsurgical retreatment as well as more discomfort.[103]

To summarize, patient symptoms were generally minor to moderate. Pain, swelling and other disabilities tended to peak within a day or two of surgery and then steadily decrease to minimal levels within a week.

Prognostic Factors

Knowledge of prognostic factors (predictors) would help the clinician in treatment planning, selecting treatment alternatives, and facilitating patient management. Most clinical studies have not reported outcome data with regard to factors that may influence healing. From a clinical perspective, prognostic factors can be divided into the following:

- Patient-related factors (eg, age, sex, health, medication, smoking)
- Tooth-related factors (eg, type of tooth, preoperative signs and symptoms, type and size of lesion, periodontal involvement, length and quality of root-canal filling, type and quality of coronal restoration)
- Treatment-related factors (eg, type of surgery, experience of the surgeon, use of magnification devices, surgical technique, root-end filling material, postoperative care)

Von Arx et al[117] published a meta-analysis on prognostic factors for apical surgeries with root-end fillings. Only studies with clearly defined healing criteria were included, and healing had to be reported for at least two categories of a specific prognostic factor (eg, male versus female). Data was extracted from 38 clinical studies. Patient-related factors (age and sex) did not influence healing. Some tooth-related factors influenced healing: Maxillary anterior teeth and mandibular anterior teeth demonstrated higher estimated healing rates than posterior teeth (85% and 88%, respectively); mandibular molars had the lowest estimated healing rate (64%). Other tooth-related factors that influenced treatment outcome included preoperative pain, preoperative signs, root canal filling density, lesion presence, and lesion size. Several treatment-related factors, including the type of surgery (first-time surgery vs resurgery) and the technique of root-end cavity preparation (ultrasonic microtips or burs) influenced healing.

Kreisler et al[40] assessed the effect of patient- and tooth-related factors on the outcome of apical surgery in a multicenter study (four private oral surgery practices and one university clinic) of 281 patients. Treatment outcomes were assessed 6 to 12 months postoperatively. Patients aged between 31 and 40 years had a significantly higher healing rate than the total study population. Sex was a significant predictor, with females showing higher success rates than males. Premolars demonstrated significantly better outcomes than molars and anterior teeth. Other significant predictors included preoperative signs and symptoms, lesion size, and presence or absence of perforating lesions.

Song et al[41] prospectively examined potential prognostic factors for apical surgery. A total of 584 teeth were included, and the evaluations were performed at least 1 year after surgery. The following preoperative factors were positively correlated with a successful outcome of apical surgery: patients younger than 40 years of age, females, anterior teeth, maxillary teeth, and simple endodontic lesions (rather than combined endodontic-periodontal lesions).

Von Arx et al[26] prospectively assessed prognostic factors of healing of apical surgery with a follow-up of 5 years. Two significant outcome predictors were identified: the mesiodistal crestal bone level measured on periapical radiographs, and the type of root-end filling material. Teeth that presented with no or minor (< 3 mm) interproximal bone loss both mesially and distally had a higher proportion of healed cases (78%) than teeth with more interproximal bone loss (53%). Furthermore, MTA (86%) was shown to be superior to SuperEBA (67%). Although the long-term prognosis of apical surgery can be broadly projected from short-term outcomes (see above), the long-term outcome predictors differed from those observed at 1 year. Preoperative pain was the sole significant prognostic factor at 1 year after apical surgery of the same cohort.[97]

Serrano-Giménez et al[118] analyzed the prognostic factors for apical surgery in a systematic review of 23 papers. The following factors were positively associated with the outcome of apical surgery: patients younger than 45 years of age, absence of preoperative signs and symptoms, maxillary anterior or premolar teeth, single-rooted teeth, lesions not surpassing 10 mm in diameter, noncystic lesions, lesions without involvement of the marginal periodontium, absence of perforating lesions, teeth with an adequate root-filling length, MTA as root-end filling material, apical resections of at least 3 mm, teeth without oroantral fistulae, and first-time surgery cases.

Tawil et al[48] identified an interesting and previously unreported prognostic factor. They studied the effect of intraoperatively detected dentinal microcracks ("root dentinal defects") on the 1- and 3-year outcomes of apical surgery. Root ends were inspected after root-end resection and cavity preparation for the presence of microcracks at the cut root face and/or inside the root-end cavity. Inspection was performed using a surgical microscope as well as transillumination of the root end with a light-emitting diode probe light. Rates of healed cases were significantly higher after 1 and 3 years in teeth without microcracks (95% and 97%) compared to teeth with microcracks (30% and 32%).

Another study retrospectively evaluated the influence of an isthmus on the outcome of apical surgery in molars.[119] A multivariate regression analysis demonstrated that the presence of an isthmus in molar roots led to a six-times higher risk of failure. Dentists must exercise considerable care to avoid weakening the root end while preparing or placing a retrograde filling in the isthmus. Isthmus management remains one of the most difficult steps in apical surgery.[119]

Although short- and long-term prognostic factors may differ, a variety of prognostic factors have been identified. Patient factors appear to have little influence on prognosis, but effects attributed to patient age and sex have been reported. Many tooth-related factors influence prognosis, including preoperative pain, preoperative signs, root canal filling density, the presence of radicular microcracks, the presence of an isthmus, lesion presence, lesion size, lesion type (simple or endo-perio or with perforation of the cortical bone, or including an oroantral fistula, or cystic), and crestal interproximal bone height. Treatment or technical factors may also influence prognosis, including first-time surgery versus resurgery, the technique of root-end cavity preparation, use of ultrasonic microtips or burs, the length of the apical resection, and the root-end filling material. Consideration of these factors will aid the dentist in understanding the likely prognosis of the tooth and in overall treatment planning.

Summary

Apical surgical outcomes are generally measured using clinical and radiographic findings according to established criteria. Generally, signs of healing are evident at the 1-year follow-up, but long-term follow-up is necessary whether initial signs are favorable or not. Long-term outcomes are very good, but a small number of failures continue to occur over time. Modern surgical techniques including microscopy, ultrasonic root-end preparation, and MTA are markedly superior to traditional techniques. The available patient-centered outcome data are good. Careful surgical techniques preserve gingiva and papillae and soft tissue esthetics. Pain is generally moderate and decreases steadily; likewise, swelling is generally minor and also decreases rapidly. A variety of prognostic indicators have been identified; these aid in treatment planning.

References

1. Torabinejad M, White SN. Endodontic treatment options after unsuccessful initial root canal treatment: Alternatives to single-tooth implants. J Am Dent Assoc 2016;147:214–220.
2. Torabinejad M, Corr R, Handysides R, Shabahang S. Outcomes of nonsurgical retreatment and endodontic surgery: A systematic review. J Endod 2009;35:930–937.
3. Hepworth MJ, Friedman S. Treatment outcome of surgical and non-surgical management of endodontic failures. J Can Dent Assoc 1997;63:364–371.
4. Nair PN, Sjögren U, Figdor D, Sundqvist G. Persistent periapical radiolucencies of root-filled human teeth, failed endodontic treatments, and periapical scars. Oral Surg Oral Med Oral Pathol Oral Radiol Endod 1999;87:617–627.
5. Torabinejad M, Landaez M, Milan M, et al. Tooth retention through endodontic microsurgery or tooth replacement using single implants: A systematic review of treatment outcomes. J Endod 2015;41:1–10.
6. Halse A, Molven O, Fristad I. Diagnosing periapical lesions—Disagreement and borderline cases. Int Endod J 2002;35:703–709.
7. Andreasen JO, Rud J. Correlation between histology and radiography in the assessment of healing after endodontic surgery. Int J Oral Surg 1972;1:161–173.
8. Molven O, Halse A, Grung B. Observer strategy and the radiographic classification of healing after endodontic surgery. Int J Oral Maxillofac Surg 1987;16:432–439.
9. Molven O, Halse A, Grung B. Incomplete healing (scar tissue) after periapical surgery—Radiographic findings 8 to 12 years after treatment. J Endod 1996;22:264–268.
10. Halse A, Molven O. Increased width of the apical periodontal membrane space in endodontically treated teeth may represent favourable healing. Int Endod J 2004;37:552–560.
11. Halse A, Molven O, Grung B. Follow-up after periapical surgery: The value of the one-year control. Endod Dent Traumatol 1991;7:246–250.
12. Burstein J, Ko B, Glick D, White SN. 18 Month clinical trial of endodontic surgical retrofilling materials [Abstract #OR 18]. J Endod 2001;27:219.
13. Chong BS, Pitt Fort TR, Hudson MB. A prospective clinical study of mineral trioxide aggregate and IRM when used as root-end filling materials in endodontic surgery. Int Endod J 2003;36:520–526.
14. Molven O, Halse A, Fristad I, MacDonald Jankowski D. Periapical changes following root-canal treatment observed 20-27 years postoperatively. Int Endod J 2002;35:784–790.
15. Frank AL, Glick DH, Patterson SS, Weine FS. Long-term evaluation of surgically placed amalgam fillings. J Endod 1992;18:391–398.
16. Mead C, Javidan-Nejad S, Mego ME, Nash B, Torabinejad M. Levels of evidence for the outcome of endodontic surgery. J Endod 2005;31:19–24.
17. Rud J, Rud V, Munksgaard EC. Effect of root canal contents on healing of teeth with dentin-bonded resin composite retrograde seal. J Endod 1997;23:535–541.
18. Rud J, Andreasen JO, Möller Jensen JE. Radiographic criteria for the assessment of healing after endodontic surgery. Int J Oral Surg 1972;1:195–214.
19. Rubinstein RA, Kim S. Short-term observation of the results of endodontic surgery with the use of a surgical operation microscope and SuperEBA as root-end filling material. J Endod 1999;25:43–48.
20. Rubinstein RA, Kim S. Long-term follow-up of cases considered healed one year after apical microsurgery. J Endod 2002;28:378–383.
21. Taschieri S, Del Fabbro M, Testori T, Francetti L, Weinstein R. Endodontic surgery using 2 different magnification devices: Preliminary results of a randomized controlled study. J Oral Maxillofac Surg 2006;64:235–242.
22. Tsesis I, Rosen E, Schwartz-Arad D, Fuss Z. Retrospective evaluation of surgical endodontic treatment: Traditional versus modern technique. J Endod 2006;32:412–416.
23. Taschieri S, Del Fabbro M, Testori T, Weinstein R. Endodontic reoperation using an endoscope and microsurgical instruments: One year follow-up. Br J Oral Maxillofac Surg 2007;45:582–585.
24. von Arx T, Jensen SS, Hänni S. Clinical and radiographic assessment of various predictors for healing outcome 1 year after periapical surgery. J Endod 2007;33:123–128.
25. Zuolo ML, Ferreira MO, Gutmann JL. Prognosis in periradicular surgery: A clinical prospective study. Int Endod J 2000;33:91–98.
26. von Arx T, Jensen SS, Hänni S, Friedman S. Five-year longitudinal assessment of the prognosis of apical microsurgery. J Endod 2012;38:570–579.
27. Kim E, Song JS, Jung IY, Lee SJ, Kim S. Prospective clinical study evaluating endodontic microsurgery outcomes for cases with lesions of endodontic origin compared with cases with lesions of combined periodontal-endodontic origin. J Endod 2008;34:546–551.

28. Saunders WP. A prospective clinical study of periradicular surgery using mineral trioxide aggregate as a root-end filling. J Endod 2008;34:660–665.
29. Taschieri S, Del Fabbro M, Testori T, Weinstein R. Microscope versus endoscope in root end management: A randomized controlled study. Int J Oral Maxillofac Surg 2008;37:1022–1026.
30. Christiansen R, Kirkevang LL, Hørsted-Bindslev P, Wenzel A. Randomized clinical trial of root-end resection followed by root-end filling with mineral trioxide aggregate or smoothing of the orthograde gutta percha root filling—1-year follow-up. Int Endod J 2009;42:105–114.
31. Kruse C, Spin-Neto R, Christiansen R, Wenzel A, Kirkevang LL. Periapical bone healing after apicectomy with and without retrograde root filling with mineral trioxide aggregate: A 6-year follow up of a randomized controlled trial. J Endod 2016;42:533–537.
32. Barone C, Dao TT, Basrani BB, Wang N, Friedman S. Treatment outcome in endodontics: The Toronto study—Phases 3, 4, and 5: Apical surgery. J Endod 2010;36:28–35.
33. Orstavik D, Kerekes K, Eriksen HM. The periapical index: A scoring system for radiographic assessment of apical periodontitis. Endod Dent Traumatol 1986;2:20–34.
34. von Arx T, Hänni S, Jensen SS. Clinical results with two different methods of root-end preparation and filling in apical surgery: MTA and adhesive resin composite. J Endod 2010;36:1122–1129.
35. von Arx T, Hänni S, Jensen SS. 5-year results comparing MTA and adhesive resin composite for root-end sealing in apical surgery. J Endod 2014;40:1077–1081.
36. Song M, Shin SJ, Kim E. Outcomes of endodontic micro-resurgery: A prospective clinical study. J Endod 2011;37:316–320.
37. Song M, Jung IY, Lee SJ, Lee CY, Kim E. Prognostic factors for clinical outcomes in endodontic microsurgery: A retrospective study. J Endod 2011;37:927–933.
38. Song M, Kim E. A prospective randomized controlled study of mineral trioxide aggregate and super ethoxy-benzoic acid as root-end filling materials in endodontic microsurgery. J Endod 2012;38:875–879.
39. Song M, Chung W, Lee SJ, Kim E. Long-term outcome of the cases classified as successes based on short-term follow-up in endodontic microsurgery. J Endod 2012;38:1192–1196.
40. Kreisler M, Gockel R, Aubell-Falkenberg S, et al. Clinical outcome in periradicular surgery: Effect of patient- and tooth-related factors—A multicenter study. Quintessence Int 2013;44:53–60.
41. Song M, Kim SG, Lee SJ, Kim B, Kim E. Prognostic factors of clinical outcomes in endodontic microsurgery: A prospective study. J Endod 2013;39:1491–1497.
42. Li H, Zhai F, Zhang R, Hou B. Evaluation of microsurgery with SuperEBA as root-end filling material for treating post-treatment endodontic disease: A 2-year retrospective study. J Endod 2014;40:345–350.
43. Lui JN, Khin MM, Krishnaswamy G, Chen NN. Prognostic factors relating to the outcome of endodontic microsurgery. J Endod 2014;40:1071–1076.
44. Friedman S. The prognosis and expected outcome of apical surgery. Endod Topics 2005;11:54–78.
45. Song M, Nam T, Shin SJ, Kim E. Comparison of clinical outcomes of endodontic microsurgery: 1 year versus long-term follow-up. J Endod 2014;40:490–494.
46. Tortorci S, Difalco P, Caradonna L, Tetè S. Traditional endodontic surgery versus modern technique: A 5-year controlled clinical trial. J Craniofac Surg 2014;25:804–807.
47. Shinbori N, Grama AM, Patel Y, Woodmansey K, He J. Clinical outcome of endodontic microsurgery that uses EndoSequence BC root repair material as the root-end filling material. J Endod 2015;41:607–612.
48. Tawil PZ, Saraiya VM, Galicia JC, Duggan DJ. Periapical microsurgery: The effect of root dentinal defects on short- and long-term outcome. J Endod 2015;41:22–27.
49. Çalişkan MK, Tekin U, Kaval ME, Solmaz MC. The outcome of apical microsurgery using MTA as the root-end filling material: 2- to 6-year follow-up study. Int Endod J 2016;49:245–254.
50. August DS. Long-term, postsurgical results on teeth with periapical radiolucencies. J Endod 1996;22:380–383.
51. Danin J, Strömberg T, Forsgren H, Linder LE, Ramsköld LO. Clinical management of nonhealing periradicular pathosis. Surgery versus endodontic retreatment. Oral Surg Oral Med Oral Pathol Oral Radiol Endod 1996;82:213–217.
52. Rud J, Rud V, Munksgaard EC. Long-term evaluation of retrograde root filling with dentin-bonded resin composite. J Endod 1996;22:90–93.
53. Rud J, Rud V, Munksgaard EC. Retrograde root filling with dentin-bonded modified resin composite. J Endod 1996;22:477–480.
54. Sumi Y, Hattori H, Hayashi K, Ueda M. Ultrasonic root-end preparation: Clinical and radiographic evaluation of results. J Oral Maxillofac Surg 1996;54:590–593.
55. Amagasa T, Nagase M, Sato T, Shioda S. Apicoectomy with retrograde gutta-percha root filling. Oral Surg Oral Med Oral Pathol 1989;68:339–342.
56. Jansson L, Sandstedt P, Låftman AC, Skoglund A. Relationship between apical and marginal healing in periradicular surgery. Oral Surg Oral Med Oral Pathol Oral Radiol Endod 1997;83:596–601.
57. Bader G, Lejeune S. Prospective study of two retrograde endodontic apical preparations with and without the use of CO_2 laser. Endod Dent Traumatol 1998;14:75–78.
58. Kvist T, Reit C. Results of endodontic retreatment: A randomized clinical study comparing surgical and nonsurgical procedures. J Endod 1999;25:814–817.
59. Reit C, Gröndahl HG. Application of statistical decision theory to radiographic diagnosis of endodontically treated teeth. Scand J Dent Res 1983;91:213–218.
60. Testori T, Capelli M, Milani S, Weinstein RL. Success and failure in periradicular surgery: A longitudinal retrospective analysis. Oral Surg Oral Med Oral Pathol Oral Radiol Endod 1999;87:493–498.
61. von Arx T, Kurt B, Ilgenstein B, Hardt N. Preliminary results and analysis of a new set of sonic instruments for root-end cavity preparation. Int Endod J 1998;31:32–38.
62. Zetterqvist L, Hall G, Holmlund A. Apicectomy: A comparative study of amalgam and glass ionomer cement as apical sealants. Oral Surg Oral Med Oral Pathol 1991;71:489–491.
63. Jesslén P, Zetterqvist L, Heimdahl A. Long-term results of amalgam versus glass ionomer cement as apical sealant after apicectomy. Oral Surg Oral Med Oral Pathol Oral Radiol Endod 1995;79:101–103.
64. Rahbaran S, Gilthorpe MS, Harrison SD, Gulabivala K. Comparison of clinical outcome of periapical surgery in endodontic and oral surgery units of a teaching dental hospital: A retrospective study. Oral Surg Oral Med Oral Pathol Oral Radiol Endod 2001;91:700–709.
65. Rud J, Rud V, Munksgaard EC. Periapical healing of mandibular molars after root-end sealing with dentine-bonded composite. Int Endod J 2001;34:285–292.
66. von Arx T, Gerber C, Hardt N. Periradicular surgery of molars: A prospective clinical study with a one-year follow-up. Int Endod J 2001;34:520–525.
67. Jensen SS, Nattestad A, Egdø P, Sewerin I, Munksgaard EC, Schou S. A prospective, randomized, comparative clinical study of resin composite and glass ionomer cement for retrograde root filling. Clin Oral Investig 2002;6:236–243.
68. Yazdi PM, Schou S, Jensen SS, Stoltze K, Kenrad B, Sewerin I. Dentine-bonded resin composite (Retroplast) for root-end filling: A prospective clinical and radiographic study with a mean follow-up period of 8 years. Int Endod J 2007;40:493–503.
69. Maddalone M, Gagliani M. Periapical endodontic surgery: A 3-year follow-up study. Int Endod J 2003;36:193–198.
70. Schwartz-Arad D, Yarom N, Lustig JP, Kaffe I. A retrospective radiographic study of root-end surgery with amalgam and intermediate restorative material. Oral Surg Oral Med Oral Pathol Oral Radiol Endod 2003;96:472–477.
71. Wesson CM, Gale TM. Molar apicectomy with amalgam root-end filling: Results of a prospective study in two district general hospitals. Br Dent J 2003;195:707–714.
72. Sahlin Platt A, Wannfors K. The effectiveness of compomer as a root-end filling: A clinical investigation. Oral Surg Oral Med Oral Pathol Oral Radiol Endod 2004;97:508–512.
73. Molven O, Halse A, Grung B. Surgical management of endodontic failures: Indications and treatment results. Int Dent J 1991;41:33–42.
74. Wang N, Knight K, Dao T, Friedman S. Treatment outcome in endodontics—The Toronto study. Phases I and II: Apical surgery. J Endod 2004;30:751–761.
75. Gagliani MM, Gorni FGM, Strohmenger L. Periapical resurgery versus periapical surgery: A 5-year longitudinal comparison. Int Endod J 2005;38:320–327.
76. Lindeboom JA, Frenken JW, Kroon FHM, van den Akker HP. A comparative prospective randomized clinical study of MTA and IRM as root-end filling materials in single-rooted teeth in endodontic surgery. Oral Surg Oral Med Oral Pathol Oral Radiol Endod 2005;100:495–500.
77. Taschieri S, Del Fabbro M, Testori T, Francetti L, Weinstein R. Endodontic surgery with ultrasonic retrotips: One-year follow-up. Oral Surg Oral Med Oral Pathol Oral Radiol Endod 2005;100:380–387.
78. de Lange J, Putters T, Baas EM, van Ingen JM. Ultrasonic root-end preparation in apical surgery: A prospective randomized study. Oral Surg Oral Med Oral Pathol Oral Radiol Endod 2007;104:841–845.
79. Peñarrocha M, Martí E, García B, Gay C. Relationship of periapical lesion radiologic size, apical resection, and retrograde filling with the prognosis of periapical surgery. J Oral Maxillofac Surg 2007;65:1526–1529.
80. von Arx T, Kurt B. Root-end cavity preparation after apicoectomy using a new type of sonic and diamond-surfaced retrotip: A 1-year follow-up study. J Oral Maxillofac Surg 1999;57:656–661.

81. Wälivaara DA, Abrahamsson P, Isaksson S, Blomqvist JE, Sämfors KA. Prospective study of periapically infected teeth treated with periapical surgery including ultrasonic preparation and retrograde IRM root-end fillings. J Oral Maxillofac Surg 2007;65:931–935.
82. García B, Peñarrocha M, Martí E, Martínez JM, Gay-Escoda C. Periapical surgery in maxillary premolars and molars: Analysis in terms of the distance between the lesion and the maxillary sinus. J Oral Maxillofac Surg 2008;66:1212–1217.
83. Martí E, Peñarrocha M, García B, Martínez JM, Gay-Escoda C. Distance between periapical lesion and mandibular canal as a factor in periapical surgery in mandibular molars. J Oral Maxillofac Surg 2008;66:2461–2466.
84. Ortega-Sánchez B, Peñarrocha-Diago M, Rubio-Martínez LA, Vera-Sempere JF. Radiographic morphometric study of 37 periapical lesions in 30 patients: Validation of success criteria. J Oral Maxillofac Surg 2009;67:846–849.
85. Shearer J, McManners J. Comparison between the use of an ultrasonic tip and a microhead handpiece in periradicular surgery: A prospective randomized trial. Br J Oral Maxillofac Surg 2009;47:386–388.
86. Wälivaara DA, Abrahamsson P, Sämfors KA, Isaksson S. Periapical surgery using ultrasonic preparation and thermoplasticized gutta-percha with AH plus sealer or IRM as retrograde root-end fillings in 160 consecutive teeth: A prospective randomized clinical study. Oral Surg Oral Med Oral Pathol Oral Radiol Endod 2009;108:784–789.
87. Wälivaara DA, Abrahamsson P, Fogelin M, Isaksson S. Super-EBA and IRM as root-end fillings in periapical surgery with ultrasonic preparation: A prospective randomized study of 206 consecutive teeth. Oral Surg Oral Med Oral Pathol Oral Radiol Endod 2011;112:258–263.
88. Villa-Machado PA, Botero-Ramirez X, Tobón-Arroyave SI. Retrospective follow-up assessment of prognostic variables associated with the outcome of periradicular surgery. Int Endod J 2013;46:1063–1076.
89. Kurt SN, Üstün Y, Erdogan Ö, Evlice B, Yoldas O, Öztunc H. Outcomes of periradicular surgery of maxillary first molars using a vestibular approach: A prospective, clinical study with one year of follow-up. J Oral Maxillofac Surg 2014;72:1049–1061.
90. Tsesis I, Faivishevsky V, Kfir A, Rosen E. Outcome of surgical endodontic treatment performed by a modern technique: A meta-analysis of literature. J Endod 2009;35:1505–1511.
91. Setzer FC, Shah SB, Kohli MR, Karabucak B, Kim S. Outcome of endodontic surgery: A meta-analysis of the literature—Part 1: Comparison of traditional root-end surgery and endodontic microsurgery. J Endod 2010;36:1757–1765.
92. Setzer FC, Kohli MR, Shah SB, Karabucak B, Kim S. Outcome of endodontic surgery: A meta-analysis of the literature—Part 2: Comparison of endodontic microsurgical techniques with and without the use of higher magnification. J Endod 2012;38:1–10.
93. Tsesis I, Rosen E, Taschieri S, Telishevsky Strauss Y, Ceresoli V, Del Fabbro M. Outcomes of surgical endodontic treatment performed by a modern technique: An updated meta-analysis of the literature. J Endod 2013;39:332–339.
94. Chindia ML, Valderhaug J. Periodontal status following trapezoidal and semilunar flaps in apicectomy. East Afr Med J 1995;72:564–567.
95. von Arx T, Salvi GE, Janner S, Jensen SS. Scarring of gingiva and alveolar mucosa following apical surgery: Visual assessment after one year. Oral Surg 2008;1:178–189.
96. Kreisler M, Gockel R, Schmidt I, Kühl S, d'Hoedt B. Clinical evaluation of a modified marginal sulcular incision technique in endodontic surgery. Oral Surg Oral Med Oral Pathol Oral Radiol Endod 2009;108:e22–e28.
97. von Arx T, Vinzens-Majaniemi T, Bürgin W, Jensen SS. Changes of periodontal parameters following apical surgery: A prospective clinical study of three incision techniques. Int Endod J 2007;40:959–969.
98. von Arx T, Salvi GE, Janner S, Jensen SS. Gingival recession following apical surgery in the esthetic zone: A clinical study with 70 cases. Eur J Esthet Dent 2009;4:28–45.
99. Velvart P, Peters CI. Soft tissue management in endodontic surgery. J Endod 2005;31:4–16.
100. von Arx T, Salvi GE. Incision techniques and flap designs for apical surgery in the anterior maxilla. Eur J Esthet Dent 2008;3:110–126.
101. Velvart P, Ebner-Zimmermann U, Ebner JP. Comparison of long-term papilla healing following sulcular full thickness flap and papilla base flap in endodontic surgery. Int Endod J 2004;37:687–693.
102. Taschieri S, Corbella S, Del Fabbro M. Do gingival soft tissues benefit from the application of a papilla preservation flap technique in endodontic surgery? J Oral Maxillofac Surg 2014;72:1898–1908.
103. von Arx T, Alsaeed M, Salvi GE. Five-year changes in periodontal parameters after apical surgery. J Endod 2011;37:910–918.
104. Hamedy R, Shakiba B, Fayazi S, Pak JG, White SN. Patient-centered endodontic outcomes: A narrative review. Iran Endod J 2013;8:197–204.
105. Kvist T, Reit C. Postoperative discomfort associated with surgical and nonsurgical endodontic retreatment. Endod Dent Traumatol 2000;16:71–74.
106. Tsesis I, Fuss Z, Lin S, Tilinger G, Peled M. Analysis of postoperative symptoms following surgical endodontic treatment. Quintessence Int 2003;34:756–760.
107. Tsesis I, Shoshani Y, Givol N, Yahalom R, Fuss Z, Taicher S. Comparison of quality of life after surgical endodontic treatment using two techniques: A prospective study. Oral Surg Oral Med Oral Pathol Oral Radiol Endod 2005;99:367–371.
108. Payer M, Jakse N, Pertl C, Truschnegg A, Lechner E, Eskici A. The clinical effect of LLLT in endodontic surgery: A prospective study of 72 cases. Oral Surg Oral Med Oral Pathol Oral Radiol Endod 2005;100:375–379.
109. Peñarrocha M, García B, Martí E, Balaguer J. Pain and inflammation after periapical surgery in 60 patients. J Oral Maxillofac Surg 2006;64:429–433.
110. García B, Peñarrocha M, Martí E, Gay-Escoda C, von Arx T. Pain and swelling after periapical surgery related to oral hygiene and smoking. Oral Surg Oral Med Oral Pathol Oral Radiol Endod 2007;104:271–276.
111. Iqbal MK, Kratchman SI, Guess GM, Karabucak B, Kim S. Microscopic periradicular surgery: Perioperative predictors for postoperative clinical outcomes and quality of life assessment. J Endod 2007;33:239–244.
112. Christiansen R, Kirkevang LL, Hørsted-Bindslev P, Wenzel A. Patient discomfort following periapical surgery. Oral Surg Oral Med Oral Pathol Oral Radiol Endod 2008;105:245–250.
113. Del Fabbro M, Taschieri S, Weinstein R. Quality of life after microscopic periradicular surgery using two different incision techniques: A randomized clinical study. Int Endod J 2009;42:360–367.
114. Georgelin-Gurgel M, Diemer F, Nicolas E, Hennequin M. Surgical and nonsurgical endodontic treatment-induced stress. J Endod 2009;35:19–22.
115. Kim SG, Solomon C. Cost-effectiveness of endodontic molar retreatment compared with fixed partial dentures and single-tooth implant alternatives. J Endod 2011;37:321–325.
116. Hasselgren G, Patel P, Alhassany H, Kunzel C. Reasons for apical surgery treatment in an underserved New York City population. N Y State Dent J 2016;82(3):31–34.
117. von Arx T, Peñarrocha M, Jensen S. Prognostic factors in apical surgery with root-end filling: A meta-analysis. J Endod 2010;36:957–973.
118. Serrano-Giménez M, Sánchez-Torres A, Gay-Escoda C. Prognostic factors on periapical surgery: A systematic review. Med Oral Patol Oral Cir Bucal 2015;20:e715–722.
119. Kim S, Jung H, Kim S, Shin SJ, Kim E. The influence of an isthmus on the outcomes of surgically treated molars: A retrospective study. J Endod 2016;42:1029–1034.

Index

Page numbers followed by "f" indicate figures; those followed by "t" indicate tables; those followed by "b" indicate boxes

A

B

C

D

E

N

O

P

R

S

T